The Fenway Guide to Lesbian, Gay, Bisexual, and Transgender Health

The Fenway Guide to Lesbian, Gay, Bisexual, and Transgender Health

Harvey J. Makadon, MD
Kenneth H. Mayer, MD
Jennifer Potter, MD
Hilary Goldhammer, MS

AMERICAN COLLEGE OF PHYSICIANS   PHILADELPHIA

Associate Publisher and Manager, Books Publishing, Tom Hartman
Director, Editorial Production, Linda Drumheller
Developmental Editor, Matthew Ray
Production Supervisor, Allan S. Kleinberg
Senior Editor, Karen C. Nolan
Editorial Coordinator, Angela Gabella
Cover Design, Flatiron Industries

Printed in the United States of America
Printing/Binding by Versa Press
Composition by Scribe Inc.

Library of Congress Cataloging-in-Publication Data

The Fenway guide to enhancing lesbian, gay, bisexual, and transgender healthcare / editors,
Harvey J. Makadon . . . [et al.].
   p. ; cm.
  Includes bibliographical references.
  ISBN 978-1-930513-95-2
  1. Gays—Medical care—United States. 2. Lesbians—Medical care—United States. 3. Transgender
people—Medical care—United States. I. Makadon, Harvey J., 1947– II. American College of
Physicians.
  [DNLM: 1. Delivery of Health Care—United States. 2. Bisexuality—United States.
3. Homosexuality–United States. W 84 AA1 F343 2007]
  RA564.9.H65F46 2007
  362.1086'6—dc22   2007025286

08 09 10 11 12 / 10 9 8 7 6 5 4 3 2 1

Contributors

Elaine J. Alpert, MD, MPH, FACP
Associate Professor of Public
  Health and Medicine,
  Department of Social and
  Behavioral Sciences, Boston
  University School of Public
  Health; Department of Medicine,
  Boston University School of
  Medicine
Boston, Massachusetts

**Jonathan S. Appelbaum, MD,
  FACP, AAHIVS**
Instructor in Medicine, Harvard
  Medical School;
Attending Physician, Brigham and
  Women's Hospital;
Medical Director, Brigham and
  Women's Physician Group
Boston, Massachusetts

Ulrike Boehmer, PhD
Assistant Professor of Social and
  Behavioral Sciences, Boston
  University School of Public
  Health
Boston, Massachusetts

Bethany A. Booth, Esq
Associate Director of Legal Services,
  AIDS Action Committee of
  Massachusetts, Inc.
Boston, Massachusetts

Deborah J. Bowen, PhD
Professor, Social and Behavioral
  Sciences, Boston University
  School of Public Health
Boston, Massachusetts

Judith B. Bradford, PhD
Director of Community Health
  Research Initiative, Center for
  Public Policy; Associate
  Professor of Epidemiology and
  Community Health, Virginia
  Commonwealth University
Richmond, Virginia;
Co-Chair, The Fenway Institute,
  Fenway Community Health
Boston, Massachusetts

Paul Burke, Esq
San Francisco, California

Staci Bush, PA-C
Medical Science Liaison, Monogram
  Biosciences
Chicago, Illinois

Michelle Cespedes, MD
Assistant Professor of Medicine,
  New York University School of
  Medicine, Department of
  Medicine, Division of Infectious
  Diseases and Immunology,
  Bellevue Hospital Center
New York, New York

Grant Colfax, MD
Co-Director, HIV Epidemiology
  Section; Director, Interventions
  Unit, San Francisco Department
  of Public Health
San Francisco, California

Demetre C. Daskalakis, MD
Assistant Professor of Medicine,
New York University School of
Medicine, Department of
Medicine, Division of Infectious
Diseases and Immunology,
Bellevue Hospital Center
New York, New York

Valerie J. Fein-Zachary, MD
Instructor of Radiology, Harvard
Medical School;
Interim Director of Breast Imaging,
Beth Israel Deaconess Medical
Center
Boston, Massachusetts

Jamie Feldman, MD, PhD
Associate Professor of Family
Medicine and Community Health,
Department of Family Medicine
and Community Health,
University of Minnesota
St. Paul, Minnesota

Deborah Fournier, Esq
Associate Director of Public Policy,
AIDS Action Committee of
Massachusetts, Inc.
Boston, Massachusetts

Marshall Forstein, MD
Associate Professor in Psychiatry,
Harvard Medical School
Cambridge, Massachusetts

Robert Garofalo, MD, MPH
Deputy Director, Howard Brown
Health Center; Director,
Adolescent HIV Services,
Children's Memorial Hospital;
Assistant Professor of Pediatrics,
Northwestern University
Chicago, Illinois

Hilary Goldhammer, MS
The Fenway Institute, Fenway
Community Health
Boston, Massachusetts

Joanne Greenfield, PhD
Private clinical practice
Lexington, Massachusetts

Robert Guzman, MPH
San Francisco Department of Public
Health, HIV/AIDS Biostatistics,
Epidemiology & Interventions
Section
San Francisco, California

Megan R. Hebert, MA
Rhode Island Hospital, Division of
General Internal Medicine
Providence, Rhode Island

Christopher P. Houk, MD
Department of Pediatrics, Backus
Children's Hospital, Mercer
University School of Medicine
Savannah, Georgia

Joyce Kauffman, Esq
Law Office of Joyce Kauffman
Cambridge, Massachusetts

Randi Kaufman, PsyD
Private practice
Cambridge, Massachusetts

John Kelleher, MD
Brown Medical School
Providence, Rhode Island

Lisa LaCava, MEd
Senior Consultant, Heller School for
Social Policy and Management,
Brandeis University
Waltham, Massachusetts

Raphael Landovitz, MD
Assistant Clinical Professor of
  Medicine, Center for Clinical
  AIDS Research & Education
  (CARE), David Geffen School of
  Medicine, University of California
Los Angeles, California

Peter A Lee, MD, PhD
Professor of Pediatrics, Department
  of Pediatrics, Milton S. Hershey
  Medical Center and Penn State
  College of Medicine
Hershey, Pennsylvania;
Professor of Pediatrics, Department
  of Pediatrics, Riley Hospital for
  Children and Indiana University
  School of Medicine
Indianapolis, Indiana

Harvey J. Makadon, MD
Associate Professor of Medicine,
  Harvard Medical School;
Director of Education, The Fenway
  Institute, Fenway Community
  Health;
Staff Physician, Beth Israel
  Deaconess Medical Center;
Vice President for Global Programs,
  Harvard Medical International
Boston, Massachusetts

Kenneth H. Mayer, MD
Medical Research Director and Co-
  Chair of The Fenway Institute,
  Fenway Community Health,
Boston, Massachusetts;
Professor of Medicine and
  Community Health, Brown
  University;
Attending Physician, Miriam
  Hospital; Director, Brown
  University AIDS Program
Providence, Rhode Island

Kelly McGarry, MD
Assistant Professor of Medicine,
  Brown University, Division of
  General Internal Medicine, Rhode
  Island Hospital
Providence, Rhode Island

Denise McWilliams, Esq
Director of Public Policy and Legal
  Affairs, AIDS Action Committee
  of Massachusetts, Inc.
Boston, Massachusetts

Emily L. Pitt, LICSW
Fenway Community Health
Boston, Massachusetts

Jennifer Potter, MD
Associate Professor of Medicine,
  Harvard Medical School;
Director, Women's Health Center,
  and Director, Women's Health
  Education, Beth Israel Deaconess
  Medical Center
Boston, Massachusetts

Matthew W. Ruble, MD
Clinical Instructor in Psychiatry,
  Harvard Medical School
Cambridge, Massachusetts

Jae M. Sevelius, PhD
Center for AIDS Prevention Studies,
  University of California, San
  Francisco
San Francisco, California

Yong S. Song, PhD
Assistant Clinical Professor,
  Department of Psychiatry,
  University of California
San Francisco, California

Contents

Section VI: LEGAL ISSUES AND THE LGBT COMMUNITY

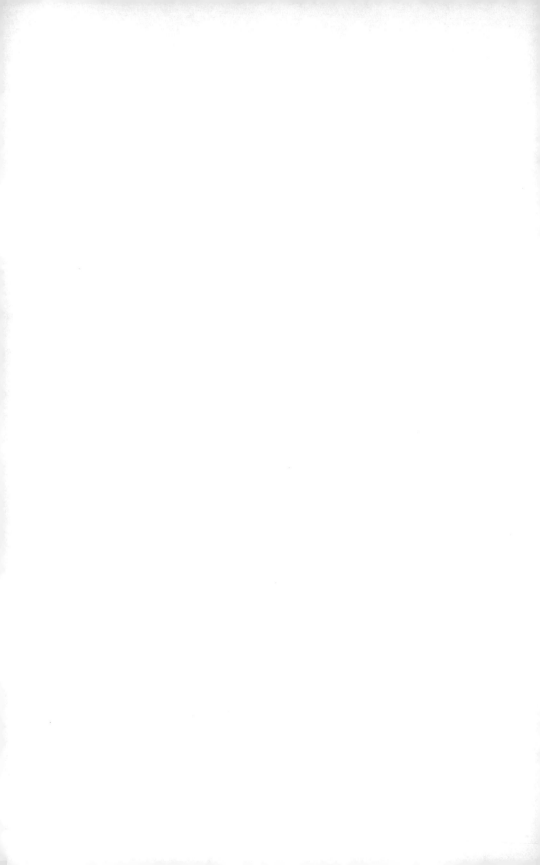

Visit http://www.acponline.org/fenwayguide *for
downloadable versions of the forms presented
in this book plus additional materials.*

Preface

While we talk about the importance of practicing evidence-based medicine, the reality is that medical science is still very much an art. This is particularly true when caring for sexual minorities, since few population-based studies have been done to document health disparities, yet stories of difficulties connecting with a caring clinician are legion. This book is dedicated to clinicians who are committed to practicing the art of medicine—learning how to form caring relationships with a wide range of patients, determine each person's unique health needs, and offer culturally relevant state-of-the-art healthcare.

Real-life experience is crucial in developing true comfort with lesbian, gay, bisexual, and transgender (LGBT) patients. Herein we describe clinical issues that are pertinent to LGBT communities and provide practical guidelines to help clinicians address these issues using a sensitive and caring approach. We hope that this information will increase clinicians' willingness to venture into new areas with patients, and thereby lead to an experiential exploration of the issues that many LGBT patients have long kept secret. Immense joy and satisfaction can be found in this work. The process of helping LGBT patients come to self-awareness and acceptance, learn how to lead healthy lives, and create strong connections with family members and friends is incredibly rewarding.

Each of us has approached this text with a unique viewpoint based on his or her own training and experience; we have worked together to include all of these perspectives in *The Fenway Guide*. We hope this work will be useful to the broad range of clinicians—nurses and nurse practitioners, physician assistants, mental health practitioners, physicians, and others—who provide primary care to LGBT patients.

Harvey J. Makadon, MD
Kenneth H. Mayer, MD
Jennifer Potter, MD
Hilary Goldhammer, MS

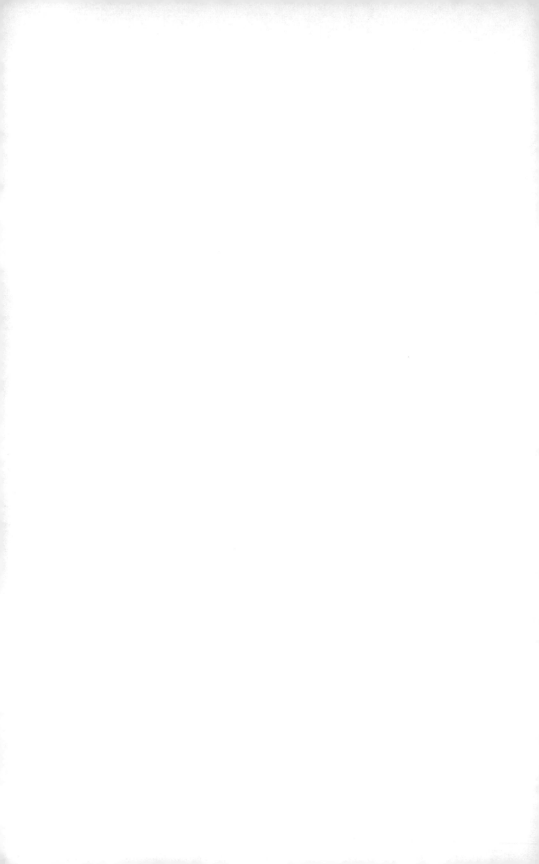

Acknowledgments

We would like to thank the American College of Physicians for publishing this ground-breaking text. We also gratefully acknowledge the individuals who have helped us along the way: Rodney Vanderwarker, Michael Cronin, Raymond Powrie, Liz Coolidge, Michele Cyr, Carol Landau, Beverly Woo, Rhonda Linde, Larry Rosenberg, Joyce Collier, Julie Ebin, Sue Johnson, Lola Wright, Serena and Marc Erickson, the Shainker-Mayer family, and Laura and Danya Potter for their invaluable insights into life as daughters with two moms and one stepmom.

In addition, we could not have undertaken this project without the pioneering efforts of the Gay and Lesbian Medical Association (GLMA), support from the Horace W. Goldsmith Foundation, and most of all, the wonderful team at the Fenway Institute and the whole Fenway Community Health family, who provide exceptional primary and behavioral healthcare and other clinical services, work tirelessly to educate the community and advocate for change to enhance LGBT healthcare, and who are creating sustainable models of care for sexual minorities and their families.

UNDERSTANDING LGBT POPULATIONS

Chapter 1

Clinicians and the Care of Sexual Minorities

JENNIFER POTTER, MD
HILARY GOLDHAMMER, MS
HARVEY J. MAKADON, MD

Elimination of health disparities among lesbian, gay, bisexual, and transgender (LGBT) individuals, also collectively called sexual minorities, was highlighted as a major goal in *Healthy People 2010*, a document prepared by the Department of Health and Human Services to serve as a roadmap for improving the health of the United States population during the first decade of this century.[1]

There is a critical need for this focus. Studies suggest that LGBT populations are disproportionately at risk for violent hate crimes, sexually transmitted infections (STIs) including HIV/AIDS, a variety of mental health conditions, substance abuse, and certain cancers. However, LGBT patients frequently encounter problems with access to quality health services, experience disparities in screening for chronic conditions, and report a lack of counseling pertinent to actual lifestyle behaviors.

Among the many factors that contribute to disparities in LGBT health, several deserve emphasis: negative societal attitudes that persist even within the medical community, lack of appropriate education for health professionals, and communication shortfalls during clinical encounters. Indeed, a major reason why clinicians do not offer appropriate guidance is that they fail to identify their LGBT patients; that is, they do not know the right questions to ask about gender identity and sexual orientation, or how to create safe environments in which patients feel comfortable volunteering this information.

Societal Attitudes and Adverse Health Effects

Societal attitudes toward homosexuality, bisexuality, and gender variance differ across cultures. However, all cultures have values regarding what is considered to be normative and appropriate with respect to both gender roles and sexual behavior. With the exception of the historical acceptance of flexible gender roles in some societies, such as among certain Native American tribes, reactions to gender variance tend to be particularly strong. We live in a society that is very conscious of and invested in gender: for example, "male or female?" is one of the first questions asked after a birth. While we can be derailed when we encounter any kind of "difference," we are often especially thrown when we make a mistake about a person's gender or when we encounter any ambiguities regarding gender. Transgender people can experience a variety of unwelcome reactions from others, such as silence punctuated by embarrassment, rejection of their gender identity (by refusing to address them with the pronoun they prefer), overt discrimination (failure to provide basic rights and services), and even frank violence.

Historically, homosexuality has also been judged quite harshly due to cultural and religious taboos against sexual openness in general, against specific sexual activities in particular (anything other than heterosexual penile-vaginal intercourse), and against the idea of sex being about pleasure, rather than just about procreation. Recent data show that much of the world is becoming more accepting of same-sex relationships between partners of legal age, although homophobia and biphobia (hostility toward lesbian/gay and bisexual people) continue to exist. The Pew Research Center's 2003 Global Attitudes Survey found that the majority of people in Western European and major Latin American countries (Mexico, Argentina, Bolivia, and Brazil) believe that homosexuality should be accepted by society, while most Russians, Poles, and Ukrainians disagreed, and people in Africa and the Middle East objected strongly. Americans are divided—a small majority (51%) believes that homosexuality should be accepted, while 42% disagree.[2] Few studies have investigated societal attitudes regarding bisexuality: existing data suggest that attitudes toward bisexuality mirror attitudes toward homosexuality.[3,4]

Stigma, prejudice, and discrimination create a stressful social environment that can lead to a variety of health problems in people who belong to minority groups.[5] *Minority stress* is a concept that researchers have begun to use when studying the health effects of chronic stress created by stigmatization. In LGBT populations, minority stress is caused by (a) an external, objective traumatic event, such as being assaulted or being fired from a job; (b) the expectation of rejection and development of vigilance in interactions with others; (c) the internalization of negative societal attitudes (also known as internalized homophobia, transphobia, or biphobia); and (d) the concealment of gender identity or sexual orientation out of shame and guilt or to protect oneself from real harm. Whatever the processes involved, minority stress produces alienation, lack of integration with the community, and problems with self-acceptance. In addition, research shows a relationship between internalized homophobia/biphobia and various forms of self-harm, including eating disorders,[6,7] high-risk sexual activity,[8] substance abuse,[9] and suicide.[9] Similar associations apply with respect to transphobia.[10]

LGBT people use a range of personal coping strategies to overcome the adverse effects of stress related to societal attitudes and their various manifestations; but many develop enhanced resilience over time. Group social structures play a critical role in this process. Affiliation with supportive community organizations permits LGBT people to experience social environments in which they are not stigmatized and to evaluate themselves in comparison with others who are like them rather than with members of the dominant culture.[5] However, it is important to realize that group solidarity and cohesiveness are not automatic outcomes, particularly for individuals who have the added challenge of managing multiple coidentities. For example, research shows that black and Latino individuals who are gay, lesbian, or bisexual frequently encounter homophobia in their racial/ethnic communities and yet also feel alienated from their racial/ethnic identity in the lesbian and gay community.[5] Though not studied, one can assume the same applies to transgender individuals. In addition, bisexuals and transgender people often experience lack of acceptance and discrimination within the lesbian and gay community. For example, male-to-female transgender and transsexual people are sometimes denied entry into women's spaces,[11] and bisexual people commonly report being shunned because they are viewed as confused, going through a phase, or in denial.[12]

Response of the Medical Profession

Homosexuality was listed as a medical disorder in the *Diagnostic and Statistical Manual of Mental Disorders* (DSM) until 1973, implying that a nonheterosexual orientation was pathological and could or should be changed. A number of purported "treatments" have been attempted, including aversion techniques, hormone administration, shock treatment, castration, and even lobotomy.[13] Despite the relatively recent proclamation by numerous professional organizations that homosexuality is not a disease and that efforts should focus on helping patients make a healthy adjustment to their sexual orientation, it is not surprising that some clinicians have been slow to change. There are still some clinicians who believe that LGBT individuals rarely face discrimination[14] or who espouse methods to prevent[15] or cure[16] homosexuality. While there is currently a movement toward removing gender identity disorder from the DSM, this designation continues to be listed as a bona fide diagnosis to this day. This inclusion is troubling, because it implies that people with gender identity issues are mentally unbalanced, contributes to a lack of willingness to consider prescribing hormone treatment, and dismisses sex reassignment surgeries as purely "elective" or "cosmetic" procedures.[17] It is, however, important to recognize that the stress of gender confusion, like any type of stress, can lead to anxiety, dysphoria, and depression as described in Chapter 12: Introduction to Transgender Identity and Health.

Until recently, the topic of human sexuality has been given short shrift in training programs for health professionals. Therefore, it is not surprising that clinicians' comfort level and skill at taking a sexual history are often not optimal. However, there is ample evidence that patients would like us to ask about sexual matters. For example, 85% of respondents in a survey of 500 men and women over age 25 expressed a desire to talk with their health providers about sexual issues; however, 68% were reluctant to raise the topic themselves, and 71% worried that their concerns would be dismissed.[18] Due to fear of negative consequences, LGBT patients are particularly unlikely to reveal information about their sexual orientation spontaneously.[19] Unfortunately, despite the need for health providers to be proactive in raising the subject, only a minority (11%-37%) of primary care clinicians obtain a sexual history routinely in encounters with new adult patients.[20] Reasons cited for this failure include fear of being intrusive; ignorance regarding clinical relevance; lack of knowledge about what and how to ask; concern about how to respond to information that is divulged; and time constraints.[20] Lack of education is largely responsible. For example, a 1999 survey of 141 North American medical schools found that the majority of undergraduate medical programs provide fewer than ten hours of education on human sexuality; over half did not offer any continuing education courses on the subject.[21] Clearly, health professions training programs need to devote more attention to the topic of human sexuality in general.

Although taking a sexual history in all patients, regardless of sexual orientation or gender identity, is crucial and often overlooked, a focus solely on the sexual behavior of LGBT persons ignores other significant health risks that deserve attention. Furthermore, this focus prevents clinicians from seeing LGBT patients as whole individuals with rich lives that are often complicated by their status as sexual or gender minorities. Clinicians need to be prepared to help their patients with a range of life issues, including the stressful process of coming out, partnership and parenting issues, and end-of-life directives for unmarried same-sex couples. Until recently, little practical information specific to the care of LGBT populations existed. This is due in large part to a lack of comprehensive research on this topic. For example, in a literature review of nearly four million English-language articles published between 1980 and 1999, only 3777 addressed LGBT issues, the majority concentrated on gay or bisexual men, and 56% of the articles focused on STIs.[22] Fortunately, there has been an increase in research on a broader variety of topics in LGBT health during the past eight years. In addition, several professional organizations[23] have declared a need for more educational resources that address LGBT health specifically. Our hope is that this book, which joins a small but growing handful of resources devoted to this topic (please see Table 1-1), will be a useful guide for clinicians who seek to enhance their care of LGBT patients.

Clinicians Have a Duty to Provide Culturally Competent Care

LGBT health is a topic of particular importance to clinicians for a number of reasons. Clinicians not only have a duty to "do no harm" but, according to the standards of care published by all of the major health professions organizations today, are obligated to educate themselves appropriately to be able to provide culturally competent health services to diverse patients, including LGBT patients.[24] The process of becoming more culturally competent requires clinicians to challenge previously held beliefs and assumptions about gender and sexuality and thereby provides an excellent

---

Table 1-1   General LGBT Health Education Resources for Clinicians

Guidelines for the care of lesbian, gay, bisexual, and transgender patients. Gay and Lesbian Medical Association.
Available at http://www.glma.org

Healthy People 2010: companion document for lesbian, gay, bisexual, and transgender health. Gay and Lesbian Medical Association.
Available at http://www.glma.org

Community standards of practice for provision of quality healthcare services for gay, lesbian, bisexual, and transgendered clients. GLBT Health Access Project.
Available at http://www.glbthealth.org/index.html.

Feldman JL, Goldberg J. **Transgender Primary Medical Care: Suggested Guidelines for Clinicians in British Columbia Vancouver Coastal Health, Vancouver, BC, 2006**.
Available at http://www.vch.ca/transhealth/resources/library/tcpdocs/guidelines-primcare.pdf.

Transgender Health Program. Trans Care Project.
Available at http://www.vch.ca/transhealth/resources/tcp.html.

The Harry Benjamin International Gender Dysphoria Association's Standards of Care for Gender Identity Disorder, 6th Version.
Available at http://www.wpath.org/soc.htm.

A Provider's Handbook on Culturally Competent Care: Lesbian, Gay, Bisexual and Transgendered Population. Kaiser Permanente National Diversity Council and the Kaiser Permanente National Diversity Department. San Francisco, 2000.
Available from:
Kaiser Permanente
National Diversity Department
One Kaiser Plaza, 22 Lakeside
Oakland, CA 94612
510-271-6663—hotline
510-271-5757—fax

opportunity for personal growth. Moreover, clinicians are likely to experience significant professional satisfaction when they realize the impact of their acceptance and support in helping LGBT patients achieve a healthy life adjustment. In addition, heightened sensitivity to the experience and needs of one population generally results in an enhanced ability to communicate more effectively with other populations and will therefore result in better care for *all* patients.

Some clinicians may sidestep becoming better educated about the needs of LGBT patients because they do not believe they provide care to any of these individuals in their practices. Health professionals frequently make incorrect assumptions about patients based on their appearance and demeanor as well as knowledge of factors such as marital and parenting status and whether they express conservative versus liberal political or religious beliefs. As mentioned previously, data suggest that the failure of clinicians to recognize their LGBT patients is an ascertainment issue (we don't ask and they don't tell) rather than a demographic issue (LGBT people do not exist). While the exact number of people who identify themselves as LGBT is not known, the best designed study of sexual behavior and orientation in the United States to date found that 1.4% of women and 2.8% of men identify themselves as bisexual or homosexual; 4.3% of women and 9.1% of men report some "same-sex behavior since puberty"; and 7.5% of women and 7.7% of men report experiencing same-sex desire or attraction.[25] There is no reliable data on the numbers of transgender people; prevalence estimates vary widely and tend to include only transsexual persons who have undergone sex reassignment surgery (SRS).[26,27] The prevalence of female-to-male postoperative transsexuals is thought to be about three times lower than that of male-to-female postoperative transsexuals.[27]

How Can We Do Better?

Understand the Dynamics of Change and Obtain Support

Failure to understand the process of change often accounts for a widespread lack of success in making educational improvements. This is particularly true when the change that is contemplated—in this case, increasing the time and attention that are devoted to instruction on LGBT health—is by its very nature bound to be unpopular among some groups. Therefore, we will briefly review factors that facilitate change before recommending strategies to help clinicians provide better care for their LGBT patients.

When people are asked to brainstorm ideas about change, they come up with a mixture of both positive and negative terms: on the one hand, *exhilaration, risk-taking, excitement, energizing, life-changing;* on the other, *fear, anxiety, loss, threat, panic.* Therefore, change can be seen as a crisis that represents both danger and opportunity. Because of the danger factor, people are often disinclined to embark on a process of change. Heifetz and Linsky describe this reluctance well in the following quote:

> Adaptive change stimulates resistance because it challenges people's habits, beliefs, and values. It asks them to take a loss, experience uncertainty, and even express disloyalty to people and cultures. Because adaptive change forces people to question and perhaps redefine aspects of their identity, it also challenges their sense of competence. Loss, disloyalty, and feeling incompetent: that's a lot to ask. No wonder people resist.[28]

Sustained behavioral change is generally accomplished only after a thorough process of self-questioning, in which a person explores his or her feelings, thoughts, and values, as well as the reasons why he or she does and does not want to change.[29] With respect to increasing competency in LGBT health, clinicians may find it helpful to start by asking: "How do I feel about learning more about LGBT health?" "What factors are motivating me?" "What factors are holding me back?" "What are my short- and long-term goals?" and "Do I have the resources and support I need to reach these goals?"

Fullan has identified three factors ("social attractors") that facilitate educational change: having a strong sense of purpose (motivation, inspiration, passion); quality ideas (content); and quality relationships (context).[30] Relationships are the crucial ingredient. Mentoring and peer support help foster and nurture purpose, knowledge is improved by sharing and critiquing information with others, and performance is strengthened by being observed and receiving constructive feedback. In essence, transformative change requires the power of people working together; by definition, this means changing the social context. Therefore, learning should take place in a setting where both teachers and learners are available to participate in this reciprocal process. For clinicians who work in isolated settings and for whom this is not possible on a day-to-day basis, we encourage connection to an external organization that can provide a similar function. Table 1-2 provides a list of organizations that sponsor regular conferences related to LGBT health and professional organizations with LGBT interest groups clinicians may be interested in joining.

Focus on the Clinician-Patient Relationship

Advances in science and technology notwithstanding, successful health outcomes continue to depend heavily on the quality of clinician-patient relationships. Good quality relationships contain several key ingredients. Empathy—the capacity of the clinician to identify with the patient and to experience his feelings vicariously—is often considered to be a core dimension.[31] Alternatively, it has been suggested that a clinician lends strength or

Table 1-2   LGBT Health: Opportunities for Learning More

Organizations Offering Conferences, Training, and Other Services

- Atlanta Lesbian Cancer Initiative (http://www.thehealthinitiative.org)
- Gay and Lesbian Medical Association (http://www.glma.org)
- GLBT Health Access Project (http://www.glbthealth.org)
- Lesbian Health Research Center (http://www.lesbianhealthinfo.org)
- LGBTI Health Summit (http://www.healthsummit2007.org)
- The Mautner Project, the National Lesbian Health Organization (http://www.mautnerproject.org)
- National Association of Lesbian and Gay Addiction Professionals, Inc. (http://www.nalgap.org)
- The National Coalition for LGBT Health (http://www.lgbthealth.net)
- Rainbow Access Initiative (http://www.rainbowaccess.org)
- The SafeGuards Project (http://www.safeguards.org)

LGBT Professional Special Interest Groups

- American Academy of Physician Assistants: Lesbian, Bisexual, Gay PA Caucus (http://www.aapa.org)
- American Medical Association: GLBT Advisory Committee (http://www.ama-assn.org)
- American Medical Student Association: LGBT Health Action Committee (http://www.amsa.org/lgbt)
- American Psychological Association: Committee on Lesbian, Gay, Bisexual Concerns (http://www.apa.org/pi/lgbc)
- American Public Health Association: LGBT Caucus of Public Health Workers (http://www.apha.org)
- Association of Gay and Lesbian Psychiatrists (http://www.aglp.org)
- Gay and Lesbian Medical Association (http://www.glma.org)
- Lavender Lamps: National Lesbian and Gay Nurses Association (718-933-1158)
- National Association of Social Workers: National Committee on Lesbian, Gay, Bisexual, and Transgender Issues (http://www.socialworkers.org/governance/cmtes/nclgbi.asp)

---

solidity to a patient whose foundation has been shaken by stress or illness.[32] Others call attention to the need for clinicians and patients to develop a shared meaning and agenda and outline specific behaviors that can facilitate the process of exchange and negotiation.[33,34] Finally, a number of writers describe caring—the personal interest a clinician feels for a patient—as the fundamental quality.[35] A productive clinician-patient relationship can have an enormous impact on patient well-being. This is perhaps best exemplified by the "placebo effect," which can be defined as the positive therapeutic effect generated by the psychosocial context in which medical care is rendered.[36]

Despite the importance of attending to the emotional aspects of healthcare, research has shown insufficient training and education in this area.[37] Fortunately, most professional organizations now have guidelines that articulate standards of care regarding optimal interaction with patients. For example, the Accreditation Council for Graduate Medical Education (ACGME) requires physician trainees to (a) demonstrate respect, compassion, integrity, and accountability to patients; (b) make a conscientious effort to exceed ordinary expectations and commit to lifelong learning; (c) adhere to ethical principles regarding confidentiality, informed consent, and providing versus withholding care; and (d) display sensitivity and responsiveness to diverse patient characteristics, including culture, age, gender, and disabilities.[38] Educational materials specifically geared toward enhancing clinician communication skills are being increasingly included in health professions curricula. The American Academy on Communication in Healthcare (http://www.aachonline.org) and the Center for Communication and Medicine (http://www.feinberg.northwestern.edu/ccm) are good overall resources.

Address All Three Domains of Learning: Attitudes, Knowledge, and Skills

Educators recognize three interrelated domains of learning—attitudes, knowledge, and skills.[39] All three domains need to be addressed to achieve maximal competence in any area of study. We therefore consider each domain separately in this section, which presents suggestions to help clinicians examine their attitudes, increase their knowledge, and enhance the skill with which they provide care to LGBT patients.

"Attitude Is Everything"
(Author unknown)

Attitudes have a major effect on health outcomes.[40] Patient attitudes toward the healthcare system and the health professionals who work in it have an enormous influence on health-seeking behaviors and adherence to healthcare recommendations. When patients have negative attitudes, they are more likely to feel disconnected, avoid the healthcare system altogether, and, in some cases, become angry or disruptive. Patients with positive attitudes, on the other hand, are more likely to develop trusting relationships, disclose complete information, respond favorably to clinical recommendations, and feel satisfied with their care. Clinicians' attitudes also drive behavior. Health professionals who harbor negative attitudes toward certain patients may avoid contact with those patients or, worse, express their negative attitudes either directly or indirectly and cause harm.

Attention to attitudes requires growth in the affective arena. For clinicians, this involves developing awareness of and respect for a patient's difference(s) and a willingness to listen empathically to that person's experience. This is not always easy to do. Negative attitudes toward LGBT people are common: clinicians—regardless of whether they are lesbian, bisexual, transgender, or heterosexual—are subject to the same influences as everyone else and are vulnerable to believing stereotypes and making assumptions. A helpful exercise in examining one's own beliefs is to quickly write down all the labels and stereotypes, both negative and positive, one associates with the terms "gay man," "lesbian," "heterosexual woman," "heterosexual man," "bisexual," and "transgender."[41] Exercises such as this can stimulate us to think about our deepest internal reactions to people of difference. It is easy to see how personal biases, even the ones we wish to dispose of, can interfere with the process of truly understanding a patient and establishing empathy during a clinical encounter.

The more "different" clinicians perceive themselves to be from their patients (and vice versa), the more likely it is that either or both parties will feel uncomfortable during clinical interactions. Numerous factors affect the quality of the clinician-patient relationship, including externally observed and internally inferred characteristics of both the clinician and the patient (gender, age, race or ethnicity, social class, education, disability, sociocultural beliefs, religious attitudes and values, and sexual orientation). Clinician-patient dyads that seek to become more comfortable with difference must attend to all of these variables. The greater the number of disconnects, the more complicated and lengthy the process is likely to be.

Depending on personal comfort level with gender and sexual diversity, clinicians may experience a wide variety of emotions when a patient discloses that they might be or are lesbian, gay, bisexual, or transgender. Surprise, anxiety, guilt, fear, confusion, anger, disgust, and delight are all possible emotional reactions. A clinician's response to the multitude of feelings that can arise can have either a negative or a positive impact on the therapeutic relationship. Clinicians who avoid acknowledging and examining their emotions are likely to have limited or incomplete understanding of their subsequent motivations and actions.[42] Avoidance also makes it more likely that these emotions will affect the patient in ways that are counterproductive or even harmful. Discriminatory reactions on the part of healthcare personnel, including hostility, denial of care, violation of confidentiality, and refusal to acknowledge a patient's partner, have been reported in the literature, though most of these studies are over ten years old.[43] On the other hand, clinicians who take the time to examine their responses in detail are more likely to be able to negotiate, accept, and perhaps even take pleasure in the differences between themselves and their patients. These clinicians are much more likely to create a trusting and nonjudgmental atmosphere in which to conduct care.

Clinicians have a professional duty to examine the basis of their emotional reactions toward patients and the assumptions they make about patients. We are trained not to casually accept the first diagnosis that pops into our heads. Instead, we ask ourselves: "What evidence supports this diagnosis?" or "Is there anything else that could be going on?" Similarly, we should not automatically accept our personal biases without question. When we have a particularly strong reaction to a patient, we might ask:

"Why am I responding this way?" "What is the evidence that my assumption is correct?" "Is there any other possible interpretation?" or "How can I take care of this patient in as nonjudgmental a manner as possible?" Materials have been developed to help clinicians-in-training examine their own beliefs and values regarding gender identity and sexual orientation.[44,45,46] Box 1-1 presents an exercise modified from these materials that can be used privately by individual readers or adapted for use in a classroom setting to assist in this process.

In addition to the value of questioning in challenging bias, stereotypical attitudes can also be changed through experience—that is, contrary to the old adage, familiarity actually breeds comfort rather than contempt. Research studies show that the more contact clinicians have with patients who are "different," the more comfortable they are likely to feel during clinical interactions and the more positive their attitudes toward these patients will become. This holds true for the majority view of various minority populations, including racial and ethnic groups as well as sexual and gender minorities.[47] Therefore, clinicians who are particularly interested in changing their attitudes about people with nontraditional gender identity and sexual orientation are advised to attend LGBT-focused continuing education conferences and to seek out training experiences in settings where they are likely to encounter large numbers of LGBT patients. Table 1-2 provides a list of professional organizations that regularly sponsor conferences, training,

---

Box 1-1 Sample Self-Assessment Exercises[44,45,46]

Personal Biases (Sample Questions):

Do you think that lesbian, gay, bisexual, or transgender people should not hold certain jobs or social positions? If so, why?

Have you ever stopped yourself from doing or saying something because you might be perceived as gay or lesbian? Or too masculine or feminine?

How do you think you would feel if a family member came out as lesbian, gay, bisexual, or transgender?

Values and Attitudes (Sample Questions):

What are your first reactions to the following statements? How strongly do you agree or disagree and why?

- I am comfortable talking with my patients about sexual behaviors other than penile-vaginal intercourse.
- Being gay or lesbian is a lifestyle choice.
- I feel uncomfortable when I see two men holding hands in public.
- I would be upset if someone thought I were gay or lesbian.
- If a child of mine came out as transgender, I would think I did something wrong as a parent.

and educational seminars, and Table 1-3 lists healthcare facilities with particular expertise in providing care to LGBT patients.

"Knowledge Is Power"
(Sir Francis Bacon, English author, courtier, and philosopher, 1561-1626)

The second educational domain—knowledge—comprises acquisition of factual data, as well as the mental capacity to question, analyze, synthesize, and evaluate this information. Progress in this domain requires that clinicians ask themselves: "What do I need to know?" and "Where can I obtain accurate information?" and "How can I, on an ongoing basis, make sure that this information is up to date?"

There are three major areas of knowledge clinicians need to master to provide optimal care to LGBT patients:

1. How to create a healthcare environment (and a trusting clinician-patient relationship) in which LGBT patients feel safe receiving care;
2. How to identify the health consequences of societal stigma, risk behaviors that are prevalent among LGBT populations (for example, alcohol use among lesbians; club drug use among gay men; and street hormone use among transgender people), and specific healthcare needs of various subpopulations (for example, the need for anatomy-appropriate and hormone-appropriate screening for a transgender patient who is in transition);
3. How to provide appropriate support, counseling, screening, treatment, and referral for patients who are (a) grappling with life-phase issues (coming out, establishing intimate relationships, parenting, aging); (b) participating in risky behaviors; or (c) have other specific healthcare needs.

Table 1-3 Healthcare Facilities with Expertise in LGBT Populations (partial listing)

- Fenway Community Health, Boston, MA (http://www.fenwayhealth.org)
- Hartford Gay and Lesbian Health Collective, Hartford, CT (http://www.hglhc.org)
- Callen-Lorde Community Health Center, New York, NY (http://www.callen-lorde.org)
- Whitman-Walker Clinic, Washington, DC (http://www.wwc.org)
- Chase-Brexton Health Services, 3 sites in MD (http://www.chasebrexton.org)
- Howard Brown Health Center, Chicago, IL (http://www.howardbrown.org)
- Montrose Clinic, Houston, TX (http://www.montroseclinic.org)
- L.A. Gay and Lesbian Center, Los Angeles, CA (http://www.lagaycenter.org)
- Magnet, San Francisco, CA (men only) (http://www.magnetsf.org)
- Pacific Pride Foundation, Santa Barbara, CA (http://www.pacificpridefoundation.org)

This chapter will not discuss these issues in great detail, as they are explored in depth in succeeding chapters in this book. However, several general observations are appropriate.

There Are Many Ways to Create a Safe Environment

There are many things clinicians can do to create a safe healthcare environment for LGBT patients. First and foremost, it is important to resist making assumptions about a person's gender identity, sexual orientation, and lifestyle behaviors based on his or her appearance, demeanor, or any other characteristics. It is important to provide nonverbal (visual and environmental) cues that signal acceptance, as well as to attend carefully and respectfully to verbal and written communication. Examples of the former include posting a nondiscrimination policy in the office; displaying educational brochures that are pertinent to LGBT populations; including demographic categories on intake forms that honor LGBT identities and lifestyles; and ensuring availability of a unisex restroom. Examples of the latter include learning how to ask sensitive, open, and direct questions about gender issues, sexual orientation, risk behaviors, and overall life adjustment and explicitly discussing and maintaining confidentiality. These measures are described in more detail in Chapter 15.

Language and Self-Definition Are Exceedingly Important

Learning how to communicate sensitively and effectively requires that we develop an appreciation for the variety of ways in which people define and express their sexuality and gender. Sexual orientation can be seen as comprising three dimensions: behavior, identity, and desire. Lesbian, gay, and bisexual populations are those who have "an orientation toward people of the same gender in sexual behavior, affection, or attraction, and/or self-identify as gay or lesbian or bisexual."[48] People who identify themselves as gay or lesbian tend to have romantic and sexual relationships with members of the same gender, while those who self-identify as bisexual have the potential for experiencing such relationships with members of any gender. Bisexuals may feel equally attracted to both men and women or have a stronger preference for one gender. It is important to note, however, that sexual identity, behavior, and attraction are fluid and may change over time, and sexual identity does not always align with sexual behavior and attraction. For example, a married man who identifies as heterosexual may be exclusively attracted to men and have sexual and emotional relationships with other men as well as with his wife. Similarly, a woman who identifies as a lesbian and has a female partner may have had relationships with men in the past.

Understanding the "T" in LGBT can be more confusing. The definition of transgender has changed over time and continues to be used inconsistently. Most broadly, the term includes anyone who does not conform to traditional gender norms for men and women. When used in this sense, it includes people who do not identify as either male or female, as well as people who experience and choose to express their gender identity as opposite to their biological (birth) sex. Cross-dressers, "drag queens," and "drag kings" are sometimes also considered transgender; however, these individuals generally do not identify as another gender and typically cross-dress for entertainment purposes or to experience erotic sensations. Importantly, transgender refers to gender identity and is therefore distinct from sexual orientation; transgender individuals may seek relationships with men, women, or other transgender individuals and may identify as gay, lesbian, straight, or bisexual.

People who are born with atypical sexual or reproductive anatomy are often referred to as intersex. The medical community has begun to use the term disorders of sex development (DSD) in place of intersex to describe the variety of conditions that involve anomalies of the sex chromosomes, reproductive ducts, gonads, and genitalia. Once considered by some to be a subgroup of transgender,[48] people with DSD are now seen as a separate group with distinct concerns regarding ethical approaches to their medical, surgical, and behavioral healthcare. Because caring for people with DSD obliges clinicians to possess greater sensitivity to the complexities of gender and sexual health, we have included a chapter on this topic (Chapter 14).

Some people object to the traditional labels of gender or sexuality and may choose to use nontraditional identity terms, such as "same-gender loving man" or "woman-loving woman." Others reject labels altogether and describe themselves as gender neutral. In recent years, the term "queer" has become increasingly popular as a term of both sexual and gender identity, especially among adolescents and young adults. Queer means many things to many people, but generally refers to anyone who does not conform to societal norms or expectations for gender or sexual orientation. Historically viewed as derogatory, queer has been embraced as an empowering self-definition by some, though not all, LGBT individuals and communities.

Finally, it is important to realize that some people who have same-gender relationships, particularly men from racial and ethnic minority communities, self-identify as heterosexual.[49] Reasons for adopting a straight rather than gay identity are multiple. Some racial or ethnic minority men view gay culture and identity as white, Western, and classist, and they do not feel welcome in the LGBT community. Others believe that to embrace a gay identity would be to reject family and religious values, or ethnic culture, and could lead to estrangement from family and community. Because of the diversity of sexual identities and behavior in different populations, much of the scientific literature on gay men's health has adopted the behaviorally focused phrase "men who have sex with men" or MSM. For similar reasons, some lesbian health research uses "women who have sex with women" or WSW. In this text, we use both LGB and MSM/WSW terminology, depending on the context. Definitions and selection of appropriate language are described in more detail in Chapters 3 and 12.

All Staff Should Receive Training

It is important to remember that a patient's experience in a healthcare facility is impacted by *all* of the individuals they encounter during the process of care. These people include the person who makes their initial appointment on the telephone, the valet in the parking garage, the receptionist who greets them on arrival, the nursing assistant who takes their vital signs, and so on. Therefore, it is vital that *everyone* who works in the healthcare arena, including administrative and janitorial staff, receive training. A physician or nurse may be very sensitive to LGBT issues, but if, for example, a receptionist makes an even remotely insensitive comment, the patient may develop a negative impression of the practice.[50] Staff development regarding LGBT-specific, culturally competent language and interactions will not only help ensure a safe, welcoming, nonjudgmental experience for patients, but may also relieve anxiety and confusion among employees who are unfamiliar with and do not feel prepared to serve LGBT patients. Table 1-2 provides a list of organizations that have developed high-quality training programs.

"Practice Is the Best of All Instructors"
(Publius Syrus, Roman author, first century BC)

The third and final educational domain—skills—consists of developing objectively measurable behaviors that demonstrate ability. For clinicians who seek to improve care for sexual and gender minorities, developing the ability to communicate sensitively and effectively with LGBT patients is the skill of paramount importance. As discussed above, attention to two areas—identification and examination of personal biases, as well as learning about cultural characteristics that impact risk factors and disease incidence—set the stage for clinicians to communicate more productively. However, attitudes and knowledge are not enough: developing skills requires practice. Clearly, the best way to practice is through actual experience interacting with LGBT patients: again, the reader is referred to Table 1-3, which provides a list of healthcare facilities where large numbers of LGBT patients receive care and where clinical internships may be available. However, since opportunities for concentrated exposure to LGBT patients are limited, it may be more practical to experiment with different communication techniques in hypothetical situations, through role-play exercises. Sample exercises are presented in Box 1-2. The educational value of both real and contrived scenarios is greatly enhanced when feedback is provided: therefore, clinicians are encouraged to ask a trusted colleague to serve as an observer.

Box 1-2 Sample Role-Play Exercises

During a routine history, a male patient tells you that he is sexually active with men and identifies as gay. He then asks how this makes you feel. How would you respond?

A patient complains of anxiety due to her adolescent daughter's recent revelation that she is bisexual. The patient worries that her daughter is sexually promiscuous and will get HIV. She has heard that bisexuality is "hip" among young people now and hopes that it is "just a stage." How would you respond?

A new patient named Lauren is waiting in the exam room for a routine checkup and Pap smear. When you walk into the room, you see a person who looks like a man. How would you respond?

During a routine history, a patient tells you that she has been feeling "real down lately" and isn't sleeping well. Later, during a sexual history, she says she had sex with another woman, but is "definitely not a lezzie." How would you respond?

A patient tells you that she and her female partner would like to start a family and want some guidance on alternative insemination techniques. How would you respond?

In the break room, you overhear two medical assistants making fun of the appearance and demeanor of a transgender patient who visited the clinic earlier in the day. How would you respond?

Strategies for Educating Others and Effecting Change

Once enlightened, some clinicians may choose to become trailblazers—to share what they have learned with others and push for more widespread change by teaching and implementing curricular reform or effecting change at the institutional or governmental (public policy) level. This section addresses some of the challenges clinician leaders are likely to encounter and suggests steps that can be taken to maximize success.

In academic medicine, "watch one, do one" and "learn one, teach one" are familiar mantras. There is an expectation that we not only continually seek to increase our own knowledge but that once we possess superior knowledge we will share it with others and use it to correct misinformation. This is surprisingly hard to do with respect to LGBT issues, since the topic is frequently judged unworthy of attention; moreover, the teacher is liable to be judged for raising it. For example, consider the small "teachable moment" that arises when a fellow student or colleague makes an antigay joke. Clinicians who decide to respond by explaining why the joke is unacceptable should anticipate reactions ranging from surprise ("I didn't know you felt so strongly about gay issues!") to ridicule ("You're taking this way too seriously—it's just a joke.") to outright denigration ("What is it with you that this matters so much—are you gay, or what?"). In essence, the experience closely resembles what it feels like to an LGBT person to come out. It is important for clinicians to feel solid before taking on this kind of challenge.

Clinicians who are themselves LGBT may consider coming out as part of the process of educating others about LGBT issues. As is true in any other arena, a number of challenges and rewards are associated with coming out as an LGBT health professional. Since bias is pervasive, LGBT clinicians who decide to be open will encounter resistance, which, in the worst case scenario, may limit opportunities for advancement. There is also a danger that once a person is known to be LGBT, other attributes are quickly forgotten, and one starts to be seen as representative of LGBT populations. On the other hand, coming out facilitates personal adjustment and can have profoundly beneficial effects on relationships with colleagues, students, and—in some cases—patients. Readers are referred to Chapter 3 for a more complete discussion. Coming out as an LGBT health professional is always a complicated decision that should only be undertaken after careful consideration of potential consequences and in the presence of sufficient support. However, we believe the results are generally positive.[51]

All clinicians, both LGBT and non-LGBT, who seek support to challenge prevailing views about gender or sexual identity, may be interested in joining a professional organization committed to improving health for sexual minority populations. A number of professional organizations are devoted to this purpose; in addition, many mainstream organizations have special interest groups that are similarly dedicated (please see Table 1-2). Clinician teachers who wish to become involved in curricular reform face additional challenges. For those who encounter a reluctant dean, mentioning the *Healthy People 2010*[1] call to action and requirements of organizations such as the ACGME regarding cultural competency[38] may be helpful. However, professional mandates are not enough. Clinician educators will be expected to explain exactly what information needs to be included in the curriculum and why, how it will be included, who will teach it, and how learning will be evaluated. Obtaining and presenting information about programs that have already been successfully implemented elsewhere is likely to be persuasive and will help facilitate the process of change without re-inventing the wheel. Educational leadership will also be more likely to respond favorably to proposals that come with funding to support the costly process of curriculum design, implementation, evaluation, and refinement. Therefore, a concerted attempt should be made to explore potential sources of funding, including individual donors, foundations, and federal grants. If all else fails, it may be helpful to remember to draw on "bottom-up" as well as "top-down" strategies; that is, look to support from the users of the curriculum—in this case, the clinician trainees themselves. Finally, external support is always valuable, and clinician teachers are encouraged to network.

Hopefully many clinicians will choose to become active at the institutional level to create an appropriate context in which to offer high quality care to LGBT patients. It is difficult to sustain an office culture that celebrates and protects diversity without having policies that clarify and support the principles of that culture. Therefore, we recommend that clinicians who are in management roles create and implement antidiscrimination policies for both employees and patients. Clinicians who do not have direct managerial responsibility themselves can advocate for adoption of these same policies with institutional leadership. Specific policy suggestions are listed in Table 1-4.

The manner in which antidiscrimination policies are disseminated has a strong influence on uptake. They should be written in languages appropriate to the populations served at the healthcare facility, posted in strategic areas, and included in informational or promotional materials about the facility. Policies geared toward employees should be discussed during the interview process, presented in the employee handbook, and reviewed during orientation programs. All staff should be aware of all policies. It is crucial to communicate clearly to all employees that discrimination in the delivery of services based on gender identity or sexual orientation violates standards of good care and will be subject to disciplinary action.

Some clinicians will also feel moved to become active in regional and national advocacy efforts. Small steps, such as starting a working group or becoming involved in an interest group, can mean a lot both to LBGT patients and LGBT employees.

Conclusion

This chapter began with a call to action, reviewed major causes of health disparities among LGBT populations, and outlined steps clinicians can take to improve the sensitivity and competence with which they care for LGBT patients. Several features of this journey deserve particular emphasis. First,

---

Table 1-4   Suggestions for Creating a Pro-Diversity Workplace

Policies

- Create a policy that prohibits discrimination in the delivery of services to all minorities, including sexual and gender minorities.
- Create a policy that prohibits discrimination and harassment of LGBT employees.
- Provide LGBT employees with the same benefits and compensation for themselves and their families as all other employees, whether they are single, married, in a civil union, or otherwise partnered.
- Put in procedures for patients to file and resolve complaints alleging violations of antidiscrimination policies.

Outreach

- Conduct patient outreach and marketing in LGBT venues, Web sites, and media.
- Post clinician contact information on the Gay and Lesbian Medical Association Web site (http://www.glma.org).
- Advertise and recruit for staff positions in LGBT media and organizations.

the importance of identifying and examining personal biases and assumptions cannot be overemphasized; Box 1-1 presented an exercise that may serve as a useful starting point. Second, it is always difficult to challenge the status quo, particularly around a topic that continues to be quite controversial. Therefore, it is crucial to find support in every corner where it exists—from students, peers, and mentors, and from within the healthcare facility where one works as well as from external sources—in order to move forward. We have tried to include a substantive list of resources to help clinicians make these connections (see Appendix A).

Lastly, but perhaps most important of all, the results of this journey can be extraordinarily gratifying. In a landmark article, "The Care of the Patient," Frances Weld Peabody wrote: "One of the essential qualities of the clinician is interest in humanity, for the secret of the care of the patient is in caring for the patient."[52] While it is inevitable that biases and assumptions will sometimes intrude in any clinician-patient interaction, diverting attention and preventing true "presence," empathy is such an integral part of the healing process that we urge clinicians to consciously and deliberately tune in to all of their patients emotionally. The power of a warm smile, a listening ear, or a kind word can be absolutely transforming.

Summary Points

- Studies suggest that LGBT populations are disproportionately at risk for a variety of medical and mental health conditions. Elimination of health disparities among LGBT populations is critical and has been highlighted as a major goal of *Healthy People 2010.*
- Negative societal attitudes toward LGBT people are diminishing but continue to persist even within the medical community.
- Stigma and discrimination, including verbal taunts and physical assault, create a stressful social environment for LGBT populations that can lead to alienation, problems with self-acceptance, and internalized feelings of shame. Research shows a relationship between internalized homophobia, biphobia, and transphobia and various forms of self-harm, including eating disorders and substance abuse.
- Clinicians need and deserve more education and training in providing a higher quality of care for their LGBT patients.
- For clinicians to achieve maximal competence in the care of LGBT patients, it is necessary to address three interrelated domains of learning—attitudes, knowledge, and skills:
    - *Attitudes* involve developing an awareness of and respect for a patient's difference(s) and a willingness to listen empathically to that person's experience. Attitude change can be achieved by examining personal beliefs and values regarding gender identity and sexual orientation, attending LGBT-focused continuing education conferences,

and seeking training experiences in settings where there are likely to be large numbers of LGBT patients.

○ *Knowledge* involves learning to create a healthcare environment in which LGBT patients feel safe and welcomed, developing an awareness and appreciation of the variety of ways in which people define and express their sexuality and gender, and ensuring that all staff in a healthcare facility receive appropriate training and support.

○ *Skills* entail actual experiences interacting with LGBT patients in a supportive learning environment or, if this is not possible, experimenting with different communication techniques in hypothetical situations through role-play exercises.

• Clinicians can play an important leadership role when they share what they have learned about LGBT health with others and push for more widespread change by teaching and implementing curricular reform or effecting change at the institutional or governmental (public policy) level. Joining a special interest group, developing and implementing antidiscrimination policies for your healthcare facility, and connecting with organizations that have developed LGBT curricula are all important steps in effecting change.

References

1. **US Department of Health and Human Services**. Healthy People 2010: Understanding and Improving Health. 2nd ed. US Government Printing Office; 2000.
2. **The Pew Global Attitudes Project**. Views of a changing world, June 2003. Pew Research Center for the People and the Press; 2003. Available at http://pewglobal.org/reports/display.php?ReportID=185.
3. **Mohr JJ, Rochlen AB**. Measuring attitudes regarding bisexuality in lesbian, gay male, and heterosexual populations. Journal of Counseling Psychology. 1999;46:353-69.
4. **Ochs R**. Biphobia: it goes more than two ways. In: Firestein BA, ed. Bisexuality: The Psychology and Politics of an Invisible Minority. Sage; 1996: 217-39.
5. **Meyer IH**. Prejudice, social stress, and mental health in lesbian, gay and bisexual populations: conceptual issues and research evidence. Psychological Bulletin. 2003;129:674-97.
6. **Kimmel SB, Mahalik JR**. Body image concerns of gay men: the roles of minority stress and conformity to masculine norms. J Consult Clin Psychol. 2005;73:1185-90.
7. **Williamson I**. Internalized homophobia and health issues affecting lesbians and gay men. Health Education Research. 2000;15:97-107.
8. **Meyer I, Dean L**. Internalized homophobia, intimacy and sexual behaviour among gay and bisexual men. In: Herek G, ed. Stigma and Sexual Orientation. Sage; 1998:160-86.
9. **Meyer I**. Minority stress and mental health in gay men, The Journal of Health and Social Behaviour. 1995; 36, 38-56.
10. **Nemoto T, Operario D, Keatley J, et al**. Social context of HIV risk behaviors among male-to-female transgenders of colour. AIDS Care. 2004;16:724-35.
11. **O'Bryan W**. Sister schism: trans debate continues at Michigan Womyn's Music Festival. MetroWeekly. August 31, 2006. Available at http://www.metroweekly.com/gauge/?ak=2275.

12. **Johnson R**. Myths about bi men. *About: Gay Life from About.com*. Available at http://gaylife.about.com/od/bisexual/a/biman.htm.

13. **Miller N**. Out of the Past: Gay and Lesbian History from 1869 to the Present. Vintage Books; 1995.

14. **Wright E**. Homosexuals are not an oppressed minority. In: Williams ME, ed. Homosexuality: Opposing Viewpoints. Greenhaven Press; 1999: 70-8.

15. **Schmierer D**. An Ounce of Prevention: Preventing the Homosexual Condition in Today's Youth. Word Publishing; 1998.

16. As espoused by organizations such as the National Association for Research and Therapy of Homosexuality (NARTH). Available at http://www.narth.com.

17. This view is described well by Madeline H. Wyndzen (pen name) in an online monograph: The Banality of Insensitivity: Portrayals of Transgenderism in Psychopathology. Available at http://www.genderpsychology.org/psychology/mental_illness_model.html.

18. **Marwick C**. Survey says patients expect little physician help on sex. JAMA. 1999;281:2173-4.

19. **Eliason MJ, Schope R**. Does "Don't ask, don't tell" apply to health care? Lesbian, gay, and bisexual people's disclosure to health care providers. Journal of the Gay and Lesbian Medical Association. 2001;5:125-34.

20. **Diamant AL, Wold C, Spritzer K, et al**. Health behaviors, health status, and access to and use of health care. Arch Fam Med. 2000;9:1043-51.

21. **Solursh DS, Ernst JL, Lewis RW, et al**. The human sexuality education of physicians in North American medical schools. Int J Imp Res. 2003;15(suppl 5):S41-S45.

22. **Boehmer U**. Twenty years of public health research: inclusion of lesbian, gay, bisexual, and transgender populations. Am J Public Health. 2002;92:1125-30.

23. For example, see the American Medical Association policy regarding sexual orientation. Available at http://www.ama-assn.org/ama/pub/category/14754.html; the American College of Obstetricians and Gynecologists: Special Issues in Women's Health, 2005. Available at http://www.acog.org/bookstore/Special_Issues_in_Women's_Health_P505 .cfm; American Medical Student Association, Lesbian, Gay, Bisexual, Transgender Health Action Committee. Available at http://www.amsa.org/lgbt/; Gay and Lesbian Medical Association. Available at http://www.glma.org.

24. For example, American Medical Association's Code of Medical Ethics. Available at http://www.ama-assn.org/ama/pub/category/2498.html; American Academy of Physician Assistants. Vision and Mission 2005-2006: AAPA Policy Manual. Available at www.aapa.org/manual/visionmission.pdf; American Psychological Association. Ethical Principles of Psychologists and Code of Conduct. Available at www.apa .org/ethics/code2002.html; American Nursing Association. Code of Ethics for Nurses. Available at http://nursingworld.org/ethics/code/protected_nwcoe303.htm.

25. **Laumann E, Gagnon J, Michael R, et al**. The Social Organization of Sexuality: Sexual Practices in the United States. University of Chicago Press; 1994: 304, Table 8.2.

26. **Conway L**. How frequently does transsexualism occur? Available at http://ai.eecs .umich.edu/people/conway/TS/TSprevalence.html.

27. **American Psychological Association**. Diagnostic and Statistical Manual of Mental Disorders. 4th ed. (DSM-IV)-TR; 2000.

28. **Heifetz R, Linsky M**. Leadership on the Line: Staying Alive Through the Dangers of Leading. Harvard Business School Press; 2002.

29. **Prochaska JO, DiClemente CC**. Stages of Change in the Modification of Problem Behaviors. Sage; 1992.

30. **Fullan M**. Change Forces with a Vengeance. RoutledgeFalmer; 2003.

31. **Spiro H**. What is empathy and can it be taught? Ann Intern Med. 1992;116:843-6.

32. **Cassell EJ**. The nature of suffering and the goals of medicine. N Engl J Med. 1982; 306:639-45.

33. **Novack DH**. Therapeutic aspects of the clinical encounter. J Gen Intern Med. 1987; 2:346-55.

34. **Irwin H**. Doctor-patient communication competency. Austr J Communication. 1991;18:14-31.
35. **Peabody FW**. The care of the patient. JAMA. 1927;88:877-82.
36. **DiBlasi Z, Kleijnen J**. Context effects: powerful therapies or methodological bias? Eval Health Prof. 2003;26:166-79.
37. **Clark PA**. What residents are not learning: observations in an NICU. Acad Med. 2001;76:419-24.
38. **Accreditation Council for Graduate Medical Education**. ACGME General Competencies Version 1.3 (9.28.99); 1999. Available at www.acgme.org/outcome/comp/compFull.asp.
39. **Bloom BS, Engelhart MD, Furst WH, et al**. Taxonomy of Educational Objectives, The Classification of Educational Goals, Handbook 1: Cognitive Domain. Longman; 1956.
40. **Goold SD, Lipkin M**. The doctor-patient relationship: challenges, opportunities, and strategies. J Gen Int Med. 1999;14(suppl 1): S26-S33.
41. **Gordon BG, Hogue HB.** Lesbian, gay, and bisexual issues in the classroom: a resource guide. Department of Social Work Education, San Francisco State University, 1993:195-98; **Linde R, The Fenway Institute, and the GLBT Health Access Project**: Gay, lesbian, bisexual, and transgender (GLBT) health access training project trainer's manual, 2003:4-6; **Office of Gay & Lesbian Health Concerns and The Community Health Project**: Giving the best care possible: unlearning homophobia in the health and social service setting, 1996:26.
42. **Pope KS, Sonne JL, Holroyd J**. Sexual Feelings in Psychotherapy: Explorations for Therapists-In-Training (Paperback). American Psychological Association; 1993.
43. **Schatz B, O'Hanlan KA**. Antigay discrimination in medicine: results of a national survey of lesbian, gay and bisexual physicians. Gay and Lesbian Medical Association; 1994.
44. **Linde R, The Fenway Institute, and the GLBT Health Access Project**: Gay, lesbian, bisexual, and transgender (GLBT) health access training project participant resource manual, 2003.
45. **Hidalgo H, Peterson TL, Woodman NJ, eds**. Lesbian and gay issues: A resource manual for social workers. National Association of Social Workers; 1985:153-5.
46. **Values Clarification Questionnaire**. AIDS Training Project, Seattle-King County Department of Public Health.
47. **Herek GM**. The psychology of sexual prejudice. Current Directions in Psychological Sciences. 2000;9:19-22.
48. **Dean L, Mayer IH, Robinson K, et al**. Lesbian, gay, bisexual, and transgender health: findings and concerns. J Gay Lesbian Med Assoc. 2000;4:101-51.
49. **Pathela P, Hajat A, Schillinger J, et al**. Discordance between sexual behavior and self-reported sexual identity: a population-based survey of New York City men. Annals of Internal Medicine. 2006;145:416-25.
50. **Makadon HJ**. Improving health care for the lesbian and gay communities. New Eng J Med. 2006;354:895-7.
51. **Potter JE**. Do ask, do tell. Annals Internal Medicine. 2002;137:341-3.
52. **Peabody FW**. The care of the patient. JAMA. 1927;88: 877-82.

Chapter 2

Demography and the LGBT Population: What We Know, Don't Know, and How the Information Helps to Inform Clinical Practice

JUDITH B. BRADFORD, PhD
KENNETH H. MAYER, MD

Introduction

In prior decades, one of the greatest challenges to accurately under-standing the specific healthcare needs of lesbian, gay, bisexual, and transgender patients was the lack of sufficient demographic data about the many subgroups within this population. However, in recent years, the inclusion of sexual orientation measures in national probability-based sur-veys, complemented by focused studies, has provided new insights about LGBT healthcare needs. Demography is the scientific study of human pop-ulation dynamics, encompassing the study of population size, structure, and distribution, as well as how populations change over time. In 1970, the first presidential commission was established to examine population growth and its future impact upon government services, the economy, national resources, and the environment.[1,2] The Commission's 1972 report, *Population and the American Future*, reviewed critical concerns that were expected to result from growth of the United States population. Although the report called attention to some concerns regarding sexual and gender minorities, such as the need to enumerate them in the census and to study their demographic trends, nearly three decades would pass before LGBT Americans were specifically acknowledged in publicly available govern-ment documents.

The term "population" refers to those individuals who live within a spec-ified geographic area, such as a country, state, or metropolitan area. The term is often used more loosely to refer to individuals who have certain social behavioral characteristics or affiliations in common. These individuals are more precisely referred to as subpopulations or population groups. The US population is counted, and its demographics reported by the decennial census, a real-time counting of all households and their inhabitants that takes place at the beginning of each decade. Although sexual orientation is not asked on the census forms, male and female same-sex partners who live in the same household have been identifiable in the US census since 1990. Gays and lesbians first became a recognized subpopulation when social scientists published census data about same-sex partnered households from the 1990 Census.[3,4] In the 2000 Census, same-sex headed households were observed in 93% of all counties in the US (see Figure 2-1). These maps have made it clear to LGBT organizations and individuals, to the general population, and to legislators that same-sex headed households can be found in

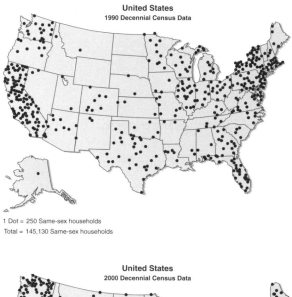

United States
1990 Decennial Census Data

1 Dot = 250 Same-sex households
Total = 145,130 Same-sex households

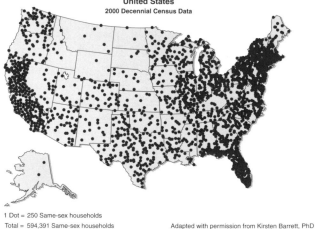

United States
2000 Decennial Census Data

1 Dot = 250 Same-sex households
Total = 594,391 Same-sex households   Adapted with permission from Kirsten Barrett, PhD

Figure 2-1   Prevalence of same-sex households in the U.S. National Census, by county.

Used with permission from Kirsten Barrett, Virginia Commonwealth University, Survey and Evaluation Research Laboratory.

virtually every county in the US and that the number and distribution of such identifiable households increased substantially from 1990 to 2000. In the 2000 Census, about one in nine respondents who were living in unmarried households (approximately 600 000) reported cohabiting with a same-sex partner, accounting for 1% of all coupled households in the US.[5]

The ability to locate same-sex partnered households within the census data also made it possible for scientists to explore the diversity within these households and to compare them to other households. Researchers' analyses of the Census 2000 data provide new insights about the characteristics of aging LGBT people, as well as LGBT households with children under the age of 18. More than one in ten same-sex couples includes a partner 65 years old or older; nearly one in four same-sex couples includes a partner 55 and older; and similar to heterosexual senior couples, same-sex senior couples live in California, New York, and Florida in significant numbers.[6] Nationally, 33% of female-partnered and 22% of male-partnered households reported living with their children under the age of 18 years old, indicating an increase over the 1990 numbers.[5,7] The 2000 Census data also provide new information about the greater racial and ethnic diversity of LGBT couples compared to heterosexual couples. Seventy-nine percent of members of opposite-sex couples racially identify as white, compared with 72% of individuals in same-sex couples, a statistically significant difference.[8] Partners in same-sex couples are more likely than individuals in married couples to identify themselves as black or of Hispanic origin. The findings suggest that same-sex parents are more likely to be from racial minorities compared to heterosexual parents and are more racially diverse than same-sex couples without children.[8-11]

The Healthy People National Program for Health Promotion and Disease Prevention was initiated by the Office of the Surgeon General during the 1970s and, like the census, is reissued with the beginning of each new decade, setting goals for the nation's health and offering recommendations about how to achieve them. Concurrently with inclusion in the census, the first official recognition of gays and lesbians within US government health policy came in 2000, when "persons defined by sexual orientation" were identified in *Healthy People 2010* as a population group experiencing health disparities.[12] Building upon an extensive review of all available literature about LGBT health,[13] the 2001 *Healthy People Companion Document for Lesbian, Gay, Bisexual and Transgender (LGBT) Health* took a more expansive view in addressing the health-related needs of sexual and gender minorities, using the inclusive terminology of lesbian, gay, bisexual, and transgender (LGBT) individuals and communities.[14] Subsequently, researchers have used existing data sets to extract information about LGBT health-related variables and probability surveys to generate population-based data on sexual and gender minorities. Through these efforts, a more accurate picture of the demographic characteristics and related health status of these increasingly visible population groups has emerged.

Measurement and Sampling Advances and Challenges for LGBT Research

Demographic analysis typically relies on large data sets, such as the census, and random sample surveys of the general population, such as the National Health Interview Survey (NHIS), to study issues of concern for the whole society or for groups defined by more specific criteria such as education, income, race, ethnicity, or religion.[15] In addition to the decennial census, the US government funds multiple recurring population-based surveys to gather demographic and specific health-related information, including the NHIS, the National Health and Nutrition Examination Survey, and the Current Population Survey.[16] Until very recently, none of these data sets incorporated any measure of sexual orientation, making it impossible to isolate group data for LGBT individuals. Since the inclusion of persons defined by sexual orientation within *Healthy People 2010*, population scientists have argued with some success for the importance of capturing this information in order to document and address perceived LGBT health disparities. At this time, measures have been incorporated in an increasing number of government surveys, and ongoing cognitive testing provides a growing body of knowledge about the best ways to word sexual and gender identity and behavioral questions for subpopulation cultural groups.[17]

Despite progress in the inclusion of sexual orientation measures, the majority of government data sets still do not include such measures, and those that do typically include only one measure for sexual orientation and none for transgender identification. Lack of more complete and more culturally sensitive measures limits the usefulness of these data sets for LGBT health planning and assessment of changes over time, making it difficult to construct interventions that are sensitive to their particular needs. Thus, existing data on LGBT health are fragmentary and inadequately integrated into medical and public health practice. With the exception of studies of the natural history and prevention of HIV disease in men who have sex with men (MSM), a limited number of surveys of gay men or sexual minority women, and longitudinal cohort studies in lesbian health, few population-based studies of LGBT people have been conducted. Additional population-based research is necessary to more fully understand the causes and consequences of health disparities among sexual minorities so that effective responses can be developed.

Although Alfred Kinsey and colleagues first conducted studies of the prevalence of homosexual behaviors in the 1940s, the first national randomized survey of adult Americans to include both accepted demographic measures and a range of theoretically derived measures of sexual orientation was conducted in 1992 by a team of researchers led by Edward O. Laumann at the University of Chicago.[18] The importance of this study cannot be overestimated in increasing awareness of the sociodemographic diversity among population groups of gay men, lesbians, and bisexual Americans. The inclusion of multiple measures of sexual orientation on a national probability survey made it clear that sexual minorities exhibit considerable diversity in how they express their same-gender sexuality and how social and geographic factors influence their choices in self-identification. Three measures of sexual orientation were used: behavior, desire/attraction, and identity. All three of these dimensions of sexuality are of direct relevance to healthcare.

The percentages of respondents who answered affirmatively to any of these measures were cross-tabulated with gender and further broken out on a range of sociodemographic variables (see Table 2-1). Clear patterns emerged from these data to show the relationships between key demographic characteristics and the degree to which respondents used sexual orientation measures to describe themselves. Men were twice as likely as women to identify as homosexual and more than twice as likely to report

Table 2-1 Percentages Reporting Various Expressions of Same-Gender Sexuality by Selected Social and Demographic Variables

| | Same-Sex Partners Since Puberty | | Desire, Attraction, Appeal | | Identity, Homo-Bisexual | |
	M	W	M	W	M	W
Total	9.1	4.3	7.7	7.5	2.8	1.4
Race/Ethnicity						
White	9.6	4.7	7.4	7.8	3.0	1.7
Black	8.0	2.8	6.7	7.0	1.5	.6
Hispanic	7.5	3.5	13.9	7.6	3.7	1.1
Asian	3.2	0.0	17.1	0.0	0.0	0.0
Place of Residence						
Top 12 central cities	15.8	4.6	16.7	9.7	9.2	2.6
Next 88 central cities	10.1	7.7	11.4	7.8	3.5	1.6
Suburbs top 12 CCs	11.9	4.1	10.3	9.0	4.2	1.9
Suburbs next 88 CCs	6.0	4.8	4.5	9.8	1.3	1.6
Other urban areas	9.7	3.4	5.3	6.9	1.9	1.1
Rural areas	2.7	2.2	7.5	2.1	1.3	0.0
Education						
Less than high school	4.7	1.8	5.8	3.3	1.6	.4
High school graduate	7.3	2.3	5.5	5.3	1.8	.4
Some college/voc.	9.8	5.1	8.9	7.3	3.8	1.2
College graduate	12.0	7.3	9.4	12.8	3.3	3.6

Data excerpted from Laumann E, Gagnon J, Michael R, et al. The Social Organization of Sexuality: Sexual Practices in the United States. University of Chicago Press, 1994:30, Table 8.2. Reprinted with permission from the University of Chicago Press.

same-sex behavior since puberty. White respondents that lived in or near major urban areas and/or had advanced education were significantly more likely to report same-sex behavior and identity. Hispanic and Asian men, however, were approximately twice as likely to report same-sex desire, attraction, or appeal compared to black or white men. These data provide a more nuanced picture of sexual and gender minorities than was apparent from census data.

Conceptual Frameworks for Understanding Sociodemographic Factors and LGBT Health

Considerable variations in income, education, race and ethnicity, cultural background, and other salient sociodemographic characteristics exist within the United States general population, and similarly, consistent differences have been found within the various population groups of sexual minorities. Contrary to earlier assumptions that gays are wealthier than heterosexuals or that gays and lesbians are mostly white and highly educated, census data and the Laumann study have shown that sexual minority population groups are as diverse as others in the general population. While sexual and gender minorities clearly have specific health-related needs associated with their unique behavioral differences, in other ways these population groups are confronted with the same socially determined challenges as other minorities within the US. Social determinants of health include socioeconomic status, stress, early life experiences, social exclusion, field of work, unemployment, social support, addiction, nutrition, and access to transport.[19] As within any subpopulation, sexual and gender minority individuals may be rich or poor, have menial or professional occupations, and experience daily lives that may be enriching or demeaning. Each of these variables may have an impact on health and access to appropriate healthcare.[20]

The emerging field of social epidemiology, with its emphasis on the social determinants of health, provides a language in which to consider how life circumstances of sexual and gender minorities may create structural, financial, and personal barriers that interfere with healthcare access. A multi-level framework that incorporates sociocultural conditions, social networks, and psychosocial mechanisms and that links these factors to health pathways has been usefully applied to understanding minority health concerns.[21,22] This framework is based upon an ecological approach that recognizes how health and well-being are affected by environmental factors beyond the control of individuals. The various ecological influences and their disproportionate impact based on individual life experience and circumstances have been described and are shown in Figure 2-2.[23] Simply put, LGBT health is not just an individual matter reflecting only personal characteristics and decisions—interpersonal, institutional, community, and

Public Policy: local, state, and federal government policies, regulations, and laws

Community: social networks, standards, and practices among organizations

Institutional/Organizational: rules, policies, procedures, and informal structures within an organization or system

Interpersonal: family, friends, peers that provide social identity and support

Individual: awareness, knowledge, attitudes, beliefs, values, preferences

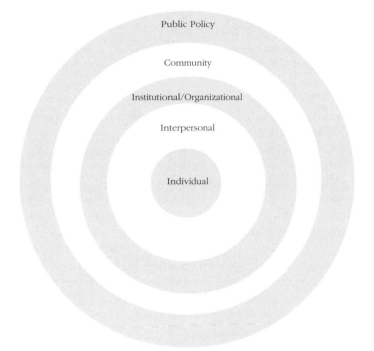

Figure 2-2   Social-Ecological Model: Spheres of Influence on Individual Health

Adapted, with permission, from McElroy K, Bibeau D, Sleckler A, et al. An ecological perspective on health promotion programs. Health Education Quarterly. 1988;15:351-377.

public policy factors all affect the health of sexual and gender minority persons. In addition to the interaction of LGBT sexual behavior and identity with demographic factors, the ways in which society has interacted with LGBT people may also have health-related ramifications. Consider the example of a gay man who becomes infected with HIV through unprotected anal intercourse with a casual partner. A model that focuses only on individual factors would simply explain this man's HIV-infected status as a consequence of his sexual behavior. A model based on an ecological framework would also recognize the larger social determinants that influence the man's sexual behavior. For example, state policies and community norms that discriminate against gay male sex create secrecy and shame; this in turn makes it more challenging for a gay man to find partners with whom he feels comfortable negotiating condom use or asking about/disclosing HIV status. Societal stigma against homosexuality can also lead to internalized homophobia. A gay man who internalizes cultural bias against his own sexual feelings may become depressed or may mask his feelings by abusing drugs or alcohol, which in turn could potentiate sexual risk-taking behavior.

Factors such as social exclusion or policy-driven discrimination negatively affect the health and well-being of LGBT individuals and communities and also create barriers to the collection of valid data. Like racial minority groups who have avoided participation in research studies in the past,[24] sexual and gender minority individuals may be unwilling to participate when self-identification of LGBT status is required. Until very recently, community surveys provided the foundation for our understanding of the health status and health-related needs of LGBT communities. The nonprobability nature, relying on convenience samples (eg, bar or gay pride surveys) of most of these studies has limited acceptance of their results within the scientific community and made it difficult to publish in the most respected journals. With broader distribution of census data and publication of results from local or regionally based randomized surveys and longitudinal cohort studies, there is a growing understanding of the specific ways in which LGBT health and related needs differ from those of the general population. The convergence of findings from several robust studies has reinforced the need to conduct more sensitive research that examines the cultural contexts of subpopulations variously self-defined as lesbian, gay, bisexual, or transgender with more careful attention to cultural differences within specific communities. For many, "gay" and "lesbian" are now conventional terms, applicable to middle-aged and older individuals. Many sexual minority youth prefer terms such as "queer" or "questioning." Individuals within transgender groups and communities report more than 100 terms that are used to convey what "outsiders" combine in the one generalized term for "transgender."

Sexual and gender identities are increasingly understood as fluid and changing over time for many individuals who engage in same-sex behaviors and who may not consistently self-identify as members of sexual or gender minorities. In repeated surveys, 40%-50% of self-identified lesbians are or have been heterosexually married, and some who have women partners continue to self-define as heterosexual.[18,25] Among men who have sex with men (MSM), Caucasians are significantly more likely to identify as gay than their African-American counterparts.[26] Within Hispanic cultures, heterosexually married and unmarried men who have sex with men typically do not interpret this behavior as indication of homosexuality.[27] Some transgender persons first identify as women, later as men; others first as men, later as women. Still others reject either of these accepted gender categories, insisting on the inclusion of transgender as a category in its own right. Government agencies are beginning to respond to this concern by considering the inclusion of transgender status measures on health surveys.

Fluidity of self-identification is related to personal and socioeconomic factors and has a generational component. As shown in Table 2-1, differences in race, education, age, and income are related to patterns of sexual orientation and disclosure. Geographic location also made a significant difference. In a southern state's HIV prevention survey, African-American men who have sex with men were less likely to disclose sexual minority status to their families as they became more educated, not wanting their parents to become ashamed or experience social disapproval.[28] Nevertheless, with broader awareness of sexual and gender minorities among the general public, such as television shows, Web sites, and public service announcements, LGBT persons are coming out in ever greater numbers throughout the United States, and recognition of sexual and gender minority status now occurs at younger ages than in previous generations. On average, today's sexual minority adult males report that their first awareness of same-sex attraction occurred at age 13, their first same-sex experience at 15, and self-identification as gay at 19-21 years of age. In contrast, contemporary sexual minority adolescent males report first sexual awareness at nine years of age, first same-sex experiences at 13-14, and self-identification at 14-16 years of age. Although females tended to be older for each of these events, the same pattern was reported: today's adult lesbians were first sexually aware at 14-16, had their first same-sex experience at 20, and self-identified at 21-23 years of age. Today's adolescent sexual minority females report first awareness at 10 years of age, first same-sex experience at 14-15, and self-identification at 15-16.[29,30]

Emergence of a New "Health Disparities Population"

On Friday evening, June 27, 1969, the New York City tactical police force raided a popular Greenwich Village gay bar, the Stonewall Inn. The backlash and several nights of protest that followed have come to be known as the Stonewall Riots. Prior to that summer there was little public discussion of the lives and experiences of gay men and lesbians beyond the references to stereotypes for entertainment. The Stonewall Riots were the first indication to many Americans that sexual minorities existed in sufficient numbers to warrant attention. In response to Stonewall, gays and lesbians organized a national effort to raise community awareness of the unique health concerns of these population groups. In major urban centers, clinical services, like Fenway Community Health, were established to meet their needs and a national organization, the Lesbian and Gay Health Foundation, was formed in 1977 to identify critical health concerns and to create linkages among responding organizations. A network of LGBT community health centers began to develop, and with the advent of HIV/AIDS, many of these programs developed excellent medical, mental health, and other services for HIV-infected persons and more broadly for diverse groups of LGBT persons.[31-33] Despite these and other initiatives, until very recently, "gay health" was equated with HIV in the minds of many Americans, and since AIDS was considered a disease of gay men, other LGBT groups were largely overlooked.

A summary of existing research about lesbian health from a 1999 Institute of Medicine (IOM) study awakened national awareness that certain negative health outcomes were more prevalent among sexual minority women compared to heterosexual women.[25] A government-sponsored scientific workshop on lesbian health was convened in 2000 to develop steps for implementing recommendations from the IOM Report on lesbian health priorities.[34] Certain recommendations were considered priorities for government action, including a focus on barriers to healthcare access; the provision of culturally sensitive information, prevention, and treatment programs; the critical need for training providers to provide culturally competent care; and the importance of conducting intervention studies on major health concerns of the population. These significant achievements in creating awareness of lesbian health concerns began to broaden the understanding that an adequate framework for sexual and gender minority health concerns would include additional health concerns and a greater diversity of population groups.

As *Healthy People 2010* documents were prepared at the end of the 1990s, community leaders and prominent national advocacy organizations had advocated successfully for inclusion of "persons defined by sexual orientation" as a subpopulation experiencing health disparities.[12] Previous studies had shown that sexual minorities more commonly experience serious physical and mental health conditions such as domestic violence and substance use, experience significant barriers to healthcare quality and access to care, and face substantial threats to their quality of life.[13] Central to the emerging discussion about LGBT health has been the need to carefully evaluate current research to better understand the unique social and legal challenges of these populations, to identify gaps in knowledge, and to formulate strategies to attain optimal information for assessing the impact of cultural and social structures on their health status and healthcare needs. Increased national attention to the existing body of knowledge about LGBT health resulted in growing awareness of its inadequacies, other than addressing HIV/AIDS risk issues and, to some extent, helping to define cancer risks in lesbians.

A convergence of findings from numerous community and other non-probability surveys and a limited number of population-based studies have made it clear that access to healthcare and provider cultural competence are substantive areas of concern for sexual and gender minorities.[14] These barriers to healthcare access are also related to racial and socioeconomic differences, further exacerbating the challenges for disadvantaged sub-groups of sexual and gender minorities.[35] Although medical associations recommend that physicians who treat HIV-infected patients have disease-specific expertise, in a national prospective cohort study, African-Americans were less likely than whites to have an infectious disease specialist, as were Alaskan natives, American Indians, Asians, Pacific Islanders, or persons of mixed racial backgrounds.[35]

In a probability sampling of sexual minority women in Boston, significantly higher percentages of lesbians and bisexual women reported negative reactions from physicians than their heterosexual counterparts.[36] In a citywide forum to establish health priorities for sexual minority women of color, the need for improved provider understanding of racial and cultural differences ranked among the top three.[37] African-American lesbian mothers have reported making thoughtful decisions about when to disclose their sexual orientation to providers, based on situational assessment of how this will affect their treatment.[38] Studies of transgender health have consistently reported that these individuals have frequent and sometimes constant exposure to discrimination and violence.[39] Forty-six percent of transgender participants in a statewide population-based study reported the need to educate their physicians about transgender health.[40]

LGBT Health Concerns

Conceptual frameworks such as the social ecological model and the social determinants of health have assisted scientists, advocates, and providers to make the connection between life experiences of sexual and gender minorities and their unique health needs, such as consistent barriers to healthcare access reported by these subpopulations. Inclusion of sexual minorities within *Healthy People 2010* also helped to underscore the need for culturally specific interventions to improve LGBT health. Among the country's ten leading health indicators that framed the national *Healthy People 2010* objectives, seven appeared to be particularly relevant for sexual minorities, including weight issues and obesity, tobacco use, substance abuse, responsible sexual behavior, mental health, injury and violence, and access to care (see Table 2-2). A thorough review of peer-reviewed publications and government-sponsored studies provided the initial scientific evidence to support the recognition of LGBT health as a matter of substantial concern within the nation's public health programs.[13] Inclusion in the discussion of *Healthy People 2010* goals for national health sparked awareness of the unique health needs of LGBT population groups. Inclusion in *Healthy People 2010* also directed national attention to the need for additional, more valid research to gather sound data that will provide a foundation for effective

Table 2-2   Leading Health Indicators

General US Population	Sexual and Gender Minorities
Physical Activity	
Overweight and Obesity	✓
Tobacco Use	✓
Substance Abuse	✓
Responsible Sexual Behavior	✓
Mental Health	✓
Injury and Violence	✓
Environmental Quality	
Immunization	
Access to Care	✓

interventions and ultimately reduce health disparities associated with sexual and gender minority status.

Priority areas of concern include tobacco use among all LGBT groups, weight issues and obesity in lesbians, exposure to social discrimination and lack of access to culturally competent healthcare for transgenders, as well as the high burden of HIV and other sexually transmitted infections among MSM and transgenders, and the high prevalence of substance abuse (ranging from alcohol to crystal methamphetamine use) among LGBT population groups. Recognizing the limitations of current terminology and research study designs, health researchers have developed and are using newer methods such as social network sampling and participatory research to investigate these and other critical issues. Peer recruitment, whereby individuals refer their social contacts for study participation, successfully yielded a higher proportion of HIV-infected persons in a testing initiative than had previously been reported.[41] This approach takes advantage of the social ties among subpopulation groups to overcome historical barriers to research participation such as lack of trust in research teams. Two statistically sound methods (respondent-driven and venue-based sampling) for developing representative samples of subpopulation groups with high prevalence of HIV infection have shown considerable promise in the National HIV Behavioral Surveillance (NHBS) Program.[42] Community-based Participatory Research (CBPR), an approach to health and environmental research meant to increase the value of studies for both researchers and the communities being studied, creates bridges between scientists and communities. Through the use of shared knowledge and valuable experiences, this method is of particular value when developing longer term research with minority and underserved groups.[43] Community methods, once criticized for lack of methodological rigor, are now valued for their ability to increase the inclusion of all population and subcultural group segments in research studies.

The Interface of Population Science and Clinical Care

Societal disapproval of minority sexual orientation and gender identity has hampered the challenging tasks of defining the healthcare concerns and needs of LGBT population groups. The generation of clinically useful data has been limited because of institutional homophobia resulting in a reticence of researchers to ask about socially unacceptable behaviors and an unwillingness of LGBT individuals to disclose their identities and behaviors to culturally insensitive interviewers. Moreover, the invisibility and fluidity of diverse homosexual populations led many clinicians to assume that patients who conformed to societal gender expectations were invariably heterosexual and that those who did not conform had deep-seated psychological or physiological problems.

The emergence of AIDS, and the recognition that sexual and substance use behaviors may have profound social consequences, led to the first significant outlays of federal research dollars to support studies of gay men and injecting drug users. Very quickly researchers learned that some men who acquired HIV through homosexual intercourse had female sexual partners; that nonparenteral substance use, as well as shared injected drugs, fueled the epidemic; and that effective prevention interventions needed to be grounded in population science and careful understanding of the diverse sexual and other subcultures that created the networks that facilitated HIV transmission. The mobilization of the LGBT communities to address the challenges of the AIDS epidemic created, or expanded, institutions focusing on LGBT health, creating the necessary environment for clinicians and investigators to seriously consider the other healthcare needs of LGBT patients.

In recent years, the evolving awareness that sexual orientation and gender identity, as well as behavior, have personal and societal health consequences has created an intellectual need and a moral imperative for population scientists to develop methodologies to more accurately assess the true prevalence of clinical conditions in sexual minority populations. Although many experts would argue that huge gaps in knowledge remain, the inclusion of measures of sexual orientation and gender identity in an increasing array of surveys and cohort studies is helping to shed new light on the healthcare disparities that remain, as well as the clinical needs of diverse LGBT population groups. Knowledgeable clinicians may be one of the best influences on optimal health outcomes, given their roles as confidantes, respected authorities, and major sources of health-promoting information for many LGBT patients. In the subsequent chapters, specific clinical topics will be addressed, but underlying each section will be the recognition that optimal clinical care for LGBT patients can be provided only if clinicians are aware of the differences in the prevalence, expression, and natural history of conditions in diverse LGBT populations and are prepared to provide culturally sensitive care, recognizing that sexual orientation and gender identity may evolve throughout the life continuum.

Summary Points

- One of the greatest challenges to accurately understanding the specific healthcare needs of LGBT patients has been the lack of sufficient demographic data about the many subgroups within this population.
- With the exception of studies of the natural history and prevention of HIV disease in MSM, a limited number of surveys of gay men or sexual minority women, and longitudinal cohort studies in lesbian health, few population-based studies of LGBT people have been conducted.
- In recent years, the inclusion of sexual orientation measures in national, probability-based surveys, complemented by focused studies of specific subpopulations has provided new insights about LGBT healthcare needs.
- In the 2000 Census, same-sex headed households were observed in 93% of all counties in the US.
- The inclusion of multiple measures of sexual orientation on a national probability survey made it clear that sexual minorities exhibit considerable diversity in how they express their same-gender sexuality and how social and geographic factors influence their choices in self-identification. Three measures of sexual orientation were used including behavior, desire/attraction, and identity. All three of these dimensions of sexuality are of direct relevance to healthcare.
- The convergence of findings from several robust studies has reinforced the need to understand the cultural contexts of subpopulations variously self-defined as lesbian, gay, bisexual or transgender, and with careful, increased attention to cultural differences within specific communities. For some, "gay" and "lesbian" are now conventional terms, applicable to middle-aged and older individuals. Many sexual minority youth prefer terms such as "queer" or "questioning."
- Sexual and gender identity are increasingly understood as fluid and changing over time for many individuals who engage in same-sex behaviors and who may not consistently self-identify as members of sexual or gender minorities. For example, several studies have documented that 40%-50% of self-identified lesbians are or have been heterosexually married, and some women who have women partners self-define as heterosexual.

- Sexual minorities more commonly experience serious physical and mental health conditions, such as domestic violence and substance use, and experience more significant barriers to healthcare quality and access to care than heterosexuals.
- Among the country's ten leading health indicators that framed the national *Healthy People 2010* objectives, seven appeared to be particularly relevant for sexual minorities, including weight issues and obesity, tobacco use, substance abuse, responsible sexual behavior, mental health, injury and violence, and access to care.
- Knowledgeable clinicians may be one of the best influences on optimal health outcomes, given their roles as confidantes, respected authorities, and major sources of health promoting information for many LGBT patients.

References

1. **Rockefeller Commission**. Population and the American future: the report of the Commission on Population and the American Future. Center for Research on Population and Security; 1969. Available at http://www.population-security.org/rockefeller/017_recommendations.htm

2. **Westoff CF**. The Commission on Population Growth and the American future its origins, operations, and aftermath. Population Index. 1973;39:491-507.

3. **Black D, Gates G, Sanders S, et al**. Demographics of the gay and lesbian populations in the United States: evidence from available systematic data sources. Demography. 2000;37:139-54.

4. **Ellis JM, Bradford JB, Honnold J, et al**. Identification and description of lesbians living in households reporting same-sex partnerships in public use micro-data samples. Paper presented at: National Lesbian Health Research Conference; 2001; San Francisco, Calif.

5. **Simmons T, O'Connell M**. Married-Couple and Unmarried-Partner Households: 2000. US Department of Commerce Economics and Statistics Administration. US Census Bureau; 2003. Census 2000 Special Reports.

6. **Bennett L, Gates G**. The Cost of Marriage Inequality to Gay, Lesbian and Bisexual Seniors. Human Rights Campaign Foundation Report; 2004.

7. **Bennett L, Gates G**. The Cost of Marriage Inequality to Children and their Same-Sex Parents. Human Rights Campaign Foundation Report; 2004.

8. **Sears RB, Gates G, Rubenstein WB**. Same-Sex Couples and Same-Sex Couples Raising Children in the United States: Data from Census 2000. The Williams Project on Sexual Orientation Law and Public Policy, UCLA School of Law; 2005:19.

9. **Ash M, Badgett MVL, Folbre N, et al**. Same-Sex Couples and Their Children in Massachusetts: A View from Census 2000. The Institute for Gay and Lesbian Strategic Studies; 2004.

10. **Gates GJ, Ost J**. A Demographic Profile of New Jersey's Gay and Lesbian Families. The Urban Institute; 2004.

11. **Smith DM, Gates GJ**. Gay and Lesbian Families in the United States: Same-Sex Unmarried Partner Households. A Preliminary Analysis of 2000 United States Census Data. Human Rights Campaign; 2001.
12. **US Dept of Health and Human Services**. Office of the Surgeon General. Healthy People 2010. US Dept of Health and Human Services; 2000.
13. **Dean L, Meyer IH, Robinson K, et al**. Lesbian, gay, bisexual, and transgender health: findings and concerns. Journal of the Gay and Lesbian Medical Association. 2000;4:101-51.
14. **Gay and Lesbian Medical Association, LGBT health experts**. Healthy People 2010 Companion Document for Lesbian, Gay, Bisexual and Transgender (LGBT) Health. Available at http://www.glma.org/_data/n_0001/resources/live/HealthyCompanionDoc3.pdf
15. **Wikipedia contributors**. Demography. Wikipedia, The Free Encyclopedia. http://en.wikipedia.org/wiki/Demography; 2006.
16. **Centers for Disease Control and Prevention, National Center for Health Statistics, Survey and Data Collection Systems**. Available at http://www.cdc.gov/nchs/express.htm.
17. **Sell R**. Gaydata.org.
18. **Laumann E, Gagnon J, Michael R, et al**. The Social Organization of Sexuality: Sexual Practices in the United States. University of Chicago Press; 1994.
19. **Marmot M, Wilkinson R**. Social Determinants of Health. Oxford University Press; 1999.
20. **Millman M**. Access to Health Care in America. National Academy of Sciences, Institute of Medicine; 1993.
21. **Berkman L, Glass T**. Social integration, social networks, social support and health. In: Berkman L, Kawachi I, eds. Social Epidemiology. Oxford University Press; 2000.
22. **Berkman L, Kawachi I**. Social Epidemiology. Oxford University Press; 2000.
23. **McElroy K, Bibeau D, Sleckler A, et al**. An ecological perspective on health promotion programs. Health Education Quarterly. 1988;15:351-77.
24. **US Dept of Health, Education, and Welfare**. Belmont report: ethical principles and guidelines for the protection of human subjects of research. DHEW Publication No. (OS) 78-0013 and No. (OS) 78-0014. US Government Printing Office; 1979.
25. **Institute of Medicine Committee on Lesbian Health Research Priorities**. Lesbian health: current assessment and directions for the future. Solarz AL, ed. Institute of Medicine, Committee on Lesbian Health Research Priorities, Neuroscience and Behavioral Health Program. Health Sciences Policy Program, Health Sciences Section; 1999.
26. **Pathela P, Hajat A, Schillinger J, et al**. Discordance between sexual behavior and self-reported sexual identity: a population-based survey of New York City men. Annals of Internal Medicine. 2006;145:416-25.
27. **Jarama S, Kennamer J, Poppen P, et al**. Psychosocial, behavioral, and cultural predictors of sexual risk for HIV infection among Latino men who have sex with men. AIDS and Behavior. 2005;9:513-23.
28. **Kennamer J, Honnold J, Bradford J**. Differences in disclosure of sexuality among African American and white gay/bisexual men: implications for HIV/AIDS prevention. AIDS Education and Prevention. 2000;12:519-31.
29. **D'Augelli A, Hershberger**. Lesbian, gay, and bisexual youth in community settings: personal challenges and mental health problems. Am J Community Psychology. 1993;21:421-48.
30. **Bradford J**. Lesbian Health in the US: Our Foundation and Our Future. Gay and Lesbian Health Association; 2005.
31. **Mayer K, Mimiaga M, VanDerwarker R, et al**. Fenway Community Health's model of integrated community-based LGBT care, education and research. In: Meyer I, Northridge M, eds. The Health of Sexual Minorities: Public Health Perspectives on Lesbian, Gay, Bisexual and Transgender Populations. Springer; 2006.

32. **Mayer K, Appelbaum J, Rogers T, et al.** The evolution of the Fenway Community Health model. Am J Public Health. 2001;91:892-4.

33. **Barrett K, Bradford J, Ellis J.** Using mapping to facilitate development of a health care infrastructure. ESRI Newsletter. 2002:1170.

34. **US Dept of Health and Human Services.** Scientific workshop on lesbian health 2000: steps for implementing the IOM report. Dept of Health and Human Services, Office on Women's Health; 2000.

35. **Heslin KC, Andersen RM, Ettner SL, et al.** Racial and ethnic disparities in access to physicians with HIV-related expertise. J Gen Intern Med. 2005;20:283-9.

36. **Bowen DJ, Bradford JB, Powers D, et al.** Comparing women of differing sexual orientations using population-based sampling. Women & Health. 2005;40:19-34.

37. **Bradford J, Norman N.** Sexual Minority Women of Color: A Summit to Develop Health Priorities. National Forum for Centers of Excellence in Women's Health. The Fenway Institute; 2003.

38. **Bradford JB, Norman N.** Barriers Faced by Pregnant and Parenting African American Lesbians. Workshop presented at the Annual Conference of Women in Medicine; July 2003; Monterrey, Calif.

39. **Xavier J, Bradford J, Hendricks M, et al.** Transgender Health Care Access in Virginia. Qualitative Health Research; 2007. In press.

40. **Bradford J, Xavier J, Hendricks M, et al.** Virginia Transgender Health Initiative survey. Virginia Department of Health, Department of Disease Prevention; 2007. Available at http://www.vdh.virginia.gov/epidemiology/DiseasePrevention/documents/pdf/THIS FINALREPORTVol1.pdf.

41. **Centers for Disease Control and Prevention.** Use of social networks to identify persons with undiagnosed HIV infection—seven US cities, October 2003-September 2004. Mortality and Morbidity Weekly Report. 2005;54:601.

42. **Gallagher K, Sullivan P, Lansky A, et al.** Behavioral surveillance among people at risk of HIV infection in the US: the national HIV behavioral surveillance system. Public Health Reports. 2007;122:32-8.

43. **Agency for Health Care Research and Quality.** Community-based Participatory Research: Assessing the Evidence. Agency for Health Care Research and Quality; 2004 Evidence Report/Technology Assessment, No. 99.

SECTION II

THE LIFE CONTINUUM

Chapter 3

Coming Out: The Process of Forming a Positive Identity

JOANNE GREENFIELD, PhD

Introduction

I n the most simple and common usage, *coming out* is the experience of becoming self-aware or the act of openly disclosing to others that one is lesbian, gay, bisexual, or transgender (LGBT). The developmental process of clarifying and accepting one's LGBT identity (*coming out to one-self*) is inextricably linked to the process of readying oneself to reveal that identity publicly (*coming out to others*). Self-acceptance and whether, when, and how to come out to others are influenced by personal history and characteristics; ethnic, cultural, and religious background; experiences of victimization and prejudice; family and societal messages that often derail rather than facilitate adjustment; and the presence or absence of community supports. These factors, combined with the inherent complexity of gender identity and sexual orientation, make coming out a challenging, dynamic, and lifelong experience.

Health professionals can play a pivotal role in supporting patients who identify or are beginning to identify as LGBT. Like everyone else, health professionals are subject to biased societal messages and often carry these prejudices into their work realms unwittingly.[1-4] For LGBT patients, access to healthcare, quality of communication during a clinical encounter, and relevance of the care that is offered are compromised when health providers are homophobic, undereducated with regard to LGBT issues, or unaware of their patients' gender or sexuality.[5-8] On the other hand, health providers who convey acceptance and affirmation can counteract the impact of confusing or negative messages LGBT patients receive elsewhere and can have an enormous influence on the development of positive self-esteem and a healthy life adjustment.

This chapter describes the nuances and complexity of the coming out process and suggests approaches clinicians can use to facilitate open and supportive communication with patients about gender identity and sexual orientation issues. The first section, *Identity Development*, describes different models of gender identity and sexual orientation, how language and stereotypes impact identity consolidation and development of self-esteem, and briefly reviews theories of identity development as they relate to LGBT populations. The second section, *Common Coming Out Patterns*, reviews models of coming out that have been described in the literature and considers the consequences—both positive and negative—of various coping strategies used by LGBT individuals. The third section, *Barriers and Benefits to Coming Out*, discusses the challenges and rewards of coming out with respect to self-esteem, relationships with family; ethnic and cultural diversity, interaction with the healthcare system, religion and spirituality, and management of daily life dilemmas, as well as coming out as a health provider. The chapter closes with *What Providers Can Do to Help*, a summary of ways in which clinicians can provide appropriate guidance and support for patients with regard to gender identity or sexual orientation issues. In addition, Appendix A consists of useful resources for both patients and clinicians who wish to learn more.

Identity Development

Child development theorist, Donald Winnicott, describes how children develop a secure sense of self and positive self-esteem in part through a process known as "mirroring," in which a child's feelings and behaviors are responded to empathically by parents and other critical role models. Through accurate mirroring, the child's experiences are validated and internalized, creating a "true self."[9] According to Winnicott, it is critical to develop a "true self" in order to achieve positive self-esteem and a sense of wholeness as a person. He states: "the true self feeling . . . requires a lived recognition of being the self one is, that this felt presence is one's true being."[10] While development of a "true self" is complicated for anyone, it is particularly challenging for LGBT individuals. Stereotypical perceptions about gender and sexuality contradict LGBT children and adolescents' true identity. Despite the fact that some parents may deem heterosexuality and stereotypical gender presentations as "more appropriate," pressure in these directions does not alter a child's or later adult's identity; rather it is confusing and destructive to the individual's positive self-development. Common language that is constrained by stereotypical conceptions frequently fails to describe the internal experience of an LGBT person accurately, which can make finding the right words to explain one's identity to others extremely challenging.

The next section examines the limitations of prevailing concepts of gender identity and sexual orientation, presents alternative models with expanded definitions, and considers possible solutions to the language problem.

Coming Out as What? Gender Identity, Sexual Orientation, and Language

Health professionals' understanding of patients' feelings, thoughts, and experiences surrounding gender and sexuality can have a large impact on patients' self-esteem and identity clarification. When clinicians confuse gender identity, gender role, and sexual orientation, patients who are in the midst of securing their identity become or remain confused, feel that aspects of their identity are blocked or degraded, and are hindered in the development of positive self-esteem. Such confusion by clinicians hinders the development of open and trusting therapeutic relations for both these patients and patients who are secure in their identity. The language we use, the questions we ask, and how we respond to patients' disclosures all determine whether we communicate bias or openness and whether we alienate patients or succeed in providing a warm welcome. Toward the goal of greater clarity, this chapter will now review and critique existing models of gender and sexuality.

Table 3-1   Common Terms Associated with Core Gender Identity, Gender Role, and Sexual Orientation

Concept	Terms
Core gender identity	man, woman, transsexual, transgender, intersex
Gender role	masculine, feminine, effeminate
	Slang:
	butch (masculine appearing or acting lesbian woman; or masculine person of any gender or sexual orientation),
	fem (feminine appearing or acting lesbian woman; or feminine person of any gender or sexual orientation),
	tomboy (masculine girl or woman),
	sissy (feminine boy or man).
Sexual orientation	heterosexual, homosexual, bisexual, gay, lesbian, straight
	Slang: used either as prejudicial insults or with pride by LGBT people:
	dyke (lesbian),
	fag (gay man),
	queer (umbrella term for any LGBT person)

According to psychobiologist J. D. Weinrich, overall gender identity consists of three main components: core gender identity, gender role, and sexual orientation.[11] *Core gender identity* consists of biological factors (such as genetics and physical anatomy) as well as psychological factors related to a person's inner experience of their gender. *Gender role* refers to social roles of males and females as defined by the society or culture at a particular time in history and can be observed in mode of dress, actions, or personal qualities. Gender role varies with historical and societal shifts and cultural differences. As with core gender identity, each person has a unique inner experience and behavioral style with regard to gender role. *Sexual orientation* refers to the propensity of a person to be romantically and/or sexually attracted to and fall in love with people of a different gender, their same gender, or both. Specific terms associated with core gender identity, gender role, and sexual orientation, are listed in Table 3-1.

Movement has been made over time from thinking of gender, gender role, and sexual orientation dichotomously or unidimensionally, toward conceptualizing the components of gender and sexuality in more complex and

Table 3-2 Binary/Unidimensional vs. Complex/Multidimensional Gender and Sexuality Models

	Binary & Unidimensional Models	*Complex/Multidimensional Models*	
Gender	Male/Female	Multiple and fluid gender constellations (male, female, transgender, intersex, transgender, ambigender, etc)	
Gender Role	Masculine/Feminine	Hi Masculinity	Hi Femininity
	Masculinity————Femininity	- -	- -
		- -	- -
		- -	- -
		- -	- -
		- -	- -
		Lo Masculinity	Lo Femininity
		Multiple and fluid gender role qualities each with their own continuum	
Sexual Orientation	Heterosexual/Homosexual Hetero/Bisexual/Homo (Freud) Hetero 0 1 2 3 4 5 6 Homo (Kinsey)	Hi Attraction to Men	Hi Attraction to Women
		- -	- -
		- -	- -
		- -	- -
		- -	- -
		- -	- -
		Lo Attraction to Men	Lo Attraction to Women
		Multiple and diverse bases on which one may be attracted to others each with their own continuum	

multidimensional ways (see Table 3-2). Insisting that individuals conform to only a male or female category of gender means that people who wish to express their true selves in expanded ways—for example, as "radical transgenderists, ambigendered or a third gender"—find no vision or reinforcement of themselves in society.[2] The perception of gender identity as nonbinary, with options that exist across a spectrum, presents a more diverse and multifaceted picture that acknowledges the existence of transgender people of all iterations. Similarly, with respect to gender role, use of a multidimensional model recognizes that people can have a variety of masculine and feminine qualities simultaneously.

Finally, sexual orientation has also been historically conceptualized according to dichotomous (heterosexual/homosexual) or unidimensional models. Examples of the latter include Freud's introduction of bisexuality in the early 1900s and Kinsey's seven-point scale with gradations from exclusively heterosexual to exclusively homosexual and degrees of bisexuality in between.[12-14] More complex/multidimensional models of sexual orientation acknowledge that each individual can have different levels of attraction to men and/or women independently.[11] For example, an exclusively gay man may be attracted only to men and not to women at all, while an exclusively lesbian woman may experience the reverse. Some individuals are attracted to both men and women to varying degrees along a continuum. While some of these people may embrace the concept of bisexuality as a description of their identity, others may use a label such as gay or lesbian rather than bisexual to describe their identity despite the fact that they have had fantasies, attractions, or experiences involving the other sex. Some people who have sex regularly or periodically with the same gender or both genders label themselves heterosexual. Finally, there are people who eschew labels as excessively constrictive or who consider sexual orientation to be fluid over time. For example:

> Mary, age 36, used to date men and was married for several years. After her divorce, she started dating women. Currently, she is single. When asked to describe her sexual orientation, she states: "When I dated men, I thought of myself as straight; when I dated women, I called myself lesbian. Some people would say I'm bisexual, but I've decided I don't really like labels."*

It is critical to find appropriate words to express oneself when trying to clarify feelings and sense of self in a confusing environment. This challenge is especially daunting when attempting to describe these aspects to another person. Clinicians who display awareness, openness, and flexibility about language options and alternative concepts of gender and sexual orientation

---

* All cases in this chapter are hypothetical.

are much more likely to be successful establishing a productive therapeutic connection. Consider the following case:

> Lee is a female-to-male transsexual who is in the process of transitioning (altering female body and gender presentation to become male, through hormone treatment and surgical interventions). Lee uses male self references despite an androgynous appearance, and sometimes refers to himself as "queer" or "trans." He presents saying: "I used to be lesbian but now I don't know what to call myself."

In addition to the fact that Lee is dealing with gender issues, he is grappling with how to discuss his sexual orientation. Instead of using labels such as lesbian, gay, or straight, it is likely to be much more fruitful to help Lee think about sexual orientation by focusing on understanding his attractions to men, women and transgender people. He may also need help exploring whether his attractions are actually changing with the move toward a male identity or whether he is simply getting bogged down in the complexities of language and labels in the transition.

For some people, a term such as "queer" is more palatable due to its gender-neutral nature. Listening to a person's language or asking them how they define or refer to themselves and using that same language not only allows for more openness about sexuality and gender between patient and health provider but also imbues more trust and safety in the relationship in general. For patients who are searching for or confused about their identity, using the models that allow for the most flexibility can be supportive and allow the patient to express or explore who they are from within rather than be constrained by stereotypes or biases of others.

Our culture's tendency is to not only categorize dichotomously (male-female, feminine-masculine, heterosexual-homosexual), but also to link up these dichotomies in culturally traditional or stereotypical ways (please see

Table 3-3   Societal Stereotypes of Gender and Sexual Orientation

Traditional/Stereotypic	*Nontraditional*
Masculine—Man—Heterosexual	Masculine—Man—Homosexual
Feminine—Man—Homosexual	Feminine—Man—Heterosexual
Feminine—Woman—Heterosexual	Feminine—Woman—Homosexual
Masculine—Woman—Homosexual	Masculine—Woman—Heterosexual

Table 3-3). For example, male is linked with masculine; female is linked with feminine. Messages that endorse the traditional view create additional identity development problems for people who do not fit these stereotypes. Consider the following example:

Sam, age 25, has been feeling panicky and is experiencing episodic chest pain and shortness of breath. He has been obsessing about his attractions to men, but says that it is impossible for him to be gay because he has always been very masculine, even playing football in college.

Similar worries might be seen in a "lipstick lesbian" who presents as very feminine and is told she can't possibly be gay; a straight, artistic, nonathletic guy who is labeled to his confusion as gay; or a big, strong, straight girl on the high school hockey team who gets labeled as lesbian. More masculine, lesbian women report being mistaken for men or being accused of wanting to be men; similarly, feminine gay men or boys are often teased or bullied for being "too much like girls." Bisexual people may feel themselves pressured (within themselves and/or by others) toward either a heterosexual or homosexual orientation based upon their gender role characteristics, thereby invalidating their bisexuality.

Misperceptions encountered by transgender people abound. For example, assuming that a masculine-looking and masculine-acting biologic female is lesbian or that a feminine biologic male is gay rather than possibly transgender misses the true identity of the individual and confuses gender identity and sexual orientation. Repeated misreading of people who present themselves in nontraditional ways can be confusing and damaging to LGBT youngsters and adults who are exploring different presentations as part of the process of clarifying who they are. Informed and supportive health providers can help by pointing out the difference between gender identity, gender role presentation, and sexual orientation, as well as by affirming the existence of hetero-, homo-, and bisexual and transgender people who have both masculine and feminine attributes.

Identity Development Models and the LGBT Population

Research indicates that the majority of lesbian, gay, and bisexual men and women realize their sexual orientation during their teens and early twenties, although some discover their orientation in early childhood or later in adulthood.[15,16] Coming out to self (self-awareness/self-identification) evolves simultaneously with the emergence of other developmental capacities and in conjunction with other developmental milestones such as the emergence of puberty. Emerging awareness of oneself as a sexual being (sexual exploration with self and others) and a relational being (developing capacities and skills for emotional intimacy) interact in complex ways with the development of one's emerging identity. Sometimes people become clearly aware of their sexual orientation prior to any sexual activity, while in other cases sexual exploration facilitates clarification of sexual orientation.[16] While there is little research on identity development among transgender people, available data suggest an incremental process beginning in early childhood, when many children attempt to communicate their gender differences to parents and others, intensifying in puberty as physical changes take place that conflict with the developing sense of self, and culminating in adulthood, when many transgender people become more fully self-aware and reveal their gender identity to others.[2,6] Transgender identity development is described in more detail in Chapter 12.

Exploration of same-sex experiences is common in adolescent development; this does not automatically infer a homosexual orientation, but it also does not mean that a youth is not gay, lesbian, or bisexual.[15] Sexual experimentation can range from being wondrous and conflict-free to an experience riddled with shame, conflict and confusion. Heterosexist or homophobic attitudes and misconceptions during this developmental phase can inhibit and disrupt a youngster's healthy exploration of sexual identity and budding sense of self. This can promote internalized homophobia, where external negative messages and experiences become transformed into self-hatred, denial, and an impaired sense of self.[17]

One problem for lesbian, gay, and bisexual (LGB) adolescents is that many adults (parents, teachers, etc) view homosexuality or bisexuality as a passing phase.[15] A young LGB child, teen, or adult working to clarify sexual identity and develop a positive sense of self can become confused, depressed, and even suicidal when faced with erroneous and invalidating messages. The stressors that promote internalized homophobia can also result in additional problems, including substance abuse, smoking, eating disorders, poor academic performance, dropping out of school, delinquency, problems with intimacy, high risk sexual behavior, prostitution, and running away.[16,18,19] These stressors do not end in early childhood, middle school, or high school; LGBT people are subject to similar prejudices and attacks and their consequences throughout their lives.[20]

People who are bisexual face certain challenges that are unique. While gay and lesbian people who are coming out experience feelings of being different from heterosexual peers, they may be able to find community more easily than bisexual people. When bisexual men and women first become aware of their attraction to or have actual sexual experiences with same-gender partners, they may feel somewhat aligned with gay and lesbian peers. However, they are also acutely aware of being different from these men and women, due to the presence of simultaneous other-gender attractions. To complicate matters, bisexual people who try to connect with gay and lesbian peers for support may find themselves accused of denying their "true homosexuality." This lack of validation, coupled with the oft-cited view that bisexuals are either "confused" or "just going through a phase," can inhibit identity clarification and result in significant isolation. The following case illustrates the challenge bisexual people face in having to contend with both homophobia and biphobia simultaneously[21]:

Bianca, age 17, dated girls for two years, and is "out" as a lesbian to her friends and parents. Her parents told her she'll "grow out of it," and to "focus on boys." She just met a boy who she feels attracted to and he feels the same way. Her lesbian and gay friends say she's in denial about being lesbian and just wants to conform. She knows she isn't straight because she still has attractions to girls. She doesn't want to identify as bisexual, because she doesn't know which group of kids to hang out with. She doesn't want to tell her parents about the new boyfriend, because they will be thrilled and think dating girls was just a phase. On the other hand, maybe her parents will be less angry with her if she pretends she is straight. It's all so weird. She doesn't know what to do, and she's starting to feel really depressed.

A healthcare appointment may be one of the few places where Bianca can discuss her concerns openly, without censorship or emotional repercussions. She needs to be told that her attractions are normal, that whoever she is in terms of sexual orientation is okay, and that she does not need to settle on a specific identity at this point in time. She also needs some guidance on how to negotiate discussion with her parents without causing harm to herself or to her family relationships. It may be helpful to provide her with a list of local and/or Web-based bisexual community resources and reading materials, so she can discover other people like herself and feel less "weird" and alone.

Loneliness and isolation are similar for transgender people. While awareness about transgender issues is increasing in gay, lesbian, and bisexual communities, misinformation and prejudice persist, and transgender people do not always feel supported by their LGB peers. In addition, even supportive LGB peers may not understand or relate to the unique challenges transgender people encounter during their process of exploration and transition. In order to work through their own internal transphobia and arrive at a positive and solid sense of self, it is critical for transgender people to find and connect with transgender communities and other knowledgeable, supportive people. Appendix A contains a list of resources where individuals who are exploring gender identity and/or sexual orientation issues can find information, affirmation, and support.

Common Coming Out Patterns

In order to be able to provide sensitive and appropriate assistance to patients who are grappling with gender or sexual orientation issues, health professionals must be able to identify where patients are in the process of self-awareness and how effectively they are coping with the challenges of coming out. While coming out is a complicated process that is unique for each individual, there are certain aspects that are common to most people's experiences. This chapter presents several coming out theories that describe the general progression of the coming out process; cases are presented that illustrate both positive and maladaptive coping styles. In addition to reading this section, it may also be useful for health professionals to read educational materials and coming out stories that demonstrate and normalize the range of possible experiences; when relevant, these readings may also be useful to patients (please see the resources listed in Appendix A).

Coming Out Theories

Early coming out theories developed in the 1970s and 1980s (please see Table 3-4)[22-25] drew heavily from life crisis literature,[26] and in particular, from models of bereavement developed by Kubler-Ross and others.[27] The lesbian or gay individual was seen as moving through specific stages— shock, denial, anger, sadness, negotiation, and acceptance—to eventually reach a healthy resolution of the life crisis. According to these early theories, coming out begins with a subconscious sense of being different, often without awareness of why. This is followed by more conscious questioning and exploration of same-sex attractions and relationships without definitive belief that one is homosexual; the process eventually progresses to clarity and acceptance of gay or lesbian identity as a fact. Initially, this definitive belief does not translate into self-acceptance, pride, or readiness to be open with others: the gay or lesbian aspect of identity is not yet integrated into the rest of one's identity or life. Achieving an open, nondefensive, and positive sense of self as a gay or lesbian person (identity synthesis or integra-

Table 3-4 Stage Theories of Coming Out [22,23,24,25]	
Theorist	*Stages*
Cass (1979)	Identity Confusion, Identity Comparison, Identity Tolerance, Identity Acceptance, Identity Synthesis
Coleman (1982)	Pre-Coming Out, Coming Out, Exploration, First Relationships, Integration
Sophie (1982)	Lesbian Feelings, Coming Out to Self, Coming Out to Others
Devine (1984)	Subliminal Awareness, Impact, Adjustment, Resolution, Integration

tion) is considered the final step in the process. While early theorists focused on developing and integrating identity as gay or lesbian rather than as bisexual, the process is easily applicable to bisexual people with regard to their same-sex attractions.

More modern theorists criticized early coming out models as excessively linear and progressive and recognized that development is a process of adaptation where growth tasks, including coming out, are creatively worked and reworked throughout the life span as new life events trigger the re-emergence of old feelings.[28,29] The following case provides a good example:

Jamal, age 47, has been happily out to everyone in his life as a gay man. Over the last two years, two of his friends developed HIV infection, and a third died of complications related to AIDS. Lately, he has been feeling anxious and worries constantly about his health even though he knows his HIV test is negative. For the first time in his life, he is dreaming of having sex with women. He is starting to believe it is unhealthy or even wrong to be gay—thoughts he has never had in the past. He ignored these thoughts initially, but is starting to think he should try being straight.

Jamal's dreams and the sudden emergence of internalized homophobia were triggered by recent traumatic events: he needs help processing his reactions to his friends' diagnoses and death. Referral to an informed and nonbiased therapist to work through his feelings is likely to be helpful. He might also benefit from a support group for gay men who are HIV-uninfected, if one is available in his area.

An LGBT person's identity is repeatedly challenged and consolidated every time they come out to a new person or in a new environment. Since this identity is often invisible, LGBT people can often make a conscious choice about whether to come out at all, when to make the announcement, and to whom they wish to share this information. It is possible to be more or less "out" or "closeted" in different situations: some LGBT people are out to everyone and everywhere, while others are selectively out to friends, but not to family, at school or work, or elsewhere. In some cases, choosing not to come out to certain people or in certain situations is a healthy decision made for reasons related to opportunity and safety, rather than self-loathing or shame.

At times, people who believe they are free of internalized homophobia (or biphobia or transphobia) find that negative feelings re-emerge when they attempt to come out to a new person or in a new realm of their life.

Sara, age 38, identifies as lesbian, has been publicly involved in gay rights issues, and has been out to friends for years. She is involved with a woman with whom she wants to make a long-term commitment, and she wants to share her joy about the relationship with her devoutly Catholic parents. As she prepares to come out to them for the first time, she notices feelings of guilt and shame about herself and her partner. She is shocked by the re-emergence of feelings she thought she worked out years ago. She can't sleep and is having heart palpitations.

Sara could be referred to an affirmative therapist to discuss her feelings about coming out to her parents and to work on her anxiety. She might benefit from reading books on coming out to parents (see resource section), and referral to her local PFLAG (Parents and Friends of Lesbians and

Gays, discussed later in this chapter) organization to attend a support group and have an opportunity to talk to some parents who have already gone through this process with their sons and daughters. All of these interventions are also likely to be helpful for her parents; in addition, educational materials that address homosexuality and religion specifically may help her parents with any religious dilemmas (please see resources in Appendix A).

Bisexual people often struggle with the question of which community they belong to and should spend time with (especially when interested in meeting eligible people with whom to develop intimate relationships). Some bisexual people initially feel that they straddle two worlds: the straight and the LGBT. While gay and lesbian people can be reasonably assured (even though it is still scary) that coming out to other gay and lesbian people will be a positive or neutral experience, bisexual people can experience negative reactions from straight, gay, and lesbian people alike. Bisexual people sometimes describe feeling incompletely seen or known by others when they are in a relationship because they are assumed to be straight when with a person of the same gender, and gay or lesbian when with a person of the opposite gender. To dispel these incorrect assumptions, a bisexual person may feel the need to come out repeatedly, even when in a stable relationship or being clear in his or her identity for a long time.

While coming out as lesbian, gay, or bisexual involves revealing a secret about oneself in terms of inner feelings and desires, coming out as transgender involves revealing one's inner sense of self as well as changes in gender, appearance, social role, and, for transsexuals, physical anatomy. Some transgender people are "forced" out of the closet by their nontraditional gender presentation or in the process of transitioning from one gender to another (if transsexual), while others have greater ability to choose the timing of their coming out to others.[6] Many transgender people, particularly transsexuals, not only come out but "cross over" to the other gender in order to remain within the binary gender system, while some transgender people come out and reject the internal, interpersonal, institutional, and societal pressures toward binary characterization of gender. Whether crossing over or not, transgender people grapple with the challenge of developing a physical (dress, manner, body, etc) presentation of themselves that is an accurate expression of their inner experience of gender identity. Sometimes this involves experimenting with a spectrum of gender expressions before settling upon one stable expression. As with LGB individuals, transgender people have to contend with shame both in the process of expressing their true selves and at times when they are hiding in order to protect themselves from attacks by others.[2]

A person's stage of life, concurrent life events and experiences, motivations for coming out, and relationship to the person(s) to whom they are coming out all create different contexts and result in a wide variety of experiences for both the person coming out and for those in whom the LGBT person confides (see Figure 3-1). Health providers who are attuned to these complexities can help patients understand their motivations for coming out;

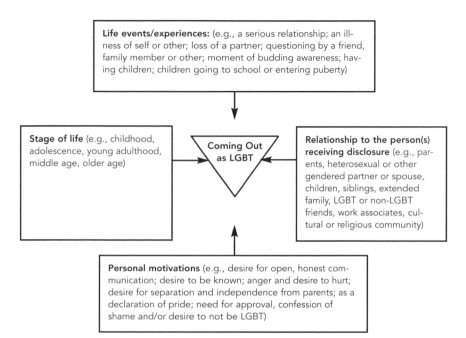

Life events/experiences: (e.g., a serious relationship; an illness of self or other; loss of a partner; questioning by a friend, family member or other; moment of budding awareness; having children; children going to school or entering puberty)

Stage of life (e.g., childhood, adolescence, young adulthood, middle age, older age)

Coming Out as LGBT

Relationship to the person(s) receiving disclosure (e.g., parents, heterosexual or other gendered partner or spouse, children, siblings, extended family, LGBT or non-LGBT friends, work associates, cultural or religious community)

Personal motivations (e.g., desire for open, honest communication; desire to be known; anger and desire to hurt; desire for separation and independence from parents; as a declaration of pride; need for approval, confession of shame and/or desire to not be LGBT)

Figure 3-1   Influences on the Coming Out Experience.

consider options for how they may wish to come out; and anticipate and ready themselves to handle people's reactions.

Common Coping Strategies

Youth and adults can employ a number of strategies to cope with internal conflicts about coming out. Some people employ the strategy of "hiding," in which they try to act and appear more stereotypically heterosexual by altering their dress, speech, or mannerisms.[15] This can be exhausting for LGB teens and adults who often, like their heterosexual peers, just want to "fit in." Some people try or pretend to be straight, dating and sometimes becoming sexually involved with peers of another gender, while others avoid the dating scene altogether and gain approval and self-worth by immersing themselves in academic achievement, extracurricular activities, sports, religious or spiritual quests, and other pursuits. Still others may try to cope by suppressing their feelings and awareness of their true selves by engaging in drug and/or alcohol abuse, sexual promiscuity, compulsive overeating, or other self-destructive behaviors that provide a diversion from unacceptable feelings and conflicts. Patients may also hide their secure or emerging gender status and sexual orientation from health providers. Creating an open and supportive atmosphere with affirmative literature in the office/clinic/waiting area, asking questions and eliciting a history in open and nonbiased ways (orally and on forms), and being open-minded, flexible and relaxed during discussions about gender and sexuality will encourage patients who hide elsewhere to consider being open in the health encounter.

Another common LGBT experience is one of *social isolation*, either through rejection by peers or dropping out of social interaction by choice. While some teens do come out, openly revealing their true selves, this can result in increased discrimination, taunting, violence, and other forms of victimization by peers, siblings, parents, and others. For LGBT youth who lack support, these negative messages can precipitate anxiety, depression, and/or suicidal behavior. Adults who are in certain geographic areas and/or who have not yet found or connected with local communities may also be isolated and suffer similar outcomes.

Social support has been found to be a buffer that mediates the stresses related to growing up "different."[18,19] Support from family, LGBT community connections, and/or a positive intimate relationship can be especially helpful. Finding and interacting with LGB or T communities and organizations can be instrumental in helping LGBT individuals develop more positive feelings about themselves and combating feelings of isolation. LGBT support groups, gay/straight alliances that exist in some high schools, books, and Web-based information can be extremely helpful. Identifying bisexual and transgender resources can be more challenging as they are less numerous and more difficult to locate. Patients may need assistance with direction to appropriate community organizations, online resources, and print materials (see resources in Appendix A).

While strategies such as hiding and isolation can be very prominent in adolescence, their impact is not exclusive to this age or period of development. Many adults who have not fully clarified or accepted their identity continue to use these coping strategies throughout life or suffer from the after effects of having "lost time" during their younger years being confused, closeted, self-hating, or isolated. Both teens and adults often need to work these issues out in therapy or through other forms of personal healing and development. Unfortunately, LGBT individuals who demonstrate gaps in development are sometimes diagnosed erroneously as having personality disturbances or other disorders. Health professionals should recognize that many LGBT patients require a "catch-up" period in which to experiment with what was missed earlier, including dating, exploring sexual likes and dislikes, and initial faltering attempts at developing intimate relationships. The following case describes a helpful intervention:

David (33) reflects on his teens and early 20s as a challenging time and recalls feeling very isolated. He found it difficult to trust others as he felt different, was afraid of getting beaten up at school and of being rejected by family and friends if he told them about his attractions to men. He avoided dating and other social activities with peers and threw himself into his schoolwork and music, excelling in those areas but missing out on some aspects of social development. Despite a successful early career life, he continued to be isolated as an adult, and began to meet men at bars for anonymous sex. He started using designer drugs such as ecstasy in the clubs, and when he got into crystal meth he spiraled downhill. His concerned health provider referred him to a gay-friendly rehab program and he is now doing 12-step work in Narcotics Anonymous and is in a gay men's support group. He feels he is gradually catching up on learning to trust other people, making friendships, and managing the dating scene. He is working avidly to overcome the shame and self-hatred he developed during years of hiding his identity. He is excited to be back at work and making new friends and feels his best years are ahead of him.

In a theory about lesbian identity "management," which also applies to GBT individuals, de Monteflores identified four types of adaptation approaches that are less than ideal: *assimilation, confrontation, ghettoization,* and *specialization* (please see Table 3-5).[30] All of these strategies are considered somewhat defensive, but de Monteflores goes on to describe a more integrated way of managing identity as follows: "The mature identity necessarily includes a recognition of sameness as well as difference. The articulation of these attributes requires a certain flexibility in boundaries, which comes out of an inner sense of security about individual identity."[30] While connection with the LGBT community is extremely important and

Table 3-5   Lesbian Identity Development Strategies[29] (de Monteflores, 1986, in Falco 1991)

Defensive Strategies	Description
Assimilation	Passing as one of the mainstream group
Confrontation	Facing up to one's difference but coming out as a form of confrontation
Ghettoization	Living almost or totally exclusively within the subculture, with energy put into avoiding intrusion by mainstream culture
Specialization	Seeing oneself and the subculture as possessing unique and superior qualities
Healthy Integration	Recognition of sameness and difference, flexibility in boundaries between gay and straight world, inner sense of security about individual identity

supportive in healthy identity development, integration of a person's identity into non-LGBT venues and aspects of life is also critical for a full acceptance of self, which includes working through gender bias and internalized homophobia.

Barriers and Benefits to Coming Out

As the coming out models describe, both self-awareness and disclosure to others are critical for development of positive self-esteem, as well as for a sense of connection in relation to others. At the same time, it is important to recognize the real and formidable difficulties associated with coming out, such as stigmatization, discrimination, and even overt violence. LGBT individuals must negotiate numerous barriers in order to attain the benefits of coming out. This section looks more closely at some aspects of this journey.

Stigmatization, Homophobia, Gender Prejudice, and Relationships with Others

While *homophobia* is the term most commonly used to describe negative attitudes towards gay men and lesbian women, terms such as *heterosexism, homonegativism, homosexism, social stigmatization, prejudice,* and *bigotry* have also been employed to capture negative societal perceptions of homosexuality and gay, lesbian and bisexual people.[31,32] Societal prejudice and stigmatization create many stresses that strongly influence LGBT people engaged in the developmental process of coming out.[18] Collectively referred to as *minority stress,* contributing factors include subtle negative attitudes and messages, insults and discriminatory language; hate crimes (including violent assault), lack of acceptance by family members, and discrimination in many realms of daily life, such as employment, housing, child custody, adoption, tax code, and marriage.[18] A parallel stigmatization occurs for people whose internal gender identity and/or external gender presentation is discordant with their biologic sex.[6] If an LGBT person recognizes they will be in danger if they reveal themselves, secrecy becomes a survival strategy rather than an act of self-hatred or a sign of incomplete personal development.[33] For example, silence may be the best option for a teen who lives with family and has reason to fear that they might be financially or physically abandoned or abused if they come out, while an adult who would lose their job if they came out at work may choose to remain hidden.

According to Herek, heterosexual peoples' ambivalent or negative impressions of lesbians and gay men are shaped by experiential, defensive, and symbolically based attitudes[34] (please see Table 3-6). Interestingly, experience is positively correlated with acceptance—that is, straight people

Table 3-6   Theory of Stigmatization/Negative Attitudes toward Homosexuals[33]

Experiential attitudes	Based upon one's past interactions with homosexual people
Defensive attitudes	Reflected by people coping with their inner conflicts or anxieties about gender and sexuality by projecting them onto gay and lesbian people
Symbolic attitudes	Expressions of abstract ideologies that are close to one's notion of self and one's social network and reference group (for example teachings of one's religion or culture)

with more gay or lesbian contact have less stereotyped and more positive attitudes toward gay and lesbian people. Defensiveness describes homophobic attitudes that some people project onto gay and lesbian (and bisexual) people in an attempt to cope with their own inner conflicts or anxieties about gender and sexuality. Symbolic attitudes refer to religious and/or cultural teachings that fuel intolerance. It is not hard to see how these concepts might also explain people's negative reactions to transgender people.

We are all subject to societal influences and are therefore vulnerable to making stereotypically based assumptions and judgments. As clinicians, we have an added duty to examine our conclusions to be sure they are soundly supported by existing data. We can check our attitudes and assumptions by asking ourselves questions like "Do I feel negatively about this person and why?" or "Are my reactions due to ideologies I've been exposed to or a personal vulnerability or defensiveness?" or "How can I learn more about LGBT populations?"

Self-esteem/Internal Issues

Herek's research not only explains the stigma and prejudice LGBT people experience from external sources, it also illuminates how internalization of these same attitudes can lead to a deep sense of shame. The need to rid oneself of shame and to challenge stereotypes about sex and gender is clearly an issue not just for LGBT people but also for many straight and traditionally gendered people. However, the process of untangling feelings about issues such as body image, participation in various sexual activities, a history of sexual abuse or assault, or expectations regarding sexual prowess is particularly complicated for a person who is simultaneously clarifying or coming out about their gender status or sexual orientation. The greater the level of internalized homophobia, biphobia, or transphobia, the more negative the impact on self-esteem.

As LGBT people encounter major life events, nontraditional gender identity and sexuality present challenges to coming out and self-esteem which may evoke a variety of emotional reactions such as a reawakening of shame or self-hatred, feelings of isolation, anger about societal prejudice, sadness or feelings of loss, and even rejecting or re-questioning a previously solid identity. The list of potential triggering events is long and includes, among others, hormonal transitions (puberty, pregnancy, and menopause), social transitions (negotiating adolescence, changes in friendships, social communities, and intimate relationships; considering parenthood and becoming a parent; experiencing one's children's life stages or career milestones; illness and death of a parent), and experiencing illness and aging. (See Figure 3-1, page 57.) The more trauma-ridden a person's history, the greater the challenge; the more support available, the better for healing and positive development. Patients with more positive self-esteem will care for their health better than patients who are filled with shame and self-hatred. LGBT people who have strong supports and who have achieved a solid, positive gender and sexual identity frequently experience feelings of pride, strength, and accomplishment as life challenges are met successfully.

Relationships with Family

Just as LGBT people's process of gaining self-acceptance and preparing for coming out to others takes months to years, it stands to reason that family members and others may require a parallel period in which to assimilate and adjust to the news after a loved one has come out to them. While LGBT people may wish for rapid integration of the news and immediate acceptance, it is helpful to guide LGBT patients toward expectations of a process for others (parents, siblings, spouses, children, friends) that is parallel to their own process. Some of these people may then take on the additional challenge of coming out to others in their own lives about their loved one's identity. This *secondary coming out* involves a process that is very similar to the one the LGBT person experiences, sometimes requiring parents and others to grapple with insecurity, trepidation, and shame.

Families with good communication and processing skills have a far easier time with the tasks of assimilation, acceptance, and secondary coming out than families with conflict and difficult family system issues. However, all families can benefit from support: PFLAG (Parents, Friends and Families of Gays and Lesbians) is an excellent resource. A national organization of parents, families, and friends of LGBT people, PFLAG offers nonjudgmental support services in every state for parents, straight spouses, other family members, and friends, as well as LGBT people (please see resources in Appendix A).

Ethnic and Cultural Diversity Issues and Coming Out

In recent years, more attention has been given to ethnic, cultural, and religious diversity issues with regard to sexual orientation, gender, and coming out. Each culture and ethnicity has its own unique nuances about gender and sexuality, the detailed examination of which is beyond the scope of this chapter. Even when speaking about what may seem to be one group, for example Latina/Latino people, there can be a multiplicity of ethnic/cultural subgroups (Puerto Rican, Dominican, Cuban, people from various South American and Central America origins, etc), racial subgroups (white, black, native, mestizos, mulattos, etc), and linguistic subgroups (English, Spanish, Portuguese, indigenous languages, "Spanglish," etc).[35] We find similar diversity among Asian,[36] African American,[37] Jewish,[38] Christian,[39] European American,[40] and other groups.[41] Class and religious differences interact with culture and ethnicity, adding further to the complexity of a person's experience of their sexual and gender identity and how they choose to communicate with others. This section highlights several well-documented, cross-cultural issues that impact the coming out process; however, readers should consult additional resources for a greater understanding of concerns and needs of LGBT individuals in specific cultures, religions, and ethnicities.

In some Asian cultures, the taboo against public discussion of anything sexual creates a barrier for any discussion that might lead to coming out.[42] Chan points out that in East Asian cultures, loyalty to the interests of family and community are dominant over the needs or wishes of the individual and that the concept of individual identity may not even exist.[42]

Different cultures have varying norms with regard to same-gender relationships: these norms are reflected in the language that exists to describe these relationships. There are no words for homosexuality or bisexuality in some cultures.[36,42] While a variety of sexual behaviors or even sustained relationships with same-gender partners may be seen as acceptable and not indicative of or described as homosexuality in some cultures, these behaviors may been seen as indicating a homosexual or bisexual identity in others.[32,36,41]

Expectations of certain gender role behaviors (for example, machismo in Latin cultures, female submissiveness in Asian cultures, and both, as in Greek culture) interact with expectations about heterosexuality, male dominance, and the family.[35,42,43] Latino or African American men may view sexual activity with other men as an acceptable part of their life while considering themselves straight, especially if they assume the "active" (dominant) rather than "passive" (receptive or submissive) position during sexual encounters, in keeping with the stereotypic masculine role. Emphasis on (heterosexual) family, child bearing and rearing, and creating future generations may also produce an intense pressure in some cultures.[35,38,42]

Many models of identity development and theories about coming out consider coming out to others, for example family of origin, to be a critical and necessary step in fighting shame, denial, and self-hatred. However, accepting this concept as universal is culturally biased, since independence and separation from family of origin is promoted as a sign of adult health and maturity in some cultures but not in others.[33] Compromise in the service of preserving multiple aspects of one's identity is quite common. There are situations in which an LGBT person can be strong and positive in their sense of self and make choices to remain closeted in some aspects of their life to preserve family connections and cultural identity. For example, in many Latin and African American cultures, close connection to family of origin is of paramount importance, and individuals may therefore choose to conceal their LGBT identity in an effort to preserve their cultural identity.[33,37]

Some families welcome, accept, and integrate significant others into the family without acknowledging openly the gay, lesbian, or bisexual family member's sexual orientation per se. In some cases, families can slowly be educated or conversations can be opened in incremental ways that do not destroy family cohesiveness or cultural ties. There are always costs involved in choosing incomplete disclosure, including lack of family support in understanding the burdens of living with oppression specific to life in a homophobic and gender-biased society. Clearly there are instances in which individuals choose to come out to the detriment of family relations and with loss of community connections. These losses must be grieved, and connection with other LGBT people from common cultural, ethnic, or religious backgrounds can be especially positive and healing in these circumstances.

Relationship with the Healthcare System

Although the medical system considered homosexuality to be an illness for many years, this designation was dropped from the *Diagnostic and Statistical Manual of Mental Disorders* (DSM) in 1973.[44] However, gender identity disorder continues to be included as a diagnostic category. The interpretation and classification of various types of transgenderism as mental illness, rather than simply as different expressions of gender or as physical variations, has a negative impact on self-esteem and efforts toward positive identity development of transgender people, much as the inclusion of homosexuality did for LGB people in the past.[6] Currently, there is movement toward removing this category from the DSM as well.

In spite of this progress, some clinicians continue to subscribe to the belief that homosexuality is a mental disorder and promote "conversion and reparative therapies"—"psychotherapeutic" interventions whose intent is the elimination of homosexual desire and behavior. These "treatments" are in direct opposition to the research findings and policy statements of all the major relevant health and mental health professional associations such as the American Psychiatric Association, American Psychological Association, National Association of Social Workers, American Academy of Pediatrics, American Counseling Association, and the American Medical Association. In 2001, the US Surgeon General's *Call to Action to Promote Sexual Health and Responsible Sexual Behavior* asserted there is "no valid scientific evidence that sexual orientation can be changed."[45]

Each of the aforementioned organizations has strong policy statements opposing conversion or reparative therapies and any approach that portrays homosexuality as a disorder. The American Psychiatric Association's position statement states in part that "The potential risks of reparative therapy are great, including depression, anxiety and self-destructive behavior, since therapist alignment with societal prejudices against homosexuality may reinforce self-hatred already experienced by the patient."[46] The American Academy of Pediatrics statement explains:

> Confusion about sexual orientation is not unusual during adolescence. Counseling may be helpful for young people who are uncertain about their sexual orientation or for those who are uncertain about how to express their sexuality and might profit from an attempt at clarification through counseling or psychotherapeutic initiative. Therapy directed specifically at changing sexual orientation is contraindicated since it can provoke guilt and anxiety while having little or no potential for achieving changes in orientation.[47]

It is not uncommon for LGBT people to experience periods in their coming out process when they wish they were not who they are. This phenomenon occurs both in people who are just beginning to explore their identity as well as in people who have been out for years and have had recent events or experiences that trigger old internal conflicts. It is critical that health professionals refrain from tacitly or openly suggesting that a patient's sexual orientation or gender status can or should be changed. All patients who are questioning should be directed to educational and therapeutic resources where internalized homophobia, biphobia, and/or transphobia can be addressed and feelings about possibly being gay, lesbian, bisexual, or transgender can be explored in a nonbiased and affirmative manner.

Religion, Spirituality, and Coming Out

The task of reconciling one's sense of self with religious and spiritual beliefs that are frequently hostile to that identity can be extremely difficult. While some religious denominations have developed policies of being "welcoming communities" for LGBT people, many religious traditions continue to convey negative messages about homosexuality and gender nonconformity, including concepts of sin, eternal damnation, religious transgression, and ostracization from the spiritual community. This can lead LGBT people who were raised in such a tradition to a religious/spiritual crisis when coming out. Some people resolve this crisis by rejecting religion altogether, some shift to more accepting religious or spiritual traditions or form their own LGBT supportive religious communities (see Appendix A), and some rework their relationship with their original spiritual or religious tradition in ways they can embrace. This can be a challenging, painful, confusing, and even frightening process. Consider the following example:

> William, age 49, is an Evangelical Christian who has always believed homosexuality is sick and sinful. Although he has had close female friends for years, he reports little sexual attraction to women. He was engaged to a woman briefly, but broke the engagement at the last minute. William has been aware of strong attractions to men since his early teens, and has anonymous sex with men periodically, with each encounter followed by a period of severe guilt, shame, and suicidal thoughts. He sought religious counsel from his minister, and was assured that he would find a spiritually healthy heterosexual life if his faith and prayer were strong enough. He has been working with a reparative therapist, but continues to desire men. Feeling desperate, William presents to his doctor saying: "I can't keep living this way. Please tell me what I can do to stop thinking about men, and shift my attraction to women."

William is caught in a serious bind between his religious beliefs and what appears to be his natural sexuality. This is a volatile situation: he needs to be urgently assessed for suicidality and should be referred to a mental health professional who has experience working in a nonjudgmental way with LGB people whose sexuality is in conflict with their religion. William needs to learn from his health provider that homosexuality is natural and healthy, that sexual orientation cannot be changed, and that there are many religious interpretations of the scriptures that are in disagreement with the concept of homosexuality as a sin. Referral to resources such as the Web site for Evangelicals Concerned, an LGBT-affirming Evangelical Christian community, and provision of written materials that address the intersection of homosexuality and spirituality may be very helpful (see Appendix A). PFLAG has developed many informative pamphlets that can be ordered and displayed in waiting areas or handed out to patients (see Appendix A).

Daily Life Dilemmas and Coming Out

As discussed earlier, numerous daily life stresses are associated with being LGBT. In instances where people are required to categorize themselves dichotomously by gender in daily life, such as on drivers license applications and other standard forms (insurance, doctor's office, hospital, marriage, and so on), a dilemma is presented for many transgender people, and coming out may be required in order to resolve the situation.[2] There are other stresses that transgender people face differently from the LGB population.

Due to stereotypes, institutional structures, and societal biases about gender, transgender people face continual challenges to their identity in public venues such as male/female restrooms, locker rooms, and dormitory sleeping arrangements.[2] Whether they select the men's or women's facility, they often encounter hostility and even violence based on their choice. Transgender people encounter discrimination in every realm, including employment, housing, medical treatment, rape crisis centers, and homeless and battered women's shelters.[6]

LGB people experience some of these problems as well. Discrimination, for example with regard to tax codes, insurance, and the completion of many forms, presents LGB people with difficult choices that often do not reflect their identities. Many forms list a limited range of relationship options (single, married, widowed, divorced): this scheme offers no viable designations for the LGB person who is in a long-term relationship with a same-gender partner and unmarried (marriage only recently being an option in a very few places). When an LGB person lists their partner as next of kin or emergency contact, the door is opened to questions about the nature of that relationship, and all of the risks of coming out (for example, to an ignorant or homophobic receptionist) ensue.

Health providers can help by creating intake forms that offer nonbiased options, signaling acceptance of LGBT lifestyles with a posted nondiscrimination policy and displays of inclusive educational materials in the waiting room, and offering sensitivity training to staff. When taking the medical history, inclusion of questions that elicit information about the entire range of gender and sexuality experiences will also promote a sense of safety and greater disclosure.

Families with children encounter numerous dilemmas and frustrations in school systems where LGBT issues are not handled affirmatively. In spite of the diversity of family structures across the United States, many teachers and school administrators continue to limit the notion of "family" to a mother, a father, and a child or children. They convey this prejudice to children and their families in insensitive or biased comments and lack of diversity of teaching materials in the classroom, exclusionary forms used by schools, and exercises such as mother's or father's day card-making. Unfortunately, more extreme instances of outright homophobic, biphobic, or transphobic comments by teachers or comments by other children that are tacitly condoned by teachers are still common. While these situations are clearly injurious to any child who does not fit the stereotype, they also pose stress for children of LGBT parents as their type of family is being ignored or attacked. Parents, both LGBT and straight, are affected by the stress being placed on their children and the assault on their family and their own self-esteem. While it is true that the judgment of peers can be brutal (as in the teasing or bullying of an LGBT youngster because they are "different"), it is also true that peer voices have incredible power to effect change (witness the success of many gay/straight alliances in the schools). Health providers can serve as catalysts for change by referring families, school teachers, and administrators to programs such as PFLAG's Safe Schools Program, which provides resources to help schools become better educated and offer safer and healthier environments for children.

Coming Out as a Health Provider

Coming out as a health provider can be a productive, educational, and rewarding experience for the clinician, patient, and colleagues[7] when the needs of the patient, the clinician's own motivations, and the costs and benefits of disclosure are all properly assessed. Reviewing all of the nuances of such an assessment is beyond the scope of this chapter; therefore, this section will highlight just a few major issues to be considered.

Clinicians may have a variety of motivations for coming out to a patient; similarly, patients may have a number of motivations for either wanting (or not wanting) to know. Patients sometimes ask personal questions simply because it makes the clinician seem a little more real or human to know a little about their lives. LGBT patients may ask about a clinician's gender status or sexual orientation because they specifically want a provider who is lesbian, gay, bisexual, or transgender; on the other hand, some patients may ask because they feel more comfortable with a provider who isn't. Reasons why clinicians may consider coming out include wanting to reassure an LGBT patient that they can provide a sense of safety and support, to serve as a positive role model for both LGBT and heterosexual patients, and to maintain an atmosphere of openness rather than secrecy. Providers may also choose to come out to colleagues in order to relieve themselves of the burdens of hiding, to have more open collegial relationships, to be a resource or role model for other providers, or to dispel stereotypes and misperceptions about LGB or T people.

When deciding whether to come out to a patient, clinicians should assess their own motivations carefully and consider both the potential positive and negative impact on the patient. Some patients (both heterosexual and LGBT) will welcome the news. On the other hand, this information might make an LGB or T patient feel pressured toward accepting a particular identity that may not be right or that they are not yet prepared to accept; a biased, heterosexual patient might feel frightened or alienated. When a patient asks about a clinician's identity, providers are able to make a better assessment of their patient's motivations and the pros and cons of coming out if they ask the patient about why they are inquiring, what they expect the answer to be, and what they would hope for and why. The provider must take the lead in helping patients to process their feelings about these issues, as patients are often inhibited in this area. While choosing not to share information is a reasonable option; lying to a patient is fraught with risks to the therapeutic relationship, and if tacitly or intentionally misleading information is discovered, it can cause breach of trust in or fracture of the entire alliance. It is important that providers, whether they come out or not, make it clear that they will accept the patient with whatever sexual orientation or gender identity the patient decides is right. Timing of any decision to come out is critical, especially in cases where a patient is unclear about their identity.

If for any reason a clinician feels confused or conflicted about how to approach these issues with a patient, the clinician should seek consultation from a qualified, nonjudgmental colleague.

What Providers Can Do to Help

Health professionals can play a pivotal role in the lives of LGBT patients who are securely established or struggling with gender identity or sexual orientation identity by providing appropriate guidance and support. The clinician-patient relationship itself can facilitate healing in that it provides a venue in which to normalize a developing LGBT person's questioning and an opportunity to "mirror" their emerging sense of self. This experience can be extraordinarily rewarding. Below are suggestions for how clinicians can create practices that are supportive of LGBT patients, particularly patients who are in the process of forming an LGBT identity.

Attitudes and Awareness

- Remain open to flexible, nonbinary models of gender and sexuality with *all* patients (not everyone initially shares their gender or sexual identity).
- Avoid assumptions based on conventional stereotypes of how LGBT people look and behave.
- Understand the coming out process; consider where in the coming out and life development process a person might be, what factors (internal and external) might be affecting their sense of self, and how that might be affecting their life choices, self-care, and other decisions.
- Develop awareness of how race, ethnicity, class, and religion can affect a patient's circumstances and perspective of their gender and sexuality and the process of coming out.
- Become aware of and sensitive to the bigotry and stigmatization that LGBT patients and their families experience in daily life and the stress it places upon them.

Skills and Practices

- Listen to how patients describe themselves and mirror their language; use nonbiased language to describe and discuss issues related to gender, sexuality, and relationships.
- Communicate that homosexuality, bisexuality, and nontraditional gender are healthy, normal, and positive expressions of gender and sexuality.
- Assess a patient's level of self-esteem and how it might be related to internalized homophobia.
- Assess a patient's connection to or isolation from LGBT resources and communities.
- Remain positive and affirming when talking to patients about their sexuality and gender identity.
- Include specific nonbinary questions about gender and sexuality on intake forms and in history-taking exams and discussions.
- Affirm the patient's true sense of self and/or their desire to find their true self-identity.
- Have available: (1) referrals to LGBT affirmative support groups, community organizations, and specialized professional mental health and health providers; (2) information on relevant LGBT community organizations and resources; (3) reading materials and/or lists of readings and Web-based materials on LGBT health issues and supportive resources; and (4) resources for friends and family members of LGBT patients. Some family members will already be very supportive and knowledgeable while others will be uninformed and/or in crisis (see Appendix A for resources).
- Coming out as a health provider can be a productive, educational, and rewarding experience. The needs of the patient, the clinician's own motivations, and the costs and benefits of a disclosure must be properly assessed.

Conclusion

Coming out is a gradual and lifelong process. Healthy adjustment requires both achieving a positive sense of self and learning how to negotiate successful relationships in a world that is filled with intolerance. Clinicians can make positive, sometimes even life-altering, impact on their patients by educating themselves about and being sensitive to the needs of LGBT patients and family members. Understanding the nuances and complexities of "coming out" as LGBT will lead to more open, productive, and communicative relationships with LGBT patients.

Summary Points

- Coming out is the process of clarifying and accepting one's identity as lesbian, gay, bisexual, or transgender, and when ready, revealing that identity to others. Self-acceptance of an LGBT identity typically evolves gradually over a period of many years.
- Gender and sexual orientation are complex and multidimensional rather than binary or unidimensional.
- Personal history and characteristics as well as the presence or absence of family and community supports all influence the experience and process of coming out. The diversity of beliefs and norms about gender and sexuality among different ethnicities, cultures, and religions also make the coming out process unique for each individual.
- Most lesbian, gay, and bisexual people realize their sexual orientation during their teens and early twenties, although some discover their orientation in early childhood or later in adulthood. Sometimes people become clearly aware of their sexual orientation prior to any sexual activity, while in other cases sexual exploration facilitates clarification of sexual orientation.
- Coming out as transgender involves revealing one's inner sense of self as well as changes in gender, appearance, social role, and, for transsexuals, physical anatomy. Some transgender people are "forced" out of the closet by their nontraditional gender presentation or in the process of transitioning from one gender to another (if transsexual), while others have greater ability to choose the timing of their coming out to others.
- Coming out to others is a dynamic and lifelong challenge. Every time an LGBT person encounters a new person or environment, they make a conscious choice about whether, when, and to whom they wish to share their identity.
- LGBT people may internalize societal prejudice and stigmatization and consequently develop a sense of shame, isolation, and loneliness affecting their coming out process. Social support from family, LGBT community connections, and/or a positive intimate relationship can help reduce the stresses related to feeling "different" and can promote formation of a positive identity.
- People who have difficulty with the process of self-acceptance and coming out cope with the challenges in a variety of ways. Some try to appear more stereotypically heterosexual; some become sexually and romantically involved with other gender peers; some avoid dating altogether and immerse themselves in academic achievement and other activities that validate their self-worth; still others engage in drug and/or alcohol abuse, sexual promiscuity, or other self-destructive behaviors that provide a diversion from unacceptable feelings.

- In order to best assist a patient who is grappling with gender or sexual orientation issues, health professionals must also be able to identify where the patient is in the process of self-awareness and how effectively they are coping with the challenges of coming out.
- Health professionals can play a pivotal role in the lives of patients who are struggling with gender or sexual identity by communicating that the patient's questioning about gender and sexuality is normal and that being LGBT is healthy and positive, by providing appropriate referrals, and by connecting patients to LGB or T communities, organizations, publications, and support groups.

References

1. **Smith EM, Johnson SR, Guenther SM**. Health care attitudes and experiences during gynecologic care among lesbians and bisexuals. Am J Public Health. 1985;75(9):1085-7.
2. **Gagne P, Tewksbury R, McGaughey D**. Coming out and crossing over: identity formation and proclamation in a transgender community. Gender and Society. 1997;11(4):478-508.
3. **Beehler GP**. Confronting the culture of medicine: gay men's experiences with primary care physicians. Journal of the Gay and Lesbian Medical Association. 2001;5(4):135.
4. **Rondahl, G, Innala S, Carlsson M**. Nursing staff and nursing students' emotions towards homosexual patients and their wish to refrain from nursing, if the option existed. Scandinavian Journal of Caring Sciences. 2004;18(1):19-26.
5. **Cole SW, Kemeny ME, Taylor SE, et al**. Elevated physical health risk among gay men who conceal their homosexual identity. Health Psychol. 1996;15(4):243-51.
6. **Gainor KA**. Including transgender issues in lesbian, gay and bisexual psychology: implications for clinical practice and training. In: Greene B and Croom GL, eds. Education, Research and Practice in Lesbian, Gay Bisexual and Transgendered Psychology: A Resource Manual. Sage Publications; 2000:131-60.
7. **Potter JE**. Do ask, do tell. Ann Intern Med. 2002;137(5 pt 1):341-3.
8. **Bonvicini KA, Perlin MJ**. The same but different: clinician-patient communication with gay and lesbian patients. Patient Education and Counseling. 2003;51(2):115-22.
9. **Winnecott DW**. Mirror-role of mother and family in child development. In: Winnecott DW. Playing and Reality. Basic Books; 1967.
10. **Winnecott DW**. Ego distortion in terms of true and false self. In: Winnecott DW. The Maturation Processes and the Facilitating Environment. International University. Press; 1965.
11. **Weinrich JD**. Sexual Landscapes. Charles Scribner's Sons; 1987.
12. **Freud S**. Three Essays of the Theory of Sexuality. Strachey J, trans-ed. Basic Books; 1962.
13. **Kinsey AC, Pomeroy WB, Martin CE**. Sexual Behavior in the Human Male. WB Saunders; 1948.
14. **Kinsey AC, Pomeroy WB, Martin CE, et al**. Sexual Behavior in the Human Female. WB Saunders; 1953.
15. **Hunter J, Mallon GP**. Lesbian, gay and bisexual adolescent development: dancing with your feet tied together. In: Greene B, Croom GL, eds. Education, Research and Practice in Lesbian, Gay, Bisexual, and Transgendered Psychology: A Resource Manual. Sage Publications; 2000:226-43.
16. **D'Augelli AR**. Lesbian, gay and bisexual development during adolescence and young adulthood. In: Cabaj RP, Stein TS, eds. Textbook of Homosexuality and Mental Health. American Psychiatric Press; 1996:267-88.

17. **Malyon AK**. The homosexual adolescent: developmental issues and social bias. Child Welfare. 1981;60:321-30.

18. **DiPlacido J**. Minority stress among lesbians, gay men and bisexuals: a consequence of heterosexism, homophobia, and stigmatization. In: Herek GM, ed. Stigma and Sexual Orientation: Understanding Prejudice Against Lesbians, Gay Men and Bisexuals. Sage Publications; 1998:138-59.

19. **Meyer IH, Dean L**. Internalized homophobia, intimacy and sexual behavior among gay and bisexual men. In: Herek GM, ed. Stigma and Sexual Orientation: Understanding Prejudice Against Lesbians, Gay Men and Bisexuals. Sage Publications; 1998:160-86.

20. **The Medical Foundation**. Health Concerns of the Gay, Lesbian, Bisexual and Transgender Community. 2nd ed. Massachusetts Department of Public Health; June 1997.

21. **Fox RC**. Bisexuality in perspective: a review of theory and research. In: Greene B, Croom GL, eds. Education, Research and Practice in Lesbian, Gay Bisexual and Transgendered Psychology: A Resource Manual. Sage Publications; 2000:161-206.

22. **Cass VC**. Homosexual identity formation: a theoretical model. J Homosex. 1979;4:219-35.

23. **Coleman E**. Developmental stages of coming out. J Homosex. 1982:31-43.

24. **Sophie J**. A critical examination of stage theories of lesbian identity development. J Homosex. 1984;12(2):39-51.

25. **Devine JL**. A systemic inspection of affectional preference orientation and the family of origin. Journal of Social Work and Human Sexuality. 1984;2(3):9-17.

26. Examples of life crisis literature are: Coelho GV, Hamburg DA. Adams JE, eds. Coping and Adaptation. Basic Books; 1974; McCubbin HI, Cauble AE, Patterson JM, eds. Family Stress, Coping and Social Support. Charles C. Thomas; 1982; and Lazarus RS, Folkman S, eds. Stress, Appraisal and Coping. Springer; 1984.

27. **Kubler-Ross E**. On Death and Dying. Collier; 1969.

28. **Weick A**. A growth-task model of human development. Social Casework. 1983;64(3):131-7.

29. **Raphael B**. The Anatomy of Bereavement. Basic Books; 1983.

30. **Falco KL**. Psychotherapy with Lesbian Clients: Theory into Practice. Brunner/Mazel; 1991. Also deMonteflores C. Notes on management of difference. In: Stein TS, Cohen CJ, eds. Contemporary Perspectives on Psychotherapy with Lesbians and Gay Men. Plenum; 1986:73-101.

31. **Herek GM**. Stigma, prejudice and violence against lesbians and gay men. In: Gonsiorek JC, Weinrich JD, eds. Homosexuality: Research Implications for Public Policy. Sage Publications; 1991:60-80.

32. **Kite ME**. When perceptions meet reality: individual differences in reactions to lesbians and gay men. In: Greene B, Herek GM, eds. Lesbian and Gay Psychology: Theory, Research and Clinical Applications. Sage Publications; 1994:25-53.

33. **Smith A**. Cultural diversity and the coming out process: implications for clinical practice. In: Greene B, ed. Ethnic and Cultural Diversity Among Lesbians and Gay Men. Sage Publications; 1997:279-300.

34. **Herek GM**. Beyond homophobia: a social psychological perspective on attitudes towards lesbians and gay men. J Homosex. 1984:1-21.

35. **Gonzalez FJ, Espin OM**. Latino men, Latina women and homosexuality. In: Cabaj RP, Stein TS, eds. Textbook of Homosexuality and Mental Health. American Psychiatric Press; 1996:583-602.

36. **Nakajima GA, Chan YH, Lee K**. Mental health issues for gay and lesbian Asian Americans. In: Cabaj RP, Stein TS, eds. Textbook of Homosexuality and Mental Health. American Psychiatric Press; 1996:563-82.

37. **Greene B**. Ethnic minority lesbians and gay men: mental health and treatment issues. In: Greene B, ed. Ethnic and Cultural Diversity Among Lesbians and Gay Men. Sage Publications; 1997:240-8.

38. **Dworkin SH**. Female, lesbian and Jewish: complex and invisible. In: Greene B, ed. Ethnic and Cultural Diversity Among Lesbians and Gay Men. Sage Publications; 1997:63-87.

39. **Haldeman D**. Spirituality and religion in the lives of gay and lesbian Americans. In: Cabaj RP, Stein TS, eds. Textbook of Homosexuality and Mental Health. American Psychiatric Press; 1996:881-96.

40. **Cerbone AR**. Symbol of privilege, object of derision: dissonance and contradictions. In: Greene B, ed. Ethnic and Cultural Diversity Among Lesbians and Gay Men. Sage Publications; 1997:117-31.

41. **Tafoya T**. Native gay and lesbian issues: two spirited people. In: Greene B, ed. Ethnic and Cultural Diversity Among Lesbians and Gay Men. Sage Publications; 1997:1-10.

42. **Chan CS**. Don't ask, don't tell, don't know: the formation of a homosexual identity and sexual expression among Asian American lesbians. In: Greene B, ed. Ethnic and Cultural Diversity Among Lesbians and Gay Men. Sage Publications; 1997:240-8.

43. **Fygetakis LM**. Greek American lesbians: identity odysseys of honorable good girls. In: Greene B, ed. Ethnic and Cultural Diversity Among Lesbians and Gay Men. Sage Publications; 1997:152-90.

44. **Greene B**. Lesbian and gay sexual orientations: implications for clinical training, practice and research. In: Greene B, Herek GM, eds. Lesbian and Gay Psychology: Theory, Research and Clinical Applications. Sage Publications; 1994:1-24.

45. US Surgeon General's Call to Action to Promote Sexual Health and Responsible Sexual Behavior. US Department of Health and Human Services. July 9, 2001.

46. **American Psychiatric Association**. Position statement: psychiatric treatment and sexual orientation. 1998. In: Just the Facts about Sexual Orientation & Youth: A Primer for Principals, Educators and School Personnel. American Psychological Association, et al; 1999: 3. The entire brochure can be viewed at the American Psychological Association Public Interest Directorate Online site: http://www.apa.org/pi/lgbc/publications/justthefacts.html

47. **American Academy of Pediatrics**. Policy statement: homosexuality and adolescence. 1993. In: Just the Facts About Sexual Orientation & Youth: A Primer for Principals, Educators and School Personnel. American Psychological Association, et al. 1999. Available at the American Psychological Association Public Interest Directorate Online site: http://www.apa.org/pi/lgbc/publications/justthefacts.html.

Chapter 4

Addressing LGBTQ Youth in the Clinical Setting

ROBERT GAROFALO, MD, MPH
STACI BUSH, PA-C

What Is Adolescence?

Adolescence is a time of change, growth, and maturation. It is recognized that young patients of this age have health and psychosocial needs requiring specific expertise by medical providers. During these tumultuous years, between the ages of 12 and 24, young people experience more than merely the physical phenomenon of puberty. Adolescents also acquire social, emotional, cognitive, and financial skills that enable them to emerge from this stage of life as autonomous adults capable of living independently. Managing the often simultaneous changes required during this transition can be especially difficult for some lesbian, gay, bisexual, transgender, and queer/questioning (LGBTQ)* youth who struggle with the widespread societal stigma associated with their emerging sexual minority identity.[1,2]

The hallmarks of adolescence are often the physical changes that accompany puberty. However, there is often a disconnect between the rapid physical development of puberty and the slower cognitive and social maturation that occur during adolescence. In many cases an adolescent may be inadequately equipped to handle situations which accompany emerging physical maturity due to developmental immaturity and childhood limitations of experience or naiveté. Youth may struggle with questions, concerns, and opinions about life in the midst of establishing their sexual and personal identities. Although LGBTQ youth face health and

---

* The term "queer," once considered pejorative, is included here because it has been reclaimed by some as a more general term denoting a broad spectrum of nonheterosexual identified people. Many of today's generation of sexual minority youth do not readily identify with traditional labels of sexual orientation (eg, lesbian or gay) and prefer "queer" as the label or terminology to describe their sexual identity.

developmental concerns common to the general adolescent population, unlike their heterosexual peers, they must also grapple with an extra layer of internal and external homophobia. Youth struggling with same-sex attraction or opposite gender identification may feel alienated from mainstream society and may clash head-on with social and familial norms. Therefore, it is the unique developmental challenge of LGBTQ youth to manage an often stigmatized identity within the constraints of a heterosexist family, society, and tradition.[2,3]

Economically and socially, adolescents are largely dependent on family and peers for support and guidance. Under these circumstances, LGBTQ youth may have limited sources of social support. They may have limited ability to contact, socialize, and communicate with individuals of similar experiences that are often unavailable in their day-to-day lives and communities.[4] As a result, some LGBTQ adolescents may feel isolated, marginalized, or alone. Such psychological and social stressors can negatively affect the health and well-being of any adolescent. When lacking peer-based or family-based opportunities for support or socialization, LGBTQ youth may seek friendship or companionship via the Internet or within the context of traditionally more adult social environments such as bars or night clubs. This can lead to potentially unhealthy behaviors such as substance use or risky sexual activity with older partners.[4] Although the vast majority of LGBTQ youth successfully navigate these inherent challenges, the unique stigma and stressors facing LGBTQ youth are undeniable and can be especially difficult when encountered in relation to family, peers, and communities of origin. Unfortunately, in too many cases, lack of acceptance, safety concerns, isolation, depression, homelessness, and antigay harassment and victimization are real-life concerns of LGBTQ youth, while other adolescents explore dating, education, and career paths largely without these additional stressors.

In order to provide the highest quality healthcare, one goal of the medical provider caring for LGBTQ youths or other youths struggling with emerging sexual identity issues is to assist the patient in making this developmental stage a time of healthy discovery, autonomy, and self-acceptance. This requires creating a welcoming clinical environment and asking nonjudgmental questions about sexuality and sexual identity as not all adolescents will describe themselves as openly LGBT or Q. It is therefore the job of the adolescent primary care provider to address concerns about sexual identity as well as social and psychological stressors that may accompany being a sexual minority with the same vigor as any physical ailment. One reason that adolescents at times create anxiety for pediatric and adult primary care providers is the complexity of their social and developmental needs and concerns that may be unfamiliar to either discipline. With all youth, including those who may be LGBTQ, the most prevalent threats to adolescent health are not typically physical complaints but are behavioral, emotional, or social issues (ie, depression, substance use, sexual activity, safety) that typically are addressed within the scope of an adolescent's medical visit. This is especially true of LGBTQ patients because the clinical setting may be the only environment in which a youth feels safe enough to seek assistance or guidance.

Why Adolescent Medicine?

Adolescents' access to care has always been influenced by the balance between patients' status as minors, their budding sexuality, and their need for confidential, culturally competent care. Traditionally, reproductive rights, access to contraception, and sexual health topped the list of topics related to adolescent medicine. In the 1960s the women's rights movement forced society to deal with young people's ability to consent to medical treatment and thereby increased their access to informed, confidential healthcare. For LGBTQ youth, the HIV epidemic to a large extent further highlighted the importance of access to culturally competent sexual healthcare for minors and adolescents. As a result, over the past few decades, adolescent medicine has become a widely accepted subspecialty of pediatrics, family practice, and internal medicine. By measuring healthcare providers' general discomfort with adolescent patients, we recognize that this is a unique population which may require a specialized clinical skill set generally neither taught nor offered by general pediatrics or adult primary care.

For example, adolescent patients often present for medical care with adult issues surrounding sex and sexuality. Even if that is not their primary concern, concerns about sexuality and/or sexual risk behaviors can be significant aspect of the adolescent medical visit. Unfortunately, many pediatric providers are uncomfortable having "adult" conversations about sexual activity or performing gynecological and rectal examinations on adolescent patients. Similarly, traditionally adult-oriented providers may not feel adequately equipped to address sexuality or the challenges inherent to the development of an LGBTQ identity in a patient they perceive as a child or adolescent. These issues can create barriers that prevent LGBTQ youth from receiving much-needed prevention education or comprehensive healthcare services despite the fact that statistics show that these youth disproportionately acquire HIV, smoke, attempt suicide, and participate in other high-risk behaviors, compared to heterosexual adolescents or LGBTQ adults.[1,2,4-6] As a result, adult and pediatric providers need specific training to become adept at covering issues such as sexuality and sexual activity with adolescents as part of routine care to guarantee that they are meeting the needs of their adolescent patients.

Goals When Treating the Adolescent Patient

Overall, the goals for LGBTQ healthcare are identical to those of any adolescent population: (1) to promote healthy development, (2) to promote social and emotional well-being, and (3) to promote and ensure physical health.[7] Thus, healthcare providers should view LGBTQ adolescents within the context of general adolescent development while maintaining a firm understanding of specific issues this population may face as a result of their sexual identity. This approach can be helpful in facilitating successful clinical encounters.

The Clinical Environment

Provider-Patient Relationship

The provider-patient relationship is pivotal to the LGBTQ youth's health maintenance and transition to healthy adulthood. A first medical visit often sets the tone for future access to care, risk reduction, help-seeking behavior, and, sometimes, adult physical and social health. While communication can be challenging, creating safe, open, and honest dialogue is the provider's primary objective with all adolescent patients, including those who may be LGBTQ. Obtaining a truthful history and making an adolescent feel comfortable within the clinical encounter are critical first steps in addressing a youth's comprehensive healthcare needs.

When clinicians deal with adolescents, in many ways the patient-provider relationship is a balancing act for both parties. The patient, caught between being a child and adulthood, is often uncomfortable discussing sensitive healthcare topics with parents or guardians in exam rooms or, conversely, accessing healthcare alone for the very first time. Youth seeing a clinician in the presence of their parents may have reasonable fears about secrecy or disclosure of their sexual orientation; this causes some to withhold information from healthcare providers until a level of trust and privacy is firmly established. For youth experiencing difficulties at home, this can be particularly distressing, and so providers need to interview adolescents without parents or others in the examination room. When accessing healthcare alone, LGBTQ youth may struggle with language and with initiating discussion with medical providers about potentially embarrassing topics such as sexual activity. They may be evasive when asked about their health, lives or their reason for the medical visit. Without the traditional buffer of having a parent or caregiver present, office procedures and exams may be uncomfortable or unfamiliar.

Ultimately, however, it is the provider who bears responsibility for carefully navigating the adolescent visit. It is important to remember that even at a very young age some LGBTQ adolescents engage in many risky behaviors that can negatively affect their health.[8] The provider serving the LGBTQ adolescent patient will need to deftly elicit a medical history while allowing the patient to feel both autonomous and comfortable during the visit. Comfort starts with making office space welcoming to LGBTQ youth with posters or flyers that are not exclusively heterosexual in nature. In addition, support staff need to be trained regarding issues that may be important to adolescent patients, such as privacy and autonomy. Once entrenched in the clinical encounter, it is then the provider, not the patient, who is charged with deciphering psychosocial assessments and healthcare needs and with constructing an appropriate plan. Providers offering comprehensive healthcare to LGBTQ youth not only need to meet youth-specific social and psychological needs but also need to manage acute and pressing medical issues to maintain health and reduce behavioral risk.

Confidentiality

As previously mentioned, confidentiality is a major concern in the LGBTQ adolescent visit. The adolescent's security regarding confidentiality sets the tone for the visit and their future access to care. Many adolescents report foregoing healthcare that they believed was necessary due in part to the fear of disclosure regarding access of care to parents.[9,10] In the LGBTQ adolescent, concerns regarding confidential care may be complicated by additional fears concerning either the advertent or inadvertent disclosure of their sexual orientation.[2] For example, even when the medical provider prioritizes patient confidentiality, other office staff or clinicians such as medical assistants, receptionists, or nursing staff can accidentally or purposefully disclose an LGBTQ youth's sexual orientation. Therefore, it is critically important that the entire medical setting be a safe and confidential environment as it may be the one place where LGBTQ youth feel safe disclosing not only health risk but also psychosocial stressors like coming out, relationship issues, peer pressure, or violence either at home or in school.

Providers need to familiarize themselves with individual state laws and the statutes which govern adolescents' right to access confidential healthcare services. In every state, statutes differ regarding consent and parental notification (see http://www.guttmacher.org/graphics/gr030406_f1.html for a summary by state); however, each allows minors to consent to treatment without parental consent under certain circumstance such as seeking family planning services, treatment for sexually transmitted infections or HIV, or emergency care. The parameters surrounding confidential healthcare services, including the exceptions to confidentiality, should be reviewed with the adolescent patient on the first visit and then regularly thereafter. It is important that whenever possible parents or guardians also be made aware of the parameters and importance of confidential care. For LGBTQ youth, confidentiality is often a major concern regarding the adolescent medical visit.[2] Neither concerns about an emerging sexual minority identity nor concerns about other sensitive topics (eg, sexual risk behaviors, substance use, depression, safety, etc) will likely be discussed openly and honestly during the medical visit without assurances regarding confidential care allowable under state law.

Access to Care

Adolescent-oriented behavioral and physical healthcare are often difficult to find and navigate. This is not unique to LGBTQ youth, but it is a major problem for many adolescents, particularly those over age 18—too old for state or federally funded health insurance programs but not yet qualified for employer-based coverage. However, for the LGBTQ adolescent, culturally competent care may seem entirely elusive. Barriers created by pervasive societal stigma, secrecy surrounding their sexual orientation or gender identity, and a lack of knowledge about where to find LGBTQ-friendly providers make access to care even more challenging for this population.[1,2] Offering comprehensive care to LGBTQ youth means establishing resources that are readily available and barrier-free. For example, LGBTQ adolescents may not be willing to use their healthcare insurance to access needed services out of concern that their sexual identities will be inappropriately disclosed to parents, guardians, or friends. When they desire confidential care, "closeted" LGBTQ youth may only be able to seek healthcare services in public health clinics, facilities catering to the uninsured, or other medical settings where they may more easily keep their anonymity.[4] Disproportionate socioeconomic factors, such as unemployment, homelessness, and lack of transportation, are also huge additional challenges for some young LGBTQ patients. For these youth, social and financial support, like case management, bus tokens, and support groups, may help promote and facilitate access to care.

The Office Visit

Chief Complaint

The chief medical complaint is frequently not the primary cause for the adolescent visit. A healthy adolescent seldom has reason for a "physical," but they trust that the questioning of an astute clinician may ultimately lead to a discussion of their true concern. Sometimes, however, the medical visit is prompted by symptoms the patient considers related to a sexually transmitted infection (STI) or to anxiety following an anonymous or otherwise high-risk sexual encounter. These represent opportunities for both medical care and significant education regarding sexual risk behaviors and family planning. In the adolescent population, even the most benign chief complaints can sometimes evolve into more complicated discussions offering the provider an opportunity for further investigation into potential areas of concern. Whether the chief complaint is acne or cold symptoms, the primary care provider should always add, "Do you have any other problems, have any questions, or want anything else checked out while you're here?"

Conducting the Patient Interview

With an adolescent, the patient interview is the most vital element of the office visit. A thorough, guided history provides more information than a youth would often give voluntarily. It fills in the chief complaint while introducing other areas of potential concern that may warrant attention or intervention. With adolescents a thorough history is not one-sided but is a dialogue of exchange that not only elicits information but also helps establish rapport between provider and patient. During the taking of a history, LGBTQ youth begin to understand what topics are relevant and important for present and future visits. Sensitive topics need to be addressed carefully and unapologetically with language easily understood by the adolescent. The goal of the medical history is not to identify all gay and lesbian youth, but rather to create an environment in which the LGBTQ adolescent is comfortable asking questions, may seek help or support, and obtain appropriate medical services as needed. In general, providers should avoid making assumptions about a patient's self-identification or the extent to which LGBTQ youth have disclosed their sexual orientation to friends or family. Providers need to allow youth opportunities for self-definition and rely on those definitions when addressing clinical issues. Terms used for self-identification may vary across racial or ethnic, gender, and socioeconomic groups. For example, some young men from communities of color or other cultures may identify as publicly "heterosexual" but engage in same-sex behavior with other men.[4] Youth from these communities may not feel comfortable disclosing their sexual identity to healthcare providers until they have fully integrated and accepted it themselves.

Although adolescents tend to be physically healthy, risk reduction regarding social and behavioral health threats is often the cornerstone of the adolescent visit. Before risk reduction can be either achieved or even attempted, providers caring for LGBTQ adolescents ought to thoughtfully and caringly assess and screen for the leading health risks of this population of youth. This is done primarily through the *social history*. As with all adolescents, social history-taking from LGBTQ youth can be guided by the acronym *HEADS*: *H*-home; *E*-education; *A*-activities; *D*-depression/drugs/ diet; *S*-safety/sexuality. Providers should be cognizant not only of social issues which arise in general adolescent populations but also be capable of addressing issues and health threats more unique to the LGBTQ experience (see Table 4-1).

Below are aspects of the social history and clinical issues that may be identified during the patient interview. Many of these issues are covered in

Table 4-1   Top Health Risks of LGBTQ Adolescents

HIV/AIDS	Stigma and Heterosexualism
Substance Abuse	Racism
Depression and Suicide	Eating Disorders and Obesity
Sexually Transmitted Infections (STIs)	Homelessness
Abuse and Victimization	Access to Care

greater detail elsewhere in this book. We focus our discussion on issues specific to the adolescent experience and offer guidance about a clinical approach to the LGBTQ adolescent patient. See Table 4-2 for examples of questions to use during the interview.

1. Sexual History and Sexual Activity

Sexual concerns or questions regarding sexuality are often a leading cause of adolescent visits to nonurgent primary care. Providers caring for adolescents need to be comfortable with the fact that experimentation with a variety of sexual behaviors and sexual partners may be part of healthy identity formation.[2] For the LGBTQ adolescent, issues and concerns regarding sexuality can be hidden behind fears of disclosure or fears of embarrassment or shame regarding engagement in same-sex sexual activity. In the LGBTQ adolescent, fluidity of sexual expression (particularly in young transgender

Table 4-2 Adolescent Patient Interview: Sample Questions

I. Sexual Activity

- Have you ever dated or gone out with someone? Are you currently dating or in a relationship with a boy or a girl?
- Do you have sex with men (boys), women (girls), or both?
- Some of my patients your age begin to find themselves attracted to other people. Have you ever been romantically or sexually attracted to men (boys), women (girls), or both?
- There are many ways of being sexual or intimate with another person: kissing, hugging, touching, having oral sex, anal sex, or vaginal sex. Have you ever had any of these experiences? Which ones? Were they with boys, girls, or both?
- How do you protect yourself against sexually transmitted diseases and pregnancy?
- When you use condoms for anal (or vaginal) sex, do you use them 5%, 50%, 75%, or 100% of the time? Are there times that you don't use condoms when you are having sex?
- Do you have sex (oral, anal or vaginal) with anyone other than your boyfriend or girlfriend? If so, how often are you using condoms in those situations?
- Has anyone ever pressured you or forced you into doing something sexually that you didn't want to do?

Table 4-2 Adolescent Patient Interview: Sample Questions (continued)

II. Sexual Identity and Disclosure

- What term (if any) do you prefer that I use to best describe your sexual orientation? For example, do you consider yourself gay, lesbian, bisexual, heterosexual (straight), or are you not sure?
- Have you ever talked to your parents, brothers or sisters, or any other adult besides me about this? Any of your friends? What did they say?
- Have you thought about disclosing your sexuality to your parents or friends? Are you concerned at all about their response or your safety?
- Was "coming out" stressful? Or, do you get stressed out thinking about "coming out?"
- It is normal for young people to sometimes be confused about their feelings and experiences. Do you have any questions you'd like to ask me or things you would like to talk about?

III. Mental Health and Depression

- Over the past few weeks, have you ever felt down or depressed? Have you had less interest in doing things that you normally enjoy?
- Have you ever thought about hurting yourself? Have you ever actually tried to hurt yourself? What did you do? What happened?
- Have you ever been treated for depression or other psychological issues? Have you ever been in the hospital for these issues or for trying to hurt yourself?
- Who do you turn to when you are down, lonely, or need someone to talk to?
- Do you have a close friend or family member who is a good source of support?
- Have you ever thought about seeing a counselor or therapist? Do you think that might be helpful?

IV. Tobacco, Alcohol, and Other Substance Use

- Do you currently smoke cigarettes? How much and for how long? Have you ever tried quitting? Do you need or want help quitting?
- Do you drink alcohol? How often? Where do you get it, and who do you drink with? How many drinks do you typically have? Do you ever get drunk?
- Have you ever used any other drugs such as marijuana, cocaine, ecstasy, GHB, crystal meth, etc? Which drugs do you currently use? How often?
- Do you think your alcohol or drug use is a problem? Would you like help in trying to quit?
- Do you have any questions about any drugs or drug use that I might be able to answer?
- Do you ever have sex while drunk or high? Have you ever done something sexually while high or drunk that you regretted or didn't really want to?
- Have you ever driven a car or motor vehicle while high or drunk? Have you ever gotten a ride from someone else who was high or drunk?

V. Safety and Violence

- How are things going at home or at school? Do you feel safe when you are at home? Do you feel safe in your neighborhood and at school?
- Has anyone ever picked on you? Can you tell me about it? Was this because you are LGBTQ?
- Who can you turn to for advice, support, or protection?

persons and young lesbian or bisexual women) and ever-evolving personal identification make sexual history-taking especially challenging and all the more important to do effectively.

When approaching the sexual history of an LGBTQ adolescent, asking straightforward questions such as, "Are you dating?" or, "Do you have sex with men (boys), women (girls), or both?" is an excellent way to initiate the discussion. Depending on the response, you may also wish to ask specifically, "Are you romantically or sexually attracted to men (boys), women (girls), or both?" as some LGBTQ-identified youth may not yet have initiated sexual activity but may welcome the opportunity to discuss their sexuality or questions related to sexual activity if given an appropriate opportunity. Providers need to be cautious when using the often asked question, "Are you sexually active?" For the adolescent, this question may be open to multiple interpretations with regard to time frame or the precise definition of sexual activity determined by the patient. A confused adolescent may inadvertently give inaccurate information to the medical provider resulting in missed opportunities for relationship-building or prevention education. For adolescent patients answering this question in the negative, follow-up questions regarding romantic attraction or more specific questions regarding sexual activity are warranted to ensure that providers are not missing these opportunities for health promotion and education.

Providers *should be careful not to make assumptions* regarding the sexual orientation, sexual activity, or sexual expression of adolescent patients. Providers may wish to ask, "Do you consider yourself gay, lesbian, bisexual, heterosexual (straight), or are you not sure?" With LGBTQ youth, operating from the premise or assumption that all young people are at risk of pregnancy or STIs can alienate some youth from healthcare and health education. Conversely, viewing youth as nonsexual because of their young age or presentation can be equally dangerous. Appropriate, unbiased, and non-judgmental questions regarding sexual activity or the need for family planning education or services are an important part of *every* adolescent clinical encounter. LGBTQ adolescents can be traumatized by providers' assumptions that bring about invasive, irrelevant, or incorrect examinations or procedures. Although some young gay men are at increased risk of acquiring sexually transmitted infections (STIs) and HIV and some young lesbian and bisexual women are at increased risk of pregnancy, it is important for providers to remember that not all LGBTQ youth are sexually active. Many may abstain from sex altogether. To assume otherwise can at times be off-putting or offensive to some youth.

Defining sexual risk for the LGBTQ adolescent patient can be in and of itself challenging for the provider. Oral sex, petting, or masturbation offer vastly different risks for the acquisition of STIs, but to youth, each may fall under the category of "not really" sex at all. Even anal sex, particularly for some young women, may not be considered "being sexually active" since it does not carry the risk of pregnancy that is often the main clinical concern.

Providers need to ask specific questions about each of these activities to get an accurate picture of the sexual risk behavior profile of each LGBTQ adolescent patient. Education and risk regarding anal and pharyngeal STIs are to be reviewed with men and women alike. Providers should use anatomically specific terminology, avoid medical jargon, and ask questions and deliver information in language easily understood by the adolescent. This is of the utmost importance when dealing with younger LGBTQ adolescent patients.

Health protective behaviors (eg, consistency of condom use), age of sexual debut, and history of sexual trauma (at any age) are important lines of questioning. With regards to condom use, providers should avoid yes or no formatted questions such as, "Do you use condoms for sexual activity?" but rather more informative, open ended questions such as, "When you use condoms for anal (or vaginal) intercourse, do you use condoms 5%, 50%, 75%, or 100% of the time?" A reporting less than 100% condom use gives providers an opportunity for more specific lines of questioning regarding the social context of inconsistent condom use. This information may assist in providing more targeted prevention education. Regarding sexual trauma, the tragic reality is that sexual abuse, incest, and rape may expose adolescents to STIs and HIV, without consent, at an early (or any) age. A history of sexual trauma is seldom identified without specific questions in this area. Adolescents with a history of sexual trauma may not report these experiences under traditional questioning of sexual activity because the abuse was neither consensual nor initiated by the patient, and therefore they do not perceive themselves as being "sexually active." Unfortunately, however, the risk of infection or pregnancy may still be present, which highlights the need for specific questioning. Youth experiencing sexual trauma may present with other confounding symptoms (eg, depression, cutting behavior, etc) and need additional support. Some research has suggested that rates of childhood sexual abuse may be higher in LGBTQ youth populations and has linked these experiences to future negative health outcomes such as high-risk sexual behaviors, substance use, or psychological distress.[11,12]

The acknowledgement of partnerships and same-sex loving relationships can also help to establish an open line of communication between the LGBTQ adolescent and the medical provider. When asking about dating, romantic, or sexual partners, providers should use gender-neutral language (eg, avoid using terms like boyfriend or girlfriend) unless instructed otherwise by the adolescent patient. This sends a subtle but important message to the LGBTQ adolescent that the provider is open to discussing same-sex relationships or concerns. This may help facilitate disclosure of same-sex feelings or behaviors when the adolescent is comfortable doing so. If a same-sex relationship is identified, acknowledgement of this may be important when the adolescent considers future healthcare options. Acknowledgement and acceptance of different sexual expressions and relationships can assist the LGBTQ youth in communicating freely with medical providers and thereby facilitate both medical history-taking and overall healthcare delivery.

The fluidity of sexual expression in the young LGBTQ population can further challenge sexual history-taking and discussions regarding sexual activity as today's youth may not identify with a binary or finite model of sexual identity. Reclaiming of the term "queer" as an affirmative and often preferred term of self-identification among some youth is a perfect example of the fluidity of sexual expression and of how this generation of youth are to a large extent dissatisfied with traditional labels of sexual orientation and sexual expression. This may make providers uncomfortable, particularly those used to thinking of "queer" as a pejorative term. Whether self-identified as gay, lesbian, or queer, it is not uncommon for a young person to have concerns about their "girlfriend" on one visit but then change this to "boyfriend" on a subsequent visit. They may either have started dating a partner of a different gender, or they may simply have become more comfortable disclosing the true gender of their partner to a trusted provider. Or, as in the case of some transgender youth, where gender differs from biologically defined sex, they or their partner may have changed their own gender identity. Overall, with the adolescent patient, nonbinary models of sexual orientation and gender identity are common, and labels are often difficult to characterize. Whether or not youth classify themselves as LGBTQ, careful and thorough history-taking, particularly with regards to the sex and gender of partners, types of sexual activity, and consistency of safe sexual activity will give the provider the necessary information they need to provide accurate and helpful preventive health education and medical advice.

Although discussions of sexual activity among LGBTQ youth are often directed toward young gay and bisexual men or transgender youth because of their disproportionate risk for acquiring HIV or other STIs, specific mention should be made of how to address sexual health issues of young lesbian and bisexual women. When young women have sex with women (WSW) or self-identify as lesbian, gay, or bisexual, their sexual behavior and identity, like other developmental constructs in adolescence, may be permanent, nonexclusive, or fluid. In all cases, when obtaining a thorough risk assessment, it is best to ask, "Have you only had sex with women, or have you ever had sex with a man? If so, when was the last time?" While lesbian and bisexual young women are often perceived as a "low risk" group, in reality adolescent WSW can be at risk for certain STIs and may engage in risky sex with male partners. In one recent study of adolescent WSWs age 16-24 in Chicago, 58% had previously had oral sex with a male partner (41% in the past year), 20% had previously been pregnant, and 26% had receptive anal intercourse with a male partner.[13] Young lesbian and bisexual women, like other adolescents, are more likely to report high-risk sexual behaviors under the influence of drugs or alcohol.[13] When caring for a young lesbian or bisexual woman, it is therefore important to take a comprehensive substance use and sexual history and to counsel about health risk, including the need for routine gynecological care as appropriate. It is also important to ask about sexual or romantic desire or attraction and to keep in mind that definitions of sexual activity may vary. See Chapters 11 and 15 for more on sexual health and taking a sexual history.

2. Psychological History and Mental Health

LGBTQ youth experience the same range of mental health concerns as all adolescents, with additional distress at times created by the need to manage stigma associated with their sexual minority identity.[2,14] Adolescence is a time when mental heath issues including depression, anxiety, psychosis, and bipolar symptoms surface. Mental health needs identified in adolescence may present in atypical ways and can either be chronic or episodic. In the case of depression, vulnerabilities and external stressors unique to adolescence or the LGBTQ adolescent experience may trigger a major or episodic depressive episode. For example, "coming out" or beginning to experiment with same-sex sexual partners can be distressing for LGBTQ youth, causing internal psychological conflict or direct or perceived conflict with family and peers.[6] (See Chapter 3 for more on the process of coming out.) In addition, life changes and transitions that by and large define adolescence are often major psychological stressors, including transition to independent living, adjusting to a new school or peer group, entering college, or finding employment. These often happen in quick succession or even simultaneously, adding to the stress experienced by some LGBTQ youth. In general, life problems that may seem minor to some adults, such as breaking up with a boyfriend or girlfriend or unhappiness with physical appearance caused by acne or obesity, can be major triggers in youth.

Suicide is a particular psychological and social concern for LGBTQ youth. It is a leading cause of death among US adolescents and has been postulated as the leading cause of death among LGBTQ youth. Much has been written about suicide risk in LGBTQ youth, and, although the data consistently supports the notion of "increased suicide risk" in this population of youth, it must be interpreted with caution.[15-17] In a Massachusetts study, lesbian, gay, and bisexual youth were more than 3 times more likely to self-report "a suicide attempt in the past 12 months" compared with their heterosexual peers.[8,15] However, the precise clinical meaning of the self-reported term "suicide attempt" is unclear when considered within the context of the broad continuum from suicidal thoughts, feelings, or behaviors including actual attempts and completions. The reality is that little is known about the actual number of youth suicides either related to distress over sexual orientation or among LGBTQ youth as data collected from death certificates and psychological autopsies cannot possibly accurately address sexual orientation issues. Many LGBTQ youth who consider or attempt suicide may not have previously discussed their sexual orientation or identity with anyone because of fear and anxiety surrounding disclosure. Providers caring for this population of youth frequently question alarming statistics frequently cited regarding LGBTQ youth suicide (eg, gay youth represent 30% of all teen suicides) that are not consistent with clinical experiences.[7,17] It remains likely, however that far too many LGBTQ youth consider or even attempt suicide in part related to stressors, isolation, or stigma surrounding their emerging sexual identities. In fact, in all adolescents, suicide risk is likely associated with a common set of predisposing influences, including family dysfunction, depression, isolation, loss of family or friends, and alcohol and other substance use—issues that may be exacerbated in LGBTQ youth, particularly those youth who lack appropriate social support.[2,15,18,19] Data shows that distressed patients frequently visit their primary care providers in the days, weeks, or months preceding the successful suicide, highlighting the importance of conducting a thorough psychological assessment in the primary care setting.[20] This will allow providers an opportunity for early intervention when needed.

One of the ways to assess LGBTQ youth psychological health and well-being is to ask about behavioral health history, psychological medication history, and history of hospitalization for issues such as clinical depression or suicidal ideation. This should be done in person, although some clinicians may use questionnaires or patient-administered self-assessment tools as adjuncts to the provider interview. It is also important to ascertain whether there is a family history of mental illness in the initial history since depression, bipolar disease, and psychosis can all have a hereditary component and may first manifest in adolescence. Taking a family history of mental illness may need to be done initially with a parent or guardian in the examination room as many adolescent patients may not be aware of these issues. Providers caring for LGBTQ youth may also wish to use general screening questions for depression such as, "Over the past two weeks have you felt down, depressed, hopeless?" or "Over the past two weeks, have you felt little interest or pleasure in doing things?" An affirmative Answer to either or both questions may warrant further assessment or intervention. Asking about available sources of support with questions such as, "Who do you turn to when you feel sad or need someone to talk to?" may help identify LGBTQ youth who are marginalized from family or peers or that feel particularly isolated or alone. In addition, specific questions regarding comfort level with their sexual minority identity or inquiries into how things are going at school, at home, or with peers may help further identify youth in need of referral to community-based support groups for LGBTQ youth (if and when available) or those in need of additional mental health support services.

3. Tobacco, Alcohol, and Other Substance Use

Alcohol and tobacco companies aggressively market products to the gay and lesbian community; youth are especially vulnerable to these efforts.[21]

With regard to tobacco, the *American Medical Association Healthy Youth 2010 Directive* states that smoking, often initiated during the adolescent years, is the single most preventable risk factor for the leading causes of death in the United States—heart disease and cancer.[22] As many as 50% of LGBTQ youth smoke cigarettes.[21] Some may report initially smoking primarily in social settings and with friends. All too frequently, LGBTQ youth who describe themselves as "social smokers" find themselves smoking on a more regular, if not daily, basis. As a result, many youth report trying but being unable to quit due to the well-documented addictive nature of nicotine. Providers caring for LGBTQ youth need to inquire about current and past smoking behavior and should be prepared to offer adolescents assistance in quitting when desired. This may include providing access to nicotine replacement medications or assisting youth in finding culturally appropriate behavioral options such as smoking cessation support groups if and when available (see Appendix A for resources).

Experimentation with tobacco, alcohol, or drugs can often be part of normal adolescent development. However, some adolescents use drugs or alcohol to self-medicate underlying depression or to relieve the pain associated with loneliness or isolation. LGBTQ adolescents are no exception to being affected by these issues. In fact, for some LGBTQ youth, this psychological distress is compounded by having few options for safe, social interaction with peers.[4] In response, LGBTQ youth may frequent bars, clubs, or other social settings that normalize the use of illicit substances or where alcohol use is ever-present. Alcohol and illicit drug use among all adolescents, including those who may be L, G, B, T, or Q, are linked to other destructive behaviors and negative outcomes including high-risk sexual behaviors, suicide attempts, or motor vehicle accidents.[23,24]

Although marijuana is the most commonly used illicit drug among adolescents, it is "club drugs" that are taking hold of the LGBTQ youth community—particularly young gay and bisexual men. Club drugs such as ecstasy, methamphetamine, gamma hydroxy butyrate (GHB), or ketamine are used by adolescents to create a sense of euphoria, social disinhibition, or heightened sexuality. There is often a perceived link between club drugs, social desirability, and popularity, resulting in limited stigma surrounding their use in some LGBTQ youth circles. Most club drugs such as ecstasy and GHB are used episodically, either alone or in combination, within specific social environments (eg, clubs, dances, or circuit parties). Others, however, such as methamphetamine can be extremely physically addictive and lead to frequent if not daily use. Methamphetamine in particular has been strongly linked to high-risk sex in young gay and bisexual men where the substance has emerged as a major risk factor for the acquisition of HIV or other STIs.[25,26] For more on substance use, see Chapter 9.

Providers assessing LGBTQ youths' use of alcohol and illicit drugs should ask specific and directed questions in a nonjudgmental and unbiased manner. As much as possible, healthcare providers need to familiarize themselves with commonly used "street terms" for various drugs but should never be afraid to ask the adolescent patient for clarification if an unknown term or substance is mentioned during the provider interview. This is an excellent opportunity to demonstrate responsiveness to the adolescent and may open up avenues for active communication and patient education. For many LGBTQ youth who use drugs or abuse alcohol, the private and confidential confines of the clinical exam room may be the only setting in which they disclose their behavior or express concerns about dependence or abuse. LGBTQ youth may ask questions regarding potential deleterious effects of alcohol or marijuana use or those associated with various club drugs such as hallucinations, seizures, hyperthermia, depression, erectile dysfunction, irritability, etc.[27] Information regarding deleterious effects of alcohol and drug use and prevention education should be delivered in a firm, knowledgeable, but nonalarmist manner, allowing youth the clear opportunity to continue the dialogue with the provider in future clinical encounters. Education should be broadbased, promoting both abstinence and harm reduction. Harm reduction strategies acknowledge that for many LGBTQ youth drug and/or alcohol use is not likely to stop at the present time. Harm reduction emphasizes personal safety (ie, consistent condom use, not driving under the influence, etc) as well as the avoidance of peer pressure that may contribute to substance use among adolescents.

4. Safety, Violence, and Victimization

Violence is a leading cause of morbidity and mortality among US adolescents, and personal safety is often a primal concern of many LGBTQ youth.[28,29] An alarming number of sexual minority youth experience violence related to their sexual orientation.[28] Safety threats can range from verbal taunts to physical or sexual harassment. Transgender youth in particular are at extreme risk for violence since, unlike sexual orientation, a transgender identity is difficult to keep hidden. Numerous studies demonstrate deleterious psychological and psychosocial effects (ie, anxiety, substance use, depression, lower self-esteem) resulting from the "antigay" harassment and violence experienced by some LGBTQ youth.[28-30] For this population of youth, violence and other threats to safety can occur within schools or within homes of origin. The perpetrators of the violence can be a range of individuals, many of whom are typically viewed as protectors of children and adolescents (eg, parents, teachers, employers, police officers, coaches).[4] Feeling unsafe can be the direct result of acts of violence resulting from a youth's presumed sexual orientation. Or it can be more subtle, such as feeling or being "different" than other youth or being alienated or unsupported from parents, family members, or peers. Being the victim of antigay violence at home or at school is profoundly difficult for LGBTQ youth to grapple with since these environments should be universally safe and nurturing. Familial or school violence may leave LGBTQ youth feeling unsure of who to turn to for advice, guidance, support, or protection.

Under these circumstances, an astute provider can be of extreme assistance. After the clinician has established rapport with an adolescent patient, including defining the parameters of the confidential clinical encounter, some LGBTQ youth may disclose concerns about their physical, emotional, or sexual safety. The healthcare provider should ask, "How are things going at home or at school?" Open-ended questions in these sensitive areas more likely yield meaningful responses, as opposed to questions offering simple yes or no response options. Providers may need to ask specifically about "being picked on by siblings, parents, or peers" or "feeling safe" within settings such as home, neighborhoods, or school. Picking up on unspoken body language can augment the oral provider history as LGBTQ youth who have experienced antigay trauma may be reticent to discuss these issues with a medical provider if a strong clinical relationship has not been previously established. It is important that adolescents know the precise legal limits of the confidentiality of the clinical encounter before beginning to answer questions regarding safety. This allows the LGBTQ adolescent to be in control of the information they provide during the patient interview. Inadvertent disclosure of abuse or violence may trigger mandatory reporting obligations on the part of the healthcare provider which the LGBTQ adolescent may not see as in their best interest. LGBTQ youth may also use the clinical setting to discuss fears or safety concerns regarding potential ramifications of self-disclosing their sexual orientation to parents or family members. LGBTQ may realistically fear expulsion from their homes if their parents or guardians become aware of their sexual orientation and may lack appropriate social support do deal with these stresses.[2] As such, LGBTQ youth are the best judges of how their parents or families may react. Providers need to use extreme caution in offering specific advice, instructions, or guidance which may be construed as encouraging "coming out." Deciding to come out is a highly personal and often frightening decision for LGBTQ youth.[2] It is not the role of the healthcare provider to give specific advice or instructions regarding timing of the coming out process. Rather, providers should offer general support, make referrals for community assistance when needed, and ensure that they are available if needed for future advice or assistance (see Appendix A for resources).

Understanding Growth and Development

There are three primary stages of adolescent growth and development. Each brings about its own physical and emotional changes and challenges. When applying these changes to the LGBTQ teen, the resulting questions and concerns are often framed within the context of gender, sexuality, and physical development. For the gay male, lesbian woman, and transgender youth, the challenges of each developmental stage may differ.

Early Adolescence: Ages 10-14

Early adolescence typically involves preoccupation and insecurity with rapid bodily changes. Peers begin to influence interests and clothing styles more than parents or guardians. Sexual curiosity may lead to the initiation of sexual experimentation with masturbation or even early sexual activity with same-gender or opposite-gender partners. LGBTQ youth, similar to other adolescents, may ask themselves, "Am I normal?" in response to early adolescence and pubertal initiation. During this stage, LGBTQ adolescents may begin to see themselves as "different" but not yet fully understand their emerging identity. For boys who are gender atypical, this may be a period of heightened psychological turmoil as they may be ridiculed or harassed by peers. Secondary sexual characteristics appear in early adolescence and, with it, accentuated gender differentiation. Young girls, particularly those who are athletic, may be somewhat uncomfortable with breast development. Some transgender youth may similarly resent or become distressed by the onset of secondary sexual characteristics which are dissonant with their gender identity. For female-to-male transgender youth, the onset of menstruation, which typically occurs during this time, may be a specific source of significant psychological unrest. Providers need to be on the look out for signs of physical self-manipulation (eg, binding, cutting) or evolving emotional distress in response to otherwise normal physical changes.

Middle Adolescence: Ages 14-17

Middle adolescents complete the physical changes of puberty and begin to have more romantic relationships typically characterized as dating or serial monogamy. They begin to distance themselves from parents and place a strong emphasis on peers. LGBTQ youth experience the same physical changes as their heterosexual peers. These warrant open discussions about normal breast development in young women and increased testicular and penile size in males. While middle adolescents often engage in risk-taking behaviors such as substance use and sexual activity, they may not yet fully appreciate the consequences of their actions. This may lead to heightened risk for HIV and STIs among sexually active middle adolescents. Providers should carefully assess sexual and substance abuse risk during these years, promoting abstinence when appropriate and offering specific health education regarding safer sexual practices. Some LGBTQ youth may disclose their sexual orientation, or consider doing so, to family or friends during this time period. This can be an obvious source of distress for many youth and their families, requiring a considerable degree of clinical support. LGBTQ youth may also have difficulty initiating romantic or sexual relationships with same-sex peers as opportunities for this type of interaction may be limited or nonexistent. Therefore some of the important milestones of middle adolescence may be delayed in this population, which can be both frustrating and upsetting to some LGBTQ youth.

Late Adolescence: Age 17 and up

With the physical changes of puberty by and large completed, late adolescents begin to have a more mature view of themselves and their sexuality. Late adolescents typically begin to prioritize romantic relationships where communication, intimacy, and support have a greater role than sexual behaviors. The delay in social maturity and lack of experience with typical dating experiences may challenge LGBTQ youth during this developmental stage. Some LGBTQ youth will be sexually active but may not have yet had opportunities for developing intimate and supportive relationships. Many adolescents will transition out of their homes and begin to live independently. Newly acquired independence can empower some youth to disclose their sexual orientation to others, which again may result in the need for clinical or emotional support. It is during this time that many LGBTQ adolescents will schedule their first independent medical appointment. It is therefore up to the healthcare provider to establish a safe and nurturing clinical environment for an often recently independent young person as well as address medical and psychosocial concerns and educate about risk reduction as appropriate.

Conducting a Physical Examination and Diagnostic Evaluation

Primary healthcare services for LGBTQ adolescents should generally follow the American Medical Association Guidelines for Adolescent Preventive Services (GAPS), including annual visits and healthcare screenings.[31] These annual visits include a comprehensive physical exam and appropriate screening for a variety of previously described health issues including sexually transmitted infections (STIs), substance abuse, mental health concerns, nutrition, etc. Screening for HIV and other STIs needs to be guided by the adolescent's sexual behavior, not orientation, and should be done whenever appropriate or indicated. For sexually active LGBTQ youth, HIV and STI screening should occur at least once per year. Cervical cytology or Pap smears should be performed in young lesbian and bisexual women at the same intervals as other young women. Providers need to be aware that young lesbian and bisexual women often delay seeking care in this area, making patient education regarding the need for routine gynecological exams of the utmost importance.[2] With regard to immunizations, all young gay and bisexual men should be vaccinated for both hepatitis A and B, given their increased risk for these diseases. Young women should be

offered the human papillomavirus (HPV) vaccine for cervical cancer prophylaxis even if they only report being sexually active with other women.
To provide prophylaxis against the development of anal warts or the development of anal cancer, the HPV vaccine may also be considered in young
gay and bisexual men, although immunological data supporting the administration of the vaccine in young men is currently not available.

For transgender individuals, the physical examination can be an unset-
tling experience. Transgender youth may be extremely uncomfortable
exposing their genitalia as part of the routine clinical encounter. This discomfort is most pronounced with the gynecological examination of female-
to-male (FTM) transgender youth. Providers should proceed slowly and use
caution when doing either an external or internal genitourinary examination. In the absence of symptoms or other clinical indications that make a
genitourinary examination important, providers may wish to defer this
aspect of the physical exam to a future visit to allow for a stronger clinical
relationship to be established.

Areas of Special Concern

HIV

No one issue threatens the well-being of young gay and bisexual men or
other young men who have sex with other men (MSM) more than HIV.
Although addressed elsewhere in this book, HIV is a major health risk for
the LGBTQ adolescent population and deserves brief mention in this chapter. One-half of all newly diagnosed HIV infections occur in persons under
25 years of age, making HIV increasingly a disease affecting adolescents
and young adults.[32] Young gay and bisexual men, particularly from communities of color, are disproportionately affected by HIV, with approximately 60% of new infections in men resulting from same-sex sexual
activity between males.[33] Male-to-female transgender youth also appear to
be at particularly high risk for HIV primarily acquired through risky sexual
behavior.[34] Despite continuing educational efforts, young MSM continue to
engage in high-risk sexual behaviors, often under the influence of alcohol
or other drugs such as methamphetamine. Whether it is fatigue from being
attentive to the known risks of HIV, lack of perceived risk due to adolescent beliefs of invulnerability, or reduced fear created by the success of
new and improved HIV medical treatments, success in achieving behavioral
change from public health campaigns promoting safer sex decades ago
now appears to be waning.[4] Use of the Internet for seeking and meeting
romantic and sexual partners, socialization in adult environments such as
bars and clubs, or sexual activity with older partners further accentuate the
increased HIV risk of young MSM.[35] Targeted, broad-based HIV prevention
efforts tailored to the unique mechanisms of HIV risk of young MSM need
to be implemented—particularly in communities of color.

The management of the HIV-infected adolescent highlights the need for healthcare delivery that is sensitive to the needs of young people. Providers caring for HIV-infected youth often need to be extremely flexible with their schedules, an often difficult task in more traditional adult-oriented health-care environments. In addition, issues such as confidentiality, lack of insurance, secrecy, shame, and stigma are enormous issues for the HIV-infected youth that can compromise clinical care. HIV education is often a time-consuming process for these patients, but it is an element of primary care that is critically necessary to maintain optimum future health. While a medical provider may wish to discuss T-cells, viral load, or other HIV-specific medical issues, many HIV-infected adolescents prefer to focus on bread-and-butter adolescent primary care issues including management of acne or seeking assistance with complex social issues such as family conflict, dating concerns, or continued engagement in high-risk sexual activity. Many face challenges to disclosing their diagnosis to others, particularly parents, family members, and romantic or sexual partners. For youth who have not disclosed either their HIV-infected status or their sexual identities, these issues seem inextricably linked. For youth financially dependent and reliant on parents or family for support, this can be an overwhelming concern. As a result, some HIV-infected youth forgo recommended medical treatment (eg, highly active antiretroviral therapy) for fear that medications will be discovered at home or at school. Others, such as youth who are homeless, may not have a safe or reliable place to store their medications. As a result, some young HIV-infected MSM may simply decide to not follow up with medical care visits at all. Adolescent HIV providers must not only be astute in the management of HIV-related disease but be adept at managing the entire range of adolescent healthcare and social concerns. Being a skilled HIV primary care provider is often not enough when dealing with the complex medical and social issues of some HIV-infected adolescents.

Homelessness

Of the estimated two million homeless adolescents living on the streets, up to 40% are estimated to be LGBTQ.[2,36,37] Conflict with parents over adolescents' sexual orientation is a major reason why the majority of LGBTQ youth find themselves living on the streets.[2,36,38] Some LGBTQ youth are asked or forced to leave their homes when parents or guardians discover or suspect a sexual minority identity.[2] Disclosure can occur directly (eg, "coming out") or inadvertently when parents discover gay or lesbian erotica, overhear phone conversations, or witness same-sex physical or sexual contact. For others, leaving home is a voluntary decision or means of escaping a volatile home situation such as verbal or physical antigay harassment or parental attempts to convince adolescents to undergo psychological counseling or reparative therapy to "become heterosexual."

Once on the streets, LGBTQ youths typically find that employment, housing, and support are temporary, precarious, or both. Lacking a means of financial independence or stability leaves them vulnerable to numerous health risks. Unable to obtain legitimate or stable employment, some homeless LGBTQ youth trade sexual activity for food, money, drugs, or shelter.[39,40] Substance use and exposure to violence or victimization further complicate the lives of many homeless youth, including those who may be LGBTQ. In addition, homeless young people are at increased risk for HIV and other STIs in large part because the primary need for shelter, food, or safety far outweighs the risks involved unsafe sexual activity. Homeless LGBTQ youth are often forced to present to the emergency room for primary medical care, where they may be further marginalized and their primary healthcare issues ignored versus management of acute physical symptoms. Access to care can be further complicated by legal constraints of young age and lack of proper identification. The bureaucracy of medicine can be difficult to navigate for the highest functioning adolescent, but for the homeless youth, culturally competent comprehensive care is all too often an elusive goal.

Conclusion

While the majority of this chapter focused on how to approach the unique health risks of LGBTQ adolescents, in many ways these youth are similar to their heterosexual peers and should be viewed broadly within the context of general adolescent health and development. LGBTQ youth face a difficult developmental phase in their lives where they confront a variety of physical, emotional, and sexual changes. For LGBTQ youth, adolescence may be complicated by the pervasive disapproval they perceive from society, family, and friends. As a result, although the vast majority of LGBTQ youth demonstrate remarkable strength and resilience and grow up to lead healthy lives as adults, there may still be too many who are victims of violence, too many who are infected with HIV, and too many who contemplate suicide as a result of their sexual identity. Health care providers need to remain aware of the unique issues and health risks facing LGBTQ adolescents but also remember to address each patient as an individual.

Summary Points

- The goal of the clinical encounter is to promote adolescents' social, emotional, and physical well-being. This includes creating an environment in which LGBTQ youth are comfortable asking questions and seeking advice, help, or support.
- It is critical that the entire medical setting be a safe and confidential environment. Security regarding confidentiality sets the tone for the

clinical encounter. For the LGBTQ adolescent, concerns about confidentiality may be complicated by realistic fears concerning the advertent or inadvertent disclosure of their sexual orientation.

- The leading health risks of LGBTQ youth are HIV/AIDS, substance abuse, depression and suicide, STIs, abuse and victimization, stigma and heterosexualism, racism, eating disorders and obesity, homelessness, and access to care.

- Adolescents tend to be physically healthy. The cornerstone of the adolescent visit is often risk reduction regarding social and behavioral health issues. Screening for the leading health threats of LGBTQ youth is done primarily through the social history, which can be guided by asking questions according to the following acronym: *HEADS*: *H*-home; *E*-education; *A*-activities; *D*-drugs/depression/diet; *S*-safety/sexuality.

- Primary care providers need to be comfortable discussing sexual activity with LGBTQ adolescent patients, including asking specific, nonjudgmental questions regarding types of sexual activity with various sexual partners and the consistency of condom use for protection against pregnancy and HIV/STIs. The fluidity of sexual expression among adolescents can further complicate sexual history-taking as some may not identify with a binary model of sexual identity.

- LGBTQ youth experience the same range of mental health concerns as all adolescents, with added stress at times created by the stigma associated with being a sexual minority. In particular, youth who are "coming out" or beginning to experiment with same-sex partners may experience internal psychological conflict or direct conflict with family and peers, requiring the assistance or support of an astute primary care provider.

- Although experimentation with alcohol, tobacco, and drugs may be a part of normal adolescence, LGBTQ youth in general smoke, drink, and use drugs more frequently than their heterosexual peers. In addition to remaining focused on primary prevention, primary care providers should educate LGBTQ youth about harm reduction strategies including refraining from driving while under the influence and avoiding risky sex while high or drunk.

- Personal safety is often a primary concern of LGBTQ youth, who may experience verbal taunts or physical or sexual harassment. Asking about "feeling safe" at home, school, and other settings is a critical aspect of the LGBTQ youth's social history, as these youth may be reticent to initiate discussion of these issues if a strong clinical relationship has not been previously established.

- LGBTQ youth are the best judges of how parents or friends will react to their "coming out." It is not the role of the provider to give specific advice regarding the timing of coming out. Rather, providers should offer general support and ensure youth that they are available for assistance if needed.

- The physical examination and diagnostic evaluation of the LGBTQ adolescent should follow the AMA Guideline for Adolescent Preventive Services (GAPS). Screening for HIV and other STIs should be guided by the adolescent's sexual behavior, not orientation.
- HIV remains an area of special concern. Young gay and bisexual men and male-to-female transgender youth are the highest behavioral risk group for adolescent or young adult HIV. These youths, particularly from communities of color, require targeted screening and HIV prevention education offered as part of routine primary care.

References

1. **Remafedi G**. Fundamental issues in the care of homosexual youth. Med Clin North Am. 1990;74:1169-79.
2. **Ryan C, Futterman D**. Lesbian and gay youth: care and counseling. Adolescent Medicine: State of the Art Reviews. 1997;8:207-374.
3. **Harper GW, Schneider M**. Oppression and discrimination among lesbian, gay, bisexual, and transgendered people and communities: a challenge for community psychology. Am J Community Psychol. 2003;31:243-52.
4. **Garofalo R, Harper GW**. Not all adolescents are the same: addressing the unique needs of gay and bisexual male youth. Adolesc Med. 2003;14:595-611, vi.
5. **Savin-Williams RC**. Verbal and physical abuse stressors in the lives of lesbian, gay male, and bisexual youths: associations with school problems, running away, substance use, prostitution, and suicide. J Consult Clin Psychol. 1994;62:261-9.
6. **Rosario M, Hunter J, Maguen S, et al**. The coming-out process and its adaptational and health-related associations among gay, lesbian, and bisexual youths: stipulation and exploration of a model. Am J Community Psychol. 2001;29:133-60.
7. **Garofalo R, Katz E**. Health care issues of gay and lesbian youth. Curr Opin Pediatr. 2001;13:298-302.
8. **Garofalo R, Wolf CR, Kessel S, et al**. The association between health risk behaviors and sexual orientation among a school-based sample of adolescents. Pediatrics. 1998;101:895-902.
9. **Klein J, McNulty M, Flatau CN**. Adolescents' access to care: teenagers' self-reported use of services and perceived access to confidential care. Arch Pediatr Adolesc Med. 1998;152:676-82.
10. **Samargia L, Saewyc EM, Elliott BA**. Foregone mental health care and self-reported access barriers among adolescents. Journal of School Nursing. 2006;22:17-24.
11. **Saewyc EM, Bearinger LH, Blum RW, et al**. Sexual intercourse, abuse and pregnancy among adolescent women: does sexual orientation make a difference? Family Planning Perspectives. 1999;31:127-32.
12. **Saewyc E, Skay C, Richens K, et al**. Sexual orientation, sexual abuse, and HIV-risk behaviors among adolescents in the Pacific Northwest. Am J Public Health. 2006; 96:1104-10.
13. **Herrick A**. Understanding the health care needs and risk behaviors of young lesbian and bisexual women. Paper presented at: Women in Medicine National Conference; 2006; Santa Fe, NM.
14. **Perrin E, Cohen KM, Gold M, et al**. Gay and lesbian issues in pediatric health care. Current Problems in Pediatric and Adolescent Health Care. 2004;34:355-98.
15. **Garofalo R, Wolf RC, Wissow LS, et al**. Sexual orientation and risk of suicide attempts among a representative sample of youth. Arch Pediatr Adolesc Med. 1999;153:487-93.

16. **Remafedi G**. Suicide and sexual orientation: nearing the end of controversy? Arch Gen Psychiatry. 1999;56:885-6.

17. **Savin-Williams RC**. A critique of research on sexual-minority youths. J Adolesc. 2001;24:5-13.

18. **Rosewater K, Burr BH**. Epidemiology, risk factors, interventions, and prevention of adolescent suicide. Curr Opin Pediatr. 1998;10:338-43.

19. **Low B, Andrews SF**. Adolescent suicide. Med Clin North Am. 1990;74:1251-64.

20. **Schulberg H, Bruce ML, Lee PW, et al**. Preventing suicide in primary care patients: the primary care physician's role. Gen Hosp Psychiatry. 2004;26:337-45.

21. **Ryan H, Pascale M, Eaton A**. Smoking among lesbian, gay, and bisexuals: a review of the literature. Am J Prev Med. 2001;21:142-9.

22. **Towey K, Fleming M**. Healthy Youth 2010: Supporting the 21 Critical Adolescent Objectives. American Medical Association; 2003.

23. **Crumley F**. Substance abuse and adolescent suicidal behavior. JAMA. 1990;263:3051-7.

24. **Remafedi G**. Predictors of unprotected intercourse among gay and bisexual youth: knowledge, beliefs, and behavior. Pediatrics. 1994;94:163-8.

25. **Mansergh G**. MSM methamphetamine use and sexual risk behaviors for STD/HIV infection. Paper presented at: Conference on Methamphetamine, HIV and Hepatitis; 2005; Salt Lake City, UT.

26. **Colfax G, Coates TJ, Husnik MJ, et al**. Longitudinal patterns of methamphetamine, popper (amyl nitrite), and cocaine use and high-risk sexual behavior among a cohort of San Francisco men who have sex with men. Journal of Urban Health. 2005;82:i62-70.

27. **Tellicr P**. Club drugs. is it all ecstasy? Pediatr Ann. 2002;31:550-5.

28. **Pilkington N, D'Augelli AR**. Victimization of lesbian, gay, and bisexual youth in community settings. Journal of Community Psychology. 1995;23:34-56.

29. **Waldo CR, Hesson-McInnis MS, D'Augelli AR**. Antecedents and consequences of victimization of lesbian, gay, and bisexual young people: a structural model comparing rural university and urban samples. Am J Community Psychol. 1998;26:307-34.

30. **D'Augelli A**. Lesbian and gay men's experiences of discrimination and harassment in a university community. Am J Community Psychol. 1989;17:317-21.

31. **Elster A, Kuznets NJ, eds**. AMA Guidelines for Adolescent Preventive Services (GAPS): Recommendations and Rationale. American Medical Association; 1994.

32. **Rosenberg P, Bigger RJ, Goedert JJ**. Declining age at HIV infection in the United States [letter]. N Engl J Med. 1994;330:789-90.

33. **Centers for Disease Control**. Cases of HIV Infection and AIDS in the United States, 2004. HIV/AIDS Surveillance Report. 2004;16.

34. **Garofalo R**. Overlooked, misunderstood and at-risk: a descriptive study of ethnic minority transgender youth. Paper presented at: Pediatric Academic Societies (PAS) Meeting; 2004; San Francisco, Calif.

35. **Garofalo R, Herrick A, Mustanski B, et al**. Tip of the iceberg: young men who have sex with men, the Internet, and HIV risk. American Journal of Public Health. 2007;97:1113-7.

36. **Kruks G**. Gay and lesbian homeless street youth: special issues and concerns. J Adolesc Health. 1991;12:515-8.

37. **Rew L, Whittaker TA, Taylor-Seehafer MA, et al**. Sexual health risks and protective resources in gay, lesbian, bisexual, and heterosexual homeless youth, Journal for Specialists in Pediatric Nursing. 2005;10:11-9.

38. **Cochran BN, Stewart AJ, Ginzler JA, et al**. Challenges faced by homeless sexual minorities: comparison of gay, lesbian, bisexual, and transgender homeless adolescents with their heterosexual counterparts. American Journal of Public Health. 2002;92:773-7.

39. **Rew L, Fouladi RT, Yockey RD**. Sexual health practices of homeless youth. Journal of Nursing Scholarship. 2002;34:139-45.

40. **Kipke MD, O'Connor S, Palmer R, MacKenzie RG**. Street youth in Los Angeles: profiles of a group at high risk for human immunodeficiency virus infection. Arch Pediatr Adolesc Med. 1995;149:513-9.

Chapter 5

LGBT Couples and Families with Children

VALERIE J. FEIN-ZACHARY, MD
LISA LACAVA, MEd

Introduction

LGBT Relationships and Families

There are many definitions of family. One that is widely accepted is the US Census Bureau's definition of a family as "a group of two or more people related to one another by blood, marriage, or adoption." However, this definition does not include many of the family relationships created by lesbian, gay, bisexual, and transgender people. The following definition by the American Academy of Family Physicians is more inclusive and therefore preferred:

> The family is a group of individuals with a continuing legal, genetic, and/or emotional relationship. Society relies on the family group to provide for the economic and protective needs of individuals, especially children and the elderly.[1]

Connection and support are crucial for healthy adjustment and development of a happy, fulfilling life. It is especially important for LGBT individuals, who often encounter societal rejection and risk becoming isolated, to surround themselves with people who accept their gender status and sexual orientation and to form nurturing relationships that provide support and love. Over time, most LGBT people develop a strong sense of connection and support by building social networks composed of friends, intimate partners, and supportive members of the families they grew up in. For LGBT people who are no longer welcomed by their families of origin, these extended social networks become family and are therefore aptly named "families of choice." Members of these families often do things for each other that are traditionally expected to occur only between biological family members or spouses. For example, a friend may serve as healthcare proxy and primary caregiver for another friend who becomes ill. In addition, an increasing number of LGBT families now include children, as more and more LGBT people are choosing to bring children into their lives through alternative insemination, surrogacy, adoption, foster parenting, or serving as a big brother/big sister for a needy youth or as a highly involved aunt or uncle to nieces and nephews. LGBT family structures are unique in that the major bond that draws family members together is an emotional rather than a biological connection. "Love makes a family" is a familiar phrase: however, given the manner in which LGBT families come together, these words ring especially true in these families.

If clinicians are to provide sensitive and effective care to LGBT adults and/or to children who are being raised by LGBT adults, it is critical that they ask about and honor family relationships and that they are willing to include family members as active participants in their patients' care when it is appropriate to do so. Unfortunately, experiences of LGBT families in the healthcare system have not always been positive. For example, there are examples of LGBT partners who were not allowed to be present during critical moments of their loved ones' care nor allowed to participate in medical decision-making or end-of-life care. LGBT parents and their children also experience barriers to smooth and effective care within the health system. For example, one third of the respondents in a survey of lesbian and gay parents (N = 255) stated that they were dissatisfied with care because of lack of understanding or acceptance of same-sex parents and generalized homophobia.[2] Clearly, there is a pressing need for clinicians to educate themselves about the experiences of LGBT couples and families and to learn to respond to their needs in a productive manner.

This chapter focuses on LGBT relationships and on families with children that are headed by at least one LGBT parent. We examine and refute common societal myths about the quality of intimate LGBT relationships, the suitability of LGBT people as parents, and the health of children raised in LGBT families, using data that have examined these questions in detail. While the field is young, available research describes rewards and challenges that LGBT couples and families encounter commonly; outlines areas where clinicians can offer support and assistance; and suggests questions for further study. Appendix A provides resources both patients and clinicians may find useful to facilitate the health and well-being of LGBT couples and families.

Healthcare Discrimination

In the early years of the AIDS crisis, thousands of gay men became sick and died. The life partners of these men were often ignored as family and denied access to hospital visitation and participation in medical decision-making.

During their time of grief, many surviving partners were excluded from planning and attending funerals or claiming the ashes of their loved one. Some were evicted from joint homes and lost precious, shared possessions-all because they were considered "legal strangers" and not recognized by the law as couples or families. At the time, few from the medical community responded to the needs of HIV/AIDS patients and their partners. Fortunately, today there are many professional medical associations and national community organizations that support LGBT couples and their rights to parent and adopt children. See Table 5-1 for a list of these organizations.

Sharon Kowalski and Karen Thompson were one of the first couples to bring serious national attention to the fight for legal recognition of lesbian and gay couples both within the healthcare system and beyond. In 1983, Sharon Kowalski was struck by a drunk driver and became comatose from a serious head injury. Her parents refused to accept her sexual orientation or to acknowledge her four-year relationship with her partner, Karen Thompson. They quickly won legal guardianship, moved Sharon to a nursing home hundreds of miles away, and fiercely prohibited Karen from visiting or caring for her. For many years, Karen fought for the legal right to visit Sharon and to help with her care. Eventually, the court allowed Karen to visit, and her tenacious care improved Sharon's condition so much that she eventually learned to communicate by typing messages. Protest rallies used the slogan "Bring Sharon Home," and after eight long years of legal battles, Karen Thompson was finally able to do so.[3]

No matter how out and accepted they are, at each step in the process of building strong relationships and loving families, LGBT couples face some form of societal rejection or discrimination. It is a testimony to the power of love and connection that so many LGBT couples and families not only survive but manage to flourish. LGBT families are common enough that almost everyone has interacted with one, though they may not know it, as not all families are open or "out." In states with laws against discrimination (in employment, housing, or places of public accommodation), the number of out LGBT families is higher than in those without them.[4] These out couples are less afraid of losing their jobs or homes because they live openly in their communities; they are also more likely to be out to their healthcare providers.

From the Closet into Activism

LGBT couples will fight fiercely to be with their partners or spouses in times of need and to protect and nurture their children. Tragedy often propels individuals to advocate for their rights and LGBT equality, as did Karen Thompson. Another such person is Nancy Walsh from New Hampshire. Nancy was the 13-year life partner of Carol Flyzik, who died on September 11, 2001, when terrorists flew the plane she was on into the World Trade

Table 5-1   Professional Associations with Policies Supportive of LGBT Parenting, Adoption, Foster Care, and/or Legal Marriage Rights*

American Academy of Child and Adolescent Psychiatry (1999)

    On gay and lesbian parenting-custody and adoption

American Academy of Family Physicians (2002)

    On gay and lesbian parenting-adoption

American Academy of Matrimonial Lawyers (2004)

    On same-sex unions—legal marriage rights

American Academy of Pediatrics (2002)

    On co-parent or second-parent adoption and legal recognition of parents

American Anthropological Association (2004)

    On same-sex unions-opposition to the federal constitutional amendment

American Bar Association (2003, 1999, and 1995)

    On gay and lesbian parenting-joint/second-parent adoption

    On gay and lesbian parenting-adoption

    On child custody and visitation

American Medical Association (2004)

    On gay and lesbian parenting, joint and second-parent adoption

American Psychiatric Association (2002, 2000, and 1997)

    On same-sex couples, joint/second-parent adoption and legal rights

    On same-sex unions-legal recognition of rights and responsibilities

    On gay and lesbian parenting, custody, adoption, and foster parenting

American Psychoanalytic Association (2002 and 1997)

    On gay and lesbian parenting-conception, custody, adoption

    On marriage-allow civil marriage rights (reaffirmed in 2004)

American Psychological Association (2004, 1998, 1998, and 1976)

    On legal benefits for same-sex couples

    On marriage rights for same-sex couples

    On parenting, adoption

Deplores discrimination against homosexuals—supports civil rights

Child Welfare League of America (1988)

    On adoption

National Adoption Center (1998)

    On adoption

National Association of Social Workers (2002)

    On adoption, second-parent adoption, foster parenting

North American Council on Adoptable Children (1998)

    On joint/second-parent adoption, foster parenting

---

*More detail can be found on the Human Rights Campaign Web site, http://www.hrc.org. Click on Family, then Marriage, then Professional Opinion.

Center. Because Carol had no will, Nancy had no legal standing to administer Carol's estate or continue to live in their home. She fought for her rights with the help of Gay and Lesbian Advocates and Defenders (GLAD). Through her activism, she eventually achieved legal recognition by the federal September 11th Victim Compensation Fund.[5]

A wrongful death suit brought by Sharon Smith provides a third example of successful activism. In 2001, Diane Alexis Whipple, a former member of the US lacrosse team and two-time member of the World Cup soccer team, was on her way home when she was attacked at her apartment door by a neighbor's dog. The owner did nothing to intervene, and the dog mauled Diane to the point that she bled to death. In response to this tragedy, Sharon Smith, her registered domestic partner, sued the owners of the dog and the apartment complex for wrongful death in the state of California. At first, the trial was denied because Sharon was not married to Diane: the court did not recognize any survivor rights for domestic partners. However, Sharon Smith's attorneys at the National Center for Lesbian Rights (NCLR) persisted, and she eventually won legal recognition as next of kin under the equal protection clause of the California Constitution.[6] Sharon donated the $1.5 million settlement to St. Mary's College, where Diane had worked as a women's lacrosse coach. Her effort to achieve recognition for her relationship gave some meaning to Diane's tragic death.

The importance of state and federal nondiscrimination laws that cover employment, housing, and public facilities cannot be overemphasized. At a very basic level, support and advocacy for nondiscrimination laws and hate-crime legislation improves the health of LGBT families. Healthcare providers can help by supporting the passage of nondiscrimination legislation and by encouraging LGBT patients to avail themselves of legal protections (such as healthcare proxies) that already exist. See Chapter 16 for more information on legal protections for LGBT individuals and families.

Intimate Relationships

Many different kinds of LGBT relationships exist: lesbian couples, gay male couples, bisexual couples, mixed-orientation couples (for example, heterosexual and bisexual and homosexual and bisexual), and couples where one or both people identify as transgender. Some couples have committed, monogamous relationships, and others choose a more open arrangement. Finally, some couples have intense emotional connections but choose to keep their relationships nonsexual.

It is impossible to obtain an accurate estimate of the number of LGBT couples in the US because fear of repercussions prevents LGBT people from voluntarily coming out on government questionnaires. Same-sex couples were intentionally counted during the 2000 US Census, which reported that there were 594 391 same-sex unmarried partner households, 301 026 gay male families, and 293 365 lesbian families).[7] Since the census did not ask any questions regarding sexual orientation or gender identity, this number does not include single LGBT-headed families or transgender couples, nor does it include LGBT couples who live at or maintain different residences. The Human Rights Campaign (HRC) estimates that same-sex couples were significantly undercounted—by about 62 percent—and suggests that the number is more likely to be over 1 568 460 families. This assessment is based on estimates that 30% of lesbians and gay men are in relationships and that approximately 5% of the adult US population is lesbian or gay.[8]

Unique Challenges

In general, LGBT individuals traverse a similar process of experimentation and exploration in the development of romantic and sexual relationships as heterosexuals. This process can be both exciting and frightening and tends to proceed most smoothly for people who feel solid in their own identity and who have strong social and family supports. As discussed in more detail in Chapters 3 and 4, because of the challenges of societal intolerance and internalized homophobia, LGBT teens and adults sometimes encounter significant obstacles to developing safe, strong, and nurturing intimate relationships.

Typically, LGBT people meet one another in the same ways that heterosexual people meet one another: at work, at school, and at play—through friends and participation in mutually enjoyable hobbies. However, since it is not always easy to identify other LGBT people, especially in some nonurban areas, LGBT people are turning increasingly to online dating services. Several generic internet dating services now serve gay and lesbian clients; in addition, a number of services cater specifically to LGBT individuals.

Established LGBT couples experience many of the same joys and challenges in their relationships as do heterosexual couples. However, most LGBT couples also have to cope with additional stressors related to a lack of family and societal support for their relationships. Acceptance from family and friends is important for a number of reasons. Emotional support enables LGBT couples to share and celebrate their lives during good times and to obtain encouragement and guidance during difficult times. Legal protections can ensure that LGBT partners are afforded equal access to health insurance and other commodities as well as equal rights in terms of taxation, child custody, inheritance, and the like.

Relationships Without Laws

LGBT individuals who are comfortable with themselves, their sexuality, and their sexual orientation often form long-lasting relationships. Most couples start by making personal commitments to one another. These commitments can range from simple promises of mutual love and support to more complex promises of commitment that include provisions for property, contingencies for illness or death, and plans for children.

Over time, many couples take their relationship responsibilities to the next level and choose to make their commitment to one another in the presence of friends and family—both families of origin and families of choice. These public commitment ceremonies mark a willingness of LGBT couples to be recognized as a new family in the context of the larger community. These couples effectively "come out as a couple," accepting the responsibilities commonly associated with being in a relationship. They are willing to take care of one another (in sickness and in health), to provide economic support if needed (for richer or poorer), and they are willing to make a long-term commitment ('til death do us part). Although all of these aspects are similar to heterosexual marriages, LGBT couples in most states are denied the use of the words "wedding" or "marriage" to describe this new level of their relationships.

Without state or federal recognition of their union, LGBT couples have none of the over 1300 legal protections or access to benefits that most heterosexual couples do. Today, most LGBT couples are considered to be "legal strangers"—no more related to one another than passengers on a train. There are a few basic documents that LGBT couples can use to protect themselves in certain, limited circumstances, such as advance directives, wills, and domestic partner agreements. Chapter 16 provides more detail about these protections.

Since most LGBT couples cannot cement their relationships with marriage or even the lesser status of a civil union, many go to great lengths for recognition of their relationships within their religious community and in the eyes of their friends, social networks, and families of origin—supportive parents and siblings. Some are able to create beautiful commitment or wedding ceremonies and are blessed by their clergy. There are several religious denominations that recognize, bless, and support same-sex couples: the Unitarian Universalist Association, the United Church of Christ, both Reconstructionist and Reform Judaism, the Society of Friends (Quakers), and the Metropolitan Community Church.[9] For LGBT families who belong to these religious denominations, acceptance and religious support affirm the dignity of their lives and gives them a place in their community where they are recognized as a couple outside of their own home.

Same-Sex Couples

Love and Commitment
Just like their heterosexual counterparts, loving same-sex couples must negotiate multiple relationship values—trust and intimacy, friends and family, work and leisure, and time and money. Committed couples develop effective communication skills and conflict resolution styles. In general,

studies comparing measures of relationship quality and satisfaction between homosexual and married heterosexual partners reveal more similarities than differences. However, Kurdock's early work (1986)[10] showed that lesbians valued autonomy and equality in their relationships and reported higher levels of intimacy when compared to heterosexual women. Gay men valued autonomy in their relationships (more than heterosexual married men). Both lesbian and gay couples were more likely to dissolve their relationships than heterosexual married couples, most likely due to the lack of institutional recognition of same-sex couples and the fact that legal marriage provides a disincentive to relationship dissolution for heterosexual couples.[11]

"Pioneers in Partnership" by Solomon, Rothblum, and Balsam[12] was the first study of same-sex couples in legally recognized relationships—civil unions in Vermont. Same-sex couples were compared to a cohort of married heterosexual siblings, as well as a cohort of friends (same-sex couples not in civil unions). Lesbian couples were more likely to form civil unions than gay male couples (2:1). Male couples were similar to their "single" friends in being out; however, lesbian couples in civil unions were more out about their sexual orientation than their friends who were not in civil unions. Same-sex couples, in general, were less traditional in their division of household chores, even when the women in heterosexual relationships worked outside the home. Same-sex couples stayed together for about 11-12 years, which was significantly less than their heterosexual siblings, who were together about 19 years. Thirty-four percent of the lesbian couples and 17.9% of the gay men in civil unions had children. This was in contrast to 80% of their married siblings* but slightly greater than their "single" lesbian and gay friends (31.3% and 9.7%).[12] The couples who entered into civil unions were successful countering societal homophobia, resolving relationship ambiguity, and developing high levels of social support from their families of origin.[13]

The next decade of research about same-sex couples will likely continue to highlight relationship diversity, and study the impact of the legal recognition of same-sex couples on their relationships and families.[14,15] According to Rostosky et al, "same-sex couples co-construct the meaning of commitment through the negotiation of boundaries, values, ideals and personal differences. . . . [They] must create new roles and new rules and modify their values and expectations for their partnership."[16]

Health
Data from the National Health Interview Survey demonstrated differences between lesbian, gay male, and heterosexual couples.[17] Lesbian couples

---

* This is higher than the national average from the 2000 Census, which was 45.6% of married heterosexual households raising children compared to 34.3% of lesbian and 22.3% of gay men raising children.

were significantly less likely than women in heterosexual couples to have health insurance. They were also less likely to have seen a healthcare provider in the previous year or to have a usual source of healthcare. In contrast, men in same-sex relationships had equivalent or greater access to healthcare when compared with their heterosexual male counterparts. It was postulated that the experience of the gay male community with HIV/AIDS has enabled gay men to interact more effectively with healthcare providers and the medical community.

As one might expect, being in a committed same-sex relationship can have a positive impact on health. In a study of 2881 gay men from San Francisco, Los Angeles, New York, and Chicago, men in domestic partnerships had decreased risk behaviors for sexually transmitted infections, including a lower prevalence of multiple partnerships, "one-night stands" and unprotected anal intercourse with a nonprimary partner.[18] Although there is not yet data to support this contention, it may well be that same-sex marriage improves the overall health of same-sex couples by increasing access to healthcare (increased availability of health insurance and decreased social stigma) and by decreasing other risk behaviors—such as high-speed driving—leading to fewer accidental deaths and injuries. Mental health would also be expected to improve, with resultant declines in depression, substance abuse, and suicide among married lesbians and gay men.

Money

Assessment of same-sex couples' income and overall financial wealth is complex as variables such as age, levels of education, location (urban or rural), and employment history must be factored into any analysis. Researchers demonstrate both higher and lower incomes for same-sex couples when compared to heterosexual married and unmarried couples due to varying data sets and statistical applications.[19-21] Because same-sex couples are not recognized by the federal government and by most states, they pay more taxes when one partner stays home and are taxed for any benefits received for their partners, such as health insurance. In addition, the lack of federal financial support in times of crisis—the lack of social security benefits to children and surviving spouses—decreases overall financial stability of same-sex couples.[8]

When comparing home ownership and joint bank accounts (measurements of economic assets) of the Vermont couples, there were similar rates of homeownership and joint bank accounts (although gay male couples not in civil unions were less likely to have joint accounts).[12] Nationally, the rate of homeownership was higher for same-sex couples with children (64.3%) when compared to unmarried heterosexual couples with children (45.4%). As expected, the rate of homeownership is the highest for legally married heterosexual couples (78.9%).[8]

Regardless of sexual orientation, couples with children have lower incomes than couples without children, since it is less likely that both partners work full-time. In one of four families with children, one parent stays at home to take care of the children. The numbers are remarkably similar for all families: 25% for heterosexual couples with children, 26% for male couples with children, and 22% for female couples with children.

Conflict and Resolution

When gay, lesbian, and heterosexual couples were studied with regard to six areas of conflict—power, social issues, personal flaws, distrust, intimacy, and personal distance—all three couple types argued most about issues related to "intimacy" and "power" in their relationships.[22] Relationship satisfaction decreased for all couples with increasing conflicts about either of these variables. Lesbian and gay couples argued more over "distrust" issues (eg, distrust regarding former lovers who were more likely to remain in the couples' social networks); whereas heterosexual couples argued more over "social issues" (presumably lesbian and gay couples share similar values regarding civil rights).[23] Coming out is another common source of conflict for many lesbian and gay couples, in which one partner often feels more comfortable than the other disclosing the nature of their relationship to family members, colleagues at work, and other people.

In a study of conflict resolution styles among four types of couples—gay, lesbian, heterosexual with children, and heterosexual without children—there was no difference between the couples in levels of ineffective arguing. Couples that reported frequent ineffective arguing also reported low relationship satisfaction.[23] Couples also evaluated their conflict resolution styles: positive problem solving, conflict engagement, withdrawal, and compliance. Analyses of the couples' responses show many similarities. For all couples, positive problem solving was associated with relationship satisfaction and withdrawal was associated with lack of satisfaction. Lesbian and gay couples rated their partners more likely to use "positive problem solving" than heterosexual married wives (with children) rated their husbands.

More recent evidence highlights differences between conflict styles of lesbian and gay couples and those of heterosexual couples. In homosexual relationships, the initiator of the conflict started the interaction in a positive manner, while in heterosexual relationships, the initiator started negatively. Not surprisingly, therefore, lesbian and gay partners tended to receive the issue positively, while heterosexual partners did not. Lesbian and gay partners tended to use more positive emotions—more humor, affection, and joy—in their interactions than their heterosexual counterparts. The researchers hypothesized that the "heightened sensitivity to equality" in same-sex relationships, makes partners less belligerent and less domineering. "These results suggest that, by analyzing observational data, homosexual relationships may be fundamentally different from heterosexual relationships."[24]

Longevity

The 2000 Census provides the most recent and reliable data comparing the longevity of unmarried same-sex versus heterosexual couples. Forty-one percent of same-sex couples who live together are in long-term relationships (defined as five years or more) compared to only 19.9% of heterosexual unmarried couples who live together.[8] Couples in Vermont who legalized their relationships with a civil union had already been together some 10-12 years.[12] A 12-year longitudinal study of heterosexual and lesbian and gay couples found that break-up rates were similar—63% for lesbian and gay couples compared to 67% for heterosexual couples.[25] In a study of 216 couples in relationships that had lasted an average of 30 years, 85% reported satisfaction with their relationships, and there were no differences between lesbians, gay men, heterosexual men, or heterosexual women. Psychologically intimate communication and minimal conflict were the most powerful factors reported for relationship satisfaction.[26]

Bisexual Couples

Bisexual couples are those in which at least one partner identifies as bisexual. Since our society continues to discriminate against bisexuals as individuals, bisexual couples may not choose to identify openly as such. Bisexual couples can be invisible to mainstream society by blending in as heterosexual couples or appearing as lesbian or gay same-sex couples. The actual number of bisexual couples in the US is not known although there are an estimated five million bisexual people living in America.[27] As the stigma of bisexuality decreases, there will be an increase in the number of couples self-identifying as bisexual couples. It is important that healthcare providers do not assume that patients who are partnered with someone of their own sex is either lesbian or gay, or that someone with an opposite-sex partner is heterosexual. These assumptions alienate members of the bisexual community and make them uncomfortable in the healthcare environment. Furthermore, it is important not to assume that someone who identifies as bisexual has multiple partners, nor that she or he is always monogamous. Bisexuals are a diverse group, and the range of their relationships reflects this.

Data on bisexual couples are scarce: those studies that do exist contain small numbers of participants. However, results from focus groups of bisexuals suggest that bisexuals in relationships have unique issues and concerns, including how to find supportive and understanding partners, coming out to partners (when in already-established relationships), and how to maintain a bisexual identity while in a relationship.[28] Focus groups data also show that bisexuals who want to be involved in monogamous relationships find that it is often difficult to get partners to believe them, while bisexuals who want to be involved with men and women simultaneously find that it is difficult to find understanding and acceptance for this lifestyle.[28]

Bisexual women in the focus groups cited several concerns regarding relationships with male partners: some men feel threatened and prefer not to talk about it; other men find female bisexuality sexy and want to be involved in threesomes with other women; and male partners are frequently unwelcome in the lesbian community. In addition, bisexual women reported encountering disinterest and resentment from some lesbians as well as pressure to identify as lesbian while involved with a lesbian partner. Bisexual men also reported challenges in their relationships. While they experienced less negative reactions from gay men than bisexual women reported from lesbians, bisexual men did report that some gay men are not accepting or not interested in them as partners. Bisexual men involved with women found that their partners struggled with their own identity and self-esteem, tended to feel insecure in their relationships, and found it hard to be supportive without having their own support network in place.[28]

Given all of these challenges, it is not surprising that many bisexual people prefer to be involved with other people who self-identify as bisexual. However, as it may be difficult to identify potential bisexual partners, especially in rural areas, it is not realistic to think that it will always be possible to find a bisexual partner. Whatever a person's circumstance, it is clear that more education and support for bisexual people and their partners are sorely needed. Safer sex information that is pertinent to people choosing both opposite and same-sex partners; coming out and support groups for bisexuals; programs and resources for non-bisexual partners of bisexuals; and referral to counselors and mental health services that are supportive of bisexuality, when appropriate, are all likely to be very helpful (see Appendix A for bisexual resources).

Transgender Couples

A transgender couple is composed of at least one partner who identifies as transgender or transsexual—nonoperative, preoperative, and postoperative. As discussed in Chapter 12, there is enormous complexity in transgender couples, since a transgender person may choose any of the following people as a potential partner: a gay/bisexual/straight man, a gay/straight/bisexual woman, or a transgender person whose sexual orientation may be defined in any number of ways.

As scant as the research literature is for gay, bisexual, and lesbian couples, research on transgender couples is essentially nonexistent. Anecdotal reports in books and movies describe the experience of female partners of transgender people. For example, Virginia Erhardt's book, *Head Over Heels*, gives voice to women who are partners to MTF (male to female) transsexuals and male cross-dressers. These women describe what it is like to discover their partners' gender variance, how they cope emotionally, and how they deal with secrecy and/or disclosure to friends, children, and other family members.[29] Similarly, the 2003 HBO feature film, *Normal*, written and directed by Jane Anderson and starring Tom Wilkinson and Jessica Lange, tells the story of the transition of a happily married man with two children, who realizes that he is a "woman trapped in a man's body." The setting (in the Bible Belt of rural America) makes the movie even more powerful as the characters learn to cope with this dramatic change in their lives.

Since transgender individuals are now identifying their gender variance and coming out at younger and younger ages, an increasing number of relationships will be formed in which both participants are already aware of one another's gender status from the outset. This younger generation of transgender people will undoubtedly encounter an entirely different set of challenges and rewards regarding their relationships and future families compared to older transgender people who came out in a more intolerant time.

Open Relationships

Just as married, heterosexual people sometimes become involved in extramarital relationships, LGBT individuals in committed relationships may do so as well. In addition, some LGBT individuals, as well as heterosexuals, believe that it is possible to love more than one other person at a time: such people call themselves "polyamorous."[30] Other LGBT people choose to be in a primary relationship but find it possible to be sexually involved with other people from time to time. In open relationships, partners acknowledge in advance that one individual cannot fulfill all of the emotional and sexual needs of another over a lifetime. By establishing some clear boundaries for what kinds of expression are acceptable, these couples recognize and accept that one or both partners will become involved with other people outside of their dyad. Common guidelines include rules such as "one-time only"; or "OK" only if out of state, across the country, or away on business, or other, similar restrictions.[31]

LGBT Families with Children

"Although I had had discussions with lesbian friends about how more lesbian couples were having children these days, I do not think I had internalized it as a reality for me. I began to ask myself, 'When had I given up the idea of having children and why? Had I decided I did not want children or did I assume that as a lesbian, it wasn't an option? What was it about seeing lesbian couples with their children that made it less of an abstract idea that other people we're doing and more of reality—something my partner and I could make happen?'"

LaCava LA. "Journeys Into Motherhood." January 13, 1994, unpublished paper, Harvard Graduate School of Education.

It is an age-old phenomenon for many people-the desire to parent, the decision to parent and the act of having and raising children. For some, it is a dream that starts young; for others it becomes clear after falling in love. For most, it is a critical developmental step of one's 20s, 30s, or 40s—filling a need for connection, for doing something beyond oneself, for connecting across generations. Whether you ask someone gay or straight, they will likely tell you similar things about their decision to parent—their hopes and fears, their dreams and expectations. However, there are some important differences to keep in mind.

First, for LGBT individuals and couples who do not have children through a previous heterosexual marriage, parenting typically does not "just happen." It is a deliberate, intentional decision that requires thought, money, and planning. Second, LGBT individuals and couples must make this decision in the context of negative societal views about LGBT people as parents. Even though research to date demonstrates that LGBT people are just as fit to parent as their heterosexual counterparts, societal disapproval can make even the most confident LGBT people wrestle with their decision in a way that heterosexual individuals and couples do not have to do. LGBT people must face their own internalized homophobia and doubts about their right and their fitness to parent: this frequently includes questioning whether they will somehow cause harm to their children because of the social stigma attached to having LGBT parents. The following sections describe the challenges faced by LGBT people who are considering parenthood and LGBT people who are actively parenting.

Trends in LGBT Parenting

In the early 1970s, many lesbians and gay men started to come out. Some had children from prior heterosexual relationships or marriages. Initially, many lesbian and gay parents were denied custody or visitation rights because of their sexual orientation; others were granted some visitation, but only if they stayed in the closet during the time spent with their children.[32,33]

Despite this discrimination, significant numbers of lesbian-headed and gay-headed families survived and began to challenge the prevailing views that LGBT people are unfit to be parents; that it is unfair to subject children to the societal stigmatization associated with having LGBT parents; and that growing up with such parents will harm a child's psychological or psychosocial development.

During the 1980s and 1990s, there was a burst of interest in parenting within the lesbian and gay community, sparked by continued momentum of the gay rights movement; a decrease in the stigma of having a child as a single woman; relaxation of restrictions against adoption by single parents and gay or lesbian parents; availability of assisted reproductive technologies; and increasing visibility of same-sex couples with children within the lesbian and gay community as well as in society in general.[34] Today, lesbians and gay men can choose to have children through a variety of different means, including alternative insemination, surrogacy, adoption, and foster parenting. The recent increased visibility of alternative families has caused the media to declare a virtual lesbian and gay "baby boom" in our society.[35,36]

Recent estimates suggest that there are between two and eight million gay and lesbian parents in the US raising somewhere between four and 14 million children.[37-39] According to the 2000 US Census, approximately ⅓ of lesbian couples and ⅕ of gay male couples are raising children. The percentages of same-sex couples raising children are highest in the South (36% of lesbian couples and 24% of gay male couples) and the Midwest (35% of lesbian couples and 23% of gay male couples). Numbers are slightly smaller and similar in the West and Northeast (33% of lesbian couples and 21%–22% of gay male couples).[8] This geographic pattern is similar to the distribution of unmarried opposite-sex partners raising children.

Parenting Options

As mentioned above, there are many ways to become a parent. Some LGBT people have children from previous heterosexual relationships. Others choose to become parents after they come out, through alternative insemination (AI) or surrogacy, adoption, or foster parenting. Whatever the method selected, achieving parenthood is generally a process that takes significant planning, time, money, and effort. Prospective parents frequently encounter significant challenges, such as the refusal of some adoption agencies to consider their candidacy. Compromise is often necessary; for example, the need to hide one's sexual orientation in order to adopt as a "single" parent, when one is actually involved in a long-term relationship with a committed prospective co-parent. Legal protections are often inadequate—for example, in states that do not offer second-parent adoption, a nonbiological lesbian mother may have few parental rights in the event that she and her partner end their relationship.

However, the act of creating a nontraditional family is also associated with incredible rewards. Prospective LGBT parents have the opportunity to "think outside the box" leading to fascinating and extraordinary parenting arrangements that are changing our understanding of what makes a family. LGBT families with children come in many shapes and sizes: single parent families, two-mom families, two-dad families, and families with a continuum of involvement of adults who may or may not be in romantic or legal relationships with each other, but who decide to parent together. This section describes the pros and cons of various parenting options for LGBT people.

Conception Using Assistive Reproductive Technologies

For years, assisted reproductive technologies (ART)—sperm and egg donation, alternative insemination (AI), *in vitro* fertilization (IVF), surrogacy, and, more recently, embryo adoption—have allowed infertile heterosexual couples to conceive and initiate a pregnancy. These same technologies are also available to LGBT individuals who wish to create a new family. However, privately run fertility clinics can refuse to offer their services to LGBT people. About 80% of clinics provide services to single women and lesbians while only some 20% will provide service to single men or male couples. Currently, no state bars lesbians and gay men from seeking ART services; hence these services should be available at state-run medical centers and other public health centers.[40]

At the most basic level, conception requires an egg, sperm, and a uterus in which gestation takes place. Therefore, conception options clearly differ depending on a person's natal sex; whether they still have the requisite reproductive anatomy; whether or not they are fertile; and whether they themselves wish to participate biologically in the creation of a child. These realities have important implications for LGBT individuals and couples. Lesbian couples who decide to use AI must decide which partner will try to conceive. Gay male couples can establish a parenting arrangement with a single woman or a lesbian couple: if a biological connection is important to them, they will need to decide which one of them will provide the sperm. All participants will need to think about what each person's roles and responsibilities will be. Gay men also have the option of hiring a woman—a surrogate—to bear their children. Transgender individuals with intact reproductive anatomy and an appropriate hormonal milieu have the same options as a person of their natal sex. In order to preserve future conception options, preoperative transgender people should always be counseled regarding the availability of banking sperm (for a MTF transsexual) or freezing embryos (for a FTM transsexual). Of course, removal of the uterus in an FTM individual means that future conception using previously stored embryos would need to involve use of a surrogate or partner with an intact uterus.

Alternative Insemination Using Donor Sperm

Lesbians and bisexual women who wish to become pregnant can choose either a known donor or an anonymous sperm donor from a sperm bank. A major advantage of a sperm bank is that donors are checked routinely for sexually transmitted infections including HIV, and sperm is quarantined until donor re-testing after a suitable window period confirms that the original sample is likely to be free of infection. Disadvantages include increased cost as compared to using a known donor, limited donor selection, limited donors of color (African-American, Latino, Asian), and decreased potency of frozen as opposed to fresh sperm. The expense can be significant: frozen sperm costs approximately $500 per cycle, and it may take a year for a woman to become pregnant. In addition, use of anonymously donated sperm from a bank can also be difficult because of discrimination against LBT women and the need to find a cooperative healthcare provider who is willing and able to store shipped sperm temporarily (many sperm banks will not ship to the customer directly) and/or to perform the insemination. Many women prefer to have a provider perform an intra-uterine insemination (IUI), since this procedure increases the likelihood of conception. An IUI is a simple procedure in which the clinician passes a small catheter through the cervix and instills the sperm directly into the uterine cavity.

Using an anonymous donor affords greater protection against possible legal challenges brought by known biologic donors or their families and can often be emotionally easier for lesbian and bisexual women creating their new family as there is no identified "father" with whom the nonbiologic mother must compete. In most cases, use of anonymous donor sperm means that it is not possible to identify a child's donor or biological father. Therefore, children conceived in this way may later raise questions about biological parentage similar to those asked by adopted children. On the other hand, some anonymous donors are willing to become "known" when the child reaches 18 years of age, when they are protected against having any legal or financial responsibilities. So called "yes-donors" are in short supply: nevertheless, some prospective parents feel strongly about choosing this option.

Use of sperm from a known donor has both advantages and disadvantages. If using a known donor, sperm can often be obtained fresh: fresh sperm is more vigorous, which increases the likelihood of conception. The cost may be less, since storage and administration fees are generally not an issue. However, it is wise to test the donor for transmissible infectious diseases, and this testing can incur significant expense. Because of concerns about possible liability when using fresh sperm, most healthcare providers will not agree to perform an insemination using known donor sperm, unless it has been frozen, and the donor re-tested according to the usual sperm bank protocol. Therefore, women using fresh sperm usually have to perform their own at-home intravaginal insemination. An example of home

insemination using fresh known donor sperm can be found at http://www
.fertilityplus.org/faq/homeinsem.html.

Psychosocial issues are also important to consider. Known donors can
have a wide variety of relationships with a child, ranging from just being
known as the donor, to having intermittent visits, to having co-parent status along a continuum of custodial and financial responsibility.
Relationships between the donor, the woman being inseminated, and her
partner can be complicated because the donor is the legal "father" until he
surrenders his rights at adoption. Without this surrender, the nonbiologic
mother cannot proceed with a second-parent adoption. In some instances,
these "parental rights" have been extended to include custody challenges
of the donor's parents to their "grandchild." In sum, the nonbiologic
mother's position is "stronger" if there is no named "father" on birth certificates and other legal documents, given the overwhelming societal belief
system that every child has one mother and one father, irrespective of their
family structure and how they are being raised. Consideration of all of these
issues in advance is wise: not surprisingly, it can be difficult to find a donor
who is willing to agree to all of the stipulations set forth. It is also important to remember that people sometimes change their minds: a donor who
genuinely believes he is not interested in having a relationship with a child
may discover that he wants to be involved after all once the child has been
born. Therefore, prospective parents who choose a known donor do so at
considerable risk and should carefully discuss expectations and hopes with
the donor. All parties can be better protected by signing a comprehensive
legal donor agreement.

Surrogacy

Surrogacy is an expensive but appealing option for some gay male couples.
It is also an option for single gay men; lesbians and bisexual women unable
to carry a pregnancy; and for some transgender couples. Using a gestational
carrier allows one partner of a same-sex couple to have a biological connection to the child. However, the costs ($50 000 to as much as $100 000)
can be prohibitive, which limits access to surrogacy for all but those with
the money to cover the agency and legal fees, as well as the surrogate's
fees and medical expenses. Surrogates are women who enjoy being pregnant and want to help others to have a child, in addition to wanting and/or
needing the payment. They will often refer to the baby they are carrying as
someone else's baby, ie, "Jim and Kevin's baby."

There are three types of surrogacy: full (also called traditional) surrogacy, gestational surrogacy, and egg-donor surrogacy. In full surrogacy, the
surrogate carries a child conceived through alternative insemination (AI)
with sperm from one of the intended parents. A traditional surrogate provides her own egg for this pregnancy: typically, she has four days after birth
before she must relinquish the child. Legally, traditional surrogacy is the

riskiest arrangement, since the surrogate may change her mind and decide to keep the baby: therefore, many agencies do not offer this option.

Some gay, bisexual men or transgender people may ask a friend or relative to serve as traditional surrogate. For example, a gay male couple might ask a sister of one partner to conceive and carry their child, while the other partner donates the sperm: this way, both men will have a biological connection to the child. Some men locate a gestational carrier through the internet, because of the prohibitive costs associated with using an agency. Surrogates typically sign an adoption surrender after the birth of the child so the intended parents can proceed with a co-parent adoption. However, many people work out complicated arrangements to permit the woman to have a relationship with the child, even though she will not have primary custodial or financial responsibility.

In gestational surrogacy, an in vitro fertilization (IVF) procedure creates embryos from the sperm and eggs of one or both of the intended parents. The next step is to implant these embryos into a woman (known as a gestational carrier) who will carry the pregnancy to term. In egg-donor surrogacy, eggs are harvested from an egg donor, fertilized through IVF, and then the resulting embryos are implanted in a woman who becomes the gestational carrier. Egg-donor surrogacy is the most common type of surrogacy used, because legally and emotionally it is the least complicated. The woman carrying the pregnancy has no biological connection to the child. An agency screens the participants and coordinates the process. Finally, embryo adoption, which occurs less frequently, involves implantation of frozen embryos into a woman who will not only carry the child but who also plans to be the parent.

Lesbian couples have created a unique kind of "surrogacy" in which one partner is the egg donor or "biological mother" and the other is the gestational mother or "birth mother." Often, the idea that both women will be physically related to the child is so desirable that a lesbian couple considers this arrangement to be most optimal. While it is wonderful to have the technology to do this, it is not a completely benign process. There are risks to each woman associated with the medications taken before harvesting eggs and before implantation of the embryo. The costs for this procedure are prohibitive for many, and health insurance will not cover this treatment unless there is proven infertility.

Second-Parent Adoption

After one partner of an LGBT couple conceives or becomes a parent through surrogacy, the couple can apply for a second-parent (also known as co-parent) adoption, which allows the nonbiological partner to become a legal parent to their child. Typically, the biological parent must relinquish their rights first, so that the couple can adopt jointly. The process of second-parent adoption can be time-consuming and expensive. One such mother from Massachusetts described her feelings about this process:

I don't remember having to put our kids in the paper prior to the adoption—we probably filed an application to waive that. What I do remember is feeling frustrated that Claire and I had to wait many months with each child to have her legal relationship established even though she (and I) intentionally brought the child into the world. The idea that the law says that a person who might not have intended to bring a child into the world and might even have not wanted the child is automatically a parent but Claire was not, really troubled me. Marriage has not cured the issue either. Most lawyers would tell you that because other states are not guaranteed to respect our marriages, the safer course still is to have the non-biological parent adopt their own child.—V. Henry[41]

Unfortunately, second-parent adoption is not yet not available everywhere. Currently, only eight states (California, Connecticut, Massachusetts, New Jersey, Illinois, New York, Pennsylvania, and Vermont) and the District of Columbia provide legal guarantees for second-parent adoptions in all counties. Currently, equal marriage rights do not replace the need for joint adoption or second-parent adoptions. See Chapter 16 for more on second-parent adoption laws.

Adoption
LGBT people often face obstacles when they pursue adoption, due to inadequate laws and regulations to protect their right to adopt, narrow definitions of family despite changing demographics about what makes a family, and societal discrimination against LGBT people.[42] In addition, there continues to be a degree of bias against men who choose to parent, particularly gay men who wish to adopt. Adoption can also be emotionally complicated. Some lesbian couples come to adoption after several years of trying to conceive on their own. These couples must grieve the losses associated with infertility and the expectation of a biological connection to their child before they are able to move from a "failed process" to the complex process of adoption, without internalizing all of these feelings and concluding that they are somehow failures as parents. Finally, while the cost of adoption varies considerably, fees at private agencies ($15 000–$50 000) can be exorbitant while public agencies are more affordable (under $10 000).[43]

Successful outcomes require creativity. While heterosexual couples can adopt as a couple, LGBT couples often cannot unless they appear to be heterosexual, as may be the case in some bisexual and/or transgender couples. Only a few US adoption agencies permit LGBT couples to adopt a child together; even when an agency is willing to work with a couple, state laws often prohibit such couples from adopting except as single people. Therefore, LGBT couples must decide which partner will apply to adopt their child, adding to the complexity of the adoption process. Couples in the numerous states that do not permit second-parent adoption face an additional stressor, since only the original adoptive parent will have a legal connection to their child. The parent who is not officially recognized may encounter numerous roadblocks navigating social, school, and healthcare environments: "Will I be permitted to pick up my child from school if he or she is sick?" "Will the emergency room allow me to make an emergency medical decision?" "What are my legal rights?"

In spite of the barriers, gay and lesbian people have continued to adopt. Although accurate numbers are hard to come by, the 2000 Census estimated that 6% of same-sex couples are raising adopted children.[8] A national survey of adoption agency policies found that approximately one third have nondiscrimination policies, and 60% of the agencies accept applications from clients who identify as lesbian or gay.[44] Overall, public agencies are more willing than private agencies to accept applications from lesbians and gay men. Religious affiliation plays a role in whether an application is accepted or not: Jewish-affiliated agencies are most likely, and Lutheran-affiliated agencies are next most likely to welcome applications from nontraditional applicants.

Almost half (47%) of the adoption agencies in the aforementioned survey provide information about the adoptive parents' sexual orientation to the potential birth parents. Interestingly, nearly 15% of agencies had requests from birth parents for placement with lesbian or gay parents, while nearly 25% said that birth parents objected to placement of their child with lesbian or gay parents. In what seems to be a growing trend favoring gay and lesbian adoption, 48% of the agencies surveyed expressed an interest in training so they could work with lesbian and gay clients.[45]

Unfortunately, even with more children unwanted and languishing in orphanages, international adoption is becoming increasingly difficult for gay men and lesbians to accomplish. Many countries have placed restrictions on single parent adoptions (all LGBT individuals must adopt as "single parents") and continue to develop other obstacles for prospective gay and lesbian parents. For example, prospective parents, applying to adopt a child from China must now sign and affidavit stating that they are not homosexual. Other barriers to international adoption include high costs— estimates vary widely from $20 000–$40 000; FBI background checks, finger printing, and immigration forms as well as the usual home study. Open corruption creates additional hassles: there is an unspoken expectation that cash payments-in $100 bills-are to be given to various officials along the way in order to ensure a smooth journey.

In addition to thinking about how to help their child adjust to life with nontraditional parents, prospective LGBT parents who are considering international adoption must also consider how they will address the cross-cultural issues raised by parenting a child whose race and/or ethnicity is often different from their own. In many multiethnic LGBT families, at least one of the parents may themselves be a source of diversity: estimates suggest that more than 10% of same-sex couples raising adopted children have one parent who was not born in the United States. Since the federal government does not allow immigration of same-sex partners, these families are at risk of fragmentation in the event that one of the parents is forced to leave the country.

Foster Parenting

Some LGBT couples choose to become loving, supportive role models as foster parents for the over 500 000 children in need of foster care. Gay and lesbian couples are permitted to become foster parents in every state in the nation. However, obstacles to foster parenting still exist. Agency workers continue to doubt the parenting skills of LGBT people, and few agencies have formal policies that support them.[46] Other LGBT people, similar to their heterosexual counterparts, become guardians or caregivers to their nieces and/or nephews when their siblings die or are unable to be adequate parents. This is also termed "relative placement." In addition, some LGBT people provide homes, financial support, and mentoring (informally, or as an official Big Brother/Big Sister) to LGBT youth who are homeless and in need of support because they have been rejected and/or disowned by their families of origin.

Blended Families or "Stepfamilies"

Individuals who end prior relationships and then find new partners or spouses, create new "blended families." Children in these families may have stepsiblings or half-siblings and may be part of both larger families on an ongoing basis, or primarily live in one family. In addition to the more typical difficulties of creating a new stepfamily (eg, unrealistic expectations, conflicts with the stepparent) these lesbian and gay stepfamilies appear to be unique as a family form.[47] If either parent was previously in a heterosexual marriage, she or he may also be dealing with a change in sexual orientation and personal identity.[48] Societal stigma of homosexuality can cause a stepparent to play more of a supportive role in the family focused on the children, rather than consolidating a mature primary relationship to her or his new partner. In the absence of legal recognition and documentation of their role in the family, stepparents are sometimes marginalized to the point of invisibility.

Other Considerations for Prospective LGBT Parents

Caring for Adults

LGBT individuals and couples frequently provide care to friends and elderly parents. Parents of heterosexual spouses are typically referred to as "in-laws." In LGBT families, these same parents are often affectionately called "out-laws," since there is no legally recognized relationship between parties. While the majority of gay men and lesbians with adult care-giving responsibilities are out to medical providers,[49] this lack of formal acknowledgment can pose challenges when visiting "out-laws" in a hospital or nursing home, adding stress to the burden associated with serving as a caregiver. Clinicians can help by encouraging LGBT individuals who have major caregiving responsibility for an "unrelated" friend or family member to obtain legal document—such as healthcare proxies—that support their role.

Language and Definitions

Once prospective parents have clarified what their family structure will be, they often begin to think about how they will describe their families to other people. The power of naming oneself (described in detail in Chapter 3), one's relationship, and one's family cannot be overestimated. LGBT people must decide what words to use to describe their partners (lover, life-partner, spouse); how to describe commitment ceremonies (blessed unions, civil unions, weddings, marriages); and how to address a partner's children, siblings, and parents (children or stepchildren, in-laws, out-laws). They often encounter insensitivity along the way. The question "who is the real mother" asked of a lesbian couple is almost illogical in today's culture in which it "takes a village" to raise a child. Similarly, the notion that same-sex couples should not "marry" seems silly when words become clichés—as merging corporations "marry" and mutual funds are bought and sold in "families."

Consequently, LGBT families are developing an entirely new language to describe their family structures (eg, "extended," "blended" or "step") and the new roles created. Some same-sex couples with children choose common (or made-up) names to describe their roles such as "mama" and "mommy," "daddy" and "papa," or "mommy J" and "daddy Bill." Younger LGBT people are using more hip terms like "dyke daddy" or "tranny pop" to refer to their new parent status. Sometimes, when parents choose terms they anticipate will be used, children simply pick the names that they like best. When communicating with patients who are children, clinicians can create a sense of inclusion by using open-ended words and phrases such as "your parents" and "family" instead of "your mom or dad."

Families created with known sperm donors or surrogates may refer to these biological (but not legal) parents simply by their names, or as "your donor," "your surrogate mother," "your birth mother," "your egg donor" and/or the "man or woman who helped make you." Because of the need to explain to others how they were conceived, children raised in LGBT-parented families typically learn about reproductive biology at a younger age than their peers raised by heterosexual parents. Legal and medical providers in the field of assisted reproductive technology are also contributing to this language expansion, using terms such as "third-party parenting" and "collaborative reproduction."

Advanced Planning and Support for Children

Prospective LGBT parents think carefully about how they will support their children, beginning during the very earliest planning stage and continuing throughout their children's lives. In addition to making sure that their children will have positive role models, LGBT parents tend to go to great lengths to enroll their children at diverse schools; to attend community events that boost respect and acceptance of LGBT people; and to help their children practice how to respond when they encounter insensitive or insulting comments. Specific resources for LGBT individuals who are considering parenthood are listed in Appendix A.

LGBT People Are "Fit" Parents

Although the field is young, an increasing body of evidence is accumulating regarding the psychological and social adjustment of children raised by same-sex couples as well as single lesbian mothers and gay fathers.[39,50-51] Children born into or adopted by bisexual or transgender parents have not been adequately studied, but one might expect the findings to be similar. To date, studies have concentrated on two populations: children born into opposite-sex families where the parents subsequently divorced or separated after one parent came out as gay, lesbian, or bisexual; and children born into or adopted by lesbian and gay families. Initial studies included toddlers[52] and young children[53,54]; studies of adolescents are emerging as early cohorts of children with lesbian and gay parents mature.[55] Specific outcomes studied include identity development (gender identity, gender role behavior, sexual orientation) and social adjustment (development of peer and extended family relationships).

Overall, research supports equivalent outcomes for children in LGBT families.[56] Lesbian and gay parents are as likely as heterosexual parents to create family environments that promote children's psychological well-being. Development is similar whether children are raised by same-sex parents or by heterosexual parents.[38,55] Currently, there is no empirical evidence that children raised by a gay or lesbian parent are in any way disadvantaged because of their parent's sexual orientation. What studies do show is that "children are more powerfully influenced by family processes and relationships than by family structure."[57] The quality of family relationships is significantly associated with adolescent outcomes, including higher self-esteem and connectedness in school (as measured by such factors as whether adolescents felt close to other students, that they were treated fairly at school and were in a safe environment), and with less "trouble in school" (eg, difficulty doing homework and problems getting along with classmates). Personal, family, and school adjustments of adolescents living with same-sex parents do not differ from those of teens who have opposite-sex parents.[55]

Notwithstanding these encouraging results, many people continue to have significant fear and trepidation about the idea of LGBT people becoming parents. This is due in large part to the ongoing presence of unsubstantiated myths. The remainder of this section examines the source of each of these myths and provides evidence to dispel the concerns they raise.

Myth #1: Gay men are more likely to molest children.

Research in the area of child sexual abuse has found that gay men are no more likely to sexually abuse children than heterosexual men.[58] An estimated 94% of all abuse is perpetrated by men who abuse both girls and boys and who abuse girls 1.5 to three times more often than boys.[59] In a study of 352 children, researchers assessed the sexual orientation of abusers and found 82% were known heterosexuals and less than 1% were identified as homosexual (17% were unknown). Thus, they estimate that, in the general population, over 97% percent of all abusers are heterosexual and only 0%–3% are homosexual.[60]

Myth #2: Lesbians hate men.

Since lesbians do not "need a man" to have emotional commitments or sex, they are often perceived as not wanting men in their lives. Some people carry this idea to the extreme and use it to argue that lesbians will therefore be unable to love and nurture male children. In fact, most lesbians develop close relationships with men during the course of their lives, and the majority of lesbian parents are delighted to raise either male or female children. In the National Lesbian Family Study (NLFS), 43 children were girls and 42 were boys. The mothers reported concerns about raising children in a homophobic world, and encouraged diversity. Seventy-six percent (76%) expressed concern about providing good, loving men as role models for their children, and 27 mothers of the 42 boys expressed dislike of policies that excluded their sons from "women only events."[52]

Myth #3: LGBT people have unstable relationships.

Many people assume, incorrectly, that LGBT individuals are promiscuous and do not choose to be in long-term, committed relationships. Biased research (often with convenience sampling conducted in gay bars) does not give an accurate picture of LGBT couples and their relationships. Today, many out LGBT people are involved in stable, committed relationships and encounter similar interpersonal challenges and rewards as their heterosexual counterparts. Like all parents, LGBT parents have both strengths and weaknesses. After three decades of research, the American Academy of Pediatrics clearly stated: "[T]here is no relationship between parents' sexual orientation and any measure of a child's emotional, psychosocial, and behavioral adjustment. These data have demonstrated no risk to children as a result of growing up in a family with one or more gay parents."[61]

Myth #4: Children need a mother and a father.
Children find role models in many places outside their homes—neighbors, teachers, grandparents, aunts, and uncles are just a few of the people who may fulfill this function. Some people might argue that the more diverse and plentiful a child's role models, the more flexible and open they are likely to be about many issues. As traditional nuclear families (with a male "provider" and a female "caregiver" and household manager) decline in numbers, so do rigid views about what it means to be male or female in our society.

Myth #5: Children raised by LGBT parents will be harmed by social stigma.
Homophobic bullying has been identified as a major reason for opposition to lesbian and gay parenting.[62] Some investigators have found that there is no difference in bullying between lesbian and gay families and other "different families"—for example, families headed by a single parent or stepfamilies. However, children with lesbian and/or gay parents do report experiencing rejection or harassment by their peers because of their family structures. By age 5, 18% of the children in the National Lesbian Family Study (NLFS) had experienced some form of homophobia.[63] By the age of 10, 43% had indicated that they had experienced homophobic comments about their moms.[64] One 9-year-old boy who has two lesbian mothers commented: "Kids are going to make fun of you for all kinds of reasons. Some kid will get picked on for having a big head—it's just a part of life. It's too bad, but it is. Maybe if more parents and grown-ups taught children to be OK with people who are different, it would stop."[65]

Not all children are this resilient: data suggest that some adolescents have difficulty with bullying.[66] The key factor in successfully facing hostility from other children and adults is a strong, loving environment where children learn how to cope with these experiences and not internalize them.[67] In supportive environments, children learn that differences in family structure are not bad, shameful, or their fault. They themselves learn not to pick on others who are different and to remember that "others may have a lot to learn."

Last, but not least, some researchers have suggested that the positive outcomes found in children of LGBT-parented families may actually be a product of their enhanced sensitivity to societal oppression:

> On the contrary, we propose that homophobia and discrimination are the chief reasons why parental sexual orientation matters at all. Because lesbigay parents do not enjoy the same rights, respect, and recognition as heterosexual parents, their children contend with the burdens of vicarious social stigma. Likewise, some of the particular strengths and sensitivities such children appear to display, such as a greater capacity to express feelings or more empathy for social diversity, are probably artifacts of marginality and may be destined for the historical dustbin of a democratic, sexually pluralist society.[66]

Myth #6: Children with LGBT parents are more likely to grow up to be LGBT themselves.
With regard to gender identity and expression, "none of the more than 300 children studied to date have shown evidence of gender identity confusion, wished to be the other sex, or consistently engaged in cross-gender behavior."[57] There is some evidence that children of gay men and lesbians are more open and tolerant of diversity and that they are more nurturing of younger siblings, which many would argue is a good outcome.[66] Included in this tolerance is a willingness to explore one's own sexuality: studies show that children of LGBT parents are more open to exploring same-sex experiences during their sexual development.[55,68] However, there is no evidence that the sexual orientation (after developmental experimentation) of these individuals is any more likely to be lesbian or gay than that of people raised by heterosexual parents.[55,69] The majority of children raised in lesbian families identify as heterosexual in adulthood.[39,66,68,70]

Helping Children Thrive

Challenges and Helpful Strategies for Children

Children can have a range of reactions to having LGBT parents: specific responses are often age-dependent or related to the age of the child when parents reveal their gender status or sexual orientation. Older children are well aware of societal homophobia: fortunately, most seem to be adept at handling this added stress. Sometimes wise beyond their years, they understand that their negative encounters at school or in the playground also hurt their parents, and they may try to protect their parents from the insults and attacks they endure, by specifically *not* telling them about incidents at school. In addition, it is likely that confident, clear parenting on these issues can help children understand that these negative encounters have nothing to do with the inherent worth or dignity of themselves or their parents. One 8-year-old child with two moms explained, "They just haven't learned enough yet, Mommy. They have more learning to do before they understand about our family."[71]

Normal developmental issues during adolescence can include shame and resentment, and it may be that some teenagers use their family structure as an "excuse" for acting out otherwise typical problems. For some teenagers, the moment their parent comes out of the closet is the moment that they go into the closet as the child of an LGBT person. They may stop bringing friends home after school or refuse to be dropped off at school by their parent's new partner, significant other, or spouse. On the other hand, some children of LGBT families are proud and accepting of their family structure and the love embodied in their families. They may also be more tolerant and open-minded about difference and more mature in their understanding of what makes a strong and loving family.

Closeted LGBT parents who live in secrecy—whether single, coupled, or divorced—can cause special problems for their children. Often, children draw their own conclusions (often correct) from the omissions; however, sometimes children concoct complex fantasies to explain the silence, such as the idea that a parent is ill. Whatever the situation, secrecy creates distance between family members, since it is clear that certain issues are "off limits" and not up for discussion. The loneliness and isolation that results is often further compounded by the fact that parents who are themselves isolated are unlikely to be able to provide adequate support to their children. There is added stress for children of LGBT parents if one of their parents actually does become ill or dies, especially if the illness is itself stigmatized, as is the case with HIV/AIDS[72]: Should they tell their friends at school? Will this news cause even greater isolation? Once again, what we may learn from future research is that societal homophobia causes most of the difficulties for children of LGBT families—not the fact that they have LGBT parents.

Just as LGBT people constantly come out in various settings and situations, the children of LGBT parents must come out regarding their parents throughout their lives—whether it is in a high school class, at summer camp, in a college dorm, at a new job, or on a romantic date. In the book *Families Like Mine*, Abigail Garner provides a fascinating portrayal of the experiences of adult children of LGBT parents, including the perception that it is important to learn the "right answers" to people's incessant questions and to appear to be perfect progeny so as to prove that LGBT families (and by extension, they themselves) are not aberrant.[73] Organizations such as COLAGE (Children of Lesbians and Gays Everywhere) and the Family Pride Coalition provide opportunities for children who are raised in LGBT households to meet one another and receive validation and support and to develop appropriate language and strategies with which to respond to people who do have questions.

In theory, children in LGBT-headed households who are themselves lesbian, gay, bisexual, or transgender ("queer kids") should have an advantage by being raised by parents who are accepting and understanding of what it means to be an LGBT person. Theoretically, the presence of an accepting and supportive environment might be expected to produce children who are closely attuned to the effects of homophobia and heterosexism and therefore better equipped to counter this negativity. Unfortunately, however, significant societal stigmatization against "queer kids" of LGBT parents persists, which perpetuates a cycle of shame related to being different.[74] LGBT communities need to work diligently to end this cycle by anticipating its occurrence, naming it as soon as it is apparent, and providing supportive intervention. As is the case for LGBT youth who have traditional parents, queer kids with LGBT parents can find support in local LGBT teen support groups, after-school Gay-Straight Alliances (GSAs), and national organizations such as COLAGE and PFLAG (Parents, Families and Friends of Lesbians and Gays).

Challenges and Helpful Strategies for Parents

When children are small, for the most part, their parents can successfully control their environments and keep them safe and happy. LGBT parents go to great lengths to enroll their children in schools that are open to or supportive of diversity; to form connections with other LGBT families; and to read books and watch movies that depict diverse families and people with whom they can identify. Appendix A provides a list of useful resources. The further children venture forth into the world, the less of a shield parents are able to provide against insensitive or insulting comments. As children mature enough to understand the meaning of "differences," LGBT parents try to prepare them for potential negative experiences by providing knowledge about societal prejudices. Parents frequently have concerns about how to discuss the issue of anti-LGBT verbal and physical harassment (homophobic bullying) with their children without raising excessive fear.

Many parents encounter schools that will not recognize their family structure and that do not value diversity. Some parents have difficulty with acceptance at parent-teacher meetings and conferences, school trips, and social events, and "invisible" parents may even encounter difficulty with simple duties such as picking their child up at school without a note from the legally recognized parent. To solve these problems, many LGBT parents become proactive in the school system, joining the Parent Teacher Organization (PTO) and working with other parents and teachers to educate them and ultimately to incorporate lesbian and gay family content in the classroom and/or curriculum. Several national organizations provide resources that can help in this process, including the Gay, Lesbian and Straight Education Network (GLSEN); Family Pride; Parents, Families and Friends of Lesbians and Gays (PFLAG); and Women's Educational Media.

When LGBT-headed families have loving and supportive parents and siblings, these individuals provide valuable extended family support. Research shows that most children raised by lesbians and gay men are in regular contact (ie, at least monthly) with their biological grandparents— more so than their nonbiological grandparents—while a few have regular contact with adults who are not biologically related but who serve as "surrogate" grandparents.[75] Grandparents can provide emotional as well as financial support for their children and their grandchildren. Grandparents, aunts, and uncles can assist with childcare and be role models. These contacts foster positive outcomes for children and fewer behavior problems.

Not surprisingly, extended family members do not always feel comfortable with their loved one's alternative family immediately. For example, in interviews of lesbian mothers with 5-year-olds, 63% reported that the children's grandparents were "out" about their grandchildren's lesbian families, while 17% refused to recognize the children as "full-fledged" grandchildren.[63] Grandparents in lesbian families with children move between mainstream heterosexual society and the often marginalized place of their daughters' lesbian community.[76] Some love and accept the grandchildren to whom they are not biologically related; others choose to distance themselves.* As mentioned previously, some LGBT parents find themselves removed from or intentionally disowned by their families of origin. Often, these parents create extended "families of choice" in which close friends serve as "aunties" and "uncles" for their children and older friends may replace absent parents as their children's "surrogate" grandparents.

In addition, numerous local and national LGBT organizations hold events for LGBT families that encourage connection and provide support. Family Pride and COLAGE are known widely for their support of families and children. Each year, Family Pride hosts "Family Week"—a series of workshops, conferences and social events—in LGBT-friendly Provincetown, Massachusetts (and also in Saugatuck, Mich) so that parents and children can experience being in the majority with their peers. COLAGE (Children of Lesbians and Gays Everywhere) is a national organization that provides a support network for children of all ages. COLAGE "engages, connects, and empowers people to make the world a better place for children of LGBT parents and families."[77] Their annual conference is concurrent with Family Week. Throughout the year, many other organizations hold educational and social events so that isolated LGBT families can come together. Other creative strategies include vacation cruises and special summer camps that cater to the children of LGBT families generally, or that include particular subsets of children raised in LGBT families—such as children adopted from China, for example.

Conclusion: Embracing Change

Today an increasing number of families in our country are no longer modeled after the traditional family, in which the man takes on the role of "breadwinner" and the woman cares for the children and maintains the home. There have been changes in family structure with new family constellations—working mothers, divorced families, single-parent families, stepfamilies, and now LGBT-headed families. It is important that healthcare providers understand these changing demographics and think about the following: What are the characteristics of these new families? How does our societal focus on the traditional family affect the children and parents in LGBT family constellations? How can the healthcare system provide support?

Prospective LGBT parents frequently look to health providers for accurate information and guidance regarding available parenting options: therefore, it is important for clinicians to be familiar with all of the options and

---

* This distinction is only made relevant because their daughters are lesbians. If their heterosexual children had adopted a child, there would be "no question" that they are the new baby's grandparents.

to be prepared to make appropriate referrals. Since the prospect of becoming a parent raises a number of unique issues that require careful attention and resolution, it is helpful for many LGBT people who are considering parenting to have an opportunity to talk with other people who are posing similar questions. Informational groups in which prospective parents can explore parenting issues are available in a number of LGBT-oriented health organizations. Finally, established LGBT families need open-minded health providers who will be supportive of their family structures and responsive to their unique needs. Therefore, it is important for clinicians to become aware of the range of family structures that exist; to learn who the key members of a patient's family are; to help patients create legal documents (such as healthcare proxies) that will protect these relationships; and to include key family members in medical decision-making when this is desired by the patient. Given the immense value of community support, it is also very useful for clinicians to have a readily available list of resources that includes local and national organizations that offer connection and support for LGBT couples and families. Appendix A provides a list of educational and legal resources that may be helpful for both clinicians and patients.

Summary Points

- Lesbian, gay, bisexual, and transgender (LGBT) people, in the course of creating relationships, getting married, and having children, are expanding what it means to be a family. This change is liberating, creating unique families and diverse communities. There is now more acceptance than ever before for LGBT inclusion in our society, despite continued objection by some.
- Legal recognition of LGBT families allows family members to care for and protect one another, especially in times of illness and tragedy. Nonetheless, in most US states, LGBT couples are still considered to be no more than "legal strangers" and have none of the over 1300 legal protections or access to benefits available to most heterosexual couples. There are currently a few documents that LGBT couples can use to protect themselves and their children in certain, limited circumstances, such as advance directives, wills, and domestic partner agreements.
- There are millions of children growing up in LGBT-parented families. Some LGBT parents have children from previous heterosexual relationships; other same-sex couples have chosen to have children through a variety of different means, including alternative insemination, surrogacy, foster-parenting, and adoption. Although many gay and lesbian people are able to successfully adopt children, adoption rights for LGBT individuals and couples are limited both domestically and internationally.
- Current peer-reviewed research supports equivalent outcomes for children with LGBT parents as compared to children with heterosexual

parents. Lesbian and gay parents are as likely as heterosexual parents to create family environments that promote children's psychological well-being.

- Many professional medical associations and national community organizations support LGBT couples and their rights to parent and adopt children.
- To provide the highest quality care to their patients, it is important for clinicians to understand the range of family structures that exist; to use inclusive language that does not assume everyone has one father and one mother; to ask their patients who the key members of their family are; and to include these family members in medical decision-making when desired by the patient.
- It is useful for clinicians to keep a readily available list of resources that includes options for prospective LGBT parents, as well as local and national organizations that offer connection and support for LGBT couples and families.

References

1. **American Academy of Family Physicians**. Policies on health issues. Available at http://www.aafp.org/online/en/home/policy/policies/f/familydefinitionof.html.
2. **Perrin EC, Kulkin H**. Pediatric care for children whose parents are gay or lesbian. Pediatrics. 1996;97:629-35.
3. **Thompson K, Andrzejewski J**. Why Can't Sharon Kowalski Come Home? Aunt Lute Books; 1989.
4. **Smith DM, Gates GJ**. Gay and lesbian families in the United States: same-sex unmarried partner households. A preliminary analysis of 2000 United States Census data. Human Rights Campaign; 2001.
5. **Gay and Lesbian Advocates and Defenders**. September 11 surviving partners: fighting for recognition. Available at http://www.glad.org/GLAD_Cases/Nancy_Walsh.shtml.
6. **National Center for Lesbian Rights**. Landmark ruling recognizes Sharon Smith's constitutional right to file wrongful death suit. Partner of dog-mauling victim Diane Whipple gains legal victory. Available at http://www.nclrights.org/releases/ssmith072701.htm.
7. **Simmons T, O'Connell M**. Married-Couple and Unmarried-Partner Households: 2000. US Department of Commerce Economics and Statistics Administration. US Census Bureau; 2003. Census 2000 Special Reports.
8. **Bennett L, Gates G**. The Cost of Marriage Inequality to Gay, Lesbian and Bisexual Seniors. Human Rights Campaign Foundation Report; 2004.
9. **Lerner D**. Why we support same-sex marriage: a response from over 450 clergy. New England Law Review. 2004;38:527-32.
10. **Kurdek L, Schmitt JP**. Relationship quality of partners in heterosexual married, heterosexual cohabiting, and gay and lesbian relationships. J Pers Soc Psychol. 1986;51:711-20.
11. **Kurdek LA**. Relationship outcomes and their predictors: longitudinal evidence from heterosexual married, gay cohabiting, and lesbian cohabiting couples. Journal of Marriage and the Family. 1998;60:553-68.
12. **Solomon SE, Rothblum ED, Balsam KF**. Pioneers in partnership: lesbian and gay male couples in civil unions compared with those not in civil unions and married heterosexual siblings. Journal of Family Psychology. 2004;18:275-86.

13. **Green RJ**. Risk and resilience in lesbian and gay couples: comment on Solomon, Rothblum, and Balsam (2004). Journal of Family Psychology. 2004;18:290-2.
14. **Lannutti PJ**. For better or worse: exploring the meanings of same-sex marriage within the lesbian, gay, bisexual and transgendered community. Journal of Social and Personal Relationships. 2005;22:5-18.
15. **Kurdek LA**. Are gay and lesbian cohabiting couples really different from heterosexual married couples? Journal of Marriage and Family. 2004;66:880-900.
16. **Rostosky SS, Riggle ED, Dudley MG, et al**. Commitment in same-sex relationships: a qualitative analysis of couples' conversations. Journal of Homosexuality. 2006;51: 199-223.
17. **Heck JE, Sell RL, Sheinfeld Gorin S**. Health care access among individuals involved in same-sex relationships. American Journal of Public Health. 2006;96:1111-8.
18. **Klausner J, Pollack L, Wong W, et al**. Same-sex domestic partnerships and lower-risk behaviors for STDs, including HIV infection. Journal of Homosexuality. 2006;51:137-43.
19. **Berg N, Lien D**. Measuring the effect of sexual orientation on income: evidence of discrimination? Contemporary Economic Policy. 2002;20:394-414.
20. **Badgett MVL**. Money, Myths, and Change: The Economic Lives of Lesbians and Gay Men. University of Chicago Press; 2001.
21. **Ash MA, Badgett MVL**. Separate and unequal: the effect of unequal access to employment-based health insurance on same-sex and unmarried different-sex couple. Contemporary Economic Policy. 2006;24:582-99.
22. **Kurdek LA**. Areas of conflict for gay, lesbian and heterosexual couples: what couples argue about influences relationship satisfaction. Journal of Marriage and the Family. 1994;56:923-34.
23. **Kurdek LA**. Conflict resolution styles in gay, lesbian, heterosexual nonparent, and heterosexual parent couples. Journal of Marriage and the Family. 1994;56:705-22.
24. **Gottman JM, Levenson RW, Swanson C, et al**. Observing gay, lesbian and heterosexual couples' relationships: mathematical modeling of conflict interaction. Journal of Homosexuality. 2003;45:65-91.
25. **Gottman JM, Levenson RW, Gross J, et al**. Correlates of gay and lesbian couples' relationship satisfaction and relationship dissolution. Journal of Homosexuality. 2003;45:23-43.
26. **Mackey RA, Diemer MA, O'Brien BA**. Relational factors in understanding satisfaction in the lasting relationships of same sex and heterosexual couples. Journal of Homosexuality. 2004;47:111-36.
27. **Burleson W**. Bi America: Myths, Truths, and Struggles of an Invisible Community. Haworth Press; 2005.
28. **Dobinson C**. Improving the access and quality of public health services for bisexuals: a position paper and resolution adopted by the Ontario Public Health Association (OPHA). Ontario Public Health Association; 2003.
29. **Erhardt VP**. Head Over Heels: Wives Who Stay with Cross-Dressers and Transsexuals. Haworth Press; 2007.
30. **Hernandez G**. Big gay love. The Advocate. May 22, 2006. Available at http://www.advocate.com.
31. **Adam B**. Care, intimacy and same-sex partnership in the 21st century. Current Sociology. 2004;52:265-79.
32. **Kleber DJ, Howell RJ, Tibbets-Kleber AL**. The impact of parental homosexuality in child custody cases: a review of the literature. Bulletin of the American Academy of Psychiatry and Law. 1986;14:81-7.
33. **Falk PJ**. Lesbian mothers: psychosocial assumptions in family law. American Psychologist. 1989;44:941-7.
34. **Martin A**. The Gay and Lesbian Parenting Handbook. HarperCollins; 1993.
35. **Gartrell N, Hamilton J, Banks A, et al**. The National Lesbian Family Study: interviews with prospective mothers. American Journal of Orthopsychiatry. 1996;66:272-81.

36. **Harakas M**. Gaby Boom. Chicago Tribune. June 12, 1998:7.

37. **Gottman JS**. Children of gay and lesbian parents. In: Bozett FW, Sussman MB, eds. Homosexuality and Family Relations. Haworth Press; 1990:177-96.

38. **Patterson CJ**. Children of lesbian and gay parents. Child Development. 1992;63:1025-42.

39. **Tasker F**. Lesbian mothers, gay fathers, and their children: a review. Journal of Development and Behavioral Pediatrics. 2005;26:224-40.

40. **Robertson JA**. Gay and lesbian access to assisted reproductive technology. Case Western Reserve Law Review. 2005;55.

41. **Henry V**. Personal communication; 2007.

42. **Ryan SD, Pearlmutter S, Groza V**. Coming out of the closet: opening agencies to gay and lesbian adoptive parents. Soc Work. 2004;49:85-95.

43. **Child Welfare Information Gateway**. Costs of adopting: fact sheets for families; 2004. Available at http://www.childwelfare.gov/pubs/s_cost/s_costb.cfm.

44. **Brodzinsky D, Patterson C, Vaziri M**. Adoption agency perspectives on lesbian and gay prospective parents: a national study. Adoption Quarterly. 2002;5:5-23.

45. **Howard J**. Expanding Resources for Children: Is Adoption by Gays and Lesbians Part of the Answer for Boys and Girls Who Need Homes? Evan B. Donaldson Adoption Institute; 2006.

46. **Brooks D, Goldberg S**. Gay and lesbian adoptive and foster care placements: can they meet the needs of waiting children? Social Work. 2001;46:147-57.

47. **Lynch JM**. Considerations of family structure and gender composition: the lesbian and gay stepfamily. Journal of Homosexuality. 2000;40:81-95.

48. **Lynch JM**. The identity transformation of biological parents in lesbian/gay stepfamilies. Journal of Homosexuality. 2004;47:91-107.

49. **Fredriksen KI**. Family caregiving responsibilities among lesbians and gay men. Social Work. 1999;44:142-55.

50. **Patterson CJ**. Lesbian and gay parents and their children: summary of research findings. Available at http://www.apa.org/pi/lgbc/publications/lgpsummary.html.

51. **Lambert S**. Gay and lesbian families: what we know and where to go from here, The Family Journal. 2005;13:43-51.

52. **Gartrell N, Banks A, Hamilton J, et al**. The National Lesbian Family Study: interviews with mothers of toddlers. American Journal of Orthopsychiatry. 1999;69:362-9.

53. **Gartrell N, Rodas C, Deck A, et al**. The USA National Lesbian Family Study: interviews with mothers of 10-year-olds. Feminism & Psychology. 2006;16:175.

54. **Chan R, Raboy B, Patterson, CJ**. Psychosocial adjustment among children conceived via donor insemination by lesbian and heterosexual mothers. Child Development. 1998;69:443-57.

55. **Wainright JL, Russell ST, Patterson CJ**. Psychosocial adjustment, school outcomes, and romantic relationships of adolescents with same-sex parents. Child Development. 2004;75:1886-98.

56. **Patterson CJ**. Family relationships of lesbians and gay men. Journal of Marriage and Family. 2000;62:1052-69.

57. **Perrin E**. Technical report of the Committee on Psychosocial Aspects of Child and Family Health: coparent or second-parent adoption by same-sex parents. Pediatrics. 2002;109:341-4.

58. **Stevenson MR**. Public policy, homosexuality, and the sexual coercion of children. Journal of Psychology & Human Sexuality. 2000;12(4):1-19.

59. **Finkelhor D**. The international epidemiology of child sexual abuse. Child Abuse & Neglect. May 1994;18:409-17

60. **Jenny C, Roesler TA, Poyer KL**. Are children at risk for sexual abuse by homosexuals? Pediatrics. 1994;94:41-4.

61. **Pawelski JG, Perrin EC, Foy JM, et al**. The effects of marriage, civil union, and domestic partnership laws on the health and well-being of children. Pediatrics. 2006;118:349.

62. **Clarke V, Kitzinger C, Potter J**. 'Kids are just cruel anyway': lesbian and gay parents' talk about homophobic bullying. Br J Soc Psychol. 2004;43:531-50.

63. **Gartrell N, Banks A, Reed N, et al**. The National Lesbian Family Study: interviews with mothers of five-year-olds. American Journal of Orthopsychiatry. 2000;70:542-8.

64. **Gartrell N, Deck A, Rodas C, et al**. The National Lesbian Family Study: interviews with the 10-year-old children. American Journal of Orthopsychiatry. 2005;75:518-24.

65. Anonymous comments from a child at a conference at Family Pride Week.

66. **Stacey J, Biblarz, TJ**. (How) does the sexual orientation of parents matter? American Sociological Review. 2001;66:159-83.

67. **Gershon T, Tschann JM, Jemerin JM**. Stigmatization, self-esteem, and coping among the adolescent children of lesbian mothers. Journal of Adolescent Health. 1999;24:437-45.

68. **Golombok S, Tasker F**. Do parents influence the sexual orientation of their children? Findings from a longitudinal study of lesbian families. Developmental Psychology. 1996;32:3-11.

69. **Bailey JM, Bobrow D, Wolfe M, et al**. Sexual orientation of adult sons of gay fathers. Developmental Psychology. 1995;31:124-9.

70. **Tasker F, Golombok S**. Adults raised as children in lesbian families. American Journal of Orthopsychiatry. 1995;65:203-15.

71. Personal communication to the author from a lesbian mother regarding her eight-year-old daughter.

72. **Garner A**. Silent panic: the impact of HIV/AIDS on children of gay parents. In: Families Like Mine: Children of Gay Parents Tell It Like It Is. HarperCollins; 2004:145-67.

73. **Garner A**. Children of LGBT parents: growing up under scrutiny. In: Families Like Mine: Children of Gay Parents Tell It Like It Is. HarperCollins; 2004:13-37.

74. **Garner A**. Second generation: queer kids of LGBT parents. In: Families Like Mine: Children of Gay Parents Tell It Like It Is. HarperCollins; 2004:168-92.

75. **Patterson CJ, Hurt S, Mason C**. Families of the lesbian baby boom: children's contact with grandparents and other adults. American Journal of Orthopsychiatry. 1998;68:390-9.

76. **Perlesz A, Brown R, Lindsay J, et al**. Family in transition: parents, children and grand-parents in lesbian families give meaning to "doing family." Journal of Family Therapy. 2006;28:175-99.

77. Quoted from the title page of the COLAGE Web site: http://www.colage.org/

Chapter 6

Late Adulthood and Aging: Clinical Approaches

JONATHAN S. APPELBAUM, MD, FACP,
AAHIVS

Introduction

With the aging of the "baby boomer" generation (those born between 1940-1960) there will be a dramatic increase in the number of adults age 65 and older living in the United States. In the year 2004, there were 36.3 million adults 65 and older; by 2030, this segment of the population will nearly double to 71.5 million.[1] The proportion of Americans adults age 65 and over will also rise markedly, from one in eight in 2004, to one in five by 2030.[1] Due to a lack of population research on all lesbian, gay, bisexual, and transgender (LGBT) persons, there is no exact data on the size of the LGBT elder population. However, if an estimated five percent of the general population is LGBT, then close to two million LGBT elders are living in the United States today. Despite their substantial numbers, LGBT elders are often "invisible" to others who matter, particularly healthcare providers and social service agencies. A fear of discrimination causes many older LGBT adults to hide their sexual orientation from their providers, while a lack of training for clinicians ensures that LGBT issues and concerns remain unspoken during the clinical encounter. The following chapter aims to provide clinicians with a better understanding of the social and health issues facing LGBT elders so they are better prepared to offer sensitive care that is supportive of their older LGBT patients. It includes clinical information pertinent to the care of aging and elderly LGBT individuals, based on the research that currently exists, and provides some context for the social and cultural aspects of the lives of LGBT elders.

Demographics and Socioeconomic Status

There is little data on the racial/ethnic and socioeconomic diversity of LGBT elders, although some evidence suggests that the racial composition of the LGBT elder population is at least as diverse as the heterosexual population.[2] The overall financial status of older Americans has generally improved, although poverty rates are higher among African-Americans and Hispanic Americans. Some studies have suggested that older homosexual men and women have a greater likelihood of living in poverty than their heterosexual counterparts; this may be because older gays and lesbians are more likely to live alone and are less likely to have family support.[3] Anecdotal reports have suggested that transgender elders are also more likely to suffer from economic disadvantage, but there is no data to support this.[3]

Some evidence suggests that sexual minorities are more likely to live in urban rather than rural areas. Exit polling data from the Voter News Service in the 1990s found that 8.8% of voters that reside in large cities self identified as gay, lesbian or bisexual, compared to 3.7% of voters in suburbs and 2.3% of voters in rural areas.[2] Because people in non-urban areas may be less likely to report their sexual orientation as gay or lesbian, the density of LGB people in these areas may be larger than the data suggests.[3] It is likely that the same holds true for transgender people, but there is no evidence to support this.

Gay and lesbian elders appear to be more likely to live alone than heterosexuals of the same age. A 1999 study of lesbian and gay elders in New York City found that 65% of survey respondents lived by themselves.[4] In comparison, only 36% of all people 65 and over in NYC are thought to live alone. This same study found that less than 20% of respondents reported living with a life partner, as opposed to about 50% of heterosexuals.[4] A study conducted in Los Angeles found that 75% of gay and lesbian elders lived alone.[5] According to census data analyses, the proportion of same-sex couples that includes a partner 65 years old or older is greater than one in 10, and nearly one in four same-sex couples includes a partner 55 and older.[6]

It is important to note that although a majority of lesbian and gay seniors do not live with partners or family members, it cannot be assumed that they are lonely. In fact, several studies have suggested that loneliness among older gay men and lesbians is less common than once thought.[3,7,8] Many LGBT elders derive social and emotional support from a rich network of friends and partners and have learned coping skills to deal with isolation. In addition, many older LGBT individuals have family members, including children and grandchildren, as well as siblings, that provide support and comfort.

In general, most elders in the US still live in homes and apartments, but more are choosing assisted living facilities. The number of seniors living in nursing homes remains stable at 4.5% for those over 65, but rises to 18.2% for people over 85.[1] With changes in acute care hospitalization leading to shorter lengths of stay, many more seniors spend some time in nursing homes, generally after discharge from a hospital.[9] In recent years, LGBT groups have begun discussing and planning long-term care, assisted living facilities, and other housing for LGBT elders. For example, Stonewall Communities (http://www.stonewallcommunities.com), a Boston-based advocacy organization, is developing a residential community of 66 condominiums for older gay men and lesbians and other active older people. The facilities will offer staffing, preventive health services, and common dining rooms.

Growing Older

As with other populations, LGBT elders tend to live out their senior years much as they did their middle years. Life experience and peer influence are more of an influence on adjustment to aging than sexual orientation.[3] However, research has shown that some gay men feel "old" at an earlier age than their biological age.[10] The perception of being "too old," often described as internalized ageism, can start as early as 30[7] and may be related to the emphasis on physical attractiveness and youth in the gay culture. Lesbians tend to approach aging differently, often with a greater sense of freedom and fulfillment. They tend to have a wider circle of friends and family than gay men.[3,10]

Some sociologists suggest that LGBT persons are better prepared for aging than their heterosexual counterparts because they have already learned to cope with life challenges and crises. By having dealt with discrimination, loss of friends and partners to AIDS, and other issues, it is thought that LGBT elders have the skills to overcome challenges related to aging.[8] Gay men and lesbians may also be better prepared for aging, having had to take more responsibility for their needs earlier in their life and being less disrupted by life-stage changes.[11]

Coming of Age Before and After the Gay Liberation Movement

The majority of LGBT elders grew up in a social climate that was highly intolerant of homosexuality. Older LGBT Americans can be seen as divided into two age cohorts, depending on whether they came of age before or after the beginning of the modern LGBT liberation movement (commonly marked as the 1969 protest event in New York City known as Stonewall).[12] Those who were born before World War II can be considered part of the *pre-Stonewall* generation, a time of widespread discrimination against LGBT people. Prior to the Stonewall uprising, there was no organized movement to protect the civil rights of LGBT persons, and there were few places for LGBT people to go for support. Those who grew up in this era often coped with their environment by keeping their sexual orientation private. Many married, had children, and did not come out as LGBT until later in life. Among those who dared to live more openly, many were subject to isolation, violence, and overt discrimination in housing, healthcare, and work. Even today, some LGBT people from this generation continue to hide their sexuality from others, and some maintain a deep mistrust of social service agencies and healthcare providers.

A 2004 article by the *Boston Globe* on the elderly in the LGBT community provided a short profile of a 63-year-old man that illustrates how some gay men and lesbians from this generation integrate their sexual identities with their private and public lives. This man, whom the article calls "Phil," has lived with his male partner for 27 years in a house in a western suburb of Boston. The partners had dated for two years prior to moving in together as a couple. Although Phil says he's "not in hiding" about his sexuality, he has also not "come out" to his family, to his friends from church, or to the veteran's community in which he is involved. The article quotes him as saying: "I'm from a generation where most of my contemporaries would be uncomfortable with it pushed in their faces. And I don't want anyone to feel uncomfortable."[13]

In contrast to Phil and his contemporaries, those considered part of the *Stonewall generation,* now in their 50s and early 60s, are more likely to have lived a greater part of their lives more openly. The HIV epidemic has had a profound effect on this group, however, due to the great loss of friends and partners to this disease, as well as the spirit of activism and advocacy inspired by it. As the Stonewall generation retire and age, they are more likely to seek services (such as long-term care facilities) and rights (such as domestic partner caregiving privileges) that are supportive of the LGBT population.[3]

Patient-Provider Communication

For LGBT individuals from the pre-Stonewall era, discrimination in healthcare was common. Many experienced overt acts of discrimination by healthcare professionals, and some were forced into outmoded psychiatric treatments to attempt to convert them to heterosexuality. It took a long time for the medical profession to recognize and accept alternative lifestyles. Until 1973, the *Diagnostic and Statistical Manual of Mental Disorders* regarded homosexuality as a pathology. Not surprisingly, many older LGBT patients, although certainly not all, continue to perceive the healthcare system and healthcare providers as unwelcoming and intolerant. Fearing discrimination, these LGBT seniors may hide their sexual orientation from their providers or decide not to access health services at all.[14] Even if they are out in their social life, older LGBT patients may remain in the closet to their healthcare provider. A consequence is that providers, including therapists, physicians, nurses, social workers, and case managers often will not realize a patient is LGBT. The invisibility of older LGBT patients to their providers further marginalizes this population and increases disparities in healthcare.

Disclosure of sexual orientation and behavior to providers, however, is critical for good health. Nondisclosure can lead to inappropriate preventive care and screening recommendations, as well as negatively affect the patient-provider rapport so important to quality healthcare. But patients will only disclose their sexuality if they feel safe doing so. Being comfortable with their provider is seen as the most important issue faced by gay men. They look for a primary care clinician who is open and relatively nonreactive to their sexual orientation.[15] Open communication with patients where no assumptions are made; intake forms that encourage reporting of the full range of sexual identity and expression; and posters and brochures that include and celebrate LGBT communities can help ensure that LGBT patients will feel safe (see Chapters 1 and 15 for more on creating a welcoming environment).

Coming Out

Providers may find that some of their older patients are in the process of coming out as LGBT. This sometimes occurs after children have grown and left the home, or after the illness or death of a spouse. It is important for healthcare providers to recognize this transition and to be as supportive as possible. For older men, ageism within the gay community (a focus on youth, attractiveness, body building) may make socializing more difficult and may increase a sense of isolation. Healthy role models and social organizations such as Prime Timers (http://www.primetimersworldwide .org) and OLE (Older Lesbian Energy) are available, but mostly only in urban areas. Health issues and infirmity among the elderly can also make coming out more difficult. To help with the process of coming out, some LGBT elders may benefit from counseling or other referrals. Appendix A provides a list of further resources that clinicians can access in helping make referrals for their LGBT elder patients.

Finally, it is important to realize that some people who have sexual relations with others of the same sex, or have sexual desires to be with someone of the same sex, do not desire to "come out" as gay, bisexual, or lesbian. Eventually some who engage in same-sex behavior will begin to describe themselves as gay, but others, particularly those from minority communities, do not choose to identify with the gay or lesbian culture or community.

Health Issues for LGBT Elders

Research on health maintenance and medical issues for older LGBT is scarce. Even the most current version of the American Geriatrics Society's *Geriatrics Review Syllabus* does not mention gay or lesbian health issues.[16] Unfortunately, this lack of attention to LGBT health is common among all medical specialties.[17] It is true that LGBT elders can suffer from all the usual geriatric syndromes of incontinence, falls, and cognitive impairment and need the same health promotion and maintenance as their heterosexual counterparts; however, there are certain issues that require particular attention in LGBT patients due to differential risk factors in these communities (as explained below). In addition, older LGBT people may be more susceptible to poor health due to the stresses associated with long-term concealment of sexual identity and many years of exposure to discrimination. Studies suggest that nondisclosure of sexual orientation can be associated with lower life satisfaction, lower self-esteem, depression and suicide, substance abuse, delay in seeking medical treatment, and increase in risk of illness.[14,18]

Finally, there is a tendency to stereotype older people as being sexless and teetotalers; these are dangerous misconceptions. Taking a history of sexual practices and substance use and providing relevant risk reduction counseling remains a critical part of care for the older population, including those who are LGBT.

Preventive Care for Older Gay and Bisexual Men

Older gay and bisexual men require the same preventive healthcare as their heterosexual peers, but with particular attention to several issues. More on preventive healthcare can be found in Chapter 7.

Sexual Health
It is important to address sexual function and sexual health in the older gay and bisexual male. Providers sometimes feel uncomfortable discussing sexual issues with their patients, particularly those who are old enough to be their parents or even grandparents. However, the majority of men over 50 can benefit greatly from regular sexual history-taking and risk reduction counseling. This is particularly true since few safer sex community outreach and education programs target the older population. Suggestions on how to talk with patients about their sexual history and provide effective risk reduction counseling can be found in Chapter 15.

Screening for HIV and other sexually transmitted infections.
Sexually active men who have sex with men (MSM) need to be routinely assessed for gonorrhea, chlamydia, syphilis, herpes simplex virus (HSV),

and human papillomavirus (HPV). HIV risk assessment should be done at the same time as other sexually transmitted infections (STIs), and the Centers for Disease Control (CDC) has recently recommended that HIV testing be a regular part of primary care.[19] With the advent of rapid testing, HIV tests (CLIA-waived) can now be done in the office, but positive tests need to be confirmed with a Western Blot Test. There are new DNA ligand techniques that allow urine samples to be collected and screened for gonorrhea and chlamydia. Depending on sexual practices, samples for gonorrhea and chlamydia screening may be obtained from anal and urethral sites, and from oral sites for gonorrhea. There is not an FDA-approved culture for chlamydia from oral and rectal sites, but some laboratories are beginning to use validated nucleic acid amplification tests (NAATs) of rectal swab specimens.[20] Routine HSV titers are not advised since many asymptomatic men have had prior exposure. Culture of suspected active lesions is a better test for active herpes virus infection. Many urban areas of the country have reported an increase in syphilis infection among MSM; therefore, routine screening of syphilis is recommended. As of this writing, the CDC does not recommend routine anal Pap tests to detect human papillomavirus (HPV)-related lesions; nonetheless, there is growing evidence that HPV disease poses a significant health risk for MSM, and many experts recommend performing yearly anal Pap smears on HIV-infected men and screening HIV-uninfected MSM who engage in receptive anal sex every two to three years. See Figure 6-1 for a risk assessment and screening flowchart. For detailed information on STI and HIV screening, see Chapter 11.

Sexual function

- *Erectile dysfunction* may be more common as men age. With direct to consumer advertising of PDE5 inhibitors, more men are willing to bring up this issue. A careful history, physical exam and directed lab studies should be done before these drugs are prescribed. Questions to ask include: Is the problem with erections (getting or maintaining) or with libido or with both? What other medications is the patient taking (prescribed and recreational), and what are the potential drug-drug interactions if prescribed a PDE5 inhibitor? Does the patient smoke or have diabetes, and is there evidence of vascular disease? The physical examination should include looking for hair distribution and testicular size. Lab examination should include prostate-specific antigen (PSA), free testosterone, thyroid-stimulating hormone (TSH), glucose, and some evaluation of pituitary function, such as prolactin. For treatment of erectile dysfunction, there are three currently approved PDE5 inhibitors. All function through similar mechanisms and differ only by onset and duration of action. Many patients prefer one to the other. All PDE5 inhibitors interact with HIV protease inhibitors as well as nitrates (nitroglycerin, isosorbide, and poppers)

Health Screening for Men who have Sex with Men

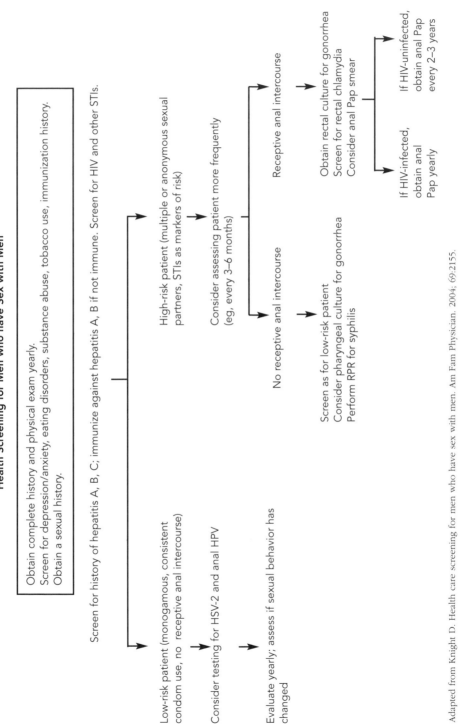

Adapted from Knight D. Health care screening for men who have sex with men. Am Fam Physician. 2004; 69:2155.

Figure 6-1   Suggested Approach to Health Screening for Men who have Sex with Men

and alpha-blockers, which can cause hypotension. For these reasons, the lowest possible dose of PDE5 inhibitors should be used.

- *Hypogonadism* is a problem in up to 20% of men over age 60 and up to 40% of men with diabetes. After careful evaluation to exclude prostate cancer, replacement therapy with physiologic doses of testosterone is appropriate. Several formulations are available including injections, transdermal patches, and topical gels. It is important to monitor and follow up patients who receive testosterone replacement therapy. Testosterone replacement does not cause prostate cancer but may unmask an indolent one. In fact lower serum levels of testosterone are associated with higher incidence of prostate cancer.[21]

Cardiovascular Health

Cardiovascular disease, despite a decline in incidence, still kills more men than cancer. Because gay men have an increased rate of recreational drug use and smoking,[22] attention to the traditional cardiovascular risk factors is important. Smoking cessation is paramount and the use of methods such as support groups, nicotine replacement products, bupropion and other medications, hypnosis, and acupuncture should be mentioned in counseling patients to stop smoking. Following blood pressure targets (below 135/85; treat hypertensive patients to a blood pressure of under 130/80) is also key, as is strict attention to the National Cholesterol Education Program-III (NCEP-III) guidelines[23] for cholesterol management.

Sexual dysfunction from antihypertensive medications is a side effect that should be mentioned and inquired about with each visit. Some medications such as calcium channel blockers may cause less sexual dysfunction, and PDE5 inhibitors may be used to counteract the erectile dysfunction caused by antihypertensive medication. Management of diabetes is beyond the scope of this chapter, but treatment goals should be a HgbA1C of under seven percent. Attention to microvascular complications of diabetes may prevent macrovascular disease.

Prostate Health

Although there are no data on the incidence of prostate cancer in gay men, it is possible that gay men's higher rates of anabolic and androgenic steroids use puts them at increased risk for prostate cancer. Screening may reduce mortality from prostate cancer, but there is not sufficient evidence to support this. Generally, the recommendation is to perform a digital rectal exam annually for men over age 50, and earlier for those at higher risk of prostate cancer (African American, one first-degree relative or two second-degree relatives with prostate cancer). The American Urologic Society and the American Cancer Society advise yearly prostate-specific antigen (PSA) testing, but the American College of Physicians does not recommend this test. The absolute value of the PSA may be important, but in younger men (less than 50) with prostate cancer, the PSA may be within the normal range. PSA velocity (the rate of rise of the PSA over time) is more useful for estimating risk, and urologists advise that a rise in PSA of greater than 0.75ng/mL in a year should be evaluated further. All patients with an abnormal rectal examination or elevated PSA levels should be referred to a urologist who might recommend ultrasound guided prostate biopsies.

Treatment of prostate cancer is beyond the scope of this chapter. However, it should be noted that gay and bisexual men may experience the social, emotional, and sexual function effects of prostate cancer and its treatments differently than heterosexual men.[24] For example, the gay patient may be more concerned about how the removal of the prostate could affect sexual response during anal sex. Internet support groups for gay men with prostate cancer and their partners are available (for example: http://www.malecare.com).

Benign prostatic hypertrophy may be less common among gay men than bisexual or heterosexual men (personal observation). Alpha-blockers and finasteride are appropriate treatments, but it is important to be aware of the potential interaction between alpha-blockers and PDE5 inhibitors, which can cause marked hypotension. Finasteride may cause sexual dysfunction but can be taken with PDE5 inhibitors.

Anal Health

For gay and bisexual men who engage in receptive anal intercourse, the anus is a sexual organ, and its dysfunction can cause the patient great distress. Anal fissures and hemorrhoids are common in gay men and are treated per usual recommendations: stool softeners, astringents, hydrocortisone creams, and suppositories. Occasionally these conditions require surgery. Proctitis is commonly associated with STIs such as chlamydia and gonorrhea. Lymphogranuloma venereum (LGV), also caused by *Chlamydia trachomatis*, may manifest as proctocolitis or inflammatory involvement of perirectal or perianal lymphatic tissues resulting in fistulas and strictures. LGV is rare in the United States, but in the last few years there has been an increase in case reports among gay urban men. Severe anal pain with urinary retention most commonly represents an acute anorectal HSV infection and should be documented by culture and then treated promptly with antiviral medication such as acyclovir.

HIV/AIDS

HIV disease remains a major health concern for older gay and bisexual men. In the 33 states with confidential name-based HIV reporting in 2005, there were an estimated 116 085 persons aged 50 and over living with HIV/AIDS. Of these, 5938 were newly diagnosed cases.[25] These numbers do not include the estimated 25% of HIV-infected people who do not know they are infected. In all age categories, including those over 50, black and Hispanic men are disproportionately affected by HIV/AIDS.[25]

The most common mode of HIV transmission in the US continues to be male-to-male sexual contact.[25] This is likely true for older adults, although it is not well studied. In a study of HIV-infected patients seen at a major urban hospital who were over age 60 at diagnosis, 38% had acquired HIV through sexual contact and 16% through injection drug use. Many also had serologic evidence of other sexually acquired diseases.[26]

Older patients tend to be diagnosed with AIDS much later in the course of the infection, primarily because the diagnosis was never considered and because older people are less likely to get tested. HIV/AIDS-related symptoms and diseases can be easily mistaken for other problems typically seen in older persons. In addition, because aging naturally weakens the immune system, and comorbidities are more likely to exist, AIDS may progress more rapidly in older persons. According to CDC estimates in 2001, only 70% of persons over 65 survived for more than 12 months after an AIDS diagnosis, versus 91% of persons aged 40-44.[25] At the same time, those over 50 who take antiretroviral medications seem to do just as well as younger persons.

Prevention of HIV transmission in older male patients requires clinicians to obtain a comprehensive sexual and substance use history, provide counseling on safer sex practices, and offer information on the use of HIV post-exposure prophylaxis (PEP). Currently the CDC recommends giving PEP (anti-HIV drugs administered to prevent infection in persons exposed to HIV after unprotected sex), as long as the treatment is begun no less than 72 hours of exposure, and preferably within 48 hours. Generally regimens that consist of two drugs are recommended.[27] Repeated exposures of this nature strongly suggest a need for counseling and educational interventions.

Cancer Risk

Gay and bisexual men may be at higher risk for certain cancers. The risks and benefits of screening should be discussed with the patient.

Anal cancer: The incidence of anal cancer among straight men is 0.8/100 000. In HIV-uninfected gay men the incidence rises to 35/100 000 and in HIV-infected gay men it approaches 70/100 000. This incidence approaches the historic levels of cervical cancer in women before the widespread use of the Pap smear. Anal cancer, like cervical cancer, is thought to be caused by infection with human papillomavirus (HPV); risk factors for anal cancer include receptive anal intercourse, number of lifetime sexual partners, and rectal insertion of recreational drugs.[28]

Lung and colon cancer: Due to increased rates of smoking and less frequent screening (colon cancer).[29]

Liver cancer: Due to a higher incidence of Hepatitis B infection.

Kaposi's sarcoma: Due to a higher incidence of HIV infection.

Prostate cancer: Although there are no data on the incidence of prostate cancer in gay and bisexual men, in the general population, prostate cancer is the 2nd leading cause of cancer deaths in men. Among gay couples, there is a 28% chance that one partner will be diagnosed with prostate cancer and a 3% chance that both partners will get the disease.[30] Risk factors include family history, African-American race, high fat diet, and possible infection.[31]

Other cancers: Lymphoma and other cancers may also be higher among those with HIV infection and may appear relatively early in the course of the illness.

Eating Disorders and Body Image

Eating disorders[32] and body image dissatisfaction[33] may be more common among gay and bisexual men than among heterosexual men. The higher risk for these disorders in the gay community is thought to be related to the emphasis on physical attractiveness that is based on the desire to attract other men. A screening tool for eating disorders can be found in Chapter 8.

See Table 6-1 for a summary of screening and history topics for gay and bisexual men.

Preventive Care for Older Lesbians

There is good evidence that lesbians of all ages receive less preventive care, access healthcare services less often, and enter the healthcare system later than heterosexual women.[34,35] Throughout the lifecourse, lesbians can face significant barriers in accessing appropriate healthcare. Women of child-bearing age tend to be asked about contraception and counseled about use of male barrier protection without consideration for sexual practices. Older women may be treated as sexually inactive. Incorrect assumptions may result in a failure to screen for cervical cancer, domestic abuse, and STIs.

Table 6-1   History and Screening Topics for Men who have Sex with Men

- Safer sex practices (use of condoms, sexual risk level)
- History of and risk for HIV, STIs. Past history of screening for these diseases
- History of and risk for testicular, prostate, colon, and anal cancer. Past history of screening for these diseases
- History of hepatitis A, B, C. History of immunization against hepatitis A and B; immunize if needed
- History of and risk for human papillomavirus infection and anal cancer. Risks and benefits of anal Pap smear
- Tobacco use and smoking cessation
- Substance use: alcohol and recreational drugs such as crystal meth
- Nutrition; weight management if needed; screen for eating disorders
- Exercise
- Screening for depression and/or anxiety

Adapted from: Ten things gay men should discuss with their health care providers. Gay and Lesbian Medical Association; 2006. Available at http://www.glma.org. Click on *Resources for Patients*; then click on "Ten things to discuss with your healthcare provider."

Clinicians can promote better healthcare for their female patients by keeping in mind that:

- Some women are sexually active with both men and women, even if they do not identify as bisexual.
- Sexual identity and behavior can change over time. For example, a woman who identifies as a lesbian and currently has sex exclusively with women, may have had sex with men in the past, or may do so in the future.
- Many lesbians have children and grandchildren, both biological and adopted, or desire and plan to have children in the future.

Older lesbian and bisexual women require the same preventive healthcare as their heterosexual peers, but with particular attention to several issues. More on preventive healthcare can be found in Chapter 7.

Coronary Heart Disease

Coronary heart disease (CHD) is the number one killer of women in the United States and therefore is likely the primary health threat for lesbians. Lesbians and bisexual women may in fact be at increased risk for CHD due to higher rates of smoking and obesity. Although CHD is commonly considered a man's disease, 25% of women over 65 have CHD, and women over 60 develop CHD at the same rate as men. In the course of a lifetime, a woman is ten times more likely to get CHD than breast cancer. Therefore, prevention of CHD in women should be as important as getting regular mammograms.[36]

Modifiable risk factors for CHD in lesbians and bisexual women include:

- **Cigarette smoking**: Studies suggest that lesbians have a higher rate of smoking than heterosexual women. The National Lesbian Health Care Survey found that about 30% of lesbians smoke[37] compared to about 23% of all women in the United States. In the Women's Health Initiative, a study of women 50-79 years old, twice as many lesbians reported themselves to be heavy smokers compared with heterosexual women.[38] It is important to provide counseling and referrals for smoking cessation programs (see Appendix A for smoking cessation resources). After smoking cessation, the risk for CHD falls within three to five years to baseline (however, the risk for lung cancer takes longer to drop).
- **Hypertension**: Reducing blood pressure into the normal range will decrease cardiovascular risk in women to the same extent as it does in men. Isolated systolic hypertension is primarily a disease of older women and is a cause of stroke as well as myocardial infarction. It is important to stress lifestyle changes such as weight reduction, salt

restriction, adequate potassium, calcium and magnesium intake, and reduction in alcohol intake.

- **Lipids**: Elevated lipids in women carry the same risk of CHD as in men. Current NCEP-III guidelines for treatment, based on low-density lipoprotein (LDL) level should be followed.

- **Diabetes mellitus**: Diabetes is a more important CHD risk factor in women than in men, and negates the later age of onset of CHD in women.[39]

- **Obesity**: Obesity is an independent CHD risk factor for women. Lesbians and bisexual women, on average, have a higher body mass index (BMI) than heterosexual women. In the Nurse's Health Study, risk for CHD was over three times higher among women with a BMI > 29, and even a moderate increase in BMI (25-28.9) was associated with a doubling of CHD risk.[40]

- **Sedentary lifestyle**: Active women have a lower risk of CHD compared to sedentary women.

- **Nonmodifiable risk factors for CHD** include age over 65, African-American race, family history of CHD, and lower socioeconomic status.

Cancer

Breast and cervical cancer screening rates have historically been lower among lesbians than heterosexual women. Recent findings from the Boston Lesbian Health Project II suggest that lesbians have increased their use of Pap smear screening and mammography, but still have not yet reached the same rate of screening as heterosexual women. In addition, lesbians continue to engage in behaviors, such as smoking and alcohol consumption, that put them at greater risk for certain cancers.[41]

Cervical cancer: Lesbians are at risk for cervical cancer and should be screened accordingly. Surveys from self-identified lesbians show that 70% have had penile-vaginal intercourse (6% within the past year), 17% have had an abnormal Pap smear, and 17% have had anal intercourse.[42] Some professional groups suggest that cervical Pap smear screening can be stopped at a certain age, but there is no consensus about this. The current recommendations are:

1. United States Preventive Services Task Force: screening may stop at age 65 if the woman has had recent normal Pap smears and is not at high risk for cervical cancer.[43]

2. American Geriatrics Society: screen at one to three year intervals to age 70, then screening may be discontinued.[44]

3. American Cancer Society: women 70 and older may elect to stop cervical Pap smear screening if they have had three consecutive normal

Pap smears and no history of abnormal Pap smears in the preceding ten years.[45]

4. American College of Obstetricians and Gynecologists: individual assessment based on risk factors and examination.[46]

Breast cancer: The primary risk factor for breast cancer is age; other risks include family history, increase in body mass, and nulliparity. Despite the presumption that the latter two factors may put lesbians at higher risk for breast cancer, there is no prospective study that shows an increased risk of breast cancer in lesbian women. Current recommendations are that lesbians receive screening according to routine guidelines.

Lung cancer: As discussed above, evidence suggests that lesbians smoke more than heterosexual women. Because smoking is still the major risk factor for lung cancer, both medical and behavioral methods for smoking cessation can benefit patients (see Appendix A for smoking cessation resources).

Ovarian cancer: Nulliparity is a risk factor for ovarian cancer, although it is important to remember that many lesbians have given birth. Family history of ovarian cancer, breast cancer, or genetic markers such as BRCA1 and BRCA2, are important indicators for high-risk patients. Ovarian cancer screening should be done routinely along with cervical exams and Pap smears.

Osteoporosis

Risk factors for development of osteoporosis include age, estrogen deficiency, smoking, family background, sedentary life style, inadequate calcium intake, and inadequate vitamin D intake. There is no data on the incidence of osteoporosis in lesbians; however some of these risk factors are seen more commonly in lesbians. Screening for risk factors, providing nutritional counseling, performing bone mineral density testing, and providing treatment to those patients who fit treatment criteria is crucial.[47]

Safer Sex for Lesbians

As noted above, many lesbians and bisexual women have been sexually active with both women and men. Therefore, taking a complete sexual history and providing sensitive risk reduction counseling is recommended (see Chapter 15). Lesbian and bisexual women can develop the same STIs as heterosexual women. In addition, lesbians have a higher incidence of bacterial vaginosis, and women can transmit candidiasis and trichomonas vaginalis to their female partners. The use of barriers ("dental dams") is recommended for oral-vaginal and oral-anal contact. Chapter 11 provides more information on STIs in lesbians and bisexual women.

See Table 6-2 for a summary of screening and history topics for lesbian and bisexual women.

Table 6-2   History and Screening Topics for Lesbians and Bisexual Women

- History of and risk for coronary heart disease; screen blood pressure, cholesterol, risk for diabetes
- History of and risk for breast cancer; mammogram for women over age 40, and earlier if a family history
- History of and risk for cervical and ovarian cancer; Pap smear and pelvic exam
- Screening for depression and/or anxiety
- Nutrition; weight management if needed;screen for eating disorders
- Exercise
- Tobacco use and smoking cessation
- Domestic violence
- Substance abuse, particularly alcohol
- Osteoporosis

Adapted from: Ten things Lesbians should discuss with their health care providers. Gay and Lesbian Medical Association; 2006. Available at http://www.glma.org. Click on *Resources for Patients*; then click on "Ten things to discuss with your healthcare provider."

Preventive Care for Older Transgender Patients

While there has been little research on the healthcare of older gay and lesbian patients, there is even less known about transgender health and the particular challenges of caring for older transgender patients. It is clear, however, that transgender people face multiple barriers to attaining appropriate healthcare. Many transgender people lack health insurance or have insurance programs that do not cover healthcare related to transgender issues, including hormone treatments. The consequence is that many transgender people use "black market" hormones, lack preventive care, and have unmet mental healthcare needs. For all of these reasons, it is crucial that clinicians be sensitive and responsive to the needs of transgender patients.

As transgender patients age, they may be more likely to encounter health issues that correspond to their biological sex; these patients may feel additional stress in coping with a disease or condition associated with the gender they have left behind. The following patient case illustrates the complexities that can arise when caring for an older transgender patient, and highlights the need for sensitive care that respects the privacy of the patient.

"Sarah Johnson" is a 60-year-old transgender woman who, at the age of 30, had both "top" (breast augmentation) and "bottom" (removal of the penis and testicles and construction of a vagina) surgery. Sarah was fortunate to have been brought up in a supportive culture and had a successful career and a happy marriage with her second husband. Her husband was not aware of her biological sex. During a routine care visit, she complained of frequent hematuria, thought to be recurrent urinary tract infections. As part of her examination, her physician felt a large anterior mass on rectal examination. Her PSA came back 256 (normal range 0-4.0 ng/mL). With the help of a supportive primary care provider and medical oncology team, this patient underwent successful radiation treatment and now has an undetectable PSA a year after diagnosis. Her husband remains unaware of the primary source of her cancer.[48]

Health Issues for Older Transgender Patients

Disease prevention and health education are key for transgender patients, who are often marginalized by society. Below is a brief list of health issues to consider when caring for transgender patients.[49] For more detailed information on the medical, surgical, and mental healthcare of transgender persons, see Chapters 12 and 13.

- **HIV/STIs**: Male-to-female (MTF) transgender persons who engage in sex work and injection drug use are at high risk for STIs and HIV. A San Francisco study found that 35% of MTF respondents were HIV-infected, with African Americans having a higher rate of HIV infection.[50]
- **Hepatitis C**: Because of the high rate of shared needles (black market hormones, cosmetic silicone injections, and drug use), transgender persons are considered at risk for hepatitis C, although the number of HCV positive transgender persons is unknown.
- **Improper hormone use**: Either due to black market use by patients or provider ignorance, many transgender persons receive improper hormone doses.
- **Sex reassignment**: For a variety of reasons, including prohibitive cost, very few transgender persons go through complete sex reassignment surgery.
- **Adverse effects from the use of hormones and other medications**: Estrogen has the potential to increase the risk of venous thromboembolism, blood pressure, blood sugar and water retention. Anti-androgen medications such as spironolactone can cause volume depletion and electrolyte abnormalities. Testosterone in high doses can cause liver function abnormalities. Oral testosterone should never be prescribed but is available on the black market and may cause severe liver toxicity.
- **Cancer**: Hormone-related cancer in transgender persons is very rare (there are case reports of breast cancer in MTFs). The major concern relates to appropriate health screening for biological sex, eg, prostate exams in MTFs and pelvic exams in FTMs.
- **Substance abuse**: Injection drug and alcohol use are common in the transgender community, particularly in MTFs. Tobacco use is also very common.

- **Mental health issues**: Depression and anxiety are of concern for transgender persons.
- **Silicone injection**: MTF transgender persons may inject silicone rather than wait for feminizing hormones to work. This silicone may migrate to other tissues and cause problems later.
- **Diet and exercise**: Lack of exercise and obesity are common among transgender persons. Proper diet counseling and exercise programs are recommended.
- **Osteoporosis**: Hormone-related osteoporosis is not seen at a higher incidence with transgender individuals[51] although there are no long-term prospective studies on this. Estrogen may have a protective effect on bone mass for MTFs.[52]

See Table 6-3 for a summary of screening and history topics for transgender persons.

Table 6-3   History and Screening Topics for Transgender Persons

- Access to appropriate healthcare
- Complete health history, including use of prescription and nonprescription hormones
- Appropriate use and doses of hormones and other medications; evaluation of risk of using these medications
- History of and use of injectable silicone
- History of and risk for coronary heart disease
- History of and risk for hormone-related cancer; appropriate cancer screening for biological sex
- Safer sex practices and screening for STIs and HIV
- Substance abuse: alcohol and injection drugs
- Tobacco use and smoking cessation
- Screening for mental health issues including depression and anxiety
- Nutrition
- Exercise

Adapted from: Ten things transgender persons should discuss with their health care providers. Gay and Lesbian Medical Association; 2006. Available at http://www.glma.org. Click on *Resources for Patients*; then click on "Ten things to discuss with your healthcare provider."

Social and Policy Issues of Aging

There are several issues that impact the healthcare of adult and older LGBT patients that are not health issues *per se*, but are important for primary care providers to consider. Chapter 16: Legal Issues of Importance to Clinicians provides more detail on these issues.

- **Advance directives**: LGBT adults should be strongly encouraged to draft advance directives. These tools include the healthcare proxy, living will, durable power of attorney, and durable power of attorney for healthcare. Lawyers may draft these or patients can download forms from online sources such as http://www.lawdepot.com or http://www.legacywriter.com. See also Appendix F and Appendix G for sample forms. These documents help clinicians direct the patient's personal wishes around healthcare in the event the patient is unable to participate in those discussions. This is particularly important when close relatives have not been an integral part of the patient's life and when the patient prefers that someone other than the person designated by common law make the decisions.

- **Legal unions**: The ability to form legal unions such as marriage (Massachusetts) and civil unions (Vermont, New Jersey, and Connecticut) provides same-sex couples with the same rights and privileges as married heterosexual couples. This has implications for healthcare, particularly concerning hospital visitation rights and medical decision-making in the absence of a living will or healthcare proxy. Marriage and civil unions provide many benefits not afforded unmarried same-sex couples. These benefits become very apparent when a member of a same-sex unmarried couple dies. According to a recent report, "widows" and "widowers" of unmarried same-sex couples have a greater risk of losing their homes and can face a loss of tens of thousands of dollars, due to higher taxes on inheritance of estates and retirement plans, and denial of social security survivor benefits.[55]

  A telemovie from HBO called *If These Walls Could Talk 2* provides a moving example of how the surviving partner of a same-sex couple can be denied the rights and privileges typically granted only to "family." In this film, Edith, the surviving partner of a lesbian couple who were together for 50 years, is refused status as family by the hospital and must grieve silently as she watches a distant relative remove her partner's belongings from their home.

- **Domestic partnership and employee benefits**: These are becoming much more available across the country. Many large and small companies offer health insurance benefits to domestic partners.

- **Long-term care**: Many long-term care facilities have not been welcoming to LGBT residents. To avoid harassment and discrimination, many elder LGBT adults have found they need to hide their identity and relationships from staff and other residents. More staff training is needed in LGBT cultural competency for existing services for the elderly. Fortunately, there are organizations that are addressing this problem by providing training and support to senior care organizations (eg, Senior Action in a Gay Environment (SAGE), http://www.sageusa .org). Prior to making referrals for LGBT patients, it is important to learn which agencies in the area provide a welcoming environment.

Summary Points

- LGBT elders came of age in an era of greater intolerance towards sexual minorities. For this reason, many LGBT elders do not "come out" to others, including healthcare providers.
- Older LGBT people face the same health challenges as other American elders, in addition to health issues specific to their sexual minority status, such as increased risk of HIV in men and an increased risk of obesity in women.
- The stereotype that LGBT elders are isolated and lonely is incorrect. Many LGBT elders have partners, rich social lives, and extended families (including children and grandchildren).
- Most LGBT elders adjust well to aging and live out their senior years much as they did their middle years. However, some gay men feel "old" at an earlier age than their biological age, possibly due to the emphasis on physical attractiveness and youth in the gay culture. In comparison, lesbians often gain a greater sense of fulfillment as they age and tend to have a wider circle of friends and family than gay men.
- As transgender patients age, they may be more likely to encounter health issues that correspond to their biological sex; these patients may need help in coping with a disease or condition associated with the gender they have left behind.
- Many LGBT social and support outlets are youth-oriented, and LGBT elders may not feel comfortable accessing these organizations. It is important to help LGBT elders locate resources geared toward the older LGBT community.
- Clinicians should familiarize themselves with later-life and end-of-life issues faced by LGBT elders and be prepared to make referrals to lawyers, elder housing, and assisted care facilities that are welcoming to LGBT people.

References

1. **US Department of Health and Human Services, Administration on Aging**. A Profile of Older Americans: 2005. Available at http://www.aoa.gov/prof/Statistics/profile/2005/profiles2005.asp.
2. **Bailey RW**. Out and Voting II: The Gay, Lesbian and Bisexual Vote in Congressional Elections, 1990-1998. Policy Institute of the National Gay and Lesbian Task Force; 2000.
3. **Cahill S, South K, Spade J**. Outing Age: Public Policy Issues Affecting Gay, Lesbian, Bisexual and Transgender Elders. The Policy Institute of the National Gay and Lesbian Task Force Foundation; 2000.
4. **Brookdale Center on Aging of Hunter College and Senior Action in a Gay Environment**. Assisted Housing for Elderly Gays and Lesbians in New York City: Extent of Need and the Preferences of Elderly Gays and Lesbians. Hunter College and SAGE; April 1999.

5. **Rosenfeld D**. Identity work among the homosexual elderly. Journal of Aging Studies. 1999;13:121-144.

6. **Bennett L, Gates G**. The Cost of Marriage Inequality to Gay, Lesbian and Bisexual Seniors. Human Rights Campaign Foundation Report; 2004.

7. **Berger R**. The unseen minority: older gays and lesbians. Social Work. 1982;27:237-8.

8. **Wahler J, Gabbay SG**. Gay male aging: a review of the literature. Journal of Gay and Lesbian Social Services. 1997;6:8-12.

9. **Burton L, Kasper JD**. Demography. In: Pompei P, Murphy JB, eds. Geriatrics Review Syllabus. 6th ed. American Geriatrics Society; 2006:1-8.

10. **Baron A, Cramer DW**. Potential counseling concerns of aging lesbian, gay and bisexual clients. In: Perez RM, DeBord KA, Bieschke KJ, eds. Handbook of Counseling and Psychotherapy with Lesbian, Gay, and Bisexual Clients. American Psychological Association; 2000:208.

11. **Kimmel DC**. Patterns of aging among gay men. Christopher Street;1977:28-31.

12. **Cohler B**. Aging, generation, and the course of gay and lesbian lives. Paper presented at: New Approaches to Research on Sexual Orientation, Mental Health, and Substance Abuse; September 1999; National Institute of Mental Health:17-19.

13. **Webber G**. Older gays still hesitant about coming out. Boston Globe; January 11, 2004. Available at http://www.boston.com/news/local/massachusetts/articles/2004/01/11/older_gays_still_hesitant_about_coming_out/.

14. **Brotman S, Ryan B, Cormier R**. The health and social service needs of gay and lesbian elders and their families in Canada. The Gerontologist. 2003;43:192-202.

15. **Beehler GP**. Confronting the culture of medicine: gay men's experiences with primary care physicians. Journal of the Gay and Lesbian Medical Association. 2001;5:135-41.

16. **Pompei P, Murphy JB, eds**. Geriatrics Review Syllabus: A Core Curriculum in Geriatric Medicine. 6th ed. American Geriatrics Society; 2006.

17. **Makadon HJ**. Improving health care for the lesbian and gay communities. N Engl J Med. 2006;354:895-897.

18. **Cole SW, Kemeny ME, Taylor SE, et al**. Elevated physical health risk among gay men who conceal their homosexual identity. Health Psychology. 1996;15:243-51.

19. **Branson BM, Handsfield HH, Lampe MA, et al**. Revised recommendations for HIV testing of adults, adolescents, and pregnant women in health-care settings. MMWR Recommendations and Reports. 2006;55:1-17; quiz CE1-4.

20. **Centers for Disease Control and Prevention**. Sexually Transmitted Diseases Treatment Guidelines 2006. MMWR Morb Mortal Wkly Rep. 2006;55:1-100.

21. **O'Donnell AB, Araujo AB, McKinlay JB**. The health of normally aging men: the Massachusetts Male Aging Study (1987-2004). Experimental Gerontology. 2004;39:975-84.

22. **Ryan H, Wortley PM, Easton A, Pederson L, Greenwood G**. Smoking among lesbians, gays, and bisexuals: a review of the literature. Am J Prev Med. 2001;21:142-9.

23. **Expert Panel on Detection, Evaluation, and Treatment of High Blood Cholesterol in Adults**. Executive summary of the third report of the National Cholesterol Education Program (NCEP) expert panel on detection, evaluation, and treatment of high blood cholesterol in adults (Adult Treatment Panel III). JAMA. 2001;285:2486-97.

24. **Perlman G, Drescher JA**. Gay Man's Guide to Prostate Cancer. Hayworth Medical Press, 2005.

25. **Centers for Disease Control and Prevention**. HIV/AIDS Surveillance Report, 2005. Vol. 17. Atlanta: US Department of Health and Human Services, Centers for Disease Control and Prevention; 2006:1-54. Available at http://www.cdc.gov/hiv/topics/surveillance/resources/reports/.

26. **Gordon SM, Thompson S**. The changing epidemiology of human immunodeficiency virus infection in older persons. Journal of the American Geriatrics Society. 1995;43:7-9.

27. **Smith DK, Grohskopf LA, Black RJ, et al**. Antiretroviral postexposure prophylaxis after sexual, injection-drug use, or other nonoccupational exposure to HIV in the United

States: recommendations from the US Department of Health and Human Services. MMWR Recommendations and Reports. 2005;54:1-20.

28. **Goldstone S**. The Ins and Outs of Gay Sex: A Medical Handbook for Men. 1999.

29. **Jalbert Y**. Gay Health: Current Knowledge and Future Actions. COCQ-SIDA and Health Canada; 1999.

30. **Santillo VM, Lowe FC**. Prostate cancer and the gay male. In: A Gay Man's Guide to Prostate Cancer. Hayworth Medical Press; 2005: 9-27.

31. **Reiter R, deKernion J**. Epidemiology, etiology and prevention of prostate cancer. In: Walsh P, Retik A, Vaughn E, eds. Campbell's Urology. 8th ed. WB Saunders; 2002:3003-24.

32. **Carlat DJ, Camargo CA, Herzog DB**. Eating disorders in males: a report on 135 patients. Am J Psychiatry. 1997;154:1127-32.

33. **Beren S, Hayden H, Wilfley D, et al**. The influence of sexual orientation on body dissatisfaction in adult men and women. Int J Eating Disorders. 1996;20:135-41.

34. **Carroll N**. Optimal gynecologic and obstetric care for lesbians. Obstetrics and Gynecology. 1999;93:611-13.

35. **White J, Levison W**. Primary care of lesbian patients. J Gen Int Med. 1993;8:41-47.

36. **Ulstad VK**. Coronary health issues for lesbians. J Gay Lesbian Med Assoc. 1999;3:59-66.

37. **Bradford J, Ryan C**. National Lesbian Health Care Survey. National Gay and Lesbian Health Foundation; 1987.

38. **Valanis BG, Bowen DJ, Bassford T, et al**. Sexual orientation and health. Arch Fam Med. 2000;9:843-53.

39. **Rich-Edwards JW, Manson JE, Hennekens CH, et al**. The primary prevention of coronary heart disease in women. N Engl J Med. 1995;332:1758-66.

40. **Manson JE, Stampfer MJ, Colditz GA, et al**. A prospective study of obesity and the risk of coronary heart disease in women. N Engl J Med. 1999;322:882-9.

41. **Roberts SJ, Patsdaughter CA, Grindel CG, et al**. Health related behaviors and cancer screening of lesbians: results of the Boston Lesbian Health Project II. Woman & Health. 2004;39:41-55.

42. **Diamant AL, et al**. Health behaviors, health status, and access to and use of health care: a population-based study of lesbian, bisexual, and heterosexual women. Archives of Family Medicine. 2000;9:1043-51.

43. **US Preventive Services Task Force**. Screening for cervical cancer. Available at http://www.ahrq.gov/clinic/uspstf/uspscerv.htm. Accessed January 10, 2007.

44. **American Geriatrics Society**. Special article, AGS position statement: screening for cervical carcinoma in older women. Available at http://www.americangeriatrics.org/products/positionpapers/cer_carc_2000.shtml. Accessed January 10, 2007.

45. **Saslow D, Runowicz CD, Solomon D, et al**. American Cancer Society guideline for the early detection of cervical neoplasia and cancer. CA Cancer J Clin. 2002;52:342.

46. **ACOG practice bulletin**. Clinical management guidelines for obstetrician-gynecologists: cervical cytology screening. Number 45, August 2003. Obstet Gynecol. 2003;102:417.

47. **Prestwood KM**. Osteoporosis and osteomalacia. In: Pompei P, Murphy JB, eds. Geriatrics Review Syllabus. 6th ed. American Geriatrics Society; 2006:210-21.

48. **Appelbaum J**. Patient case; 2006.

49. **Lombardi E**. Enhancing transgender health care. Am J Public Health. 2001;91:869-72.

50. **Clements-Nolle K, Marx R, Guzman R, et al**. HIV prevalence, risk behaviors, health care use, and mental health status of transgender persons: implications for public health interventions. Am J Public Health. 2001;91:915-21.

51. **Schlatterer K, Auer DP, Yassouridis A, et al**. Transsexualism and osteoporosis. Exp Clin Endocrinol Diabetes. 1998;106:365-8.

52. **Van Kesteren P, Lips P, Gooran IJG, et al**. Long-term follow up of bone mineral density and bone metabolism in transsexuals treated with cross-sex hormones. Clinical Endocrinology. 1998;48:347-54.

HEALTH PROMOTION AND DISEASE PREVENTION

Chapter 7

Health Promotion and Disease Prevention

ULRIKE BOEHMER, PhD
DEBORAH J. BOWEN, PhD

Health Promotion: Opportunities and Challenges

Health promotion and disease prevention activities happen in diverse environments, including primary care and public health settings. Clinicians have multiple opportunities to improve the health of lesbian, gay, bisexual, and transgender (LGBT) populations during the primary care encounter. But despite these opportunities, research indicates that prevention services for LGBT people are not routinely available and that multiple barriers to LGBT health promotion continue to exist.[1]

Although there is no single proven strategy to optimize health promotion,[2,3] a growing literature points to the importance of cultural competency in the physician-patient relationship[4,5] and of providing patients with evidence-based information during the clinical encounter.[6] This chapter discusses several recommended evidence-based preventive services and how they can be applied to LGBT populations, with the understanding that most clinician training on the care of LGBT individuals is limited.[7-9] (For a discussion of cultural competency, see Chapters 1 and 15). Within healthcare it is widely recognized "that providing high quality, evidence-based preventive care is a critical factor in helping people live healthier lives. We also know from research that the best way to ensure that preventive services are delivered appropriately is to make evidence-based information readily available at the point of care."[6]

Disparities in the delivery of health promotion services to some underserved populations have been recognized, and the federal government has responded by funding programs to reduce these disparities (eg, the Breast and Cervical Cancer Mortality Prevention Act). Nonetheless, funding to evaluate the scientific evidence on the health of the LGBT population and to present recommendations for their preventive care has been minimal. Subsequently, evidence-based, culturally specific interventions that increase health promotion activities in LGBT populations are limited. This chapter will attempt to address this information gap and provide helpful information for physicians and other providers caring for LGBT patients.

National Standards

This chapter uses two frameworks established by national policy bodies. First, *The Guide to Clinical Preventive Services: Recommendations of the US Preventive Services Task Force (USPSTF)* (http://www.ahrq.gov/clinic/uspstfix.htm), provides guidelines for use of evidence based clinical care.[6] Many primary care providers are familiar with this tool. To create the guide, *USPSTF* systematically evaluated scientific evidence and subsequently derived recommendations about preventive care.[6] A second national policy guide, *The Guide to Community Preventive Services* (http://www.the communityguide.org) helps providers and healthcare organizations keep up-to-date with approved clinical tests and behavioral practices. This guide summarizes interventions that have been proven to increase health promotion in the general population.

Table 7-1 presents a summary of *The Guide to Clinical Preventive Services* along with LGBT-specific information relevant to each preventive service. The body of the chapter provides more detail on these recommended services and how they can be applied to LGBT adult patients (note that certain topics, such as sexually transmitted infections and prevention of substance abuse are covered in other chapters and therefore not included here). The chapter lists the services in the order of the magnitude of net benefit assigned by USPSTF.

Screening and Counseling for Tobacco Use

Tobacco use remains the leading cause of avoidable morbidity and mortality in the United States.[10] Smoking or exposure to secondhand smoke has been attributed to an estimated 259 494 deaths annually among men and 178 408 deaths among women in the United States.[11] Of these 438 000 annual premature deaths, 39.8% are attributed to cancer, 34.7% to cardiovascular diseases, and 25.5% to respiratory diseases.[11] Since 1996, when the Agency for Health Care Policy and Research released its first comprehensive clinical practice guidelines on smoking cessation, it has been recommended that clinicians screen all adults for tobacco use and provide tobacco cessation interventions.[6,12] Although recent national data suggest that 55% of daily smokers and 43% of nondaily smokers receive smoking cessation advice from their provider, Hispanic smokers receive smoking cessation advice significantly less often compared to all other racial groups.[13]

Table 7-1   *USPSTF Clinical Preventive Services[6] and their application in LGBT Populations*

Rank	Service	Description	What is known about LGBT populations	What should be done in LGBT populations
A	**Tobacco Use and Tobacco-Caused Disease, Counseling to Prevent**	Screen all adults and provide tobacco cessation interventions for those who use tobacco products.	Evidence shows higher prevalence of tobacco use in LGBTs.	Screen for tobacco use, offer standard or LGBT cessation opportunities
A	**High Blood Pressure, Screening**	Screen adults 18 years of age and older.	Evidence suggests higher risk of cardiovascular disease (CVD) in LGBTs.	Screen for blood pressure (BP), offer standard care
A	**Aspirin for the Primary Prevention of Cardiovascular Events**	Discuss aspirin chemo-prevention with adults who are at increased risk for coronary heart disease. Address the potential benefits and harms of aspirin therapy.	Evidence suggests increased risk of CVD in LGBTs.	Offer standard care
A	**Lipid Disorders in Adults, Screening**	Routinely screen men 35 years of age and older and women 45 years of age and older. Treat abnormal lipids in people at increased risk for coronary heart disease.	Evidence suggests increased risk of CVD in LGBTs.	Offer standard care
A	**Cervical Cancer, Screening**	Screen women who have been sexually active and have a cervix.	LBT risk of cervical cancer possibly same as heterosexual women; evidence suggests lower screening rates in LBs.	Screen for cervical cancer, offer standard care

Table 7-1   *USPSTF Clinical Preventive Services*[6] and their application in LGBT Populations (continued)

Rank	Service	Description	What is known about LGBT populations	What should be done in LGBT populations
A	**Colorectal Cancer, Screening**	Screen men and women 50 years of age or older.	Evidence suggests lower screening rates in LGBTs.	Offer standard CRC screening opportunities
A	**HIV, Screening**	Screen for human immuno-deficiency virus (HIV) all adolescents and adults at increased risk for HIV infection and all pregnant women.	See Chapter 11	
A	**Syphilis Infection, Screening**	Screen persons at increased risk and all pregnant women.	See Chapter 11	
A	**Chlamydial Infection, Screening**	Routinely screen all sexually active women 25 years of age and younger, and other asymptomatic women at increased risk for infection.	See Chapter 11	
A	**Hepatitis B Virus Infection, Screening**	Screen pregnant women at their first prenatal visit.	See Chapter 11	
A	**Rh (D) Incompatibility, Screening**	Perform Rh (D) blood typing and antibody testing for all pregnant women during their first visit for pregnancy-related care.	Many LBT women have pregnancies (see Chapter 5).	Offer standard screening

Table 7-1   *USPSTF Clinical Preventive Services[6] and their application in LGBT Populations (continued)*

Rank	Service	Description	What is known about LGBT populations	What should be done in LGBT populations
A	**Bacteriuria, Screening for Asymptomatic**	Screen all pregnant women, using urine culture, at 12–16 weeks' gestation.	Many LBT women have pregnancies (see Chapter 5).	Offer standard screening
B	**Obesity in Adults, Screening**	Screen all adult patients. Offer intensive counseling and behavioral interventions to promote sustained weight loss for obese adults.	Evidence shows higher prevalence of obesity in lesbians.	Screen for obesity
B	**Behavioral Counseling in Primary Care to Promote a Healthy Diet**	Intensive behavioral dietary counseling for adult patients with hyperlipidemia and other known risk factors for cardio-vascular and diet-related chronic disease. Intensive counseling can be delivered by primary care clinicians or by referral to other specialists, such as nutritionists or dietitians.	Evidence suggests LB women have poorer diet.	Screen for obesity; refer to dietary change program
B	**Diabetes Mellitus in Adults, Screening for Type 2**	Screen adults with hyper-tension or hyperlipidemia.	Evidence suggests increased risk of CVD in LGBTs.	Screen for diabetes, risk factors; refer to dietary change and activity programs

Table 7-1   *USPSTF Clinical Preventive Services[6] and their application in LGBT Populations (continued)*

Rank	Service	Description	What is known about LGBT populations	What should be done in LGBT populations
B	**Lipid Disorders in young adults, Screening**	Routinely screen younger adults (men 20 to 35 years of age and women 20 to 45 years of age) if they have other risk factors for coronary heart disease. Include measurement of total cholesterol and high-density lipoprotein cholesterol.	Evidence suggests increased risk of CVD in LGBTs.	Screen for lipids, offer standard care
B	**Breast Cancer, Screening**	Screening mammography, with or without clinical breast examination, every 1-2 years for women 40 years of age and older.	Evidence shows lower screening rates in LBTs.	Offer breast screening, LBT specific interventions
B	**Breast Cancer, Chemoprevention**	Discuss with women at high risk for breast cancer and at low risk for adverse effects of chemoprevention. Inform patients of the potential benefits and harms.	Lesbians have more behavioral risk factors for breast cancer.	Offer standard care
B	**Breast and Ovarian Cancer Susceptibility, Genetic Risk Assessment and BRCA Mutation Testing**	Refer women whose family history is associated with an increased risk for deleterious mutations in *BRCA1* or *BRCA2* genes for genetic counseling and evaluation for BRCA testing.		Offer standard care

Table 7-1   *USPSTF Clinical Preventive Services*[6] and their application in LGBT Populations (continued)

Rank	Service	Description	What is known about LGBT populations	What should be done in LGBT populations
B	**Abdominal Aortic Aneurysm, Screening**	One-time screening for abdominal aortic aneurysm (AAA) by ultrasonography in men aged 65 to 75 who have ever smoked.	Evidence suggests higher prevalence of tobacco use in LGBTs	Screen GB men, 65–75 years, who have ever smoked
B	**Osteoporosis in Postmenopausal Women, Screening**	Routinely screen women 65 years of age and older. Begin at age 60 for women at increased risk for osteoporotic fractures.	See Chapter 6	
B	**Gonorrhea, Screening**	Screen all sexually active women, including those who are pregnant, for gonorrhea infection if they are at increased risk for infection (that is, if they are young or have other individual or population risk factors).	See Chapter 11	
B	**Depression, Screening**	Screen adults in clinical practices that have systems in place to assure accurate diagnosis, effective treatment, and follow-up.	See Chapter 8	
B	**Alcohol Misuse, Screening and Behavioral Counseling Interventions in Primary Care to Reduce**	Use screening and behavioral counseling to reduce alcohol misuse by adults, including pregnant women.	See Chapter 9	

Table 7-1　*USPSTF Clinical Preventive Services[6] and their application in LGBT Populations (continued)*

Rank	Service	Description	What is known about LGBT populations	What should be done in LGBT populations
B	**Chlamydial Infection, Screening of pregnant women**	Routinely screen all asymptomatic pregnant women 25 years of age and younger and others at increased risk.	See Chapter 11	
B	**Rh (D) Incompatibility, Screening**	Repeated Rh (D) antibody testing for all unsensitized Rh (D)-negative women at 24–28 weeks' gestation, unless the biological father is known to be Rh (D)-negative.	Many LBT women have pregnancies (see Chapter 5).	Offer standard screening
B	**Breastfeeding, Behavioral Interventions to Promote**	Recommend structured breastfeeding education and behavioral counseling programs.	Many LBT women have biological children (see Chapter 5).	Offer standard counseling and education
I	**Prostate cancer, Screening**	Screening for prostate cancer using prostate specific antigen (PSA) testing or digital rectal examination (DRE).	Risk of prostate cancer assumed to be comparable to heterosexual men.	Discuss risks and benefits of screening
None	**Anal cancer, Screening**		Higher risk of anal cancer in GB men, some T.	Consider screening (Pap test)

Table 7-1   *USPSTF Clinical Preventive Services[6] and their application in LGBT Populations (continued)*

Rank	Service	Description	What is known about LGBT populations	What should be done in LGBT populations
None	**Penile Cancer, Screening**		Evidence suggests possiblity of higher risk in GBs.	Consider screening
D	**Testicular Cancer, Screening**	Recommendation against routine screening for testicular cancer in asymptomatic adult males.	Men with HIV/AIDS at increased risk for testicular cancer.	Consider screening HIV-infected GB men

Explanation of Ranking; USPSTF has assigned a letter grade that reflects the magnitude of net benefit (balance of benefits and harms) and the strength of the evidence supporting the provision of a preventive service. Preventive services are graded from "A" (strongly recommended) to "D" (recommended against). A grade of "I" means the evidence is insufficient to determine net benefit. "None" indicates that the USPSTF has not assigned a rank.

Adapted, with permission, from "Health Care Screening for Men Who Have Sex with Men," May 1, 2004, American Family Physician. Copyright © 2004 American Academy of Family Physicians. All Rights Reserved.

Counseling LGBT patients about smoking cessation is of great importance because the existing evidence suggests that adult sexual minorities have higher smoking rates than the general population. Recent studies indicate that sexual minority women's smoking rates are almost twice those of heterosexual women[14]: 29.8% of sexual minority women smoked compared to 17.0% of heterosexual women.[15] Higher smoking rates have also been reported for sexual minority men.[16] One study found gay men were more than twice as likely to smoke as heterosexual men.[14] Data on smoking rates for transgender individuals are not available, but it has been hypothesized that smoking is prevalent in this population.[17]

The Guide to Community Preventive Services points to considerable evidence for the effectiveness of interventions to decrease tobacco use that can be implemented by healthcare systems and providers of different specialties.[18] Screening for tobacco use and providing brief smoking-cessation counseling (lasting 3 minutes or less) have shown an increase in cessation rates, although there is a dose-response effect between quit rates and more intense counseling.[6] Provider reminder systems including flow sheets, stickers attached to patients' medical charts, etc have been determined effective at increasing providers' advice to patients to quit smoking.[18] Scientific evidence also supports the effectiveness of the combination of reminder systems and provider education in achieving increases in providers' tobacco-related counseling and patient cessation rates.[18] Strong evidence exists for the effectiveness of telephone counseling as well, indicating that supportive telephone contact can assist patients in quitting smoking and can help patients who recently stopped smoking. In the clinical setting, telephone counseling has typically been implemented as follow-up to other interventions, such as provider counseling and other cessation-related activities.[18]

A few smoking cessation interventions have been developed specifically for LGBT populations. In the early 1990s, the Coalition of Lavender Americans on Smoking and Health (CLASH) created The Last Drag program in San Francisco, an educational program that targeted LGBT communities. This program was based on volunteer models of smoking cessation supported by the American Lung Association and American Cancer Society (http://www.lastdrag.org).[17] A second LGBT-focused smoking cessation program called Out & Free uses the Stages of Change theory to help people quit. Although many smoking cessation programs for the general population have been based on Stages of Change theory, Out & Free made it relevant to LGBT persons by comparing the stages of quitting to the stages of the LGBT "coming out" process. In this program, LGBT smokers hoping to quit are asked to draw on the same skills, inner strength, and resources they developed during the coming out process.[19] A third program called QueerTip uses elements of both of these programs, and delivers them in a group format.[19] (See Appendix A for resources on LGBT smoking cessation programs.)

It is not yet known whether LGBT individuals enrolled in culturally specific programs are more likely to quit smoking than those in standard smoking cessation programs. It is also not known whether LGBT persons respond differently to pharmacological management of smoking cessation than other individuals. Moreover, the long-term effectiveness of LGBT-focused smoking interventions has not been sufficiently evaluated. Ideally, future programs will conduct more rigorous evaluation studies to determine the benefits of LGBT-focused interventions. Additional research is also needed to explore the reasons why LGBT populations smoke; for example, psychosocial factors such as coping with discrimination due to sexual orientation may play a role in smoking initiation. Information on such factors can lead to more effective programs.

Finally, older gay and bisexual male patients with a history of smoking can also benefit from screening by ultrasound for abdominal aortic aneurysms (AAAs)—a condition in which the primary artery in the abdomen expands and ruptures. The USPSTF recommends one-time screening for AAA by ultrasonography in men aged 65 to 75 who have ever smoked.[6]

Prevention of Cardiovascular Events

Heart disease is the leading cause of mortality for men and women in the United States, accounting for nearly 40% of all annual deaths.[20] All adults, beginning with age 18, should be routinely screened for high blood pressure, and men aged 35 and older, as well as women aged 45 and older, for lipid disorders.[6] It is recommended that screening for lipid disorders include measurement of total cholesterol and high-density lipoprotein cholesterol. Blood lipid screening is also recommended for younger adults (eg, men aged 20 to 35 and women aged 20 to 45) if they have other risk factors for coronary heart disease.[6] Clinicians should discuss aspirin chemoprevention with adults who are at increased risk for coronary heart disease, and these discussions should address both the potential benefits and harms of aspirin therapy.[6]

Sexual minority populations have more risk factors for heart disease than the general population. Some sexual minority men's cardiovascular risks may be increased due to their use of either anabolic steroids[21] or club drugs,[22] which have both been linked to hypertension. Transgender individuals' risk of cardiovascular disease may be elevated due to use of estrogen or testosterone. Data suggest that an increased rate of polycystic ovarian syndrome in female-to-male transgender individuals may also affect cholesterol and blood pressure.[23] Others hypothesize that sexual minority populations are at increased risk of hypertension due to other factors; the stress that could result from concealing one's sexual orientation may increase the risk for hypertension.[24] Additionally, experiences of discrimination based on one's sexual orientation or race and ethnicity have been linked to higher blood pressure.[25-27] Heart disease has been found to be more prevalent in lesbian and bisexual than in heterosexual women.[28] It has also been suggested that bisexual women are less likely than heterosexual women to undergo appropriate cholesterol screening.[29] Routine screening of LGBT populations to identify risk factors to prevent cardiovascular events is advised in light of the suggested greater prevalence of risk factors and the greater prevalence of heart disease in sexual minority women.[28]

State-funded and federally funded studies have indicated that providers can play an invaluable role in decreasing cardiovascular risk factors. For example, a CDC-funded state program in Utah implemented electronic reminder messages to alert doctors in community health centers to patients' preventive service needs, and as a result the proportion of patients who had their blood pressure under control increased to 58% from a baseline level of 33%.[20] To reach underserved populations, a federally funded demonstration project entitled WISEWOMAN[30] screened women who were already participating in a breast and cervical cancer screening program for heart disease. The cardiovascular component sought to increase the utilization of prevention activities, such as assessing blood pressure and lipid levels.[31]

Heart disease prevention programs that specifically focus on sexual minority populations have yet to be developed or evaluated. In the interim, clinicians should adhere to established guidelines for cardiovascular prevention activities and implement health promotion programs that have been proven effective in the general population.

Screening for Cervical Cancer

With the widespread use of the Papanicolaou test (also called Pap smear, Pap test), the mortality of cervical cancer considerably decreased. Cervical cancer is linked to an infection with oncogenic strains of human papillomavirus (HPV). With the recent availability of a vaccine that prevents cervical cancer caused by HPV, the prevalence and mortality due to cervical cancer should be greatly reduced in the future, but currently available vaccines will not protect HPV-infected women from clinical progression. The USPSTF strongly recommends screening all women regularly for cervical cancer within 3 years of the start of sexual activity or age 21, whichever comes first.[6]

There are no data on HPV vaccination rates in different communities yet, since the vaccine has only been recently introduced. Cervical cancer screening rates are lower for sexual minority compared with heterosexual women, raising concerns that vaccination disparities may occur in sexual minorities, putting their health further at risk. Sexual minority women should undergo screening as has been recommended for women in general.[32-35] While few population-based data are available, studies suggest that sexual minority women have lower Pap test rates than heterosexual women[36-39] and that the time interval between Pap tests is almost three times longer for lesbians compared to heterosexual women.[40] There are no existing data on screening rates in transgender persons. However, female-to-male transgender persons who have cervixes remain at risk for cervical cancer and require routine Pap tests.

Although, provider recommendation has been strongly linked to screening compliance of women in the general population,[41-45] population-based studies of the likelihood of sexual minority women receiving a physician's recommendation for screening are lacking. There is some evidence that physician recommendation increases the likelihood of accepting screening for cervical cancer among sexual minority women.[34] Some healthcare providers have been shown to harbor the false assumption that if lesbians are not currently sexually active with men, they are not at risk for HPV, and therefore these providers may not routinely screen sexual minority women.[46] Moreover, studies have suggested that sexual minority women perceive themselves to be at lower risk for sexually transmitted infections and believe they do not need to engage in sexual risk reduction behaviors.[47]

A few interventions have been developed to help increase Pap testing and other cancer screening in sexual minority women. In Seattle and King County, an educational campaign entitled Lesbian Health Matters reached out to both healthcare providers and the general public by placing paid advertisements on radio stations and in newspapers. After listeners complained about hearing the word "lesbian" on the radio, the radio stations cancelled the ads. When some community members demanded the campaign be completed, associated publicity increased the campaign's educational reach.[48]Another intervention consisted of two one-hour lesbian-specific educational sessions led by a lesbian physician. This pilot study explored the impact of these sessions on the cancer screening behaviors of lesbians aged 50-81 and found a limited increase in Pap testing. They also found that some of the lesbian participants who had not had a mammogram for two or more years, obtained mammograms, and some began performing monthly breast self-examinations.[49]

Screening for Colorectal Cancer

Annually, more than 148 000 new cases of colorectal cancer are diagnosed in US men and women and more than 55 000 men and women succumb to this disease.[50] It is therefore strongly recommended that both men and women undergo screening for colorectal cancer, starting at age 50 at least every decade until about age 80, and those with a family history of colorectal cancer should begin screening at an earlier age. Potential screening options for colorectal cancer include home fecal occult blood testing (FOBT) (to screen for asymptomatic gastrointestinal bleeding), flexible sigmoidoscopy, the combination of home FOBT and flexible sigmoidoscopy, colonoscopy, and double-contrast barium enema.[6]

There are limited data about colorectal screening in LGBT populations. HIV-infected patients are less likely to be screened for colorectal cancer compared to controls without HIV, despite the more intense healthcare utilization of HIV-infected individuals.[51] Results from a sample of sexual minority women participating in the Women's Health Initiative suggested that higher proportions of sexual minority women reported histories of colon cancer compared to heterosexual women,[52] emphasizing the need for screening in this population.

For the general population, there are a number of effective interventions to increase cancer screening rates, including community-based initiatives, individual-based initiatives, and programs that focus on clinician behavior. (Some research-tested intervention programs can be found at: http://cancercontrol.cancer.gov/rtips). The Task Force on Community Preventive Services has concluded that reminders to patients that they are due for screening is an effective means to promote colorectal cancer screening.[53] Reducing structural barriers (eg, changing the location where the screening is performed, hours of operation, and availability of child care) has also been shown to increase colorectal cancer screening.[54]

Patients who are screened for colorectal cancer and have an abnormal result need follow-up, including a complete diagnostic evaluation consisting of colonoscopy or flexible sigmoidoscopy and barium enema X-ray. An intervention that provided feedback to physicians about patients who had a positive fecal occult blood test resulted in an increase in completed diagnostic evaluations of these patients.[55]

Currently, there have not been any targeted interventions to increase the screening rates for colorectal cancer in sexual minorities. The previously mentioned pilot study that used education by a lesbian physician to increase cancer screening behaviors in sexual minority women did not demonstrate an increase in women's colorectal cancer screening.[49] It is possible that an educational program for sexual minority women that primarily addresses colorectal cancer screening would be more effective, but this remains to be proven.

Screening for Breast Cancer

In 2006, an estimated 212 920 women were expected to receive a diagnosis of breast cancer, the most prevalent cancer in women. In the same year, an estimated 40 970 women were expected to die of breast cancer.[50] The prevention goal for breast cancer is screening to detect it early. It is recommended that providers discuss chemoprevention with women at high risk for breast cancer and refer women whose family history is associated with an increased risk for deleterious mutations in the *BRCA1* or *BRCA2* genes for genetic counseling and evaluation for *BRCA* testing. US prevention guidelines suggest that women over the age of 40 should receive a screening mammogram with or without a clinical breast examination every one to two years.[6]

Data suggest that mammography, the best proven method of breast cancer screening to date, occurs less frequently among sexual minority women. Recent population-based data indicate that lesbians are 4 times less likely to have undergone mammography in the past two years compared to heterosexual women,[39] confirming earlier surveys of sexual minority women that suggested lower mammography rates.[52,56,57] One study of lesbians with a family history of breast cancer found that perception of susceptibility to breast cancer was linked to greater mammography screening adherence.[58] Another study found that 75% of lesbian and bisexual participants had heard relatively little about genetic testing for breast and ovarian cancer risk; however, 88.1% said they were interested in testing, and 77.4% believed they were candidates for testing. Perception of risk of developing cancer as well as cancer worry were significant predictors of interest in genetic testing.[59]

The screening rates for transgender individuals are unknown, but it has been suggested that male-to-female individuals who use or have used hormone replacement therapy may be at increased risk for breast cancer.[23]

In 1990, the US Congress passed the Breast and Cervical Cancer Mortality Prevention Act to increase medically underserved women's access to mammograms and Pap tests. While this Centers for Disease Control and Prevention (CDC)-funded program, called the National Breast and Cervical Cancer Early Detection Program (NBCCEDP), has generally been applauded as an important step in increasing the utilization of cancer screening, it has also been recognized that only 15 percent of all eligible low-income women are reached by this program.[60,61] Many call for an expansion of this program, so more underserved women will be screened.[60,61]

Only one study has designed a breast health program for healthy sexual minority women and tested it in a rigorous research design to determine its effects on screening behaviors.[62] The intervention consisted of breast health counseling by a trained health counselor who led 4 weekly 2-hour sessions of groups with five to eight women. Each of the 4 sessions had a different theme, consisting of: risk assessment and education, breast cancer screening, stress management, and social support. The sessions included information about breast cancer risk, group discussion, and skills training.[62] The study showed that the breast health educational program was effective in changing sexual minority women's screening behaviors: women in the intervention group had a higher rate of mammography screening and performed breast self-examinations more frequently compared to women in the control group. This study suggests that sexual minority women's perception of breast cancer risk and their screening behaviors could be modified through counseling. Healthcare providers should consider offering sexual minority women similar culturally sensitive programs to increase breast cancer awareness and screening.

Screening for Obesity

Obesity has reached epidemic proportions in the US.[63,64] Negative implications of obesity include the substantial increased risk of morbidity from hypertension; dyslipidemia; type 2 diabetes; coronary heart disease; stroke; gallbladder disease; osteoarthritis; sleep apnea and respiratory problems; as well as endometrial, breast, prostate, and colon cancers[65] leading to preventable deaths.[66] It is recommended that clinicians screen all adult patients for obesity, offer counseling, and behavioral interventions to achieve a healthy weight.[6]

Evidence derived from cohort and convenience samples suggests that lesbians have higher rates of being overweight and obese.[52,57,67-70] One recent population-based study confirmed that lesbian women differed from all other women in being more likely to be overweight and obese.[71] Similar assessments of weight issues in sexual minority men do not exist. Lesbians' body image and perceptions of physical attractiveness are thought to differ from heterosexual women, and their exercise behavior may not be as tied to thinness compared to bisexual and heterosexual women.[68,72-78]

Culturally specific interventions to prevent and treat obesity in sexual minorities have yet to be developed. However, interventions for the general population could be adapted for LGBT patients. One randomized control intervention tested a practice-tailored approach to enhance providers' preventive service delivery.[79] After a one-day assessment of their needs, primary care practices received assistance from a nurse facilitator in choosing and implementing individualized tools and approaches for prevention. Practices were then followed at 6-month intervals and evaluated on their use of preventive services. Study results showed that the practices that received the intervention had increased rates of screening (including height and weight measurement) and health habit counseling (including advice on nutrition and exercise) compared to control practices.

Behavioral Counseling in Primary Care to Promote a Healthy Diet

Adult patients with hyperlipidemia and other known risk factors for cardiovascular and diet-related chronic disease can benefit from intensive dietary counseling. This is of particular relevance for lesbian women given their higher risk for obesity. Recommendations for improving dietary quality are available,[80,81] as are healthy diet models for clinical nutrition counseling in a primary care setting. Evidence indicates that including such counseling in the context of primary care has the potential to improve health.[82,83] A few studies suggest that sexual minority women may make less healthful food choices.[52] However, the extent of this disparity is unknown. Two relatively recent reviews[82,83] discussed interventions available to primary care clinicians, including interventions that can be undertaken in the primary care setting and those that require provider referral. These reviews document that primary care interventions have proven successful in increasing healthy eating behaviors. Several interventions involve an encouraging message from the provider, paired with take-home printed materials that discuss eating choices. Referrals to programs in workplaces, voluntary organizations, churches, and other community settings can also support and enhance primary care interventions.[84] At this time there are no published LGBT interventions that focus on healthy eating.

Screening for Type 2 Diabetes Mellitus

The CDC reported that in 2004, about 1.4 million adults between 18 and 79 years of age were diagnosed with diabetes mellitus. From 1997 through 2004, the number of new cases of diagnosed diabetes increased by 54%.[85] Given the growing diabetes rates, adults with hypertension or hyperlipidemia are recommended to undergo routine screening for type 2 diabetes.[6]

Currently there are no studies that prove that the prevalence of diabetes differs by sexual orientation.[28,26] However, increased risk factors for diabetes in the sexual minority population have been documented. In transgender individuals, diabetes risks may be elevated due to the use of administered hormones to assist in their transition.[23] Lesbian women may be at increased risk of diabetes due to higher levels of obesity.[71]

The Task Force on Community Preventive Services points to both disease management and case management interventions at the healthcare system level as effective means in improving the care of individuals with diabetes.[87] Disease management is an organized, proactive, and multicomponent approach to healthcare delivery that includes the use of care guidelines or performance standards for diabetes patients and the use of tracking and monitoring systems to improve health outcomes.[87] Case management refers to assigning a case manager (who is a professional, but not the primary provider) to individuals with diabetes to oversee and coordinate their healthcare use. These case management interventions can be delivered either alone or in combination with disease management (for instance, in combination with a tracking system). Case management has been shown to be an effective means to improve the provision of care to diabetes patients, thereby reducing their risk of poor outcomes.[87] No research to date has shown the effectiveness of these interventions in sexual minority populations, nor is there any documentation of interventions developed specifically for LGBT people with diabetes.

Screening for Genital and Rectal Cancers

Prostate cancer is the most prevalent male cancer, accounting for 33% of all cancer diagnoses in men.[50] In 2006, an estimated 232 090 men were estimated to have been diagnosed with prostate cancer and an estimated 30 350 men were expected to die of this malignancy, the second most common cancer mortality in men.[50] Prostate cancer screening using prostate specific antigen (PSA) testing and digital rectal examination (DRE) has been suggested as a possible means for prostate cancer detection. However, the availability of these two tests has not been clearly linked to a decrease in mortality due to prostate cancer. Further, neither PSA testing nor a DRE are 100% accurate. Prostate cancer screening has become a controversial issue because some men may have had unnecessary prostate biopsies and possibly disabling side effects from prostate cancer treatments.[88,89] Although prostate cancer screening has been discussed as a means of primary prevention for men who are 50 years and older and younger men who have an increased risk due to a family history of prostate cancer, the USPSTF concluded that the evidence was insufficient to recommend for or against routine screening for prostate cancer using PSA testing or a DRE.[6] In the absence of an affirmative recommendation, men are advised to discuss prostate cancer screening with their primary care providers.

The lack of clarity in screening guidelines for prostate cancer are similar for sexual minority men as for heterosexual men; therefore sexual minority men should discuss the pros and cons of screening with their providers. It is important to remember that male-to-female transsexuals may not be perceived as being at risk for prostate cancer, given their female gender presentation, but after gender realignment surgeries, they may have retained the prostate. Cases of prostate cancer have been reported in male-to-female individuals using feminizing hormones. However, the existing data are limited, and it is unclear how the rate of prostate cancer compares to natal men.[23] Male-to-female transgender persons should be considered for screening as appropriate for natal men.[23,90]

In 2006, an estimated 8010 men were expected to have been diagnosed with **testicular cancer** and 1470 men with **penile cancer**.[50] An estimated 390 men were expected to have died of testicular and 270 of penile cancer.[50] The USPSTF recommends against routine screening for testicular cancer in asymptomatic adult males. Clinical examination by a clinician during routine physical exams and monthly self-examination are the potential screening options for testicular cancer. There is insufficient evidence to assess the accuracy, yield, and benefit of these screenings. The low incidence of testicular cancer and favorable outcomes in the absence of screening argue against a routine screening recommendation.[6] However, some evidence exists that HIV-infected men may be at increased risk for testicular cancer,[91-94] suggesting that routine screening of HIV-infected sexual minority men should be considered. There are no data on transgender individuals with respect to risk factors or incidence of testicular cancer.

There are no particular screening procedures or recommendations for **penile cancer**. Patients with growths or sores on the penis, abnormal penile discharge, or bleeding should be evaluated for penile malignancies if relevant sexually transmitted infections are excluded. Limited research studies suggest that infection with HPV may be a risk factor for penile cancer.[95] This deserves some consideration in the clinical encounter with sexual minority men (see Chapter 11 for more detail). Similarly, male-to-female transgender persons who have undergone penile-inversion vaginoplasty (the procedure designed to create a vagina) with penile tissue retained as a neocervix should be offered neocervical Pap tests because of the risk of HPV-associated penile cancer in this group.[96]

An estimated 3990 new cases of **anal cancer** will have been diagnosed in 2006, 2240 of them in women and 1750 in men.[50] As with other diseases that have low incidence in the general population, the Preventive Service Guidelines do not recommend routine screening for anal cancer.[6] However, sexual minority men who engage in receptive anal intercourse are thought to be a high-risk group for anal cancer,[97] and it has been recommended to screen sexual minority men with anal Pap smears to detect anal dysplasia and preinvasive anal cancer.[98-100] While reliable population-based data are missing because cancer registries do not collect information on sexual orientation,[101,102] several studies suggest that gay and bisexual men are at an excess risk for anal cancer.[103-105] Thus although anal cancer is uncommon in the general population, it has been suggested that its incidence is approximately 80 times higher in homosexual and bisexual men[100] or comparable to the rate of cervical cancer in women prior to the implementation of screening programs.[106] Studies have also demonstrated increased rates of anal cancer in HIV-infected sexual minority men, perhaps because of their compromised immune system making them more susceptible to HPV progression, resulting in anal cancer.[91,98] However, HIV-uninfected sexual minority men also have an excess of anal cancer compared to the general population, suggesting that the main causal link is HPV infection.[106] The higher incidence of anal cancer and HPV infection has been linked to receptive anal intercourse and high number of lifetime sexual partners.[97,107] This cumulative evidence leads to the recommendation to screen HIV-infected and HIV-uninfected homosexual and bisexual men engaging in anal sex with anal Pap tests. Data are not available concerning anal cancer rates in transgender individuals. Although the Preventive

Service Task Force has not recommended routine anal Pap tests, it has been stated that the recommended screening offers quality-adjusted life expectancy benefits at a cost comparable with other accepted clinical preventive interventions.[108,109] Please see Chapter 11 for further information on anal HPV infection.

Despite the higher risk of HPV-associated anal disease in MSM,[105,106,111-113] it is unclear whether physicians routinely discuss HPV prevention and screening with their gay or bisexual male patients. Prior research suggests that clinicians may feel uncomfortable with male homosexuality and avoid frank discussions in the clinical encounter.[113-115] There is great need for increased research into factors that may facilitate clinicians' ease in counseling and advising sexual minority men on health promotion. Currently, professional organizations such as the Gay and Lesbian Medical Association (http://www.glma.org) provide guidelines on the care of sexual minority patients (see also Chapters 1 and 15).[116]

Conclusion

All health promotion activities of relevance to LGBT patients have to be considered in the context of LGBT health services utilization patterns. Studies indicate that LGBT patients who are younger or are racial and ethnic minorities are less likely to have a regular source of care and are less likely to be insured.[39,117] Recent population-based data confirmed the long-standing hypothesis that sexual minority women are less likely to use health services than heterosexual women.[39,117-119] However, a recent population-based study found sexual minority men use healthcare services more than heterosexual men.[117] The reasons for sexual minority men's increased healthcare use are poorly understood and could be biased by HIV screening and care visits.[117] These utilization patterns suggest differences in the number of opportunities clinicians have for disease prevention in LGBT compared to heterosexual patients, and within LGBT patient populations. In any case, it is clear that clinicians need to have information on relevant LGBT health prevention readily available.

Effective strategies to increase the delivery of preventive services to the general population have focused on the system level and the individual level (clinicians and patients). When applying these strategies to improve health promotion in LGBT populations, a number of considerations should be taken into account. Office systems, such as electronic reminders, flagging charts, etc, have been shown to be cost-effective, successful strategies to improve health promotion. Implementing these systems is a good starting point. Detailed steps on how to implement office-based systems are available online at http://www.ahrq.gov/ppip/manual/; cancer screening programs can be found on the National Cancer Institute (NCI) Web site: http://cancercontrolplanet.cancer.gov/. Since research suggests that physicians believe they are providing more health promotion than they are, it may be helpful to conduct an internal audit of medical charts to determine if these system-level activities are reaching LGBT patients.

Screening recommendations by providers have been shown to have a strong impact on patients' receipt of prevention services. It is likely that this has the same effect on LGBT screening behavior, but not enough research has been done to measure how often physicians recommend screening or provide counseling to LGBT populations. More research on the physician-sexual minority patient relationship is also needed to understand appropriate ways for physicians to communicate with sexual minority patients to improve patient adherence to health promotion recommendations. A limited number of attempts have been made to increase health promotion among sexual minority patients; however most have been small pilot projects that have not always included a thorough evaluation component or have not been conducted with the appropriate scientific rigor to draw firm conclusions. Therefore, it is still unclear which intervention methods to use to improve sexual minorities' health behaviors. Also, without an increased commitment to fund well-designed studies of sexual minority populations, the mechanisms for behavior change in sexual minority populations will remain unexplored. It is clear that our understanding of appropriate health promotion activities in sexual minorities is only in the beginning stages and many questions remain to be addressed.

Summary Points

- Clinicians have multiple opportunities to improve the health of LGBT populations during the primary care encounter.
- Evidence suggests that LGBT populations have a higher prevalence of tobacco use and may be at increased risk for obesity, cardiovascular disease, diabetes, breast cancer, colorectal cancer, and anal cancer. Screening for these conditions in LGBT patients, and providing relevant primary prevention services is recommended.
- Effective strategies to increase the delivery of preventive services to the general population have focused on the system level and the individual level, (both provider and patient).
- Little is known about effective strategies to improve health promotion in LGBT populations.
- In the absence of guidelines on how to implement prevention services for LGBT populations, clinicians with LGBT patients should consider adapting programs and strategies that have been effective in the general population.

References

1. **Gay and Lesbian Medical Association and LGBT health experts**. Healthy People 2010 companion document for lesbian, gay, bisexual, and transgender (LGBT) health. Gay and Lesbian Medical Association; 2001.

2. **Grimshaw J, Eccles M, Thomas R, et al**. Toward evidence-based quality improvement. Evidence (and its limitations) of the effectiveness of guideline dissemination and implementation strategies 1966-1998. J Gen Intern Med. 2006;21:S14-20.

3. **Ellis P, Robinson P, Ciliska D, et al**. A systematic review of studies evaluating diffusion and dissemination of selected cancer control interventions. Health Psychology. 2005;24:488-500.

4. **Anderson LM, Scrimshaw SC, Fullilove MT, et al**. Culturally competent health care systems. A systematic review. Am J Prev Med. 2003;24:68-79.

5. **Flores G**. Culture and the patient-physician relationship: achieving cultural competency in health care. Journal of Pediatrics. 2000;136:14-23.

6. **United States Preventive Services Task Force**. The Guide to Clinical Preventive Services, 2005. Recommendations of the US Preventive Services Task Force. Agency for Health Care Research and Quality; 2005.

7. **Harrison AE**. Primary care of lesbian and gay patients: educating ourselves and our students [see comment]. Family Medicine. 1996;28:10-23.

8. **Sanchez NF, Rabarin J, Sanchez JP, et al**. Medical students' ability to care for lesbian, gay, bisexual, and transgendered patients. Family Medicine. 2006;38:21-7.

9. **McGarry, KA, Clarke JG, Cyr M, et al**. Evaluating a lesbian and gay health care curriculum. Teaching and Learning in Medicine. 2002;14:244-8.

10. **Office of the Surgeon General**. The health consequences of smoking: a report of the Surgeon General. Dept. of Health and Human Services, Centers for Disease Control and Prevention, National Center for Chronic Disease Prevention and Health Promotion, Office on Smoking and Health; 2004.

11. **Centers for Disease Control and Prevention**. Annual smoking-attributable mortality, years of potential life lost, and productivity losses—United States, 1997-2001. MMWR Morb Mortal Wkly Rep. 2005;54:625-8.

12. **Anderson JE, Jorenby DE, Scott WJ, et al**. Treating tobacco use and dependence: an evidence-based clinical practice guideline for tobacco cessation. Chest. 2002;121:932-41.

13. **Lopez-Quintero C, Crum RM, Neumark YD**. Racial/ethnic disparities in report of physician-provided smoking cessation advice: analysis of the 2000 National Health Interview Survey. Am J Public Health. 2006; 96:2235-9.

14. **Tang H, Greenwood GL, Cowling DW, et al**. Cigarette smoking among lesbians, gays, and bisexuals: how serious a problem? (United States). Cancer Causes and Control. 2004;15:797-803.

15. **Burgard SA, Cochran SD, Mays VM**. Alcohol and tobacco use patterns among heterosexually and homosexually experienced California women. Drug and Alcohol Dependence. 2005;77:61-70.

16. **Greenwood GL, Paul JP, Pollack LM, et al**. Tobacco use and cessation among a household-based sample of urban men who have sex with men (MSM) in the US. American Journal of Public Health. 2005;95:145-51.

17. **American Lung Association**. Lung disease data in culturally diverse communities: 2005. American Lung Association; 2005. Available at http://www.lungusa.org.

18. **Hopkins DP, Briss PA, Ricard, CJ, et al**. Reviews of evidence regarding interventions to reduce tobacco use and exposure to environmental tobacco smoke. Am J Prev Med. 2001;20:16-66.

19. **QueerTip**. Manual: QueerTIPs for LGBT Smokers, A Stop Smoking Class for LGBT Communities. San Francisco, CA: University of California San Francisco & Progressive Research Training for Action; 2002.

20. **Centers for Disease Control and Prevention**. Chronic Disease Prevention: Preventing Heart Disease and Stroke. 2005. Available at http://www.cdc.gov/nccdphp/publications/factsheets/Prevention/cvh.htm.

21. **Bolding G, Sherr L, Elford J**. Use of anabolic steroids and associated health risks among gay men attending London gyms. Addiction. 2002;97:195-203.

22. **Freese TE, Miotto K, Reback CJ**. The effects and consequences of selected club drugs. Journal of Substance Abuse Treatment. 2002;23:151-6.

23. **Feldman J, Goldberg J**. Transgender Primary Medical Care: Suggested Guidelines for Clinicians in British Columbia. Vancouver Coastal Health, Transcend Transgender Support & Education Society, and the Canadian Rainbow Health Coalition: Vancouver, BC Canada; 2006.

24. **Cole SW, Kemeny ME, Taylor SE, et al**. Elevated physical health risk among gay men who conceal their homosexual identity. Health Psychology. 1996;15:243-51.

25. **Krieger N, Sidney S**. Prevalence and health implications of anti-gay discrimination: a study of black and white women and men in the CARDIA cohort. Coronary artery risk development in young adults. International Journal of Health Services. 1997;27:157-76.

26. **Krieger N**. Racial and gender discrimination: risk factors for high blood pressure? Social Science and Medicine. 1990;30:1273-81.

27. **Krieger N, Sidney S**. Racial discrimination and blood pressure: the CARDIA Study of young black and white adults. American Journal of Public Health. 1996;86:1370-8.

28. **Diamant AL, Wold C**. Sexual orientation and variation in physical and mental health status among women. Journal of Women's Health. 2003;12:41-9.

29. **Koh AS**. Use of preventive health behaviors by lesbian, bisexual, and heterosexual women: questionnaire survey. Western Journal of Medicine. 2000;172:379-84.

30. **Centers for Disease Control and Prevention**. WISEWOMAN: a crosscutting program to improve the health of uninsured women. Available at http://www.cdc.gov/wise-woman.

31. **Will JC, Farris RP, Sanders CG, et al** Health promotion interventions for disadvantaged women: overview of the WISEWOMAN projects. Journal of Womens Health. 2004;13:484-502.

32. **Marrazzo JM, Koutsky LA, Kiviat NB, et al**. Papanicolaou test screening and prevalence of genital human papillomavirus among women who have sex with women. American Journal of Public Health. 2001;91:947-52.

33. **O'Hanlan K, Crum CP**. Human papillomavirus-associated cervical intraepithelial neoplasia following lesbian sex. Obstetrics and Gynecology. 1996;88:702-3.

34. **Rankow EJ, Tessaro I**. Cervical cancer risk and Papanicolaou screening in a sample of lesbian and bisexual women. Journal of Family Practice. 1998;47:139-43.

35. **Robertson PA**. Offering high-quality ob/gyn care to lesbian patients. Available at http://www.lesbianhealthinfo.org/research/obgyn_lesbian.htm. Accessed September 10, 2005.

36. **Diamant AL, Wold C, Spritzer K, et al** Health behaviors, health status, and access to and use of health care: a population-based study of lesbian, bisexual, and heterosexual women. Archives of Family Medicine. 2000;9:1043-51.

37. **Matthews AK, Brandenburg DL, Johnson TP, et al**. Correlates of underutilization of gynecological cancer screening among lesbian and heterosexual women. Preventive Medicine: An International Journal Devoted to Practice and Theory. 2004;38:105-13.

38. **Powers D, Bowen DJ, White J**. The influence of sexual orientation on health behaviors in women. Journal of Prevention and Intervention in the Community. 2001;22:43-60.

39. **Kerker BD, Mostashari F, Thorpe L**. Health care access and utilization among women who have sex with women: sexual behavior and identity. J Urban Health. 2006; 83:970-9.

40. **Robertson P, Schachter J**. Failure to identify venereal disease in a lesbian population. Sexually Transmitted Diseases. 1981;8:75-6.

41. **MacDowell NM, Nitz-Weiss M, Short A**. The role of physician communication in improving compliance with mammography screening among women ages 50-79 in a commercial HMO. Managed Care Quarterly. 2000;8:11-9.

42. **Fox SA, Stein JA**. The effect of physician-patient communication on mammography utilization by different ethnic groups. Med Care. 1991;29:1065-82.

43. **Halabi S, Skinner CS, Samsa GP, et al**. Factors associated with repeat mammography screening. J Fam Pract. 2000;49:1104-12.

44. **Lerman C, Rimer B, Trock B, et al**. Factors associated with repeat adherence to breast cancer screening. Prev Med. 1990;19:279-90.

45. **Coughlin SS, Breslau ES, Thompson T, et al**. Physician recommendation for Papanicolaou testing among US women, 2000. Cancer Epidemiology, Biomarkers and Prevention. 2005;14:1143-8.

46. **Marrazzo JM**. Barriers to infectious disease care among lesbians. Emerging Infectious Diseases. 2004;10:1974-8.

47. **Marrazzo JM, Coffey P, Elliott MN**. Sexual practices, risk perception and knowledge of sexually transmitted disease risk among lesbian and bisexual women. Perspectives on Sexual and Reproductive Health. 2005;37:6-12.

48. **Phillips-Angeles E, Wolfe P, Myers R, et al**. Lesbian health matters: a Pap test education campaign nearly thwarted by discrimination. Health Promotion Practice. 2004;5:314-25.

49. **Dibble SL, Roberts SA**. Improving cancer screening among lesbians over 50: results of a pilot study. Oncology Nursing Forum Online. 2003;30:E71-9.

50. **Jemal A, Siegal R, Ward E, et al**. Cancer statistics, 2006. CA: A Cancer Journal for Clinicians. 2006;56:106-30.

51. **Reinhold JP, Moon M, Tenner CT, et al**. Colorectal cancer screening in HIV-infected patients 50 years of age and older: missed opportunities for prevention. American Journal of Gastroenterology. 2005;100:1805-12.

52. **Valanis BG, Bowen DJ, Bassford T, et al**. Sexual orientation and health: comparisons in the women's health initiative sample. Archives of Family Medicine. 2000;9:843-53.

53. **The Task Force on Community Preventive Services**. Promoting Colorectal Cancer Screening in Communities: Task Force Recommendations on the Use of Client Reminders. 2005. Available at http://www.thecommunityguide.org/cancer/screening/ca-screen-int-cc-client-remind.pdf.

54. **The Task Force on Community Preventive Services**. Promoting Colorectal Cancer Screening in Communities: Task Force Recommendations on Reducing Structural Barriers. 2005. Available at http://www.thecommunityguide.org/cancer/screening/ca-screen-int-cc-reduce-barriers.pdf.

55. **Myers R, Turner B, Weinberg D, et al**. Impact of a physician-oriented intervention on follow-up in colorectal cancer screening. Preventive Medicine. 2004;38:375-81.

56. **Bowen DJ, Bradford JB, Powers D, et al**. Comparing women of differing sexual orientations using population-based sampling. Women and Health. 2004;40:19-34.

57. **Case P, Austin SB, Hunter DJ, et al**. Sexual orientation, health risk factors, and physical functioning in the Nurses' Health Study II. Journal of Women's Health. 2004;13:1033-47.

58. **Burnett CB, Steakley CS, Slack R, et al**. Patterns of breast cancer screening among lesbians at increased risk for breast cancer. Women and Health. 1999;29:35-55.

59. **Durfy SJ, Bowen DJ, McTiernan A, et al**. Attitudes and interest in genetic testing for breast and ovarian cancer susceptibility in diverse groups of women in western Washington. Cancer Epidemiology, Biomarkers and Prevention. 1999;8:369-75.

60. **Freeman H, Wingrove B**. Excess Cervical Cancer Mortality: A Marker for Low Access to Health Care in Poor Communities. Rockville, MD: National Cancer Institute, Center to Reduce Cancer Health Disparities; 2005.

61. **Hewitt M, Devesa SS, Breen N**. Cervical cancer screening among US women: analyses of the 2000 National Health Interview Survey. Preventive Medicine. 2004;39:270-8.

62. **Bowen DJ, Powers D, Greenlee H**. Effects of breast cancer risk counseling for sexual minority women. Health Care for Women International. 2006;27:59-74.

63. **US Department of Health and Human Services**. Healthy People 2010: Understanding and Improving Health. Conference Edition. Washington, DC: US Dept of Health and Human Services; 2000. Also available at http://www.health.gov/healthypeople/default.htm.

64. **US Department of Health and Human Services**. The Surgeon General's Call to Action to Prevent and Decrease Overweight and Obesity. US Department of Health and Human Services, Public Health Service, Office of the Surgeon General; 2001.

65. **National Heart Lung and Blood Institute**. Clinical Guidelines on the Identification, Evaluation, and Treatment of Overweight and Obesity in Adults: The Evidence Report. NIH Publication NO. 98-4083. National Institutes of Health; 1998.

66. **Flegal KM, Graubard BI, Williamson DF, et al**. Excess deaths associated with underweight, overweight, and obesity. JAMA. 2005;293:1861-7.

67. **Cochran SD, Mays VM, Bowen D, et al**. Cancer-related risk indicators and preventive screening behaviors among lesbians and bisexual women. American Journal of Public Health. 2001;91:591-7.

68. **Aaron DJ, Markovic N, Danielson ME, et al**. Behavioral risk factors for disease and preventive health practices among lesbians. Am J Public Health. 2001;91:972-5.

69. **Dibble SL, Roberts SA, Robertson PA, et al**. Risk factors for ovarian cancer: lesbian and heterosexual women. Oncology Nursing Forum. 2002;29:E1-7.

70. **Roberts SA, Dibble SL, Nussey B, et al**. Cardiovascular disease risk in lesbian women. Women's Health Issues. 2003;13:167-74.

71. **Boehmer U, Bowen DJ, Bauer GR**. Overweight and obesity in sexual minority women: evidence from population-based data. American Journal of Public Health. 97. In press.

72. **Smith CA, Stillman S**. What do women want? The effects of gender and sexual orientation on the desirability of physical attributes in the personal ads of women. Sex Roles. 2002;46:337.

73. **Bergeron SM, Senn CY**. Body image and sociocultural norms: a comparison of heterosexual and lesbian women. Psychology of Women Quarterly. 1998;22:385-401.

74. **Cogan JC**. Lesbians walk the tightrope of beauty: thin is in but femme is out. Journal of Lesbian Studies. 1999;3:77-89.

75. **Cohen AB, Tannenbaum AJ**. Lesbian and bisexual women's judgments of the attractiveness of different body types. Journal of Sex Research. 2001;8:226-32.

76. **Heffernan K**. Lesbians and the internalization of societal standards of weight and appearance. Journal of Lesbian Studies. 1999;3:121-7.

77. **Strong SM, Williamson DA, Netemeyer RG, et al**. Eating disorder symptoms and concerns about body differ as a function of gender and sexual orientation. Journal of Social and Clinical Psychology. 2000;19:240-55.

78. **Bowen DJ, Balsam K**. A review of obesity issues in sexual minority women. Obesity Research. Under review.

79. **Goodwin MA, Zyzanski SJ, Zronek S, et al**. A clinical trial of tailored office systems for preventive service delivery. The Study to Enhance Prevention by Understanding Practice (STEP-UP). Am J Prev Med. 2001;21:20-8.

80. **US National Research Council, Committee on Diet and Health**. Diet and Health: Implications for Reducing Chronic Disease Risk. National Academy of Sciences; 1989.

81. **US Department of Health and Human Services**. Healthy People 2000: National Health Promotion and Disease Prevention Objectives. US Government Printing Office; 1990.

82. **Bowen DJ, Beresford SA**. Dietary interventions to prevent disease. Annual Review of Public Health. 2002;23:255-86.

83. **Ammerman AS, Lindquist CH, Lohr KN, et al**. The efficacy of behavioral interventions to modify dietary fat and fruit and vegetable intake: a review of the evidence. Prev Med. 2002;35:25-41.

84. **Barefoot JC, Brummet BH, Clapp-Channing NE, et al**. Moderators of the effect of social support on depressive symptoms in cardiac patients. American Journal of Cardiology. 2000;86:438-42.

85. **Centers for Disease Control and Prevention**. Data & Trends: National Diabetes Surveillance System. 2005. Available at http://www.cdc.gov/diabetes/statistics/index.htm.

86. **Mays VM, Yancy AK, Cochran SD, et al**. Heterogeneity of health disparities among African American, Hispanic, and Asian American women: unrecognized influences of sexual orientation. American Journal of Public Health. 2002;92:632-9.

87. **Zaza S, Briss PA, Harris KW, Task Force on Community Preventive Services, eds**. The Guide to Community Preventive Services. What Works to Promote Health? Oxford University Press; 2005.

88. **Barry MJ**. The PSA conundrum. Arch Intern Med. 2006;166:7-8.

89. **Briss P, Rimer N, Reilley B, et al**. Promoting informed decisions about cancer screening in communities and health care systems. American Journal of Preventive Medicine. 2004;26:67-80.

90. **van Kesteren PJM, Asscheman H, Megens, JA, et al**. Mortality and morbidity in transsexual subjects treated with cross-sex hormones. Clinical Endocrinology. 1997;47:337-42.

91. **Cooley TP**. Non-AIDS-defining cancer in HIV-infected people. Hematology/oncology clinics of North America. 2003;17:889-99.

92. **Frisch M, Biggar RJ, Engels EA, et al**. Association of cancer with AIDS-related immunosuppression in adults [see comment]. JAMA. 2001;285:1736-45.

93. **Hentrich MU, Brack NG, Schmid P, et al**. Testicular germ cell tumors in patients with human immunodeficiency virus infection. Cancer. 1996;77:2109-16.

94. **Dieckmann KP, Pichlmeier U**. Clinical epidemiology of testicular germ cell tumors. World J Urol. 2004;22:2-14.

95. **van der Snoek EM, Neisters HG, Mulder PG, et al**. Human papillomavirus infection in men who have sex with men participating in a Dutch gay-cohort study. Sexually Transmitted Diseases. 2003;30:639-44.

96. **Lawrence AA**. Vaginal neoplasia in a male-to-female transsexual: case report, review of the literature, and recommendations for cytological screening. The International Journal of Transgenderism. 2001;5. Available at http://www.symposion.com/ijt/ijtvo05no 01_01.htm.

97. **Gee R**. Primary care health issues among men who have sex with men. Journal of the American Academy of Nurse Practitioners. 2006;18:144-53.

98. **Friedman HB, Saah AJ, Sherman ME, et al**. Human papillomavirus, anal squamous intraepithelial lesions, and human immunodeficiency virus in a cohort of gay men. Journal of Infectious Diseases. 1998;178:45-52.

99. **Goldstone SE, Welton ML**. Anorectal sexually transmitted infections in men who have sex with men—special considerations for clinicians. Clinics in Colon and Rectal Surgery. 2004;17:235-39.

100. **Knight D**. Health care screening for men who have sex with men [see comment]. American Family Physician. 2004;69:2149-56.

101. **Bowen DJ, Boehmer U**. The lack of cancer surveillance data on sexual minorities and strategies for change. Cancer Causes and Control; in press.

102. **Clarke CA, Glaser SL**. Population-based surveillance of HIV-associated cancers: utility of cancer registry data. Journal of Acquired Immune Deficiency Syndromes. 2004;36:1083-91.

103. **Koblin BA, Hessol NA, Zauber AG, et al**. Increased incidence of cancer among homosexual men, New York City and San Francisco, 1978-1990. American Journal of Epidemiology. 1996;144:916-23.

104. **Chin-Hong PV, Vittinghoff E, Cranston RD, et al**. Age-related prevalence of anal cancer precursors in homosexual men: the EXPLORE study. Journal of the National Cancer Institute. 2005;97:896-905.

105. **Chin-Hong PV, Vittinghoff E, Cranston RD, et al**. Age-specific prevalence of anal human papillomavirus infection in HIV-negative sexually active men who have sex with men: the EXPLORE study. Journal of Infectious Diseases. 2004;190:2070-6.

106. **Dunleavey R**. The role of viruses and sexual transmission in anal cancer. Nursing Times. 2005;101:38-41.

107. **Dean L, Meyer IH, Robinson K, et al**. Lesbian, gay, bisexual, and transgender health: findings and concerns. Journal of the Gay and Lesbian Medical Association. 2000;4:101-51.

108. **Goldie SJ, Kuntz KM, Weinstein MC, et al**. Cost-effectiveness of screening for anal squamous intraepithelial lesions and anal cancer in human immunodeficiency virus-negative homosexual and bisexual men. American Journal of Medicine. 2000;108:634-41.

109. **Goldie SJ, Kuntz KM, Weinstein MC, et al**. The clinical effectiveness and cost-effectiveness of screening for anal squamous intraepithelial lesions in homosexual and bisexual HIV-positive men. JAMA. 1999;281:1822-9.

110. **Chiao EY, Giordano TP, Palefsky JM, et al**. Screening HIV-infected individuals for anal cancer precursor lesions: a systematic review. Clinical Infectious Diseases. 2006;43:223-33.

111. **Chin-Hong PV, Palefsky JM**. Human papillomavirus anogenital disease in HIV-infected individuals. Dermatologic Therapy. 2005;18:67-76.

112. **Palefsky JM, Holly EA, Efirdc JD, et al**. Anal intraepithelial neoplasia in the highly active antiretroviral therapy era among HIV-positive men who have sex with men. AIDS. 2005;19:1407-14.

113. **Bonvicini KA, Perlin MJ**. The same but different: clinician-patient communication with gay and lesbian patients. Patient Education and Counseling. 2003;51:115-22.

114. **Hinchliff S, Gott M, Galena E**. 'I daresay I might find it embarrassing': general practitioners' perspectives on discussing sexual health issues with lesbian and gay patients. Health & Social Care in the Community. 2005;13:345-53.

115. **Kiss A**. Does gender have an influence on the patient-physician communication? The Journal of Men's Health and Gender. 2004;1:77-82.

116. **Gay and Lesbian Medical Association**. Guidelines for care of lesbian, gay, bisexual and transgender patients. Available at http://www.glma.org/pub/GLMA_Guidelines.pdf. Accessed October 27, 2005.

117. **Heck JE, Sell RL, Sheinfeld Gorin S**. Health care access among individuals involved in same-sex relationships. American Journal of Public Health. 2006;96:1111-8.

118. **Diamant AL, Schuster MA, Lever J**. Receipt of preventive health care services by lesbians. American Journal of Preventive Medicine. 2000;19:141-8.

119. **Institute of Medicine Committee on Lesbian Health Research Priorities**. Lesbian Health. Current Assessment and Directions for the Future. Institute of Medicine, Committee on Lesbian Health Research Priorities, Neuroscience and Behavioral Health Program. Health Sciences Policy Program, Health Sciences Section; 1999.

Chapter 8

Mental Health: Epidemiology, Assessment, and Treatment

MATTHEW W. RUBLE, MD
MARSHALL FORSTEIN, MD

Homosexuality is assuredly no advantage, but it is nothing to be ashamed of, no vice, no degradation, it cannot be classified as an illness
—Sigmund Freud, "Letter to an American Mother," 1935

Introduction

As with all patients, a basic mental health assessment is an important aspect of primary care for lesbian, gay, bisexual, and transgender (LGBT) patients. In order to offer the most appropriate care for LGBT patients, it is critical for clinicians to familiarize themselves with the particular vulnerabilities to mental illness in LGBT populations, as well as the most effective assessment techniques and treatment approaches available. Generations of gay, lesbian, and bisexual individuals still remember a time when the medical professions pathologized their sexual identity and behavior. Despite the fact that three decades have passed since the American Psychiatric Association removed homosexuality as a diagnostic category, lingering stigma remains a barrier to accessing mental healthcare. By presenting the differences in epidemiology, presentation, diagnosis, and treatment of common mental health disorders affecting lesbian, gay, and bisexual (LGB) communities (note that transgender mental health needs are addressed in Chapter 12), this chapter aims to prepare clinicians to break down these barriers and offer the best care possible to their patients. It is not meant to be a complete text on psychiatric evaluation and treatment, but to provide a primer on the role of the primary care clinician in mental healthcare. The relationship between a healthy mind and a healthy body is clear, highlighting the need for primary care providers and mental health professionals to collaborate in the total care of patients.

Epidemiology

Background

The prevalence of mental health disorders among LGB populations is not yet well understood. Relatively few studies have applied higher quality research methodologies to this area. In the book *Sexual Orientation and Mental Health*,[1] Cochran and Mays describe "three major transformations" in the epidemiologic research on LGB mood disorders over the last 50 years. First, during the years in which homosexuality was pathologized, epidemiologic research was conducted with cohorts of patients presenting only to mental health clinics, resulting in overestimates of the prevalence of mood and anxiety disorders among gay men and lesbians. The second transformation in epidemiologic research reflected the removal of homosexuality as a psychopathology diagnosis in 1973. Researchers began to sample populations from settings outside the medical and mental health arenas, resulting in studies involving healthier and less stigmatized individuals. The research from this period revealed that homosexual men and women had relatively equal rates of psychopathology as those of heterosexuals. The third and most recent transformation in research has focused on healthcare disparities related to social status, HIV status, ethnicity, and race, in addition to gender and sexual orientation, and has led to more valid research, given the multiple social determinants of mental health. In addition, LGB research has expanded to try to understand the influence of harassment, discrimination, and victimization on the prevalence of mental health disorders. These studies, although still limited in size and scope, have found that LGB populations have similar rates of many mental health disorders compared to the general population but may be more at risk for mood disorders, anxiety disorders, and suicidal behavior.

Mood Disorders, Anxiety Disorders, and Suicidal Behavior

It is projected that, by 2020, mental illness will be the fourth largest cause of morbidity and mortality around the world.[2] LGB populations may be particularly vulnerable to some mental health disorders. A recent Dutch population-based study[3] found that gay and lesbian participants reported more acute mental health symptoms, poorer general mental health, more acute physical symptoms, and more chronic conditions than heterosexuals. In their analysis of psychiatric and sexual behavior data from the 1996 National Survey of Midlife Development in the United States, Cochran and Mays[4] found that the prevalence of panic attacks and major depression was greater in gay or bisexual men than in heterosexual men (17.9% vs. 3.8% and 31% vs. 10.2%, respectively, p < .05). Lesbian or bisexual women had a significantly greater 12-month prevalence of generalized anxiety disorder (14.7%) compared with heterosexual women (3.8%, p < .05).

This study also found that gay or bisexual men and lesbian or bisexual women used one or more mental healthcare services at a significantly higher rate in the last 12 months compared to heterosexual men and women. The four treatment services measured were (1) attending an appointment with a mental health provider; (2) attending an appointment with a primary care provider for a mental health reason (3) attending a self-help group; and (4) taking psychiatric medication. Lesbian or bisexual women used one or more of these treatment services (66%) at a greater rate than heterosexual women (35.8%, p < .05); gay or bisexual men also had a greater rate of use (56.7%) compared to heterosexual men (24.9%, p < .05). In addition, 17.8% of gay or bisexual men in this study rated their overall mental health at age 16 as "fair" or "poor," compared to only 6.1% of heterosexual men (p < .05); they also rated their current overall mental health less favorably (20.4% "fair" or "poor") compared to heterosexual men (7.7% "fair" or "poor", p < .05). Differences in overall mental health ratings between heterosexual and lesbian or bisexual women were not significant.[4] It should be noted that most mental health studies group individuals who report bisexual orientation with those reporting gay or lesbian orientation, making it difficult to separate out rates specifically for bisexual mental health.

A review of multiple studies[5] found an increased lifetime prevalence of suicidal ideation for gay or bisexual men and lesbians compared to the general population,[5] but studies of completed suicides found no evidence for elevated rates in LGB populations.[5] Data from the Chicago Health and Life Experiences of Women study (1997) and the National Study of Health and Life Experiences of Women (2003) also suggested that lesbians may be at heightened risk for suicidal ideation.[6]

The National Longitudinal Study of Adolescent Health found that boys with same-sex or bisexual attractions or behaviors tended to have higher rates of self-assessed anxiety and depression, and adolescent girls with same-sex or bisexual attractions or behaviors reported lower levels of self-esteem and were more likely to describe themselves as depressed.[7] LGB youths appear to have higher rates of suicide attempts and ideation compared with heterosexual youths.[8] It has not been established whether the elevated risk for suicidal ideation in LGB adolescents evolves from the same underlying psychiatric stress and disorders as their heterosexual counterparts, along with the additional stress of growing up with same-sex feelings in a homophobic society, or if isolation, stigma, and shame in certain personality constellations affect the emergence of psychiatric stress and disorder that leads to suicidal ideation. The complex interaction of individual personality traits (that evolve out of the interplay of temperament and parental/sibling relationships); genetic predispositions for psychiatric disorders; cognitive coping strategies; antihomosexual societal attitudes and internalized homophobia, as well as vulnerabilities to abuse, complicates the interpretation of LGB adolescent mental health research findings. It does appear that LGB youth are at higher risk for suicidal ideation, attempts, and completions than their non-LGB counterparts. It also appears that, for some, this risk declines after adolescence.

Environmental, Cultural, and Social Factors

It is not clear why LGB populations have higher rates of mood disorders, anxiety disorders, and suicidal ideation. However, there are theories that the higher rates are not due to some inherent risk in being LGB but due to the environmental and social factors surrounding LGB patients. One study[9] found higher rates of depression, hopelessness, and present suicidality among LGB youths compared to heterosexual peers. However, when they controlled for other predictors of these issues, such as negative stress, poor social supports, poor coping techniques, and barriers to social supports, the differences based on sexual orientation disappeared. This study suggests that sexual orientation alone cannot account for the higher levels of distress but rather the lack of social supports and internal self-esteem that result from living in a culture intolerant to homosexuality. A 2004 study[10] with a household probability-based sample of 2881 men who have sex with men (MSM) found that 17.2% of the sample were depressed and 12.1% were distressed. Both depression and distress were associated with a history of victimization by antigay violence; not self-identifying as gay or homosexual; a high level of alienation from the LGBT community; and not having a current domestic partner. Being HIV-infected was also correlated with distress and depression, but the association was no longer significant after controlling for other factors, such as demographic characteristics, substance use, and current social context. Depression (but not distress) was associated with being abused as a child and recent sexual dysfunction.[10] Studies of lesbian mental health suggest that suicidal behavior and depression among lesbian and bisexual women may be related to a history of physical abuse or childhood sexual abuse.[11]

As suggested above, a lack of social supports appears to be correlated with poorer mental health in LGB individuals, particularly men. Additional studies have supported these findings. For example, two studies found that gay male subjects who reported social isolation later experienced significantly more adverse mental health outcomes.[12,13] Internalized homophobia may also be a risk factor for mental health problems in LGB individuals, including substance abuse, eating disorders, self-mutilation, and suicidal behavior.[14]

Assessment and Diagnosis: The Initial Interview

Primary care providers often see patients who present with symptoms of depression, anxiety, and other mental health issues. These symptoms may or may not be explicitly stated by the patient. In order to provide an environment conducive to high-quality assessment, diagnosis, and treatment of mental health conditions, it is critical for providers to establish a good alliance with their patients, to conduct a thorough initial clinical interview, and to ask evidence-based screening questions for potential mood or anxiety disorders. This is true for all patients, regardless of sexual orientation; however, with LGB patients, it is especially important to assess additional factors, including their comfort with sexual identity and orientation, their sexual and substance use risk behaviors, and the extent of their social networks and supports. How to approach these areas during the initial clinical interview is explored in more detail below. (See Chapter 12 for a discussion of transgender mental health evaluation and management; see Chapters 9, 11, and 15 for information on assessing substance use and sexual risk behaviors).

Sexual Identity

The initial clinical interview with LGB patients who have mental health concerns is similar in most ways to those for other patients, whether in primary care or when referred to a mental health specialist. However, when caring for LGB patients, it is important to understand how the patient self-identifies his or her sexual orientation, and to assess the patient's acceptance of his or her orientation. This is particularly important for LGB patients for whom a lack of social acceptance and opportunities to discuss complex issues of sexuality may have exacerbated underlying psychological problems. Clinicians should also keep in mind that sexual identity is to be distinguished from sexual behaviors or fantasies. Some people fantasize or behave homosexually, but do not self-identify as a homosexual. Others may accept their same-sex orientation, but do not publicly identify as gay or lesbian, because of general society's negative perceptions of stereotypic behaviors associated with sexual minorities (eg, effeminate gay men, aggressive lesbians, etc), or because of perceived social stigma.

During the interview, clinicians can begin by asking what the most pressing concerns are for the patient, and then let the patient lead the discussion; based on what the patient says, the clinician can then assess how much the rest of the interview should focus on sexual orientation and identity issues. Clinicians should avoid making assumptions about how sexual orientation may influence the patient's well-being. By attending to what is, and what is not said (eg, anxiety when discussing a relationship), the provider may be able to assess the key issues that should be explored in future sessions.

To assess the patients' degree of comfort with their sexual orientation in a thorough manner, several key questions can be addressed at the outset. The primary care provider might choose a few of the following critical questions for the first visit, and then revisit the others at future visits.[15]

- At what age did you become aware of your sexuality? How?
- At what age did you identify yourself with that sexuality? How did you describe the identity you gave yourself?
- At what age did you disclose this information to another person? Who was that person, and what was the outcome of the disclosure?
- At what age did you have your first sexual experience? What was the behavior you engaged in?
- Do you engage, or have you engaged, in heterosexual activity? With whom? When? What is/was the behavior?
- With whom are you sexually active now?
- How "out" are you now? Who knows about your sexual identity?
- Who are the most important people in your life at this time? What is the nature of those relationships?
- What were/are the negative aspects of coming out?
- What were/are the positive aspects of coming out?

Asking questions in the vernacular used by patients may be particularly helpful in establishing rapport and may strengthen the alliance between the patient and provider, enhancing the disclosure of relevant clinical information.

Assessment of Social Factors

Sociological assessment in conjunction with psychological assessment is vital in any evaluation of mental health disorders. As discussed in the epidemiology section above, there are specific environmental, cultural, and social factors that may influence the mental health of LGB individuals. For example, social stigma, victimization, fear of "coming out," loneliness, and inability to find a partner may lead to depression, anxiety, and/or suicidality. Therefore, it is critical for clinicians, when doing a mental health assessment, to ask about social isolation, social supports, and current and historic trauma, including victimization by hate crimes or other discriminatory acts. Furthermore, clinicians should evaluate the coping styles of patients by asking questions such as, "Do you talk about your problems?" "Are you able to be distracted during times of stress ("do something fun")?" "Are you able to confront the factors that cause you stress?" and "Do you use exercise to deal with stress?"[11] These simple questions have diagnostic value and provide an entry to more advanced psychotherapeutic treatment techniques. A summary of the psychological, sociological, and biopsychosocial factors that should be assessed in every LGBT patient is provided in Table 8-1.

Probing to learn about positive mentors, role models, and supports that are currently present or have been present in the patient's life may also be helpful in eventually developing a therapeutic plan. The presence of positive role models seems to have a protective effect for LGB youth, and one

Table 8-1   Psychological, Sociological, and Biopsychosocial Factors to Include in Assessment of LGB Patients

Psychological Factors	Sociological Factors	Biopsychosocial Factors
• Negative life stress • Coping techniques—how one deals with stress • Loneliness • Personal identification as LGB • History of abuse, neglect, abandonment, or rejection • History of suicidal ideation • "Out" status (public awareness of homosexual behavior)	• Lack of social supports or events • Stigmatization • Community alienation • Presence of a significant other or ability to find one if desired • Barriers to social supports	• Exercise and other physical activity • HIV status • History of suicide attempt • Medical illness • Alcohol / Drug use or abuse

would assume this effect would persist into adulthood.[16] It may be helpful to ask if the person has ever had someone they really admired or if they know about any openly gay LGB people.

Clinician-Patient Communication

Although not well studied specifically in LGB populations, alliance formation between patient and clinician may be the key critical factor to a positive outcome in mental healthcare. Patients do best when their provider is supportive and empathic.[17-18] Given the historical factors related to psychiatry's past view of LGB patients and given the fact that some patients may have experienced neglect, discrimination, or violence at the hands of strangers, healthcare professionals, or their own families, it is particularly important that all clinicians should focus on establishing trust and encourage candor early in the initial encounter.

Clinicians should also be prepared at the first encounter to answer question from LGB patients, such as "Do you have other gay, lesbian, or bisexual patients?" "What do you believe about same-sex relationships?" and "Are you gay?" Clinicians should take the time in advance to think about their own biases and perspectives on sexual orientation so they can comfortably answer these questions. Self-disclosure of sexual orientation by the provider depends on the reason an individual is seeking care, provider type, and treatment goals as well as individual choice. Mental health providers may want to explore the meaning of those questions more thoroughly even while agreeing to answer them at the beginning of treatment.

For example, in psychotherapy it is appropriate to address the patient's query as to the sexual orientation of the therapist at the outset of therapy, but that same question takes on a significantly different meaning six months into the treatment, as it may be bound up with subconscious and unconscious fantasies and projections on the part of the patient. Primary care providers might more easily answer the question directly at the initial request, disclosing their sexual orientations but little else that is not relevant to the development of an alliance, in order to assure patients that their concerns will be understood. Some patients only feel comfortable seeing LGB providers. While there may be many reasons for this, the choice may suggest deeply seated issues of shame and low self-esteem that reflect a sense of rejection from the non-LGB people in their life.

Even in primary care practice, at times, it is useful to answer the question, "Are you gay?" with a statement like: "I'll tell you the answer in a few minutes, but it might be worthwhile for us to explore this question first to see if we can learn anything that might be helpful to me as your provider." The clinician can then follow-up a question such as, "What will it mean to you if I am gay, lesbian, or bisexual?" The answer to this question could help the provider recognize what is important to the patient and evaluate the patient's level of internalized homophobia or degree of comfort with his or her own identity. LGBT healthcare providers may have experienced their own degree of victimization and struggled with their own internalized homophobia or self-hatred. Gay and lesbian physicians in training have invested "considerable energy and emotion navigating training programs, which may be, at best, indifferent and at worst, hostile" towards their sexual orientation.[19] So, it is important for the clinician to be sure that he or she has addressed these personal issues prior to caring for vulnerable populations.

Tools for Assessment of Mood and Anxiety Disorders

To date, no studies suggest that depression, anxiety, or suicidal ideation manifest in a significantly distinct manner in LGBT patients. The objective assessment for mood and anxiety disorders should therefore follow the same structure as for the general population. The following assessment tools can prove useful in assessing depression and bipolar disorder:

- Beck Depression Inventory II, revised[20]
- Mood Disorders Questionnaire to assess bipolar disorder[21]
- Cornell Dysthymia Rating Scale[22]

These objective rating scales, the first two involving patient self-assessment, can be accessed at https://www.familyaware.us/moodtest/questionnaire .php, the Web site for the nonprofit group Families for Depression Awareness. These scales are thorough in scope, quick, and easy to use and interpret and can guide treatment, especially if psychopharmacologic management is needed.

An assessment for anxiety disorders should first include a review of the three A's of anxiety (acute anxiety, anticipatory anxiety, and avoidance) and a standardized rating tool to measure the critical features of the baseline degree of illness. Examples of these tools include:

- Beck Anxiety Inventory,[23]
- Self-rating Anxiety Scale,[24]

Both of these can be accessed at http://www.anxietyhelp.org/index.html. None of these scales have been specifically validated in LGB populations, but clinical experience has shown them to be effective for sexual minority patients.

After completing a comprehensive initial history and assessment, it will be appropriate to refer some patients for further evaluation and therapies by clinicians trained in these modalities. The primary care provider should evaluate for the general disorders, such as depression or anxiety disorder, but should have a low threshold for consulting a psychiatrist or other mental health professional for specialist care.

Risk Behaviors, Comorbidities, and Cofactors of Concern

When performing mental health assessments, clinicians should also be aware that LGB patients may experience certain risk behaviors, comorbidities, and cofactors that can complicate, or have a causal role in, mental illness. These are explained below.

Issues for Gay and Bisexual Men

Methamphetamine Use

Crystal methamphetamine use appears to be on the rise among gay and bisexual men who live in urban areas. Several studies have shown methamphetamine to have a causative role in depression, mania, and psychosis.[25-26] In addition, these same studies suggest that gay and bisexual men may also "self-medicate" their mental health illnesses with methamphetamine. These worrisome facts, in addition to the data showing gay and bisexual men who use methamphetamine are more likely to engage in high-risk sexual activity, suggest primary care providers should screen for this substance use in all gay and bisexual men. Please see Chapter 9 to learn more about substance abuse and treatment for LGBT patients.

Anabolic Steroid Use

The psychological effects of anabolic steroids have been well-known and documented for decades.[27] Researchers in the United Kingdom have found an alarming rate of anabolic steroid abuse among gay men sampled from local London gyms. This data has not been replicated in the United States, but this trend supports the suggestion to screen all gay men for anabolic steroid abuse and possible mental health sequelae, such as depression, mania, and psychosis.[28]

Sexual Desire and Behavior

It is commonly thought that depression can lower sexual desire and safer sex competency. In one study, gay men with dysthymia disorder were found to be two times more likely to have unprotected anal sex with casual partners than gay men who were not depressed. [29] Also in this study, gay men with major depressive episode, not dysthymia, were less likely to have any type of sex overall.[29]

HIV/AIDS

It is beyond the scope of this chapter to comment on all of the mental health implications of HIV and AIDS. Untreated mood disorders, and likely untreated anxiety disorders, have an impact on adherence to medication management and progression of HIV/AIDS. A recent review by Olatunji et al summarizes the psychological and psychopharmacological treatments of mood disorders for patients with HIV/AIDS.[30] Perhaps of greatest importance to the primary care clinician is the fact that there are many drug interactions between medications used to treat HIV and medications for anxiety and depression that must be considered before starting any HIV patient on a psychopharmacologic regimen. Key interactions to be aware of are highlighted in Table 8-2. For more details of other drug interactions with antiretrovirals, please see: http://www.hopkins-hivguide.org.

Syphilis

Reports of increasing rates of syphilis infection in gay and bisexual men should prompt primary care clinicians to screen for serum markers and neurological signs of tertiary syphilis. Common mental and cerebrospinal health symptoms would include personality change, mood lability, depression, psychosis, and mania.

Issues for Lesbian and Bisexual Women

Reproductive Health and Pyschological Well-being

Within the spectrum of mood disorders, all women should be screened for premenstrual dysphoric disorder. The trend of increasing pregnancy rates for lesbian women should prompt primary care clinicians to screen for

Table 8-2   Types of Drug Interactions of Psychotrophics with HIV/AIDS Antiretrovirals

ANTIRETROVIRALS	DRUG-DRUG INTERACTION
Efavirenz: Reverse transcriptase inhibitor; Cytochrome P450 inhibitor/inducer	Use caution with midazolam, triazolam.
Nevirapine: Reverse transcriptase inducer; Cytochrome P450 inducer	Use caution with midazolam, triazolam, oral contraceptives.
Protease Inhibitors (PI)	Do not prescribe with midazolam, triazolam, pimozide, St. John's wort.
Ritonavir: the most potent enzyme inhibitor	Use caution with carbamazepine, clonazepam, antipsychotics, stimulants, SSRIs and TCAs (monitor levels if able).
	PI levels may be increased by fluvoxamine and nefazodone.
	PI levels may be decreased by carbamazepine, phenobarbital, phenytoin, venlafaxine.
	Do not use with alprazolam, clozapine, diazepam, flurazepam, meperidine, zolpidem.
	Use caution with maprotiline, nefazodone, trazodone, venlafaxine.

mood disorder complications due to fertility medications or pregnancy itself. A recent study found that pregnancy does not necessarily ameliorate mood disorders and that depressed women who are currently on antidepressants should likely continue the medication to prevent relapse during pregnancy.[31] Data collected from the National Birth Defects Prevention Study found one class of antidepressant medication, the SSRIs (selective serotonin reuptake inhibitors), were not associated with significantly increased risks of most catagories of birth defects.[32] This fact must be balanced with new findings about paroxetine, an SSRI antidepressant, and fetal malformations[33] and another study that reveals a risk of persistent pulmonary hypertension for a newborn with SSRI use during pregnancy and delivery.[34]

There are suggestions that LGB teens are more likely than heterosexual teens to become pregnant or father a pregnancy during adolescence, sometimes in response to denying sexual orientation, identifying with peers, or feeling extreme loneliness.[35] Decisions regarding parenting choices may have significant mental health implications. Screening should be done with all lesbian and bisexual women for current and past pregnancies, terminations, and the situations surrounding these events.

Issues for All LGB Patients

Body Image and Eating Disorders

Research in this area presents conflicting data. One recent study found that gay men diet more, fear becoming fat more, and are more dissatisfied with their body image and muscularity compared to heterosexual men.[36] In the same study, however, it was found that gay and straight men exercise with the same frequency and have the same degree of guilt when missing a workout. [36] Another recent study of body image in gay men found that gay men and heterosexual men had rated their body image similarly.[37]

For lesbian and bisexual women, there is also variable data on eating disorders. The most recent self-assessment questionnaire suggests that "out" bisexual women have at least a two times greater prevalence of an eating disorder compared to "out" lesbians and heterosexual women.[38] An earlier study suggested that being a lesbian was "protective" from eating disorders.[39]

Given the current evidence, primary care providers should consider screening LGB patients for both general satisfaction with body image and eating disorders. A simple and memorable tool such as the SCOFF can be helpful for evaluating eating disorders.[40]

SCOFF	
SICK	Do you make yourself Sick because you feel uncomfortably full?
CONTROL	Do you worry you have lost Control over how much you eat?
ONE	Have you recently lost more than One stone in a three month period?
	(One stone is 14 pounds)
FAT	Do you believe yourself to be Fat when others say you are too thin?
FOOD	Would you say that Food dominates your life?

*One point for every "yes"; a score of ≥ 2 indicates a likely case of anorexia nervosa or bulimia

Aging

LGB individuals may be at risk for mental illness in later life. In addition to the typical developmental milestones for this age group: integrity and pleasure with a life well-lived versus despair for a life wasted or purposeless, LGB people may struggle with negative self-image and self-hatred; self-imposed or societal isolation; and, if coming out late in life, despair for time wasted. A recent study of gay and lesbian adults aged 60-91 revealed that these older adults had more favorable ratings of their own mental health if they had a higher sense of self-esteem, greater supports (friends and family or socialization), and a lower level of internalized homophobia. Older lesbians reported less internalized homophobia, lower rates of alcohol abuse, and lower levels of suicidality than heterosexual women.[41] A complete review of social supports and the patient's own self-concept could preemptively alert the primary care provider to risks for late life depression, anxiety, and suicide.

Spirituality

Exposure to religious teachings and values often begin before the awakening of sexual identity. Integrating spiritual beliefs with being LGB can be challenging and can evolve over time. Limited and inconsistent data exists on the benefits and drawbacks of religious affiliation for LGB people. One study suggests that having a religious affiliation may be a source of protection and support for mental and medical health.[42] A conflicting study suggests that some religious affiliations may be a source of alienation and lower self-esteem for LGB people.[43] In either case, it may be useful for clinicians to take a spiritual history by asking initial questions such as, "Are you a spiritual person?" or "What do you think (the patient's word for spirituality, eg, "God," "the spirit," etc) thinks of you?" The patient's answers to these questions could be considered a projective assessment of their own superego or identity and will help determine if their view of religion is either a support or a source of condemnation.

Treatments

It is commonly known that the best practices for treatment of the mental health illnesses discussed in this chapter include psychotherapy, somatic treatment, or a combination of the two. Among LGB populations, in addition to these treatment modalities, it is especially critical to help patients achieve a positive identity, establish supports, and consider unique needs (for example a dual diagnosis of depression and methamphetamine abuse) and to be vigilant about potential medication interactions (for example, the interaction of antiretroviral drugs with psychotropics). The following sections review some of the options for both psychotherapy and somatic treatments and refer the reader to more thorough discussions of these modalities, as the general principles and medications are similar for LGB, as well as heterosexual, patients. This section concludes with suggestions for improving the social supports of LGB patients.

Biologic/Somatic Treatment

To date, no psychopharmacologic evidence suggests a different medication treatment algorithm for depressed, anxious, or suicidal LGB patients compared to heterosexual patients. A general text in psychiatry, such as *Synopsis of Psychiatry: Behavioral Sciences/Clinical Psychiatry* by Benjamin J. Sadock and Virginia A. Sadock will provide an overview of the routine management of all psychiatric illnesses. Even in HIV-infected patients with depression, very little pharmacologic information exists that focuses on sexual orientation. One small study exploring the use of sertraline in 27 depressed, HIV-infected men and one HIV-infected woman showed that 14 participants (52%) responded to the medication.[44] Another small study of 27 HIV-infected individuals with depression compared the efficacy rates and time to improvement using methylphenidate and desipramine. The study found each medication was equally effective, and there was no difference in the time to improvement.

Most current approaches to the medical treatment of depression begin with a gradual dosing of selective serotonin reuptake inhibitors or SSRIs. Unfortunately, less than one-third of individuals with major depressive disorder (MDD) who are treated with a representative SSRI will achieve remission.[45] For patients with MDD, using the Sequenced Treatment Alternatives to Relieve Depression (STAR*D), developed for a large population-based National Institutes of Mental Health study,[46] could prove effective. To date, this study provides the greatest degree of evidence for depression treatment with medication, although it may not be the most appropriate treatment for all patients. The STAR*D treatment algorithm included multiple phases. In Phase I, all patients are started with citalopram (an SSRI) treatment. Phase II randomized patients who did not achieve remission to either augmentation with either buspirone (a type of SSRI), buproprion (a norepinepherine/dopamine agent), or cognitive therapy, or switched citalopram to sertraline (an SSRI), buproprion, venlafaxine (an SNRI-serotonin/norepinepherine reuptake inhibitor) or cognitive therapy. Phase III suggests nonremitters either switch to mirtazapine (a novel agent) or nortriptyline (a TCA), or that their current antidepressant is augmented by either lithium or thyroid hormone. Phase IV suggests nonremitters switch to either a combination treatment with both mirtazapine and venlafaxine xr, or switch to tranylcypromine (an MAOI). Although the study findings do not provide specific information for LGB patients, they do provide evidence for primary care providers that aggressive management of depression can lead to total remission of depression even in patients with comorbid medical illness. At the same time, this study reveals that a significant proportion of patients seen in the primary care setting will not respond to conventional psychopharmacologic treatments and will require appropriate referral. For more details, see http://www.nimh.nih.gov/healthinformation/stard.cfm.

Primary care providers who are treating patients with depression should seek consultation from a mental health professional in the following situations:

1. *If the patient fails to achieve remission after initiating therapy using an SSRI.* For example, if the patient does not improve with a trial of a generic SSRI and does not improve after a subsequent switch or augmentation strategy.

2. *If the patient has a significant disability from the mental illness.* For example, if the patient is having difficulty at work, in interpersonal relationships, with comorbid substance abuse/dependence, with comorbid mental illness (such as posttraumatic stress disorder or PTSD, panic disorder, pain disorders, somatization disorders, or personality disorders), or with hopelessness or suicidal ideation.

3. *If the patient has a comorbid medical illness that might cause or worsen the mental health issues.* For example, if the patient has HIV/AIDS, diabetes, postpartum depression, or hypothyroidism, a psychiatrist who will consider both the medical and mental illnesses in guiding treatment, is needed to provide optimal care.

4. *If the patient has an objective response to medical treatment and social situations seem positive, but the patient continues to experience a sense of dissatisfaction.* For example, if the patient seems to have a pervasive negative sense of self-esteem relating to his or her LGBT status, this would suggest a form of psychotherapy is necessary.

In addition, electro-convulsive therapy must be kept in mind as an alternative treatment for depression and suicidality related to mood disorders, especially if multiple medications have been tried.

There are no algorithms similar to the STAR*D for standardized medication treatments for anxiety disorders or suicidal patients. In these cases, it can be helpful to use an evidence-based medicine approach to define treatment approaches for each of these areas.[47-49]

Psychotherapeutic Treatment

It is beyond the scope of this chapter to review the specific practice of psychotherapeutic techniques. Rather, we provide general features of psychotherapeutic treatments that are relevant to LGB patients. In all cases, we suggest following the American Psychological Association's Guidelines for Psychotherapy with LGB clients, summarized in Table 8-3.

Conversion Therapy

Currently there is one putative psychotherapeutic technique that is contraindicated—the Food and Drug Administration (FDA) equivalent of a black box warning—for all LGB patients. This is conversion or "reparative" therapy (realistically it cannot be considered a therapy), as labeled by the American Psychiatric Association (APA), a technique focused on changing someone's sexual orientation from homosexual or bisexual to heterosexual. There has been no published evidence to support the efficacy or safety of such techniques. The medical community has uniformly strongly advised against conversion therapy, as detailed in the following statement from the APA:

Table 8-3   American Psychological Association's Guidelines for Psychotherapy with Lesbian, Gay, and Bisexual Clients

Attitudes Toward Homosexuality and Bisexuality	**Guideline 1**. Psychologists understand that homosexuality and bisexuality are not indicative of mental illness.
	Guideline 2. Psychologists are encouraged to recognize how their attitudes and knowledge about lesbian, gay, and bisexual issues may be relevant to assessment and treatment and seek consultation or make appropriate referrals when indicated.
	Guideline 3. Psychologists strive to understand the ways in which social stigmatization (ie, prejudice, discrimination, and violence) poses risks to the mental health and well–being of lesbian, gay, and bisexual clients.
	Guideline 4. Psychologists strive to understand how inaccurate or prejudicial views of homosexuality or bisexuality may affect the client's presentation in treatment and the therapeutic process.
Relationships and Families	**Guideline 5**. Psychologists strive to be knowledgeable about and respect the importance of lesbian, gay, and bisexual relationships.
	Guideline 6. Psychologists strive to understand the particular circumstances and challenges facing lesbian, gay, and bisexual parents.
	Guideline 7. Psychologists recognize that the families of lesbian, gay, and bisexual people may include people who are not legally or biologically related.
	Guideline 8. Psychologists strive to understand how a person's homosexual or bisexual orientation may have an impact on his or her family of origin and the relationship to that family of origin.
Issues of Diversity	**Guideline 9**. Psychologists are encouraged to recognize the particular life issues or challenges experienced by lesbian, gay, and bisexual members of racial and ethnic minorities that are related to multiple and often conflicting cultural norms, values, and beliefs.
	Guideline 10. Psychologists are encouraged to recognize the particular challenges experienced by bisexual individuals.
	Guideline 11. Psychologists strive to understand the special problems and risks that exist for lesbian, gay, and bisexual youth.
	Guideline 12. Psychologists consider generational differences within lesbian, gay, and bisexual populations, and the particular challenges that may be experienced by lesbian, gay, and bisexual older adults.
	Guideline 13. Psychologists are encouraged to recognize the particular challenges experienced by lesbian, gay, and bisexual individuals with physical, sensory, and/or cognitive/emotional disabilities.
Education	**Guideline 14**. Psychologists support the provision of professional education and training on lesbian, gay, and bisexual issues.
	Guideline 15. Psychologists are encouraged to increase their knowledge and understanding of homosexuality and bisexuality through continuing education, training, supervision, and consultation.
	Guideline 16. Psychologists make reasonable efforts to familiarize themselves with relevant mental health, educational, and community resources for lesbian, gay, and bisexual people.

See http://www.apa.org/pi/lgbc/guidelines.html for the full set of guidelines.

In December of 1998, the Board of Trustees issued a position statement that the American Psychiatric Association opposes any psychiatric treatment, such as "reparative" or conversion therapy, which is
based upon the assumption that homosexuality per se is a mental disorder or based upon the a priori assumption that a patient should
change his/her sexual homosexual orientation. In doing so, the APA
joined many other professional organizations that either oppose or
are critical of "reparative" therapies, including the American Academy
of Pediatrics, the American Medical Association, the American
Psychological Association, the American Counseling Association, and
the National Association of Social Workers.[50]

LGB-Affirmative Therapy

In contrast to conversion therapy, LGB-affirmative therapy supports the
medical community's current view that homosexuality is a normal variant
of human behavior. This modality attempts to directly address issues of
internalized homophobia that may contribute to the development of mental health disorders, such as anxiety and depression. Although formal studies do not exist, we support the use of LGB-affirmative therapy in
combination with these methods. Many authors of textbooks on psychotherapy with LGB patients suggest a similar technique (see Appendix A
for resources). The psychotherapeutic treatments that have been determined to be "beneficial" or "likely to be beneficial" per the evidence-based
medicine method of clinical evidence for both depressive and anxiety disorders are listed in http://www.clinicalevidence.com.

Community Supports

It is a central argument of this book that all clinicians, to the extent possible and no matter the type of practice, should be trained and educated to
feel competent and knowledgeable in LGBT health. In a few areas of the
country, specialized health facilities already exist with services developed
specifically for the mental health needs of LGBT patients. These clinics may
be either stand-alone facilities where the mental and physical health and
social service needs of LGBT communities are gathered under one roof,
such as Fenway Community Health (FCH) in Boston, Mass (http://
www.fenwayhealth.org) or the Howard Brown Health Center in Chicago,
Ill (http://www.howardbrown.org), or may include a group of individuals
with expert training and interest in LGB health who work within a larger
facility (eg, the Psychiatry Department of Cambridge Hospital in
Massachusetts). For LGBT patients with mental health needs, these types of
facilities can be affirming and therapeutic, particularly since perceived
social support can have a positive influence on mental health. Mental
health referrals to these types of organizations can be helpful for patients
who seek care in an environment that is knowledgeable about the health

needs of LGBT communities. Appendix A has a list of resources for finding such facilities.

In-person support groups with other LGB people may also prove beneficial, particularly for those who feel isolated. Patients who live in more remote areas without these kinds of services or seek additional sources of social support may find help from LGBT hotlines and Web sites, such as the GLBT National Help Center (http://www.glnh.org, 1-888-The-GLNH); and Fenway Community Health Center's (http://www.fenwayhealth.org) LGBT Helpline (1-888-340-4528) and Peer Listening Line (1-800-399-PEER).

Conclusion

This chapter has reviewed the epidemiologic evidence that supports a greater vulnerability to mental illness in LGB populations and has made suggestions for initial screening, assessment, and treatment of depressive and anxiety disorders and suicidal ideation and risk. While culturally sensitive screening and assessment can be developed for the LGB patients in a helpful and health-promoting manner, the somatic or biological treatments for these illnesses are unlikely to vary from treatment methods employed for all patients with these disorders. However, psychotherapeutic interventions, social interventions, and educational programs seem to have the greater potential for narrowing the gap seen in the greater rates of these illnesses in LGB populations. Further research is needed in all areas of assessment and treatment of LGB patients with mental illness, including specific studies on the differences in treatment between heterosexual and homosexual patient's responses to somatic and psychotherapeutic treatments. Also, new theories exploring the development of one's sexual identity and the new theories regarding the fluidity of sexuality should influence the construction of these studies and subsequently, the clinical approach to assessment and treatment.

Summary Points

- LGB patients report more acute mental health symptoms and poorer general mental health than heterosexuals. Lesbian or bisexual women may be at higher risk for generalized anxiety disorder, gay or bisexual men for depression and anxiety disorders, and both for comorbid illnesses.
- LGB people, particularly LGB adolescents, are at increased risk for suicidal ideation and attempts.
- The higher rates of these mental health disorders are likely due to environmental and social factors surrounding LGB patients, rather than some inherent risk in being LGB. For example, the lack of social

supports and low internal self-esteem that result from living in a culture intolerant to homosexuality can confer risk for these illnesses.

- Primary care providers should provide a catered assessment that focuses on these greater risks for LGB patients and, in parallel, affirms the LGB patient's sexual identity. The provider must be prepared to create a safe, supportive professional relationship and to answer questions about his or her own experience with LGB issues.

- Assessment for mood and anxiety disorders should follow the same structure as for the general population. Assessment tools for these disorders have not been specifically validated in LGB patients, but seem to be equally effective.

- LGB patients should also be screened for risk behaviors, comorbidities, and other factors that could complicate or have a causal role in mental health disorders. For gay or bisexual men, this includes: anabolic steroid use, methamphetamine abuse, syphilis, and HIV/AIDS; for lesbian or bisexual women, this includes: menstruation, pregnancy, and menopause. For both LGB men and women, this includes: eating disorders, issues related to aging; and spirituality.

- New psychopharmacological treatment algorithms, such as STAR*D, have been developed to treat these illnesses in the general population; at this time there is little evidence to suggest alternative biological treatments for LGB patients. Primary care providers should seek consultation from mental health professionals in certain situations.

- Psychotherapy is a valuable treatment modality for LGB patients as long as the clinician supports the view that homosexuality is a normal variation of human behavior. The American Psychological Association's Guidelines for Psychotherapy with LGB Clients provides a starting point for clinicians. In LGB-affirmative therapy, the clinician addresses issues of internalized homophobia that may contribute to the development of mental health disorders.

- LGB patients with mental health conditions can benefit greatly from connecting with LGBT community resources, such as support groups, hotlines, or LGBT-specific health facilities.

- Future clinical research specific to LGB patients with mental health issues will need to focus on validating assessment tools for LGB patients and examining which treatment options are most effective in LGB patients.

References

1. **Cochran SD, Mays VM**. Estimating prevalence of mental and substance using disorders among lesbians and gay men from existing national health data. In: Omoto AM, Kurtzman HS, eds. Sexual Orientation and Mental Health: Examining Identity and

Development in Lesbian, Gay, and Bisexual People. American Psychological Association; 2006: 143-65.

2. **Murray CJL, Lopez AD, eds**. The Global Burden of Disease: A Comprehensive Assessment of Mortality and Disability from Diseases, Injuries, and Risk Factors in 1990 and Projected to 2020. Harvard University Press; 1996.

3. **Sandfort TGM, Bakker F, Schellevis FG, et al**. Sexual orientation and mental and physical health status: findings from a Dutch population survey. Am J Public Health. 2006;96:1119-25.

4. **Cochran SD, Mays VM, Sullivan JG**. Prevalence of mental disorders, psychological distress, and mental health services use among lesbian, gay, and bisexual adults in the United States. J Consult Clin Psychol. 2003;71:53-61.

5. **Dean L, Meyer IH, Robinson K, et al**. Lesbian, gay, bisexual, and transgender health: findings and concerns. Journal of the Gay and Lesbian Medical Association. 2000;4:102.

6. **Hughes TL, Wilsnack SC, Johnson TP**. Investigating lesbians' mental health and alcohol use: what is an appropriate comparison group? In: Omoto A, Kurtzman H, eds. Sexual Orientation and Mental Health: Examining Identity and Development in Lesbian, Gay, and Bisexual People. American Psychological Association, 2006.

7. **Resnick MD, Bearman PS, Blum RW, et al**. Protecting adolescents from harm. Findings from the National Longitudinal Study on Adolescent Health. JAMA. 1997;278:823-32.

8. **D'Augelli AR, Grossman AH, Salter NP, et al**. Predicting the suicide attempts of lesbian, gay, and bisexual youth. Suicide Life Threat Behav. 2005;35:646-60.

9. **Safren SA, Heimberg RG**. Depression, hopelessness, suicidality, and related factors in sexual minority and heterosexual adolescents. J Consult Clin Psychol. 1999;67:859-66.

10. **Mills TC, Paul J, Stall R, et al**. Distress and depression in men who have sex with men: the Urban Men's Health Study. Am J Psychiatry. 2004;161:278-85.

11. **Matthews AK, Hughes TL, Johnson T, et al**. Prediction of depressive distress in a community sample of women: the role of sexual orientation. Am J Public Health. 2002;92:1131-9.

12. **Lackner JB, Joseph JG, Ostrow DG, et al**. A longitudinal study of psychological distress in a cohort of gay men. Effects of social support and coping strategies. J Nerv Ment Dis. 1993;181:4-12.

13. **Hays RB, Turner H, Coates TJ**. Social support, AIDS-related symptoms, and depression among gay men. J Consult Clin Psychol. 1992;60:463-9.

14. **Williamson I**. Internalised homophobia and health issues affecting lesbians and gay men. Health Education Research: Theory and Practice. 2000;15:97-107.

15. **D'Augelli AR**. Coming out, visibility, and creating change: empowering lesbian, gay, and bisexual people in a rural university community. Am J Community Psychol. 2006; 37:203-10.

16. **Rotheram-Borus MJ, Fernandez MI**. Sexual orientation and developmental challenges experienced by gay and lesbian youths. Suicide Life Threat Behav. 1995;25: 26-34; discussion 35-9.

17. **Stiles WB, Agnew-Davies R, Hardy GE et al**. Relations of the alliance with psychotherapy outcome: findings in the Second Sheffield Psychotherapy Project. J Consult Clin Psychol. 1998;66:791-802.

18. **Vogel PA, Hansen B, Stiles TC, et al**. Treatment motivation, treatment expectancy, and helping alliance as predictors of outcome in cognitive behavioral treatment of OCD. J Behav Ther Exp Psychiatry. 2006;37:247-55.

19. **Risdon C, Cook D, Willms D**. Gay and lesbian physicians in training: a qualitative study. CMAJ. 2000;162:331-4.

20. **Beck AT, Steer RA, Ball R, et al**. Comparison of Beck Depression Inventories -IA and -II in psychiatric outpatients. Journal of Personality. 1996;67:588-97.

21. **Hirschfeld RM, Calabrese JR, Weissman MM, et al**. Screening for bipolar disorder in the community. J Clin Psychiatry. 2003;64:53-9.

22. **Kocsis, J.H., Friedman RA, Markowitz JC, et al**. Maintenance therapy for chronic depression. A controlled clinical trial of desipramine. Arch Gen Psychiatry, 1996. 53: p. 769-74; discussion 775-6.

23. **Beck AT, Epstein N, Brown G, et al**. An inventory for measuring clinical anxiety: psychometric properties. J Consult Clin Psychol. 1988;56:893-7.

24. **Zung WW**. The Depression Status Inventory: an adjunct to the Self-Rating Depression Scale. J Clin Psychol. 1972;28:539-43.

25. **Shoptaw S**. Methamphetamine use in urban gay and bisexual populations. Topics in HIV Medicine. 2006;14:84-7.

26. **Peck JA, Reback CJ, Yang X, et al**. Sustained reductions in drug use and depression symptoms from treatment for drug abuse in methamphetamine-dependent gay and bisexual men. Journal of Urban Health. 2005;82:i100-8.

27. **Hartgens F, Kuipers H**. Effects of androgenic-anabolic steroids in athletes. Sports Med. 2004;34:513-54.

28. **Bolding G, Sherr L, Elford J**. Use of anabolic steroids and associated health risks among gay men attending London gyms. Addiction. 2002;97:195-203.

29. **Rogers G, Curry M, Oddy J, et al**. Depressive disorders and unprotected casual anal sex among Australian homosexually active men in primary care. HIV Medicine. 2003; 4:271-5.

30. **Olatunji BO, Mimiaga M, O'Cleirigh C, et al**. Review of treatment studies of depression in HIV. Topics in HIV Medicine. 2006;14:112-24.

31. **Cohen LS, Altshuler L, Harlow B, et al**. Relapse of major depression during pregnancy in women who maintain or discontinue antidepressant treatment. JAMA. 2006;295: 499-507.

32. **Alwan S, Reefhuis J, Rasmussen SA, et al**. Use of selective serotonin-reuptake inhibitors in pregnancy and the risk of birth defects. N Engl J Med. 2007. 356: 2684-92.

33. **Morag I, Batash D, Keidar R, et al**. Paroxetine use throughout pregnancy: does it pose any risk to the neonate? J Toxicol Clin Toxicol. 2004;42:97 100.

34. **Hallberg P, Odlind V, Sjoblom V**. Selective serotonin-reuptake inhibitors and persistent pulmonary hypertension of the newborn. N Engl J Med. 2006;354:2188-90. Author reply 2188-90.

35. **Saewyc EM, Bearinger LH, Blum RW, et al**. Sexual intercourse, abuse and pregnancy among adolescent women: does sexual orientation make a difference? Fam Plann Perspect. 1999;31:127-31.

36. **Kaminski PL, Chapman BP, SD Haynes SD, et al**. Body image, eating behaviors, and attitudes toward exercise among gay and straight men. Eat Behav. 2005;6:179-87.

37. **Hausmann A, Mangweth B, Walch T, et al**. Body-image dissatisfaction in gay versus heterosexual men: is there really a difference? J Clin Psychiatry. 2004;65:1555-8.

38. **Koh AS, Ross LK**. Mental health issues: a comparison of lesbian, bisexual and heterosexual women. J Homosex. 2006;51:33-57.

39. **Siever MD**. Sexual orientation and gender as factors in socioculturally acquired vulnerability to body dissatisfaction and eating disorders. J Consult Clin Psychol. 1994;62: 252-60.

40. **Luck AJ, Morgan JF, Reid F, et al**. The SCOFF questionnaire and clinical interview for eating disorders in general practice: comparative study. BMJ. 2002;325:755-6.

41. **D'Augelli AR, Grossman A, Hershberger S, et al**. Aspects of mental health among older lesbian, gay, and bisexual adults. Aging Ment Health. 2001;5:149-58.

42. **Woods TE, Antoni MH, Ironson G, et al**. Religiosity is associated with affective and immune status in symptomatic HIV-infected gay men. J Psychosom Res. 1999;46: 165-76.

43. **Greenberg JS**. A study of the self-esteem and alienation of male homosexuals. J Psychol. 1973;83:137-43.

44. **Rabkin JG, Wagner G, Rabkin R**. Effects of sertraline on mood and immune status in patients with major depression and HIV illness: an open trial. J Clin Psychiatry. 1994;55:433-9.

45. **Trivedi MH, Rush AJ, Wisniewski SR, et al**. Evaluation of outcomes with citalopram for depression using measurement-based care in STAR*D: implications for clinical practice. Am J Psychiatry. 2006;163:28-40.

46. **Fava M, Rush AJ, Wisniewski SR, et al**. A comparison of mirtazapine and nortriptyline following two consecutive failed medication treatments for depressed outpatients: a STAR*D report. Am J Psychiatry. 2006;163:1161-72.

47. **Stein DJ**. Guidelines and algorithms for anxiety disorders: evidence-based excellence or garbage in, garbage out? Current Psychiatry Reports. 2006;8:253-5.

48. **Baldwin DS.** Evidence-based guidelines for anxiety disorders: can they improve clinical outcomes? CNS Spectrums. 2006;11:34-9.

49. **Frierson RL, Melikian M, Wadman PC**. Principles of suicide risk assessment. How to interview depressed patients and tailor treatment. Postgrad Med. 2002;112:65-66, 69-71.

50. **American Psychiatric Association**. COPP Position Statement on Therapies Focused on Attempts to Change Sexual Orientation (Reparative or Conversion Therapies); 2000. Available at http://www.psych.org/psych_pract/copptherapyaddendum83100.cfm

Chapter 9

Substance Use and Abuse

YONG S. SONG, PhD
JAE M. SEVELIUS, PhD
ROBERT GUZMAN, MPH
GRANT COLFAX, MD

Introduction

Substance abuse is a problem that affects every segment of our society. According to the most recent National Survey on Drug Use and Health (NSDUH), more than half of Americans 12 years or older reported current alcohol use, with more than one fifth engaging in binge drinking behaviors.[1] In addition, over 19 million Americans reported illicit drug use in the past 30 days, representing over 8% of the national population. Substance use has been referred to as the number one health problem in the United States.[2] Available studies indicate that certain lesbian, gay, bisexual, and transgender (LGBT) subpopulations exhibit higher rates of lifetime alcohol and other drug use than their heterosexual counterparts.[3-5] In addition, substance use among these populations may be closely linked to other important healthcare issues requiring clinical attention, such as sexual risk taking behaviors[6-7] and mental health disorders.[8-10] This chapter will provide the clinician with a general overview of substance use-related factors as they affect the diverse community of LGBT persons. The various drugs of abuse within the LGBT communities will be reviewed, as well as the associated social, medical, and psychiatric factors clinicians should consider when assessing substance use matters with their LGBT patients.

Epidemiology of Substance Use and Abuse

Early epidemiological studies of LGBT persons showed alarmingly high rates of alcohol use and abuse among gay men and lesbians. These well-cited early studies suggested that upwards of a third of gay men and lesbians reported excessive alcohol use or abuse behaviors.[11-12] However, due to methodological issues in these early studies (eg, oversampling of individuals recruited because of high-risk behaviors), these rates are higher than the prevalence of substance use problems in the overall LGBT population. Given the stigma attached to homosexuality, representative samples of LGBT individuals to study were often difficult to find in the 1960s and 1970s, thus these early studies relied upon convenience samples. For example, the Fifield study[11] surveyed patrons of gay and lesbian bars in the metropolitan Los Angeles area, significantly limiting generalizablity to other populations of gay men and lesbians (eg, individuals from rural areas who may not frequent gay or lesbian bars). Although mainstream American culture has come to better accept LGBT persons, stigma and discrimination against LGBT persons persist. Thus, many LGBT persons remain "invisible" citizens even today, making it difficult to obtain representative samples for such epidemiological studies. For these reasons, reliable estimates of alcohol and drug use among the LGBT subpopulations are still difficult to determine. Even among the limited number of studies focusing on LGBT substance use, there are discrepancies in how substance use is measured and studied. Substance use falls within a wide spectrum of use, abuse, and dependence, as well as everything in between, and there is no consistent standard in how substance use and misuse are measured within the LGBT communities. Furthermore, there are differences in the way homosexual identity is defined. Some studies rely upon the self-reporting of homosexual or bisexual identity whereas other studies use gender and sexual behavior to approximate sexual orientation. In addition, the main epidemiological studies report substance use in diverse ways and focus only on use patterns indicative of substance use or dependence disorder diagnoses. Other studies report lifetime use and may not be studying problematic use patterns. Therefore, these findings should be interpreted with caution.

Although recent studies indicate that substance use and abuse rates are substantially lower than initially reported by Fifield et al[11] and Saghir and Robbins,[12] available research suggests that LGBT persons may use alcohol and drugs more than the general population.[13] Below is a selected review of the existing literature measuring either problematic substance use behaviors or indices of problematic substance use behaviors among LGBT persons. Given the relative paucity of research in this topical area for LGBT persons, this should not be considered definitive, but it can be a general review of the patterns of substance use and abuse within the diverse LGBT communities.

Lesbians: One study utilizing a sample of 748 lesbian women recruited in the metropolitan Chicago area found them to be less likely to abstain from alcohol than heterosexual women; only 15% of lesbians reported complete abstinence from alcohol compared to 35% of the heterosexual sample.[14] Similarly, they found lesbians to be more likely to report moderate alcohol use (76% versus 59% of heterosexual women) and almost three times more likely to report alcohol use problems than heterosexual women (23% versus 8%, respectively). In addition, this study also found higher rates of marijuana and cocaine use when compared with the general population. Another large study of lesbians (N = 1925), the National Lesbian Health Care Survey,[15] revealed that 25% of the sample reported drinking alcohol several times a week, with 6% reporting daily drinking. 47% reported lifetime use of marijuana, and 19% reported lifetime cocaine use. In addition, 14% of respondents reported being worried about their alcohol use and 16% had previously been in treatment for alcohol or drug-related problems. When homosexually active women who participated in the 1996 National Household Survey on Drug Abuse (NHSDA) were compared to heterosexually active women, the homosexually active women reported significantly higher lifetime use rates of marijuana, cocaine, hallucinogen, inhalant, sedative, and stimulant use than heterosexually active women.[4] When this same sample was asked about dysfunctional substance use patterns in the past year, homosexually active women were more likely to report greater rates of dysfunctional marijuana, cocaine, and hallucinogen use than heterosexually active women. Although the available research suggests higher rates of problematic drinking among lesbians, more population-based research is needed to confirm problematic drug use patterns, particularly in relevant and culturally diverse subpopulations.

Gay men: Homosexually active men who participated in the NHSDA also showed patterns of greater lifetime use of several substances (ie, cocaine, hallucinogens, inhalants, analgesics, and tranquilizers) than heterosexually active men.[4] One probability-based telephone sample of urban gay men from four large metropolitan US cities (Chicago, Los Angeles, New York, and San Francisco) found that 85% of gay men reported alcohol use and that 52% reported some recreational drug use within the past six months.[5] Another random household sample of gay men in San Francisco revealed alcohol use patterns similar to their heterosexual counterparts; however, gay men were significantly more likely to report use of many drugs, including marijuana, poppers, MDMA (also known as ecstasy), psychedelics, barbiturates, and amphetamines,[16] with another San Francisco sample noting relatively high levels of substance use among gay men (eg, 64% using marijuana, 24% using cocaine, 25% using amphetamines, and 31% using ecstasy).[17] Relatively high rates of alcohol and other drug use were also noted in a large multisite sample (N = 3212) of HIV-uninfected men who have sex with men (MSM) enrolled in a multisite HIV vaccine preparedness trial, where alcohol was used by 89% of participants, marijuana by 49%, inhalants by 29%, amphetamines by 21%, cocaine by 14%, and hallucinogens by 14%.[18] In addition to urban samples, other studies suggest that certain subpopulations within the gay male community, eg, circuit party participants, may exhibit higher rates of drug and alcohol use than the general population of gay men.[19]

Bisexual men or women: Few studies have specifically looked at rates of substance use among bisexual men and women. Many studies have combined gay and bisexual men together, as well as lesbian and bisexual women.[17,20] Furthermore, the existing literature sometimes make assumptions that bisexual men and women share more in common with their homosexual counterparts than they do with heterosexual men and women.[13] This may or may not be the case, but the scant number of representative studies investigating substance use patterns among bisexual men and women leave this assumption untested. Therefore, better-substantiated rates of alcohol and drug use among bisexual men and women are difficult to ascertain. One recent study suggested that bisexually identified women were more likely to report illicit drug use and experience adverse alcohol-related consequences than heterosexual women.[21] However, further studies are needed to ascertain whether bisexual men and/or women are indeed at greater risk for developing substance use problems.

Transgender men or women: Almost all the existing literature on substance use among transgender populations focuses on male-to-female (MTF) transgender sex workers, where HIV risk taking is the primary focus and substance use variables are collected as cofactors that affect HIV and sexually transmitted infection (STI) risk. As such, these studies are not representative of all transgender populations, including nonsex workers and female-to-male (FTM) transgender individuals. However, the existing studies with MTF sex workers suggest high rates of drug use in certain transgender communities. In one report of HIV prevalence among transgender individuals in San Francisco, Clement et al[3] reported high rates of lifetime injection drug use (IDU) among transgender individuals (ie, 34% IDU use among MTF and 18% among FTM). In another study of MTF transgender individuals in Los Angeles, Reback and Lombardi[22] reported that 35% were sex workers. Furthermore, 37% of MTF individuals reported using alcohol, 13% marijuana, 11% crack, 11% methamphetamine, 7% cocaine, and 2% heroin in the past month. These figures are greater than the 1996 NHSDA figures of prior use for men who have sex with women with the following rates of use in past month (8% marijuana, 1% cocaine, 1% other stimulants, and 0.1% heroin). Therefore, these limited studies with targeted samples of MTF sex workers suggest elevated substance use rates; however, no reliable data exists to suggest problematic substance use rates among the diverse subpopulations of transgender persons.

Social and Cultural Context of Substance Use

For LGBT persons, substance use must be considered within the context of social and cultural settings. Bars have historically been gathering places for LGBT people, facilitating both social and sexual connections with others in one's own community, and providing opportunities to develop these networks and establish an LGBT identity.[23] A national household survey in 2000 found that gay men, lesbians, and bisexual women spent more time in bars than heterosexuals of the same sex.[24] For lesbians, having bars as a primary social setting has been shown to be the most significant factor associated with alcohol use.[25]

Particularly for gay and bisexual men, bathhouses and sex clubs have also been settings for both substance use and meeting new partners. A recent study of gay and bisexual men who attend different gay venues found that those who attended sex clubs or bathhouses reported the highest levels of unprotected anal sex, and those who attended circuit parties reported the highest levels of unprotected anal sex with partners of different or unknown HIV status.[7] Another study found that men who use "party drugs" (eg, methamphetamine, GHB, poppers, etc) were more likely to visit bathhouses and public cruising areas.[26]

The Internet has emerged not only as a meeting place for social support but also as a way to meet sex partners who may be interested in using similar substances. The Internet also provides a way for rural men to connect with the larger society of gay and bisexual men, and along with bars, it is the most common way for these men to meet sex partners.[27-28] However, several studies have shown that gay and bisexual men who seek partners over the Internet report higher levels of risky sex, sexually transmitted infections (STIs), and use of drugs and alcohol during sex.[29-30]

Substance Abuse and Identity

The stress experienced by stigmatized and marginalized minority groups is often cited as a significant contributing factor to higher levels of drug and alcohol abuse among these groups.[31-32] Negative attitudes toward LGBT people certainly abound in society and can be a major source of stress among LGBT people. The term *homophobia* has been used to describe negative attitudes about homosexuality generally, while *internalized homophobia* is often used to describe LGB people's acceptance of those negative attitudes. Other similar terms include *heterosexism, internalized heterosexism*,[33] and *internalized homonegativity*.[34] Similarly, negative attitudes about transgender people have been referred to as *transphobia*,[35] and when that negativity is internalized by transgender people, it is referred to as *internalized transphobia*. Whether a person is "out" as LGBT or not, dealing with these types of stressors on a daily basis has been theorized to contribute to the higher rates of alcohol and drug use sometimes found in studies of LGBT communities.[31] However, the links between homophobia or transphobia and substance use have not been clearly demonstrated. Some studies have found partial support for this link,[12,33,36] but others have not.[32,37] The few empirical studies that have been conducted on this topic focus exclusively on gay men and lesbians, so the effect of homophobia or transphobia on bisexual and transgender individuals' patterns of substance use is not known. Additional research is needed to adequately investigate these relationships.

Drugs of Abuse

Alcohol

Ethyl alcohol (ethanol) is a general nonselective central nervous system (CNS) depressant similar to other sedative-hypnotic substances; its use results in states of relaxation, sedation, and euphoria. It is both absorbed and metabolized quickly by the body and acts on the GABA inhibitory neurotransmitter system.[38] The harmful effects of alcohol are well documented and include elevated risk of cancers affecting the liver, esophagus, throat, and larynx.[38] Additionally, alcohol use increases risk of death from motor vehicle accidents, workplace and other unintentional injuries, suicide, and homicide.[39] While there is evidence that low to moderate use of alcohol is associated with decreased risk of coronary artery heart disease (CHD), risk is actually increased with greater consumption and even binge drinking among otherwise moderate users.[40]

Alcohol is the most commonly used and abused recreational drug in available samples of LGBT populations.[5,41] For example, a household sample of urban MSM found that 85% used some alcohol in the past six months.[5] In general, compared to gay and bisexual men, there is more evidence of elevated levels of alcohol use and abuse among lesbian and bisexual women. For example, lesbians have been shown to be more likely than heterosexual women to have a history of alcohol treatment[41] and are more likely than the general population of women to report any and heavy alcohol use.[42] Another national survey of lesbians found higher rates of drinking, heavy alcohol intake, and self-reported alcoholism than in national studies of women in general.[43] Some studies that have found higher rates of alcohol-related problems among lesbians and bisexual women have not found differences among men by sexual orientation.[44]

Marijuana

Marijuana, also known as *cannabis* (pot, weed, grass, and chronic are other common terms), is the most commonly used illicit drug in the general population, and the same pattern appears present among LGBT people.[4-5] Marijuana consists of the dried leaves and flowers of the hemp plant, sometimes also containing the stems and seeds.[38] It is usually smoked in cigarette form or in a tobacco or water pipe but can also be ingested. The primary active agent in marijuana is delta-9-tetrahydrocannabinol, or THC, and the level of THC in marijuana determines the strength of its effect on the user. Other stronger forms of marijuana include "Sinsemilla," hashish, and hash oil. All forms of marijuana alter brain function, which produces various mind-altering effects. Desired effects include feeling high or euphoric, relaxed, and creative. Adverse effects include anxiety, paranoia, problems with memory and learning, distorted perceptions, loss of motor coordination, and increased heart rate.

Estimates of the prevalence of lifetime marijuana use range from 24%-36% for lesbians,[45-46] 18%-37% for gay men,[45] and 13% for transgender women.[22] Lesbians and gay men have reported higher levels of marijuana use than heterosexual women and men across a number of studies, with less difference between gay men and lesbians than between men and women in the general population.[4,14] Youth may be especially likely to use marijuana, with rates as high as 79% reported.[46] Few studies have reported specific prevalence rates of marijuana use among bisexual and transgender people, but there is good reason to believe it is at least as high as lesbians and gay men. Among one sample of MTF ethnic minority youth, 71% reported having used marijuana in the last year.[47]

Cocaine

Cocaine (also known as coke, blow, snow, "nose candy," and crack) is a psychoactive stimulant derived from the leaves of the coca plant indigenous to the Andean region of South America. It serves as a vasoconstrictor and as other stimulants in its class (eg, amphetamine) increases central nervous system activity for the user.[38] Common routes of administration include nasal (snorting), smoking (crack or rock, freebase), and intravenous (IV). Cocaine acts primarily by augmenting the dopamine neurotransmitter system, blocking neuronal presynaptic reuptake.[48] The clinical presentation of cocaine intoxication varies and is often dependent upon dosage, pattern, administration mode, and duration of use. Powder cocaine snorted provides major effects lasting 60-90 minutes, while smoking it in the freebase format (crack) provides a shorter more euphoric peak lasting approximately five minutes.[38]

Intoxication from cocaine often occurs with moderate to high dosages, and short-term physical effects include increased heart rate and blood pressure, constricted blood vessels, increased temperature, and dilated pupils. Persons on cocaine often report feeling euphoria, increased energy, mental alertness, hypersexuality, and decreased appetite. Cocaine intoxication may also include increased psychomotor agitation, hyperawareness, and hypervigilance behaviors, resembling symptoms of mania, which may or may not be perceived as pleasant for the user. Long-term effects of chronic cocaine use include irritability, persistent restlessness, paranoid ideation, mood disturbances (eg, dysphoric mood and depression), perceptual disturbances (eg, auditory and tactile hallucinations), and addiction. Cocaine is often used in binges lasting days.

Existing epidemiological studies show that cocaine abuse is prevalent among LGBT communities. McKirnan and Peterson reported higher lifetime prevalence rates of cocaine use among gay men.[14] Specifically, gay men over 35 years were more likely to be frequent cocaine users than the general population of men of the same age. Similarly, Cochran et al found homosexually active men and women (37% and 39%) were significantly more likely to have reported lifetime cocaine use than heterosexually active men and women (20% and 12%).[4] A study by Crosby et al revealed that 25% of the young gay men in a San Francisco sample reported cocaine use.[17] Similarly, some transgender populations (mostly MTF) have also been shown to exhibit increased rates of cocaine use. Reback and Lombardi reported that 19% of the sampled MTF transgender persons in West Hollywood reported use of cocaine and/or crack.[22] When sex work was factored in, sex workers were more likely to report crack cocaine use (25% versus 3% for nonsex workers).

Given the reported hypersexual effects of cocaine, studies indicate that gay men are using cocaine during sex activity, with associated increased HIV or STI risk behaviors.[6,10] Colfax and colleagues revealed in their sample of 4295 gay men from six major metropolitan US cities that cocaine users were more likely to engage in unprotected anal intercourse than non-cocaine users.[6] Hirshfield et al also found similar associations between cocaine use and unprotected anal intercourse among gay men in a national online survey.[49] Thus, in addition to the increased risk of developing substance abuse and dependence problems associated with cocaine use, gay men and MTF transgender individuals who use cocaine may be at increased risk for HIV and other STIs.

Methamphetamine

Methamphetamine (also known as meth, speed, crystal, ice, crank, and Tina) is a powerful stimulant that can be synthesized from the cold and sinus medications ephedrine and pseudoephedrine; it is similar to amphetamine.[38] The drug is generally sold in powdered form; users administer it by smoking, snorting, injecting, swallowing, or inserting into the rectum. Effects can last two to 12 hours or more, depending on dosage, and it is often used as part of multi-day binges.[50-51] Because methamphetamine is less expensive and longer lasting than cocaine and is widely available, users of the drug have a greater potential for abuse and addiction. People use methamphetamine to experience increased energy, feelings of euphoria, loss of appetite, increased self-esteem, and sex that can be prolonged and less inhibited. Methamphetamine increases extracellular dopamine levels through the release of dopamine from vesicular stores and through inhibiting dopamine reuptake transporters, which has been considered the main contributor to the desirable effects.[52] Methamphetamine also causes increases in release of epinephrine and serotonin.[53]

On the downside, methamphetamine also results in many short-term and long-term health effects. Prolonged exposure to methamphetamine is associated with decreased dopamine levels, which are thought to be due to reductions in dopamine transporter activity and degeneration of dopamine nerve terminals.[52] Severe weight loss can result from appetite suppression in frequent users.[52] Methamphetamine has effects on the cardiovascular system, including increased heart rate and blood pressure, atypical heart rhythms, and tachycardia.[54] Another negative effect of methamphetamine use is excessive scratching and picking behaviors that can cause severe dermatologic lesions.[55] Methamphetamine is also associated with severe dental disease, due to decreased oral hygiene during periods of methamphetamine use, xerostomia (persistent dry mouth attributable to methamphetamine's sympathomimetic properties), and bruxism (excessive teeth grinding).[56] Other effects of acute methamphetamine intoxication or overdose include rhabdomyolysis,[57] ischemic episodes including stroke,[58] myocardial infarction,[59] and severe hyperthermia and convulsions.[60] The prevalence of methamphetamine and other stimulant use among gay and bisexual men is ten times higher than among the general population.[5] Although little is known about methamphetamine use among the transgender population, lesbians and bisexual women also report higher levels of lifetime history of methamphetamine use than heterosexual women.[61]

Opioids

Opioids are a category of narcotic analgesics; they are either naturally (opium, heroin, morphine) or synthetically derived (eg, oxycodone, fentenyl). One commonly abused illicit opioid is heroin, which is a naturally derived narcotic drug derived from the opium poppy plant. Heroin appears in either powder (white or brown) or "black tar" form. The type of heroin largely depends on geographic location and local drug trafficking patterns (eg, powder available in New York City, and "black tar" prevalent in San Francisco). The effects of heroin, similar to other short-acting opioids (eg, morphine, oxycodone, and hydrocodone), include analgesia (pain relief) and euphoria.[38] Physical effects include slowed cardiac functioning, decreased respiration, drowsiness, dry mouth, and skin flushing. Long-term effects of chronic opioid use include tolerance and dependence, as well as associated medical complications associated with injection drug use (IDU), including infectious diseases (eg, HIV, hepatitis B, and hepatitis C), vascular disorders (eg, collapsed veins), and bacterial infections (eg, abscesses, cellulitis, endocarditis).

The existing epidemiological data suggests that heroin use among LGBT populations is low. Cochran et al found no significant differences in either lifetime prevalence or use in the past month between homosexually active men and women and their heterosexually active counterparts.[4] Similarly, Woody et al reported low prevalence rates of heroin or injection drug use (< 2%) among their large multisite sample of men who have sex with men (MSM),[18] which is less than the 1996 NHSDA lifetime rates of heroin use (2.2%) for heterosexually active men.[4] However, the scant literature on transgender individuals suggests that MTF transgender persons who engage in sex work and are at high risk for HIV might be at increased risk for heroin and/or injection drug use. One sample of ethnically diverse street-recruited MTF transgender persons in San Francisco revealed high prevalence rates of IDU, where 18% reported injecting "street drugs" in the past six months.[9] More studies are needed to further quantify heroin use among MTF transgender persons associated with the sex trade.

Overall, use of heroin is low among LGBT communities. However, there appears to be a growing national epidemic of increasing prescription opioid use, abuse, and dependence. The National Survey on Drug Use and Health, the Monitoring the Future Study, and the Drug Abuse Warning Network Report, all national indicators of drug use, showed significant increases in prescription opioid use over the past five years, with young people showing increased use.[1,62-63] The limited available data with LGBT populations indicate that gay men and lesbians might be using prescription analgesic medications at higher rates than their heterosexual counterparts.[4] When compared with heterosexually active men, Cochran and his colleagues found homosexually active men to report lifetime use of analgesics with use rates twice as high. Similarly, homosexually active women were significantly more likely to have reported analgesic use within the last month than heterosexually active women. Furthermore, with the proliferation of Internet-based commerce and offshore pharmacies selling prescription medications through the Internet without prescriptions, people can obtain large quantities of prescription analgesics without leaving their own homes. A recent study showed how easily prescription opioids could be obtained by doing simple Internet searches on target words.[64] By using target words such as "codeine" and "vicodin," over half of the Internet links were commercial sites classified as "no prescription Web sites" (NPW). Given the availability of prescription opioids and given some indication of increased use patterns among gay men and lesbians, ongoing studies are needed to better quantify prescription opioid use and/or misuse among LGBT persons.

Hormones

Because hormones have such a powerful effect on the way a person's body looks and feels, they are an essential part of many (but not all) transgender people's ability to feel comfortable with their bodies. Given that many transgender people, especially MTFs, have difficulty finding employment and thus do not have health insurance or a reliable means of accessing healthcare, many obtain hormones on the street, from friends, or through other nonmedical providers.[3] In one large San Francisco-based study, 73% of transgender women and 53% of transgender men were using hormones.[3] Of these, 42% of the transgender women and 97% of the transgender men were using injection hormones, specifically. The majority of the sample were obtaining their hormones from a medical provider (71%

MTF, 97% FTM), but almost one-third (29%) of the transgender women had obtained their hormones from the streets, the "black market," or friends, compared to only 3% of the transgender men.[3] For youth, it is even harder to obtain hormones from a medical source. Among a sample of ethnic minority transgender female youth in Chicago, 61% used hormones, and only 29% of those using hormones obtained them from a medical provider.[47]

Recent research suggests that gay men are also abusing illicitly obtained steroids.[65] Some gay men use anabolic steroids to enhance physical appearance through increased muscle growth. One recent study surveyed 772 gay men from six gyms in London and found that 15% of the sampled men reported steroid use in the past 12 months, where 12% reported injecting steroids.[65] Almost all the reported steroid users in this study reported some adverse side effect from steroid use, including testicular atrophy, insomnia, depression, and hypertension. It should be noted that the health consequences of illicit hormone use have not been fully explored, and more studies are needed to further characterize the full risks associated with steroid use among gay men and transgender persons.

Club Drugs

"Club drugs," sometimes called "party" drugs, refer to a category of drugs used by adults and teens who are part of a nightclub, bar, or "rave" scene. However, club drugs are not just taken in these contexts. Club drugs have become popular among young adults and urban MSM. As "raves" and dance clubs are all-night events in many cities, club drugs are typically used to increase energy to dance for prolonged periods of time and to decrease social inhibitions. As most club drug users describe their use as "recreational," there is a common misperception that these drugs are relatively harmless. The following sections will describe common club drugs, as well as their associated risks.

MDMA

MDMA (3,4-methylenedioxymethamphetamine, also known as ecstasy, X, XTC, Rolls, Adam) is usually ingested as a pill. MDMA has euphoric, empathogenic, and stimulant effects that last for three to six hours.[39] It is chemically similar to the hallucinogenic drug mescaline, as well as amphetamine.[39] MDMA is believed to affect users by both increasing serotonin release and inhibiting its reuptake.[66-67] MDMA users often take part in long dance marathons. This activity, along with the subsequent volume depletion that occurs, may contribute to MDMA-associated morbidity and mortality.[68] Although the most serious medical consequences of MDMA use are infrequent, the effects of MDMA include problems regulating temperature and blood pressure, resulting in hyperthermia, hypertension, tachycardia, hyponatremia (low blood sodium), rhabdomyolysis (muscle breakdown), liver failure, and death.[69-72] Additionally, MDMA pills may contain other substances, including methamphetamine and pseudoephedrine, that may either have additional medical effects or compound the effects of MDMA.[73] Acute MDMA intoxication is treated by restoration of fluid and electrolyte balance and careful evaluation and management of hepatic function.[69]

While there is some evidence of potential for MDMA dependence, typical use is intermittent.[74] In animal studies, exposure to MDMA results in reduced serotoninergic activity, potentially due to the down-regulation (decreasing presence) of the serotoninergic neurons caused by MDMA-associated toxicity.[75-76] While some, but not all, studies report high rates of impaired cognitive performance, insomnia, depression, and anxiety among MDMA users,[69,74,77-78] there is also some evidence that there are clinically significant neurological consequences of MDMA use.[79] Studies have shown that large numbers of gay men who attend "circuit parties" (ie, weekend-long dance events targeted for gay men similar to all-night "rave" events) report MDMA use. For example, 80% of Colfax et al's sample from San Francisco reported MDMA use during their most recent out-of-town "circuit" party.[19]

Ketamine

Ketamine (also known as K or special K) is a dissociative anesthetic used in veterinary medicine; ketamine for recreational use is typically illicitly obtained from medical sources.[69] A derivative of an anaesthetic, phencyclidine hydrochloride, ketamine exerts strong hallucinogenic and euphoric effects, and it is often combined with other club drugs.[19,69] It may be snorted, injected, or ingested.[80] The drug's effects have a rapid onset (1-30 minutes, depending on the route of administration used) and last 30 to 180 minutes.[69] With too large of a dose, users may fall into a "k-hole," a catatonic, dissociative state that typically resolves as the drug wears off. Additional adverse effects include agitation, amnesia, hypertension, delirium, depression, tachycardia, rhabdomyolysis, vomiting, and respiratory depression.[39,69] Treatment for acute complications involves supportive care, including volume repletion. Treatment with benzodiazepines may be indicated for cases of severe agitation.[69]

Ketamine is thought to affect users primarily through its effects on a brain receptor known as the N-methyl-D-aspartate receptor (NMDA), where it competes with other neurochemicals for binding sites.[81] N-methyl-D-aspartate dysfunction has been associated with psychoses and schizophrenia; similar symptoms are seen in among ketamine users.[69] Although data are inconclusive, some studies suggest that memory deficits and perception distortions from acute ketamine use may persist.[82] Ketamine dependence has been reported, with symptoms of craving and tolerance but with no physiological withdrawal symptoms reported.[83-84] Prevalence of ketamine use among LGBT populations is unknown, although in one study of MSM who attended circuit parties, where club drugs are commonly used, found that 58%-66% reported ketamine use during their most recent circuit party weekend.[19]

GHB

Gamma hydroxy butyrate (GHB) is a metabolite which occurs naturally in the human brain. Synthetic GHB and its precursors are used for their euphoria-inducing effects.[85] It is a controlled substance which has been used to treat alcohol withdrawal and narcolepsy.[86] GHB is manufactured using readily available industrial chemicals and instructions available on the Internet. GHB is generally taken orally as a liquid, affects users within 10-20 minutes, and has effects that can last for up to four hours.[39] GHB has a narrow safety index, with small increases in dosages resulting in a switch from a euphoric, relaxed state to a drug-induced coma and respiratory depression in users.[69] This is particularly concerning because the potency of GHB preparations can vary by as much as 10-fold, and persons may inadvertently overdose by taking the same volume of drug they have taken previously without incident. These variations in drug concentrations, along with the fact that the safety index narrows considerably when alcohol is used in conjunction with GHB, probably account for the numerous GHB-related emergency department admissions. Because of these effects, GHB has been implicated as a date-rape drug.[39] Other adverse effects of GHB include amnesia, depression, confusion, alternating states of agitation and coma, syncope, hypotonia, ataxia, nystagmus, random clonic movements of the face and extremities, and seizures.[87-90] GHB-related deaths have been attributed to aspiration, respiratory depression, and pulmonary edema. Treatment for acute GHB intoxication involves mainly supportive care, and may require intubation for airway support.[69] GHB binds to both GHB and g-aminobutyric acid receptors, which modulate sleep and memory; the drug-induced effects of exogenous GHB likely occur primarily as a result of its interaction with g-aminobutyric acid type B receptors.[91] GHB has been associated with changes in dopaminergic activity in the CNS, and there is evidence that GHB causes increases in dopamine levels in brain tissue.[92]

Users may become dependent, with acute withdrawal symptoms (vomiting, tremors, and insomnia) lasting up to two weeks and prolonged withdrawal (characterized by anxiety, dysphoria, and memory problems) lasting several months.[85,91] Benzodiazepines and supportive care are provided to treat withdrawal.[91] Little is known regarding prevalence of GHB among the greater LGBT populations, although it is used frequently by MSM during circuit party weekends, with 25%-29% reporting use during local and out-of-town parties.[19]

Poppers

Although they are not always included in the definition of club drugs, inhaled nitrites, also known as "poppers," are included here because they are frequently used in party settings and by MSM at risk for, or infected with, HIV.[93] These inhalants may consist of various forms of amyl, alkyl, or butyl nitrites. Poppers are often sold as cleaning products on the Internet, although more clearly promoted as a recreational drug on some web sites. Nitrites are usually inhaled nasally and cause rapid onset of vasodilation, resulting in light-headedness and euphoria that may progress to severe headaches; these symptoms are accompanied by tachycardia and decreased blood pressure.[94] Other negative effects of popper use include allergic reactions, hemolytic anemia, and methemoglobinemia.[95] Poppers are rapidly metabolized, with their effects generally lasting less than a few minutes.

Poppers are typically used in sexual settings because of their orgasm-enhancing effects and because users report they relax the anal sphincter and make receptive anal sex more comfortable.[94] Coadministration of poppers with phosphodiesterase inhibitors, such as sildenafil citrate (ie, Viagra® by Pfizer) is contraindicated, as the combination of these vasodilators may cause cardiovascular collapse.[94] Popper use has also been associated with an increased risk of human herpes virus 8 infection,[96] likely due to sexual practices associated with popper use.[94]

Sexual Risk Behavior and Drug Use

Among Gay Men

Sex under the influence of drugs and alcohol is one of the most commonly cited risk factors for HIV, as it often leads to unsafe sex practices.[97] However, drawing conclusions about the links between various drugs and increased sexual risk behavior for HIV and STIs is limited by several factors. In studies that are cross-sectional, studies demonstrating associations between substance use and sexual risk do not always distinguish between any use and use that occurs specifically during sexual episodes. This may also be the case in longitudinal studies, thereby making unclear the causal pathway. For example, substance use may be a coping mechanism for dealing with anxiety over having engaged in risky sex. Even when temporal factors are accounted for, other potentially unmeasured factors, such as depression, degree of sensation-seeking as a goal in and of itself, multiple drug use, partner type, and sexual and substance use setting may complicate interpretation of associations found between and single substance and high-risk sexual behavior.

Despite such limitations, most, but not all, studies show significant associations between increased sexual risk behavior and the use of both poppers and methamphetamines, two drugs which have also been independently associated with HIV infection and other STIs.[98-102] Several studies show a doubling of the risk for HIV infection among popper users;

similarly, an increased risk for HIV infection has been noted in association with methamphetamine use.[103-105] A recent study of MSM seeking HIV testing found that HIV seroincidence was 6.3% among methamphetamine users, compared with 2.1% among nonusers.[106] MDMA use has been associated with unprotected anal sex and a greater number of sexual partners in some, but not all, studies.[6,19,107-110] Ketamine and GHB use have also been associated with sexual risk behaviors in some, but not all studies.[109-111]

Methamphetamine used specifically in association with sex has been found to be more common among HIV-infected men than HIV-uninfected men.[112-113] Several studies of MSM (largely consisting of gay-identified men) have found that users are two to three times more likely than nonusers to engage in unprotected anal sex, have condoms break or slip off, acquire a sexually transmitted infection, or become infected with HIV than nonusers.[19,114-115] Such risks are elevated among both frequent and occasional users.[19] One recent study found an elevated risk of HIV infection among methamphetamine users even after adjusting for specific sexual risk behaviors such as unprotected anal sex with HIV-infected partners.[114] This suggests methamphetamine use contributes to HIV infection above and beyond increasing likelihood that users will engage in risky behavior, perhaps due to prolonged intercourse in which condom breakage and increased mucosal trauma occurs.

Alcohol (typically heavy use) has been also been linked to high-risk sexual behavior among MSM in many, but not all, studies.[49] Heavy drinking has been associated with unsafe sex, as has use of alcohol prior to sex,[6] and alcohol use may variously affect sexual risk depending on the type of sexual partner (eg, casual versus primary).[102,116] For example, one study found that HIV-uninfected men who reported having six or more drinks prior to sex were 2.4 times more likely to engage in unprotected anal sex with a recent partner.[6] Some of the potential explanations for the relationship between alcohol and sexual risk behavior include the disinhibitory effects of alcohol, lowered perceptions of risk after drinking, and excusing behavior that is otherwise perceived as unacceptable, or increased use by MSM with risk-taking personalities.[117]

Increased levels of risk behavior and increased risk of HIV and STI due to drug use are believed to be due largely to the disinhibitory effects of these substances. However, other factors, including prolongation of sexual encounters while on drugs, decreased pain thresholds leading to increased mucosal trauma, and the possible immunosuppressive effects of drugs have been suggested as additional factors that may account for these increased risks, even after controlling for sexual behavior.[118] Some drugs have also been associated with increased rates of condom failure, suggesting that even when safer sex practices are attempted, drug use may lead to increases in sexual risk.[115]

Among Transgender Persons

HIV rates have been found to be consistently high among MTF transgender women, especially among Latinas and African Americans. HIV prevalence among transgender women has been reported in the ranges of 14% to 68%, depending on the subgroup of transgender women that was sampled,[119-120] with rates ranging from 35% in San Francisco,[9] 32% in Washington, DC,[121] 27% in Houston,[122] and 22% among MTF ethnic minority youth in Chicago.[47] Less is known about rates of HIV among FTM transgender people. Their rates have been reported to be as low as 2% to 3%.[9,121] More research needs to be done on gay-identified FTMs who are believed to be at higher risk.

HIV has been consistently linked to substance abuse in the transgender community. In San Francisco, those who reported intravenous drug use were 2.69 times more likely to be HIV-infected than nonsubstance users.[9] In Washington, DC, transgender people who had a self-reported substance abuse problem were more then twice as likely to be HIV-infected than those who did not report substance abuse.[121] Unsafe sex under the influence of substances seems to be especially prevalent with primary partners.[35,122] Transgender women have also been found to be more likely than gay or bisexual males and heterosexual females to have a steady sex partner who injected drugs.[35]

Impact of Drug Use on HIV Disease

Evidence of the impact of various substances on HIV disease is limited. While methamphetamine, MDMA, and poppers have all been shown to affect cellular immune responses, the clinical implications of these effects are unknown.[123-126] Methamphetamine use has been found to increase cytokine levels, suggesting that it may play a role in enhancing the immune activation seen in chronic HIV disease.[127-129] In animal models, feline immunodeficiency virus, a retrovirus closely related to HIV, undergoes enhanced replication and mutation rates in the presence of methamphetamine.[130-131] However, most natural history studies do not report significant associations between drug use and HIV disease progression. One study found that weekly hallucinogen use (including MDMA) was independently associated with progression to AIDS and death.[132] Another study found that methamphetamine users had higher viral loads and worse responses to antiretroviral therapy (ART) than nonusers, even after controlling for self-reported medication adherence.[133] These studies are limited and do not establish definitive links between substance use and HIV disease progression but support the need for further research in this area.

Patients who use drugs and alcohol while taking antiretroviral therapy present specific challenges, both because of the potential impact of substance use on adherence, and also because of potential interactions with anti-HIV drugs. In general, substance users report less adherence to ART than nonusers, although data is limited.[134-136] For methamphetamine users in particular, binges may be specific periods of decreased adherence.[134] Such inconsistent patterns of adherence could lead to the development of drug-resistant HIV strains and eventual treatment failure.

The combination of certain drugs with ART may produce serious and even fatal interactions. Patients on antiretroviral therapy should be advised that their typical drug doses may be less safe when coadministered with ART. Methamphetamine, ketamine, MDMA, and GHB are all at least partially cleared through the cytochrome p450 (CYP-450) system, a major system for liver metabolism of many drugs, including antiretroviral medications, particularly protease inhibitors.[94] Thus, concomitant use of these drugs and antiretrovirals can delay clearance and increase blood levels of these drugs to dangerous levels, leading to adverse events. Ritonavir has been implicated in increasing both GHB and MDMA levels, with at least one fatality attributed to the effect of ritonavir on increasing blood levels of MDMA.[137-138] Interactions between various recreational drugs and nucleoside reverse transcriptase inhibitors and nonnucleoside reverse transcriptase inhibitors remain less understood, although ketamine levels may be elevated in the setting of protease inhibitors (PIs) and non-nucleoside reverse transcriptase inhibitors (NNRTIs).[139]

Co-occurring Disorders

Mental Illness

The National Comorbidity Study (NCS) reported information on co-occurring mental and substance use disorders in a sample of 8098 Americans between the ages of 15 and 54 and found that approximately 4.7% of the US population had a coexisting mental disorder and substance abuse or dependence.[140] Similarly, the 2002 National Survey on Drug Use and Health (NSDUH) reported that approximately four million adults met the criteria for a serious mental illness (SMI) and substance dependence and abuse.[1] This survey revealed that people with SMI were more likely to also have a coexisting substance use disorder. While only 8% of the persons without SMI had a substance abuse problem, over 23% of persons with SMI had a substance abuse problem. Similarly, SMI was associated with increased rates of binge drinking, with 29% with SMI versus 13% without. Thus, for significant proportions of individuals with substance abuse disorders, they might also be dealing with a severe mental disorder as well, making their treatment course more difficult.

In addition to higher alcohol and substance use prevalence rates, some studies suggest that LGBT persons may also have higher prevalence rates of mental disorders than heterosexuals[9,141-142] (see Chapter 8). Several

LGBT cohorts demonstrated the co-occurrence of mood and substance use disorders.[9,142-147] These studies also show high rates of depression and histories of suicidal thoughts. Elevated levels of depression, suicidal thoughts, and anxiety disorders have been repeated patterns in studies with LGBT populations.[8-10] Therefore, for some LGBT persons presenting with substance use disorders, treatment might also include evaluation for, and treatment of, other mental disorders.

The impact of substance abuse on psychiatric disorders appears to be additive, illustrated best by the effects of alcohol on worsening depression and increased risk for suicide for dually diagnosed individuals.[148] Not only do persons with dual diagnoses often struggle with the serious symptoms characteristic of substance use disorders, but these symptoms are often amplified or exacerbated by their psychiatric disorders. For example, dysphoric or depressed mood is commonly a withdrawal symptom of certain substances (eg, cocaine or methamphetamine), but for an individual with a pre-existing major depressive disorder, the dysphoric state could be so severe that it might lead to suicidal thoughts or gestures. Furthermore, prolonged chronic use of several substances can lead to clinically significant substance-induced mood, anxiety, and psychotic disorders. Current data about the natural history of substance use disorders among those with co-occurring severe mental illnesses suggests that treatment outcomes may be quite poor when individuals receive treatment that is not integrated to meet the needs of both disorders.[149] There are some good treatment models that address the focused treatment needs of dual-diagnosed individuals.[149] Therefore, it is important that all individuals being evaluated for a substance use disorder should also be evaluated for the presence of a coexisting mental disorder so that optimal treatment can be provided for such individuals.

Trauma and Abuse

Experts estimate that interpersonal violence in same-sex relationships occur at rates comparable to heterosexual relationships.[150-151] Rates of same-sex intimate partner violence have been shown to vary between 8% and 46%.[152] Furthermore, studies suggest that LGBT persons with substance use problems experience sexual abuse at higher rates than the general public.[153] Ratner et al found in a study of gay men and lesbians enrolled in a residential substance abuse program that 37% of the gay men and 67% of the lesbians had been sexually abused. Given these exposures to trauma and abuse, LGBT persons may be at increased risk for developing other mental illnesses, such as posttraumatic stress disorder (PTSD), and further complicate treatment for their substance use disorders.[154] (See Chapter 10 for more on trauma and abuse in LGBT populations.)

Special Considerations for Lesbians

Research suggests that substance use among lesbians does not decrease as dramatically with age as it does in the general population.[45,155] Although very few studies have explored ethnic differences in patterns of substance use among lesbians, one did find that African American women were more likely to identify themselves as heavy drinkers and to report adverse consequences as a result of alcohol use.[155] Whereas substance use among women in the general population may be influenced over time by changing social contexts and roles such as employment, parenthood, and marriage, lesbians are less likely to experience the protective qualities of these factors. Lesbians are often not as restricted by gender role socialization as women in the general population and may be more likely to choose jobs that are nontraditional for women, a factor that has been linked to increased alcohol consumption.[156]

Special Considerations for Gay Men

Circuit parties are large, often multiday, dance events attended primarily by gay and bisexual men. Several studies have shown that MSM attending these events report extremely high levels of substance use, including combining substances and high rates of overuse episodes.[19,93,109] One study found that party attendees used a median of four substances during their most recent out of town circuit party weekend; 80% used MDMA, 66% used ketamine, 58% used alcohol, 43% used methamphetamines, 29% used GHB, and 27% used cocaine on this weekend.[19] Thus, frequent substance use is likely to potentiate sexual risk behavior during circuit party weekends.

Special Considerations for Bisexual Men and Women

There is a dearth of research on bisexual men and women. Bisexual persons represent a wide spectrum of individuals with diverse genders, identities, and sexual behavior patterns. Many studies have classified individuals based upon reported sexual activity with same-gender partners. Therefore, many bisexual persons are included with "homosexuals," as they engage in same-gender sexual activity, and as a result not much is known about bisexual individuals other than research extrapolated from gay men or lesbians.[13] To further complicate things, many gay men and lesbians report looking back upon their own identify formation and indicate that at one point in their "coming out" process, they might have self-identified as bisexual.[157] This transitory identity formed during a fluid developmental "coming out" process, however, does not account for the distinct crystallized sexual orientation many ascribe. Nevertheless, bisexual individuals may experience some particular issues when it comes to substance abuse treatment.

Some bisexual individuals may be misunderstood by others, with the often mistaken beliefs that they are confused about their sexual orientation or homosexual identity and that they are not willing to commit to being "fully gay" due to not wanting to experience the social stigma and discrimination faced by gay men and lesbians.[157] Therefore, some bisexual individuals may feel marginalized by society, not fully accepted by the mainstream heterosexual community, but also not fully accepted by gay men or lesbians. This marginalization may have an impact in the recovery process from alcohol and drugs. For example, often 12-step fellowship (eg, Alcoholics Anonymous, Narcotics Anonymous, etc) participation is encouraged as an adjunct to formal treatment for persons with addictive disorders. Many 12-step fellowship programs have gay, lesbian, and transgender groups. However, often there are no such groups for bisexual persons. Bisexual individuals may or may not relate with other gay men or lesbians, opting instead to participate in such fellowship programs with heterosexual peers. Just as other forms of identity formation are varied, bisexual persons also vary in terms of their identification with the homosexual and heterosexual aspects of their identities. As such, clinicians should carefully assess the sexual identity of their bisexual patients and make referrals to fellowship or adjunctive community supports that are most appropriate to the individual's self-identity and treatment needs.[157]

Special Considerations for Transgender Individuals

Research on transgender communities is extremely limited, as public health research related to LGBT issues has focused least often on transgender issues.[158] Many large studies that focus on LGBT issues include very few transgender participants.[159-160] Much of the literature that is available focuses on MTF transgender people and is often specific to sex workers.

Within the literature on LGBT substance use, transgender people are often overlooked or rendered invisible by discussions that focus exclusively on heterosexism and homophobia. Because sexual orientation is separate from gender identity, transgender people can and often do identify as heterosexual. Transgender people who identify as homosexual may experience homophobia in addition to transphobia when seeking treatment for substance use. Because so many of the issues that transgender people face are distinct from those faced by the LGB community (eg, legal gender change, medical issues surrounding transition, etc), it has proved difficult for treatment services set up to be "one-stop shopping" for the LGBT community to adequately serve the transgender community. Those organizations that have expanded to include the "T" in their name often are not adequately equipped with the proper resources, staff, and knowledge to be truly inclusive. Transgender people may thus feel misunderstood and isolated within the LGB community, which might contribute to transgender people underutilizing services meant to include them.

Sex work: Many transgender people endure transphobia from a very young age, including conflict with their families and at school. Young transgender women are especially vulnerable to harsh treatment in our society, where feminine men are often targets of ridicule and abuse. Subsequently, many young transgender people, especially young transgender women, end up dropping out of school and living on the streets, leaving them with few job skills and a need to survive. Young transgender women in particular may become sex workers as a means of surviving, receiving much needed support from older transgender people, and being validated in their chosen gender identity. In Chicago, 63% of a sample of MTF ethnic minority youth reported having trouble finding a job, and more than half (59%) reported trading sex for money, drugs, or shelter at some point in their lives.[47] In a sample of transgender women in Houston, 51% had traded sex for money, and 26% had traded sex for drugs.[122] In fact, sex work has been consistently linked with substance use, particularly methamphetamines, as a means both of coping with the stress of sex work and of maintaining stamina.[22,35] Drug use can then in turn increase MTF sex workers' risk of acquiring HIV through needle sharing and sex under the disinhibiting influence of drugs.

Treatment provision: The need for substance abuse treatment for transgender people is well-documented.[161-162] However, the knowledge and sensitivity levels of treatment providers lag well behind the need in the community.[163-164] Providers who feel uncomfortable or who are not competent to address issues of gender identity in treatment result in largely unsuccessful treatment with transgender clients.[161] One treatment recovery program in San Francisco geared specifically toward transgender women has reported high rates of client retention and successful sensitivity training for its staff.[164] This program describes its key elements as affirmation of transgender identity, peer staff, and community building among MTF women and other clients, as well as the larger community. Substance abuse treatment programs striving to better serve their transgender clients may benefit from adopting a similar model.

Assessment

Many substance use disorders are undetected and may go undiagnosed in clinical settings; therefore, a thorough assessment of substance use patterns is recommended for all patients receiving any kind of clinical care. As candid discussions about substance use can lead to discussions about behaviors and acts that may be associated with stigma and shame, it is important that clinicians have a nonjudgmental attitude and express genuine empathy for their patients. Often, it is difficult for patients to divulge their substance use or associated behaviors. For example, it may be hard for a gay man to discuss his sexual risk behaviors while using "crystal meth." Some people might have difficulty disclosing other problematic behaviors associated with drug use, such as legal problems, interpersonal problems, employment problems, etc. Providers need to understand that the stigma attached to illicit substance use is quite prevalent. Like the stigma many LGBT persons face in relation to their sexual or gender identity, shame and guilt associated with their substance use may result in nondisclosure. That said, clinicians should be aware that patients might have some internal defenses related to acknowledging substance use behaviors. For example, individuals may minimize their drug use, or they may go to extreme lengths to rationalize why they use. In addition, it is not uncommon for patients to deny or externalize blame to someone else for their drug use. Therefore, it is important for the clinician to acknowledge this difficulty by not challenging the patient's resistance but by conducting assessments without directly confronting patients. It is recommended that clinicians ask questions in a straightforward and nonleading manner.

Continuum of Substance Use, Abuse, and Dependence

Although many people have tried alcohol and other drugs, both licit and illicit, the vast majority of persons who have used substances do not develop any significant problems associated with substance use. In addition, there are also many individuals, both within the LGBT and larger population, who use alcohol or other drugs on a regular basis but do not experience any significant impairment or problems associated with use. Most "recreational users" never experience any social, vocational, educational, medical, and psychological consequences often associated with problematic substance use patterns.

However, when an individual begins to experience any of the above consequences directly related to his or her use of alcohol or drugs, problematic use and/or substance use disorders might be present. There are two broad diagnostic categories for substance use disorders according to the *Diagnostic and Statistical Manual for Mental Disorders*, 4th Edition, Text Revision (DSM-IV-TR).[165] They include substance abuse and substance dependence. Individuals can have abuse or dependence diagnoses for any psychoactive substance, or they can have problems with several substances. In order for an individual to receive a DSM-IV-TR diagnosis of *substance abuse*, an individual must exhibit a "maladaptive pattern of substance use leading to clinically significant impairment or distress, as manifested by *at least one* of the following within a 12-month period:

- Recurrent use resulting in failure to meet obligations of work, school, or home
- Recurrent use in situations in which it is physically hazardous
- Recurrent substance-related legal problems
- Continued use despite having persistent social or interpersonal problems caused or exacerbated by use (182-183)

Substance dependence, a more severe diagnostic category, involves "a maladaptive pattern of substance use leading to clinically significant impairment or distress, as manifested by *three or more* of the following occurring at any time in the same 12-month period:

- Tolerance
- Withdrawal
- Substance taken in larger amounts over a longer period than intended
- Persistent desire or unsuccessful efforts to stop or cut down on use
- Great deal of time spent in activities necessary to obtain substance, use the substance, or recover
- Disruptions in important social, occupational or recreational activities
- Continued use despite knowledge of having persistent physical or psychological problems likely caused or exacerbated by substance use (181)

Table 9-1 outlines some useful diagnostic questions that clinicians might ask patients in assessing substance use problems.

Table 9-1   Diagnostic Questions for Assessing Substance Use Disorder[180]

1. Have you often ended up consuming much more than you intended to?

2. Have you found it difficult to limit or stop your use?

3. Have you ever spent so much time using and/or recovering from the effects that you had little time for anything else?

4. Has your use caused you to neglect responsibilities at work or home?

5. Has your use ever led you to give up or greatly reduce important activities and/or time with family/friends?

6. Have you continued to use despite being aware of these negative consequences?

7. Do you ever get tolerant to the effects so that you need to take larger doses?

8. Do you experience any withdrawal or other physical discomfort when you try to cut down on your use or stop all together?

9. Have you ever taken alcohol or drugs to avoid having withdrawal or to relieve withdrawal symptoms you were already experiencing?

Screening Instruments

There are short screening instruments that clinicians can administer to their patients to screen for substance use. There are alcohol use screening measures that have been used in many primary care settings, including the CAGE Questionnaire,[166] the Alcohol Use Disorders Identification Test (AUDIT),[167] and the Michigan Alcohol Screening Test (MAST).[168] These scales are quite short and often have good sensitivity, but they vary in specificity, needing a more thorough clinical interview to rule out the presence of substance use disorders.[166-168]

A very brief and sensitive measure commonly used to screen for the presence of alcohol use disorders is the CAGE questionnaire.[166] (See Table 9-2.) An affirmative response to any of the CAGE items indicates the likelihood of an alcohol use problem, which needs to be followed up with a more thorough clinical interview to rule out the presence of a substance use disorder.

Table 9-2   CAGE Questionnaire for Alcohol Use Problems[166]

1. "Have you ever felt you should **C**ut down on your drinking?"

2. "Have you ever felt **A**nnoyed by criticism of your drinking?"

3. "Have you ever felt bad or **G**uilty about your drinking?"

4. "Have you ever taken a drink first thing in the morning (**E**ye-opener) to steady your nerves or get rid of a hangover?"

Clinical Interview

In addition to the use of screening measures, conducting a thorough clinical interview can be helpful in identifying the presence of substance use disorders or understanding an individual's patterns of use and the context in which it occurs. Thorough clinical interviews should address multiple domains of an individual, as substance use disorders often affect many aspects of an individual's life. Table 9-3 presents some elements that might be helpful to address when conducting a thorough clinical assessment of substance use.

Table 9-3   Domains to Assess During Clinical Substance Abuse Assessment

Substance use history

1. Age at first use

2. Frequency of use

3. Amount of substance taken during an episode of use

4. Route of administration

Table 9-3   Domains to Assess During Clinical Substance Abuse Assessment (cont.)

5. Patient perceived consequences of use

6. Drug abuse treatment history

7. Descriptions of periods of abstinence

8. Relapse histories

9. Family history of alcohol/drug abuse

Psychiatric history

1. Are there any co-occurring psychiatric problems?

2. If so, inquire about relationship between two.

3. Inquire about emergence (which one predated the other?).

4. Do psychiatric symptoms occur during periods of abstinence?

5. Does substance use trigger psychiatric or vice versa?

6. Does substance use exacerbate the psychiatric problem?

Medical History

1. Look for medical conditions associated with substance use (eg, cirrhosis related to alcohol use).

2. Look for medical conditions related to increased risk behaviors while using substances (eg HIV or STIs related to increased sexual risk behaviors).

Social Developmental History

1. Provides factors that may have influenced the development and perpetuation of substance use disorders

2. Sexual identity formation

3. Relationships with significant others

4. Role of substance use in families

5. Role of substances in social activities

6. Role of substances in sexual activities

7. Does the individual have any abstinence support systems?

8. Educational or vocational achievement

9. Is there a history of physical, sexual, or emotional abuse?

Functional Impairment Associated with Substance Use

1. Social problems

2. Health problems

3. Educational or vocational problems

4. Psychological distress

5. Legal issues

6. Leisure activities

7. Family and friends

8. Spiritual disengagement

Substance Abuse Treatment

Currently, there is very little available research focused on targeted treatment approaches for the diverse and unique needs of LGBT populations. When available, existing research on effective treatment approaches and innovative treatment programs specializing in the care of LGBT populations are described below. The following is a very brief overview of the various types of treatments available for substance use disorders, types of settings in which they occur, as well as a discussion of some treatment models or programs with a specifically LGBT focus. A basic understanding of the available continuum of substance abuse treatment options in one's community can equip the clinician in providing better resources and appropriate treatment referrals for their patients experiencing substance use disorders.

Treatment Options

Drug addiction is a complex, and for some a chronic, disorder. As one treatment is not effective for all individuals, there are a variety of effective treatment modalities, including pharmacotherapy and behavioral treatments.

Pharmacotherapy

There are a variety of effective medications used in the treatment of addictive disorders.[169] Medications are effectively used as treatments for detoxification or maintenance therapies or used to prevent individuals from relapsing to a particular substance.

Detoxification: When an individual has become physiologically tolerant to a substance (eg, alcohol, benzodiazepine, opioid, etc), treatment might include medically assisted detoxification. Medically assisted detoxification involves use of a medication that is cross-tolerant to the substance of dependence and given in decreasing amounts under close medical supervision. For some substances, the withdrawal syndrome can be quite noxious, physically taxing, and, in some instances, dangerous. Withdrawal from substances like alcohol or benzodiazepines can result in clinically significant problems (eg, seizures, delirium, etc); therefore, an appropriately supervised detoxification can avoid these adverse effects. A medical detoxification, however, is the first step in a comprehensive treatment plan, often most effective when paired with behavioral treatments in order to assist with sustained abstinence.

Maintenance therapies: A subpopulation of opioid dependent persons has difficulty maintaining abstinence from illicit drug use without the continuous aid of certain medications to aid them in maintaining abstinence. Some populations of opioid dependent persons benefit from prolonged opioid agonist treatments to prevent relapse. Methadone and buprenorphine are two demonstrated effective pharmacotherapies for the treatment of opioid dependence.[170-171] Although the settings in which methadone (eg, narcotic treatment programs) and buprenorphine (eg, office-based) are provided differ, effective outcomes of methadone and buprenorphine treatment include a combination of pharmacotherapy and behavioral counseling. The use of opioid antagonists can also be used to prevent relapse to illicit opioid use. Naltrexone is an opioid antagonist that works by blocking the positively reinforcing euphoric effects of opiates. After a successful medical detoxification, naltrexone is another maintenance medication that can be used to support continued abstinence.[172] Finally, disulfiram (antabuse) is another medication used to maintain abstinence from alcohol. It works by blocking the oxidation of alcohol at the adetaldehyde stage, resulting in a noxious aversive physiological state when an individual consumes alcohol.

Behavioral Treatments

Research has identified several effective behavioral treatment approaches. *Individualized drug counseling* has been shown to be quite effective in reducing illicit drug use.[173] The effective elements of this treatment includes the use of short-term behavioral goals that help patients develop appropriate coping strategies that help them abstain from alcohol or drug use. This approach is often used in conjunction with group counseling and community support groups (eg, 12-step groups such as Alcoholics Anonymous, Narcotics Anonymous, etc). *Motivational enhancement therapy* has also been shown to be an effective behavioral intervention approach.[174] This client-centered approach tries to help patients engage in behavior change through use of therapeutic techniques aimed at resolving the ambivalence often faced by individuals struggling with addictions. *Relapse prevention therapy* is another empirically validated behavioral treatment approach.[175] Relapse prevention therapy employs a cognitive-behavioral framework that is based on the theory that maladaptive behavioral patterns (ie, drug abuse) are shaped by learning processes. Therefore, this approach aims to help individuals identify and correct maladaptive behavioral patterns. The Matrix model is another clinically useful treatment developed especially for stimulant users.[176] This model employs a comprehensive, highly structured treatment approach that integrates individual, group, education, family, and community support modalities with the goal of supporting positive behavior change. This model has been tailored for use with gay men by integrating culturally appropriate elements applicable to gay men.[177] Another effective behavioral treatment is the use of *contingency management,* which is a purely behavioral intervention that provides increasingly valuable reinforcers in the form of vouchers for negative urine drug test samples documenting drug abstinence.[178] Taken together, there exist a number of effective behavioral treatments that are used by many drug treatment programs aimed at reducing drug use and helping the individual make sustained changes associated with drug use to effect continued abstinence. Greater research is needed in identifying specific culturally appropriate behavioral drug treatments for the diverse LGBT community, with their different treatment needs.

Treatment Settings

Pharmacological and behavioral treatments for alcohol and drug abuse come in differing treatment settings. Most treatment programs can be categorized as residential or outpatient treatment settings. The following is an overview of these types of treatment settings.

Residential Treatment

Residential treatments are intensive inpatient programs offering protective settings where the patient is removed from their drug using environments so they may focus on complete rehabilitation without the environmental triggers and cues that might distract individuals from effective treatment. Residential treatments vary in type (therapeutic community, medical detoxification units, social model recovery homes, etc). These highly structured programs often provide a multidisciplinary approach to care, many of which are based upon the 12-step model of addiction. Residential programs provide recovering people with alternative social environments that support recovery, with a particular focus on changing maladaptive "lifestyles."[179] There are some residential programs that focus exclusively on the LGBT community. The Van Ness Recovery House (http://www.vnrh.org) in Los Angeles, Calif, is one example of a comprehensive residential program that provides culturally sensitive and appropriate substance abuse treatment for the diverse LGBT community.

Outpatient Treatment

Outpatient programs vary in content, intensity, and duration. They are typically less intensive than inpatient programs and often incorporate individual and group counseling, as well as adjunctive self-help (ie, 12-step) treatment methods. Many outpatient programs employ a variety of empirically validated treatment approaches mentioned above, depending on the treatment population and the presenting problems, from medication-assisted treatment for opioid dependence (eg, use of opioid agonist treatment, such as methadone or buprenophine) to use of other empirically validated psychosocial treatment approaches, including motivational enhancement therapy,[174] cognitive behavioral relapse prevention therapy,[175] contingency management,[178] individualized drug counseling,[173] Matrix model,[176] and specific treatments aimed at improving targeted skills including social skills training, stress management, assertiveness skills training, and anger management. Similarly, several notable outpatient programs nationwide provide substance abuse treatment targeted for the special treatment needs of LGBT individuals. Examples include the Fenway Community Health programs in mental health and addiction services located in Boston,

Mass (http://www.fenwayhealth.org). The Fenway program provides a full range of addiction treatment services for the entire LGBT community. Furthermore, other programs offer more specialized treatment for targeted subpopulations within the LGBT communities. The Stonewall Project (http://psych.ucsf.edu/sfgh.aspx?id=472) in San Francisco, Calif, offers a harm-reduction model of care specially addressing the unique treatment needs for MSM methamphetamine users. These model programs strive to provide culturally specific and LGBT affirming treatments that attempt to take into account the unique social and identity-related factors often inter-twined in problematic alcohol and drug use patterns.

As the treatment needs of LGBT persons are as diverse as the individuals comprising the LGBT communities, one chapter cannot adequately address all the various factors facing LGBT persons. In 2001, the Center for Substance Abuse Treatment (CSAT) published *A Provider's Introduction to Substance Abuse Treatment for Lesbian, Gay, Bisexual, and Transgender Individuals*.[154] In an effort to provide both evidence-based and consensus-based treatment (when the empirical evidence is lacking), CSAT developed this guide, which provides a review of the best practices approaches in the treatment of LGBT persons with substance use disorders. It is available free of charge from the Substance Abuse and Mental Health Services Administration by contacting their National Clearinghouse for Alcohol and Drug Information (NCADI: 1-800-729-6686 or via the Internet at http://www.ncadi.samhsa.gov). It can also be downloaded from the Internet at the following link: http://kap.samhsa.gov/products/manuals/pdfs/lgbt.pdf.

Conclusions

Just as the many subgroups that comprise the LGBT community are diverse in many ways, so are the various factors that contribute to substance use and misuse among LGBT persons. Although further research is needed to better understand the degree, nature, and complex contexts of substance use and abuse problems within the diverse LGBT community, the available research suggests that some LGBT persons are at risk for the many negative multifactorial consequences frequently associated with problematic substance use. As such, healthcare providers can better support their LGBT patients by achieving a better understanding of the unique social, psychological, physical, and medical factors that may contribute to the maladaptive substance use patterns. Through this understanding, clinicians can better assess and provide appropriate resources and referrals for care when necessary.

Summary Points

- There exists a wide continuum of substance use within the LGBT communities. Most persons who use alcohol or drugs (licit and illicit) do not exhibit problematic use patterns warranting intervention. However, clinicians should systematically screen for problematic alcohol and/or drug use for all persons under their clinical care in order to provide timely interventions or resources when necessary.

- As gay, lesbian, and transgender bars typically are the primary social settings for many LGBT persons to make social and sexual connections with other LGBT persons, clinicians should understand the social and cultural contexts of alcohol and drug use within LGBT communities. Clinicians can better support LGBT persons in recovery by assisting them to identify alternative means and venues of socialization that do not include alcohol and/or drugs.

- Available studies suggest increased rates of problematic drinking among lesbians compared to other populations. Therefore, alcohol use screenings should be included as part of a comprehensive assessment for lesbians accessing any healthcare system.

- Gay men in urban areas report high rates of alcohol and drug use. Although most gay men who report drug and alcohol use do not exhibit problematic substance use patterns, "recreational" use of certain drugs (eg, methamphetamine and poppers) have been associated with increased HIV and STI risks. Thus, clinicians should assess both recreational drug use and co-occurring sexual risk behaviors for gay men.

- Male-to-female transgender persons from large urban centers have shown increased rates of commercial sex work, with accompanying substance use and risky sexual behaviors placing them at risk for HIV disease. Clinicians working with MTF transgender persons should be aware of these risk factors, which can assist in better assessment and referral for appropriate prevention and treatment services.

- Substance use in certain subpopulations of LGBT persons (eg, circuit party participants, MTF transgender persons) has been associated with increased risk for HIV and STIs. Therefore, clinicians should include substance abuse assessments that include sexual risk behaviors in the context of substance use for these populations at risk.

- Substance use has been shown to impact HIV disease in several ways. Certain drugs have been shown to affect immune system response, have serious drug interaction profiles with certain antiretroviral therapies (ARTs), and are associated with poor ART medication adherence. Therefore, clinicians should assess for the interplay between substance use and HIV disease for HIV-positive patients.

- LGBT persons with substance use disorders can benefit from substance abuse treatment in a variety of settings. Some urban settings have culturally appropriate treatment services targeted for LGBT persons. Clinicians should know the appropriate drug treatment resources in their communities in order to better provide resources and direct appropriate treatment referrals.

References

1. **Substance Abuse and Mental Health Services Administration**. National Survey on Drug Use and Health: National Findings 2002. Office of Applied Studies; 2003.
2. **Robert Wood Johnson Foundation**. Substance Abuse: The Nation's Number One Health Problem, Key Indicators for Policy. Robert Wood Johnson Foundation; 2001.
3. **Clements K, Wilkinson W, Kitano K, et al**. HIV prevention and health service needs of the transgender community in San Francisco. International Journal of Transgenderism. 1999;3:1-2.
4. **Cochran SD, Ackerman D, Mays V, et al**. Prevalence of non-medical drug use and dependence among homosexually active men and women in the US population. Society for the Study of Addiction. 2004;99:989-98.
5. **Stall R, Paul JP, Greenwood G, et al**. Alcohol use, drug use and alcohol-related problems among men who have sex with men: the Urban Men's Health Study. Addiction. 2001;96:1589-601.
6. **Colfax G, Vittinghoff E, Husnik MJ, et al**. Substance use and sexual risk: a participant- and episode-level analysis among a cohort of men who have sex with men. American Journal of Epidemiology. 2004;159:1002-12.
7. **Xia Q, Tholandi M, Osmond DH, et al**. The effect of venue sampling on estimates of HIV prevalence and sexual risk behaviors in men who have sex with men. Sex Transm Dis. 2006 Sep;33:545-50.
8. **Bradford J, Ryan C, Rothblum ED**. National Lesbian Health Care Survey: implications for mental health care. Journal of Consulting and Clinical Psychology. 1994;62: 228-42.
9. **Clements-Nolle K, Marx R, Guzman R, et al**. HIV prevalence, risk behaviors, health care use, and mental health status of transgender persons: implications for public health intervention. American Journal of Public Health. 2001;91:915-21.
10. **Colfax G, Coates TJ, Husnik MJ, et al**. Longitudinal patterns of methamphetamine, popper (amyl nitrite), and cocaine use and high-risk sexual behavior among a cohort of San Francisco men who have sex with men. Journal of Urban Health. 2005;82:i62-i70.
11. **Fifield L, Latham JD, Phillips C**. Alcoholism in the Gay Community: The Price of Alienation, Isolation and Oppression. Gay Community Services Center; 1977.
12. **Saghir M, Robins W**. Male and Female Homosexuality. Williams & Wilkins; 1973.
13. **Hughes TL, Eliason M**. Substance use and abuse in lesbian, gay, bisexual, and transgender populations. The Journal of Primary Prevention. 2002;22:263-298.
14. **McKirnan DJ, Peterson, PL**. Alcohol and drug use among homosexual men and women: epidemiology and population characteristics. Addictive Behaviors. 1989;14:545-53.
15. **Bradford JB, Ryan, C**. National Lesbian Health Care Survey: Mental Health Implications for Lesbians. Report No. PB88-201496/AS. National Institute of Mental Health; 1987.
16. **Stall R, Wiley J**. A comparison of alcohol and drug use patterns of homosexual and heterosexual men: the San Francisco Men's Health Study. Drug and Alcohol Dependence. 1988;22:63-73.
17. **Crosby GM, Stall RD, Paul JP, et al**. Alcohol and drug use patterns have declined between generations of younger gay-bisexual men in San Francisco. Drug and Alcohol Dependence. 1998;52:177-82.

18. **Woody GE, Donnell D, Seage GR, et al**. Non-injection substance use correlates with risky sex among men having sex with men: data from HIVNET. Drug and Alcohol Dependence. 1999;53:197-205.

19. **Colfax GN, Mansergh G, Guzman R, et al**. Drug use and sexual risk behavior among gay and bisexual men who attend circuit parties: a venue-based comparison. J Acquir Immune Defic Syndr Hum Retrovirol. 2001;28:373-9.

20. **Bloomfield K**. A comparison of alcohol consumption between lesbians and heterosexual women in an urban population. Drug and Alcohol Dependence. 1993;33:257-69.

21. **McCabe SE, Hughes TL, Boyd CJ**. Substance use and misuse: are bisexual women at greater risk? Journal of Psychoactive Drugs. 2004;36:217-25.

22. **Reback CJ, Lombardi EL**. HIV risk behaviors of male-to-female transgenders in a community-based harm reduction program. International Journal of Transgenderism. 1999;3: 1+2.

23. **Parks KA, Zetes-Zanatta LM**. Women's bar-related victimization: Refining and testing a conceptual model. Aggressive Behavior. 1999;25:349-64.

24. **Trocki KF, Drabble L, Midanik L**. Use of heavier drinking contexts among heterosexuals, homosexuals and bisexuals: results from a National Household Probability Survey. J Stud Alcohol. 2005 Jan;66:105-10.

25. **Heffernan K**. The nature and predictors of substance use among lesbians. Addict Behav. 1998 Jul-Aug;23:517-28.

26. **Binson D, Woods WJ, Pollack L, et al**. Differential HIV risk in bathhouses and public cruising areas. Am J Public Health. 2001;91:1482-6.

27. **Horvath KJ, Bowen AM, Williams ML**. Virtual and physical venues as contexts for HIV risk among rural men who have sex with men. Health Psychol. 2006 Mar;25:237-42.

28. **Williams ML, Bowen AM, Horvath KJ**. The social/sexual environment of gay men residing in a rural frontier state: implications for the development of HIV prevention programs. The Journal of Rural Health. 2005 Winter;21:48-55.

29. **McKirnan D, Houston E, Tolou-Shams M**. Is the Web the culprit? Cognitive escape and Internet sexual risk among gay and bisexual men. AIDS Behav. 2007; 11:151-60.

30. **Klausner JD, Wolf W, Fischer-Ponce L, et al**. Tracing a syphilis outbreak through cyberspace. JAMA. 2000 Jul 26;284:447-9.

31. **Savin-Williams RC**. Verbal and physical abuse as stressors in the lives of lesbian, gay male, and bisexual youths: associations with school problems, running away, substance abuse, prostitution, and suicide. Journal of Consulting and Clinical Psychology. 1994; 62:261-9.

32. **McKirnan, DJ, Peterson, PL**. Psychosocial and cultural factors in alcohol and drug abuse: an analysis of a homosexual community. Addictive Behaviors. 1989;14:555-63.

33. **Amadio DM**. Internalized heterosexism, alcohol use, and alcohol-related problems among lesbians and gay men. Addictive Behaviors. 2006;31:1153-62.

34. **Reilly A, Rudd NA**. Is internalized homonegativity related to body image? Family and Consumer Sciences Research Journal. 2006;35:58-73.

35. **Nemoto T, Luke D, Mamo L, et al**. HIV risk behaviours among male-to-female transgenders in comparison with homosexual or bisexual males and heterosexual females. AIDS Care. 1999;11:297-312.

36. **DiPlacido J**. Minority stress among lesbians, gay men, and bisexuals: a consequence of heterosexism, homophobia, and stigmatization. In: Herek GM, ed. Stigma and Sexual Orientation: Understanding Prejudice Against Lesbians, Gay Men, and Bisexuals. Thousand Oaks, CA: Sage;1998:138-59.

37. **Amadio DM, Chung YB**. Internalized homophobia and substance use among lesbian, gay, and bisexual persons. Journal of Lesbian and Gay Social Services. 2004;17:83-101.

38. **Inaba DS, Cohen WE**. Uppers, Downers, All Arounders: Physical and Mental Effects of Psychoactive Drugs. 5th ed. CNS Publications; 2004.

39. **National Institute on Drug Abuse (NIDA)**. NIDA Community Drug Alert Bulletin-Club Drugs. Vol. 2005. Bethesda, MD: NIDA, 2005.

40. **Rehm J, Gmel G, Sempos CT, et al**. Alcohol-related morbidity and mortality. Alcohol Research & Health. 2002;27:39-51.

41. **Hughes TL**. Lesbians' drinking patterns: beyond the data. Subst Use Misuse. 2003 Sep-Nov;38:1739-58.

42. **Aaron DJ, Markovic N, Danielson ME, et al**. Behavioral risk factors for disease and preventive health practices among lesbians. Am J Public Health. 2001;91:972-5.

43. **Roberts SJ, Grindel CG, Patsdaughter CA, et al**. Lesbian use and abuse of alcohol: results of the Boston Lesbian Health Project II. J Subst Abus. 2005 Dec;25:1-9.

44. **Drabble L, Midanik LT, Trocki K**. Reports of alcohol consumption and alcohol-related problems among homosexual, bisexual and heterosexual respondents: results from the 2000 National Alcohol Survey. J Stud Alcohol. 2005;66:111-20.

45. **Skinner WF**. The prevalence and demographic predictors of illicit and licit drug use among lesbians and gay men. American Journal of Public Health. 1994;84:1307-10.

46. **Skinner WF, Otis MD**. Drug and alcohol use among lesbian and gay people in a Southern US sample: epidemiological, comparative, and methodological findings from the trilogy project. Journal of Homosexuality. 1996;30:59-91.

47. **Garafalo R, Deleon J, Osmer E, et al**. Overlooked, misunderstood and at-risk: exploring the lives and HIV risk of ethnic minority male-to-female transgender youth. Journal of Adolescent Health. 2006;38:230-6.

48. **Julien RM**. A Primer of Drug Action. 6th ed. W.H. Freeman & Co; 1992.

49. **Hirshfield S, Remien RH, Humberstone M, et al**. Substance use and high-risk sex among men who have sex with men: a national online study in the USA. AIDS Care. 2004;16:1036-47.

50. **Cretzmeyer M, Sarrazin MV, Huber DL, et al**. Treatment of methamphetamine abuse: research findings and clinical directions. Journal of Substance Abuse Treatment. 2003;24:267-77.

51. **Guzman R, Wheeler S, Colfax G**. An Event-Specific Analysis of Methamphetamine Use and Sexual Risk Behavior Among Men Who Have Sex With Men. XVI International AIDS Conference. Toronto, Canada: August, 2006.

52. **Nordahl TE, Salo R, Leamon M**. Neuropsychological effects of chronic methamphetamine use on neurotransmitters and cognition: a review. J Neuropsychiatry Clin Neurosci. 2003;15:317-25.

53. **Ellinwood EH, King G, Lee TH**. Chronic amphetamine use and abuse. In: Psychopharmacology: The Fourth Generation of Progress CD-ROM. Edited by Watson SJ. Philadelphia, PA: Lippincott, Williams & Wilkins; 1998.

54. **Hardman JG, Limbird L, Gilman AG, eds**. The Pharmacologic Basis of Therapeutics. New York: McGraw Hill; 2001.

55. **Peck JA, Reback CJ, Yang X, et al**. Sustained reductions in drug use and depression symptoms from treatment for drug abuse in methamphetamine-dependent gay and bisexual men. Journal of Urban Health. 2005;82:i100-8.

56. **McGrath C, Chan B**. Oral health sensations associated with illicit drug abuse. Br Dent J. 2005;198:159-62.

57. **Lan KC, Lin YF, Yu FC, et al**. Clinical manifestations and prognostic features of acute methamphetamine intoxication. J Formos Med Assoc. 1998, 97:528-33.

58. **Perez JA Jr, Arsura EL, Strategos S**. Methamphetamine-related stroke: four cases. J Emerg Med. 1999;17:469-71.

59. **Hong R, Matsuyama E, Nur K**. Cardiomyopathy associated with the smoking of crystal methamphetamine. JAMA. 1991;265:1152-54.

60. **Buffum JC, Shulgin AT**. Overdose of 2.3 grams of intravenous methamphetamine: case, analysis and patient perspective. Journal of Psychoactive Drugs. 2001;33:409-12.

61. **Parsons JT, Kelly BC, Wells BE**. Differences in club drug use between heterosexual and lesbian/bisexual females. Addict Behav. 2006 Dec;31:2344-9.

62. **Johnston LD, O'Malley PM, Bachman JG, et al**. Monitoring the Future: National Results on Adolescent Drug Use: Overview of Key Findings, 2003. NIH Publication 04-5506. Bethesda, MD: National Institute on Drug Abuse; 2004.

63. **Substance Abuse and Mental Health Services Administration, Office of Applied Studies**. The DAWN Report: Trends in Drug Related Emergency Visits, 1994-2002. 2003.

64. **Forman RF, Woody GE, McLellan T, et al**. The availability of web sites offering to sell opioid medications without prescriptions. The American Journal of Psychiatry. 2006;163:1233-8.

65. **Bolding G, Sherr L, Elford J**. Use of anabolic steroids and associated health risks among gay men attending London gyms. Addiction. 2002;97:195-203.

66. **Freese TE, Miotto K, Reback CJ**. The effects and consequences of selected club drugs. J Subst Abuse Treat. 2002;23:151-6.

67. **Gudelsky GA, Nash JF**. Carrier-mediated release of serotonin by 3,4-methylene-dioxymethamphetamine: implications for serotonin-dopamine interactions. J Neurochem. 1996;66:243-9.

68. **Graeme KA**. New drugs of abuse. Emerg Med Clin North Am. 2000;18:625-36.

69. **Lin M**. The underappreciated dangers of "club drugs": what clinicians need to know. Advanced Studies in Medicine. 2004;4:191-8.

70. **Patel MM, Wright DW, Ratcliff JJ, et al**. Shedding new light on the "safe" club drug: methylenedioxymethamphetamine (ecstasy)-related fatalities. Acad Emerg Med. 2004;11:208-10.

71. **Vuori E, Henry JA, Ojanpera I, et al**. Death following ingestion of MDMA (ecstasy) and moclobemide. Addiction. 2003;98:365-8.

72. **Beitia G, Cobreros A, Sainz L, et al**. 3,4-Methylenedioxymethamphetamine (ecstasy)-induced hepatotoxicity: effect on cytosolic calcium signals in isolated hepatocytes. Liver. 1999;19:234-41.

73. **Baggott M, Heifets B, Jones RT, et al**. Chemical analysis of ecstasy pills. JAMA. 2000;284:2190.

74. **Thomasius R, Petersen KU, Zapletalova P, et al**. Mental disorders in current and former heavy ecstasy (MDMA) users. Addiction. 2005;100:1310-9.

75. **Ricaurte GA, Yuan J, McCann UD**. 3,4-Methylenedioxymethamphetamine ('Ecstasy')-induced serotonin neurotoxicity: studies in animals. Neuropsychobiology. 2000;42:5-10.

76. **Mechan A, Yuan J, Hatzidimitriou G, et al**. Pharmacokinetic profile of single and repeated oral doses of MDMA in squirrel monkeys: relationship to lasting effects on brain serotonin neurons. Neuropsychopharmacology. 2005;31:339-50.

77. **Sumnall HR, Cole JC**. Self-reported depressive symptomatology in community samples of polysubstance misusers who report ecstasy use: a meta-analysis. J Psychopharmacol. 2005;19:84-92.

78. **Hanson KL, Luciana M**. Neurocognitive function in users of MDMA: the importance of clinically significant patterns of use. Psychol Med. 2004;34:229-46.

79. **Kish SJ**. How strong is the evidence that brain serotonin neurons are damaged in human users of ecstasy? Pharmacol Biochem Behav. 2002;71:845-55.

80. **Swanson J, Cooper A**. Dangerous liaison: club drug use and HIV/AIDS. IAPAC Monthly. 2002;8:330-8.

81. **Haas DA, Harper DG**. Ketamine: a review of its pharmacologic properties and use in ambulatory anesthesia. Anesthesia Progress. 1992;39:61-68.

82. **Morgan CJ, Monaghan L, Curran HV**. Beyond the k-hole: a 3-year longitudinal investigation of the cognitive and subjective effects of ketamine in recreational users who have substantially reduced their use of the drug. Addiction. 2004;99:1450-61.

83. **Pal HR, Berry N, Kumar R, et al**. Ketamine dependence. Anaesth Intensive Care 2002;30:382-4.

84. **Jansen KL, Darracot-Cankovic R**. The nonmedical use of ketamine, part two: a review of problem use and dependence. J Psychoactive Drugs. 2001;33:151-158.

85. **Miotto K, Darakjian J, Basch J, et al**. Gammahydroxybutyric acid: patterns of use, effects and withdrawal. Am J Addict. 2001;10:232-41.

86. **Dupont P, Thornton J**. Near-fatal gamma-butyrolactone intoxication—first report in the UK. Hum Exp Toxicol. 2001;20:19-22.

87. **Mamelak M**. Gammahydroxybutyrate: an endogenous regulator of energy metabolism. Neurosci Biobehav Rev. 1989;13:187-98.

88. **Gibson KM, Hoffmann GF, Hodson AK, et al**. 4-Hydroxybutyric acid and the clinical phenotype of succinic semialdehydedehydrogenase deficiency, an inborn error of GABA metabolism. Neuropediatrics. 1998;29:14-22.

89. **Lettieri J, Fung HL**. Improved pharmacological activity via pro-drug modification: comparative pharmacokinetics of sodium g-hydroxybutyrate and gamma-butyrolactone. Research Communications in Chemical Pathology and Pharmacology. 1978;22:107-18.

90. **Li J, Stokes SA, Woeckener A**. A tale of novel intoxication: a review of the effects of g-hydroxybutyric acid with recommendations for management. Ann Emerg Med. 1998;31:729-36.

91. **Snead OC III, Gibson KM**. G-hydroxybutyric acid. N Engl J Med. 2005;352:2721-32.

92. **Teter CJ, Guthrie SK**. A comprehensive review of MDMA and GHB: two common club drugs. Pharmacotherapy. 2001;21:1486-513.

93. **Mansergh G, Colfax GN, Marks G, et al**. The Circuit Party Men's Health Survey: findings and implications for gay and bisexual men. Am J Public Health. 2001;91:953-8.

94. **Romanelli F, Smith KM, Thornton AC, et al**. Poppers: epidemiology and clinical management of inhaled nitrite abuse. Pharmacotherapy. 2004;24:69-78.

95. **Newell GR, Adams SC, Mansell PW, et al**. Toxicity, immunosuppressive effects and carcinogenic potential of volatile nitrites: possible relationship to Kaposi's sarcoma. Pharmacotherapy. 1984;4:284-91.

96. **Pauk J, Huang ML, Brodie SJ, et al**. Mucosal shedding of human herpes virus 8 in men. N Engl J Med. 2000;343:1369-77.

97. **Xavier J, Bobbin M, Singer B, et al**. A needs assessment of transgender people of color living in Washington, DC. International Journal of Transgenderism. 2005;8:31-47.

98. **Wong W, Chaw JK, Kent CK, et al**. Risk factors for early syphilis among gay and bisexual men seen in an STD clinic: San Francisco, 2002-2003. Sex Transm Dis. 2005;32:458-63.

99. **Molitor F, Truax SR, Ruiz JD, et al**. Association of methamphetamine use during sex with risky sexual behaviors and HIV infection among non-injection drug users. West J Med. 1998;168:93-7.

100. **Myers T, Rowe CJ, Tudiver FG, et al**. HIV, substance use and related behaviour of gay and bisexual men: an examination of the Talking Sex project cohort. British Journal of Addiction. 1992;87:207-14.

101. **Ostrow DG, VanRaden MJ, Fox R, et al**. Recreational drug use and sexual behavior change in a cohort of homosexual men: the Multicenter AIDS Cohort Study (MACS). AIDS. 1990;4:759-65.

102. **Purcell DW, Moss S, Remien RH, et al**. Illicit substance use, sexual risk, and HIV-positive gay and bisexual men: differences by serostatus of casual partners. AIDS. 2005;19:S37-47.

103. **Page-Shafer K, Veugelers PJ, Moss AR, et al**. Sexual risk behavior and risk factors for HIV-1 seroconversion in homosexual men participating in the Tricontinental Seroconverter Study, 1982-1994. Am J Epidemiol. 1997;146:531-42.

104. **Buchbinder SP, Vittinghoff E, Heagerty PJ, et al**. Sexual risk, nitrite inhalant use, and lack of circumcision associated with HIV seroconversion in men who have sex with men in the United States. J Acquir Immune Defic Syndr. 2005;39:82-9.

105. **Seage GR III, Mayer KH, Horsburgh CR Jr, et al**. The relation between nitrite inhalants, unprotected receptive anal intercourse, and the risk of human immunodeficiency virus infection. Am J Epidemiol. 1992;135:1-11.

106. **Buchacz K, McFarland W, Kellogg TA, et al.** Amphetamine use is associated with increased HIV incidence among men who have sex with men in San Francisco. AIDS. 2005;19:1423-4.

107. **Tardieu S, Poirier Y, Micallef J, et al.** Amphetamine-like stimulant cessation in an abusing patient treated with bupropion. Acta Psychiatr Scand. 2004;109:75-8; discussion 77-8.

108. **Klitzman RL, Pope HGJ, Hudson JI.** MDMA ("Ecstasy") abuse and high-risk sexual behaviors among 169 gay and bisexual men. Am J Psychiatry. 2000;157:1162-4.

109. **Mattison AM, Ross MW, Wolfson T, et al.** Circuit party attendance, club drug use, and unsafe sex in gay men. J Subst Abuse. 2001;13:119-26.

110. **Purcell DW, Parsons JT, Halkitis PN, et al.** Substance use and sexual transmission risk behavior of HIV-positive men who have sex with men. J Subst Abuse. 2001;13:185-200.

111. **Rusch M, Lampinen TM, Schilder A, et al.** Unprotected anal intercourse associated with recreational drug use among young men who have sex with men depends on partner type and intercourse role. Sex Transm Dis. 2004;31:492-8.

112. **Semple SJ, Patterson TL, Grant I.** Motivations associated with methamphetamine use among HIV+ men who have sex with men. Journal of Substance Abuse Treatment. 2002;22:149-56.

113. **Halkitis PN, Shrem MT, Martin FW.** Sexual behavior patterns of methamphetamine-using gay and bisexual men. Substance Use & Misuse. 2005;40:703-719.

114. **Koblin BA, Husnik MJ, Colfax G, et al.** Risk factors for HIV infection among men who have sex with men. AIDS. Mar 21 2006;20:731-9.

115. **Stone E, Heagerty P, Vittinghoff E, et al.** Correlates of condom failure in a sexually active cohort of men who have sex with men. J Acquir Immune Defic Syndr Hum Retrovirol. 1999 Apr 15 1999;20:495-501.

116. **Vanable PA, McKirnan DJ, Buchbinder SP, et al.** Alcohol use and high-risk sexual behavior among men who have sex with men: the effects of consumption level and partner type. Health Psychology. 2004;23:525-32.

117. **Irwin TW, et al.** Alcohol and sexual HIV risk behavior among problem drinking men who have sex with men: an event level analysis of timeline followback data. AIDS and Behavior. 2006;10:299-307.

118. **Colfax G, Shoptaw S.** The methamphetamine epidemic: implications for HIV prevention and treatment. Current HIV/AIDS Reports. 2005;2:194-9.

119. **Rodriquez-Madera S, Toro-Alfonso J.** An exploratory study regarding social vulnerability, high-risk sex conduct, and HIV/AIDS in Puerto Rico's transgender community. Roundtable paper presented at: The 2000 United States Conference on AIDS; Atlanta, GA; 2000.

120. **Elifson KW, Boles J, Posey E, et al.** Male transvestite prostitutes and HIV risk. American Journal of Public Health. 1993;83:260-2.

121. **Xavier J, Bradford J.** Transgender Health Access in Virginia: Focus Group Report. Virginia HIV Planning Committee, Virginia Department of Health; 2005.

122. **Risser JMH, Shelton A, McCurdy S, et al.** Sex, drugs, violence, and HIV status among male-to-female transgender persons in Houston, Texas. International Journal of Transgenderism. 2005;8:67-74.

123. **Soderberg LS, Barnett JB.** Inhalation exposure to isobutyl nitrite inhibits macrophage tumoricidal activity and modulates inducible nitric oxide. J Leukoc Biol. 1995;57:135-40.

124. **Connor TJ.** Methylenedioxymethamphetamine (MDMA, "Ecstasy"): a stressor on the immune system. Immunology. 2004;111:357-67.

125. **Nunez-Iglesias MJ, Castro-Bolano C, Losada C et al.** Effects of amphetamine on cell mediated immune response in mice. Life Sci. 1996;58:PL 29-33.

126. **Pacifici R, Zuccaro P, Farre M et al.** Effects of repeated doses of MDMA ("ecstasy") on cell-mediated immune response in humans. Life Sci. 2001;69:2931-41.

127. **Yamada K, Nabeshima T**. Pro- and anti-addictive neurotrophic factors and cytokines in psychostimulant addiction: mini review. Ann N Y Acad Sci. 2004;1025:198-204.

128. **Kubera M, Filip M, Basta-Kaim A et al**. The effect of amphetamine sensitization on mouse immunoreactivity. J Physiol Pharmacol. 2002;53:233-42.

129. **Rofael HZ, Turkall RM, Abdel-Rahman MS**. Immunomodulation by cocaine and ketamine in postnatal rats. Toxicology. 2003;188:101-4.

130. **Phillips TR, Billaud JN, Henriksen SJ**. Methamphetamine and HIV-1: potential interactions and the use of the FIV/cat model. J Psychopharmacol. 2000;14:244-50.

131. **Gavrilin MA, Mathes LE, Podell M**. Methamphetamine enhances cell-associated feline immunodeficiency virus replication in astrocytes. J Neurovirol. 2002;8:240-9.

132. **Vittinghoff E, Hessol NA, Bacchetti P, et al**. Cofactors for HIV disease progression in a cohort of homosexual and bisexual men. J Acquir Immune Defic Syndr Hum Retrovirol. 2001;27:308-14.

133. **Ellis RJ, Childers ME, Cherner M, et al**. Increased human immunodeficiency virus loads in active methamphetamine users are explained by reduced effectiveness of antiretroviral therapy. J Infect Dis. 2003;188:1820-6.

134. **Reback CJ, Larkins S, Shoptaw S**. Methamphetamine abuse as a barrier to HIV medication adherence among gay and bisexual men. AIDS Care. 2003;15:775-85.

135. **Metsch LR, Pereyra M, Brewer TH**. Use of HIV health care in HIV-seropositive crack cocaine smokers and other active drug users. J Subst Abuse. 2001;13:155-67.

136. **Zaccarelli M, Barracchini A, De Longis P et al**. Factors related to virologic failure among HIV-positive injecting drug users treated with combination antiretroviral therapy including two nucleoside reverse transcriptase inhibitors and nevirapine. AIDS Patient Care and STDS. 2002;16:67-73.

137. **Henry JA, Hill IR**. Fatal interaction between ritonavir and MDMA. Lancet. 1998;352:1751-2.

138. **Harrington RD, Woodward JA, Hooton TM, et al** Life-threatening interactions between HIV-1 protease inhibitors and the illicit drugs MDMA and gamma-hydroxybutyrate. Arch Intern Med. 1999;159:2221-4.

139. **Antoniou T, Tseng AL**. Interactions between recreational drugs and antiretroviral agents. Ann Pharmacother. 2002;36:1598-1613.

140. **Kessler RC, McGonagle KA, Zhao S, et al**. Lifetime and 12-month prevalence of DSM-III-R psychiatric disorders in the United States: results from the National Comorbidity Survey. Archives of General Psychiatry. 1994;51:8-19.

141. **Meyer IH**. Prejudice, social stress, and mental health in lesbian, gay, and bisexual populations: conceptual issues and research evidence. Psychological Bulletin. 2003;129:674-97.

142. **Nemoto T, Operario D, Keatley J, et al**. HIV risk behaviors among male-to-female transgender persons of color in San Francisco. American Journal of Public Health. 2004;94:1193-9.

143. **Atkinson JH, Grant I, Kennedy, et al**. Prevalence of psychiatric disorders among men infected with human immunodeficiency virus: a controlled study. Archives of General Psychiatry. 1988;45:859-64.

144. **Cochran SD, Mays VM**. Relation between psychiatric syndromes and behaviorally defined sexual orientation in a sample of the US population. American Journal of Epidemiology. 2000;151:516-23.

145. **Ferguson DM, Horwood JL, Beautrais AL**. Is sexual orientation related to mental health problems and suicidality in young people? Archives of General Psychiatry. 1999;56:876-80.

146. **Gillman SE, Cochran SD, Mays VM, et al. Risks** of psychiatric disorders among individuals reporting same-sex sexual partners in the National Comorbidity Survey. American Journal of Public Health. 2001;91:933-9.

147. **Sandfort TG, deGraaf R, Bijl RV, et al**. Same-sex sexual behavior and psychiatric disorders: findings from the Netherlands Mental Health Survey and Incidence Study (NEMESIS). Archives of General Psychiatry. 2001;58:85-91.

148. **Bartels SJ, Drake RE, McHugo G**. Alcohol use, depression, and suicidal behavior in schizophrenia. American Journal of Psychiatry. 1992;149:394-395.

149. **Mueser KT, Noordsy DL, Fox L, et al**. Disulfiram treatment for alcoholism in severe mental illness. The American Journal on Addictions. 2003;12:242-52.

150. **Island D, Letellier P**. Men Who Beat the Men Who Love Them. Harrington Park Press; 1991.

151. **Lobel K**. Naming the Voice: Speaking Out About Lesbian Battering. Seal Press; 1986.

152. **Elliot P**. Shattering illusions: same sex domestic violence. Journal of Gay and Lesbian Social Services. 1996;4:1-8.

153. **Ratner EF, Kosten T, McLellan AT**. Treatment outcome of PRIDE institute patients: first wave-patients admitted from September 1988 through February 1989. In: McLellan AT, ed. Outcome Report. PRIDE Institute; 1991.

154. **Center for Substance Abuse Treatment**. A Provider's Introduction to Substance Abuse Treatment for Lesbian, Gay, Bisexual, and Transgender Individuals. Substance Abuse and Mental Health Services Administration; 2001.

155. **Hughes TL, Wilsnack SC, Szalacha LA, et al**. Age and racial/ethnic differences in drinking and drinking-related problems in a community sample of lesbians. Journal of Studies on Alcohol. 2006;67:579-90.

156. **Wilsnack SC**. Patterns and trends in women's drinking: recent findings and some implications for prevention. In: Women and alcohol: Prevention throughout the lifespan (19-63). National Institute on Alcohol Abuse and Alcoholism (NIAAA), Research Monograph Series. Department of Health and Human Service. American Psychological Association; 1996.

157. **McVinney D**. Clinical issues with bisexuals. In: A Provider's Introduction to Substance Abuse Treatment for Lesbian, Gay, Bisexual, and Transgender Individuals. Substance Abuse and Mental Health Services Administration, Center for Substance Abuse Treatment; 2001.

158. **Boehmer U**. Twenty years of public health research: inclusion of lesbian, gay, bisexual, and transgender populations. American Journal of Public Health. 2002;92:1125-30.

159. **Cochran B, Cauce AM**. Characteristics of lesbian, gay, bisexual, and transgender individuals entering substance abuse treatment. Journal of Substance Abuse Treatment. 2006;30:135-46.

160. **Cochran BN, Stewart AJ, Ginzler JA, et al**. Challenges faced by homeless sexual minorities: comparison of gay, lesbian, bisexual, and transgender homeless adolescents with their heterosexual counterparts. American Journal of Public Health. 2002;92:773-7.

161. **Sperber J, Landers S, Lawrence S**. Access to health care for transgendered persons: results of a needs assessment in Boston. International Journal of Transgenderism. 2005;8:75-91.

162. **Kenagy GP, Bostwick WB**. Health and social service needs of transgender people in Chicago. International Journal of Transgenderism. 2005;8:57-66.

163. **Eliason MJ, Hughes T**. Treatment counselors' attitudes about lesbian, gay, bisexual, and transgendered clients: urban vs. rural settings. Substance Use & Misuse. 2004;39: 625-44.

164. **Oggins J, Eichenbaum J**. Engaging transgender substance users in substance use treatment. International Journal of Transgenderism. 2002;6. Available at: http://www.symposion.com/ijt/ijtvo06no02_03.htm.

165. **American Psychiatric Association**. Diagnostic and Statistical Manual for Mental Disorders 4th ed. APA Press; 2004.

166. **Mayfield D, McLeaod G, Hall P**. The CAGE questionnaire: validation of a new alcoholism instrument. American Journal of Psychiatry. 1974;131:1121-3.

167. **Babor TF, Kranzler HR, Lauerman RJ**. Early detection of harmful alcohol consumption: comparison of clinical, laboratory, and self-report screening procedures. Addictive Behaviors. 1989;14:139-57.

168. **Selzer ML**. The Michigan Alcoholism Screening Test: the quest for a new diagnostic instrument. American Journal of Psychiatry. 1971;127:1653-8.

169. **National Institute on Drug Abuse (NIDA)**. Principles of Drug Addiction Treatment: A Research Based Guide. Bethesda, MD: NIDA; 1999.

170. **Ball JC, Ross A**. The Effectiveness of Methadone Maintenance Treatment. Springer-Verlag; 1991.

171. **Johnson RE, Chutuape MA, Strain EC, et al**. A comparison of levomethadyl acetate, buprenorphine, and methadone for opioid dependence. The New England Journal of Medicine. 2000;343:1290-7.

172. **Resnick RB, Schuyten-Resnick E, Washton AM**. Narcotic antagonists in the treatment of opioid dependence: review and commentary. Comprehensive Psychiatry. 1979;20:116-25.

173. **McLellan AT, Arndt IO, Metzger DS, et al**. The effects of psychosocial services in substance abuse treatment. JAMA. 1993;269:1953-9.

174. **Miller WR, Rollnick S**. Motivational Interviewing: Preparing People for Change. 2nd ed. Guilford Press; 2002.

175. **Marlatt GA, Donovan DM**. Relapse Prevention: Maintenance Strategies in the Treatment of Addictive Behaviors. 2nd ed. Guilford Press; 2005.

176. **Rawson RA, Shoptaw SJ, Obert JL, McCann MJ, Hasson AL, et al**. An intensive outpatient approach for cocaine abuse treatment: the Matrix model. Journal of Substance Abuse Treatment. 1995;12:117-27.

177. **Rawson RA, Gonzales R, Brethen P**. Treatment of methamphetamine use disorders: an update. Journal of Substance Abuse Treatment. 2002;23:145-50.

178. **Higgins ST, Budney AJ, Bickel WK, et al**. Achieving cocaine abstinence with a behavioral approach. The American Journal of Psychiatry. 1993;150:763-9.

179. **Margolis RD, Zweben JE**. Treating Patients with Alcohol ad Other Drug Problems: An Integrated Approach. APA Press; 1998.

180. **Washton AM, ed**. Psychotherapy and Substance Abuse: A Practitioner's Handbook. Guilford Press; 1995.

Chapter 10

Violence and Trauma: Recognition, Recovery, and Prevention

EMILY L. PITT, LICSW
ELAINE J. ALPERT, MD, MPH

Introduction

Trauma is an all too common experience that generally proves to be an isolating event for the individual, whether victimized directly or affected indirectly. Trauma can be physical or emotional and can lead to psychological or behavioral problems.[1] Traumatic events cause disruptions in arousal, attention, perception, and emotion.[2] Effective and sensitive recognition, intervention, and prevention are key to optimal care for all patients, including those who are lesbian, gay, bisexual, and transgender (LGBT). Although any type of physical or psychological trauma can happen to an LGBT patient, this chapter focuses on three specific causes of trauma: hate crimes, domestic violence, and sexual assault. The first part of the chapter describes the clinical presentation of trauma; then, suggestions are provided for the evaluation, management, and prevention of anti-LGBT hate crimes, domestic violence, and sexual assault.

Presentation of Trauma

Understanding the presentation of trauma allows the clinician to both fully understand the range of symptoms with which patients may present and to know how to intervene in an efficient, sensitive, and prevention-focused manner. Additionally, survivors of trauma often engage in behavioral patterns that are maladaptive, such as substance abuse, suicidal ideation, cutting, and sexual risk-taking.[3] Because many survivors of trauma do not have mental healthcare, they may present to a clinician with somatic symptoms that indicate a diagnosis of posttraumatic stress disorder (PTSD). Survivors of trauma typically experience symptoms that result from adaptive responses that may occur during a traumatic event, but these symptoms become maladaptive once the immediate threat is gone.

The amygdala, part of the limbic system of the brain, facilitates the body's ability to respond instantaneously to violent stimuli. When danger is perceived, the amygdala allows for the evaluation of the incoming stimulus. The subsequent release of hormones, suppression of heart rate, increased breathing rate, and release of adrenaline and norepinephrine allows the organism to be more sensitive to incoming stimuli and thus respond faster.[4] This is typically referred to as the "fight or flight" response. The secondary response occurs in the cerebral cortex, providing for the release of cortisol to turn off the stress response and allow the organism to stop and consider options.

The repeated release of hormones that provide biological safety for organisms that need to flee quickly from danger can eventually interfere with the body's ability to respond quickly. If a traumatic experience is encoded in the amygdala, the fight/flight response can be triggered repeatedly and reflexively, resulting in hypervigilance and other signs and symptoms of early PTSD. Altered levels of hormones and neurotransmitters lead to intrusive trauma symptoms. Reminders of trauma (also known as 'triggers') can cause heightened activity in the right visual cortex, which can cause the patient to re-experience the trauma in a visual manner (typically referred to as a flashback). Even moderate stress can interfere with pre-frontal cortical function, which can lead to distraction, disorganization, and memory difficulties, as well as other impairments in cognitive functioning. Because of this, many trauma survivors may feel as though they are "going crazy."

Three types of trauma symptoms predominate in survivors of hate crimes, domestic violence, and sexual assault:[2]

1. **Hyperarousal**: Because trauma creates autonomic arousal, traumatized individuals develop a permanently aroused state. The normal baseline of arousal is no longer relaxed but rather is vigilant and acutely alert. As a consequence, the autonomic system becomes constantly alert and reacts excessively to minor disturbances. Such a sequence typically results in symptoms such as exaggerated startle response, irritability, sleep disturbances, anxiety, and panic attacks.

2. **Intrusion or re-experiencing**: Memories of traumatic events can continue to intrude involuntarily into the patient's consciousness. Because traumatic memories are not encoded in the same way as other memories, they are often not recalled in a linear fashion. Thus, intrusive memories can be triggered by everyday events, such as sights, smells, sounds, or sensations. It is often difficult for patients to assign a verbal narrative to these memories, so the memory is experienced as an unanticipated, unwelcome, frightening, and intrusive emotional flood, rather than as a linear narrative that can be

controlled and acknowledged in proper perspective. Patients who experience these symptoms are often fearful of evoking intrusive memories and therefore may feel endangered in environments that are actually safe. The ensuing autonomic arousal can trigger unwanted conscious memories of the trauma and can interfere with the patient's psychological comfort, ranging from ill-defined unease to panic.

3. **Constriction or avoidance**: Often during a traumatic event, a patient escapes by experiencing an alteration of her or his state of conscious awareness, resulting in a dissociative episode. Dissociation is especially common if the trauma is severe or recurrent and if the victim perceives no means of escape, feels especially helpless, and/or senses a threat to his or her life. In this case, feelings of terror, rage, or pain are suddenly replaced by a sense of numbness or altered reality. While events may continue to register with the patient, those events, as well as perceptions of time, become disconnected from their original meaning. Once a dissociative response arises in connection with trauma, overt or even unconscious reminders of the trauma can trigger similar dissociative responses, which may cause patients to dissociate long after the trauma is no longer present. Similarly, patients may attempt to produce similar numbing effects by using alcohol or drugs or other compulsive behaviors.

All medical providers need to understand the sequelae of trauma and the effects on the brain, behavior, and cognitive functioning. For more information on trauma, refer to the resources listed in Appendix A.

Hate Crimes

A hate crime is an incident that is perpetrated specifically because of a person's race, ethnicity, religion, gender, disability status, or sexual orientation. This type of crime is different from others because of its severity, as well as its effects on both the victim and others in the community. Some, but not all, states have laws that prosecute hate crimes as distinct categories of crime (see http://www.adl.org for a comprehensive list; see also Chapter 16 for more on hate crime laws). Regardless of state or local statutes, the effects of hate crimes on victims are the same. Anti-LGBT hate crimes that include physical violence are often more severe than similar hate crimes perpetrated against members of other minority or marginalized groups.[5] Some common reactions to hate crimes include:[6]

- Personal targeting: Although the incident may have been random, victims often feel as though they have been personally targeted.
- Crisis of identity: The incident may cause victims to question their own sense of personhood and place in the world.

- Internalization: Victims may experience feelings of shame, guilt, self-blame, and internalized homophobia.
- Loss of trust: Victims may experience a diminution or loss of trust in law enforcement officers and other service providers, including medical providers.
- Perception of personal vulnerability: Victims may experience an increased sense of vulnerability as well as a view of the world as a dangerous place. Perceptions such as these may cause some victims to alter their appearance and behavior as a coping strategy.
- Mental health effects: Victims may experience increased and long-lasting symptoms of depression, stress, and anxiety.

Hate crimes often engender a condition known as *vicarious trauma*—emotional effects felt by bystanders and others not directly victimized by the trauma. Since a hate crime typically targets an individual victim or vulnerable group to send a message of fear and control to all members of that group, it is often other community members who, upon hearing about the occurrence of a hate crime, experience symptoms of trauma themselves.

The first large-scale study of hate crime prevalence in gay men and lesbians (N = 2074) was performed in 1984 by the National Gay and Lesbian Task Force. This study, conducted in eight US cities, found that 19% of respondents had experienced physical assault, 44% were threatened with violence, and 83% lived with the fear of being victimized because of their sexual orientation. In addition, 45% had modified their behavior to reduce the risk of an antigay attack.[7] Although conducted over two decades ago, these data have been corroborated by more recent prevalence studies of hate crimes.[8] The FBI Uniform Crime Report for 2005 shows that 7160 hate crimes were reported to law enforcement that year, 1017 (14.2%) of which were specifically anti-LGBT.[9]

The National Coalition of Anti-Violence Programs, a network of local programs in several regions of the country that provides services for LGBT survivors of hate crimes, sexual assault, and domestic violence and collects surveillance data from those survivors, reported 1962 anti-LGBT incidents in 2005.[10] This number represents cases that were reported to anti-violence programs, which is usually somewhat higher than criminal justice statistics, due to widespread underreporting to criminal justice authorities. Because of the vicarious traumatization and triggering that occurs in the context of hate crimes, at some point during the life span, most LGBT patients will experience either direct or indirect victimization, or at least legitimate fear of being the target of a hate crime.

In 1998, Matthew Shepard was murdered in a highly publicized antigay hate crime incident. In the years that followed, much was written about this horrific homicide. Numerous media sources reported stories about the tragedy and its aftermath, movies and plays were written and performed, books were written, and the phenomena following his death were closely followed by many in the LGBT community. Many members of the LGBT community were strongly affected by Matthew Shepard's murder even though they did not personally know him. Reported symptoms included increased feelings of vulnerability, changes in behavior to reduce the possibility of being targeted, perceived decreased sense of self-worth, and reports of negative effects on overall mental health status.[5] It is important to note that patients who experience decreased self-worth and increased vulnerability often turn to adverse coping behaviors such as substance abuse and sexual risk-taking as a response to trauma.[11]

The clinical presentation of LGBT patients who experience victimization by hate crimes may be similar to that seen in other types of trauma. The exceptional nature of hate crimes, including those that target the LGBT population, requires clinicians to be knowledgeable and understanding about the specific responses brought out by hate crimes. LGBT patients are best served by medical care that is sensitive to their particular experiences, needs, and vulnerability to hate crimes.

Domestic Violence

Domestic violence should be thought about broadly as intentionally violent acts or controlling behavior in a current or concluded dating or romantic relationship. The spectrum of domestic violence includes, but is not limited to the following:

- physical attacks
- sexual assault
- threats
- psychological abuse
- economic control
- social isolation
- destruction of a victim's property or personal possessions
- abuse of animals or pets
- spiritual abuse or misuse of scripture

Although each of the above manifestations can occur singly or in any combination in both LGBT and heterosexual relationships, additional elements of the spectrum of domestic violence in the LGBT community include the following:

- threats of being "outed" to friends, family, colleagues, and coworkers
- use of homophobia to deter the victim from getting help by telling the victim that authorities will not help a LGBT person
- attempts to persuade the victim that leaving the relationship is akin to admitting that LGBT relationships are deviant

- suggestions to the victim that to involve law enforcement would mean a betrayal of the entire LGBT community
- the assertion that women cannot be violent
- the assertion that men are naturally violent and therefore domestic violence should be expected
- frequently inadequate law enforcement response
- homophobia on the part of providers
- difficulty distinguishing abuser from victim
- elevated risk of identity theft-type behavior when victim and perpetrator are the same sex

Figure 10-1 is a graphic representation of the spectrum and dynamics of abuse, often used in educational and patient care venues.

In most abusive relationships—whether heterosexual or LGBT—the abusive dynamics represent efforts by the perpetrator to assert power and maintain control in the relationship. Abusive relationships generally are not violent when they begin but tend to become increasingly so over time, as the perpetrator exerts progressive control over increasing dimensions of the victim's life. Therefore, although primary prevention is ideal, and early intervention once abuse has begun is key, providers often do not identify victims until the abuse has progressed substantially to the point of serious physical or psychological injury.

Although victims may strike back in self-defense, abuse is generally one-way, with one partner "calling the shots" while the other makes repeated attempts to adjust to a confusing maze of changing rules and restrictions. The abuser holds the majority of the power and control in the relationship, while the victim tends to shape his or her life around the needs of the abuser.

Physical violence is often cyclical and recurrent.[12] Apologies and promises of hope and change often follow a physically violent incident. There is then a variable period of increasing tension, culminating in a subsequent episode of violence. Especially following a violent incident, victims may feel hopeful that caring behavior, apologies, and promises herald an end to the abuse and that the situation will improve. Because of this, patients often make excuses for an abuser's behavior and/or return to an abusive partner even after initially leaving the relationship.

Many victims are fearful of their partners but may not feel comfortable disclosing this fear to medical providers. Male victims in particular may feel an increased sense of shame about feeling fearful of an intimate partner. In addition, patients often minimize the threat of violence, and therefore it may be difficult for providers to know the true level of risk for some patients. Finally, the patient may also believe that clinicians do not know about or understand domestic violence at all, especially in LGBT relationships. The patient may worry that the clinician will not take the situation seriously or that the clinician may not believe, or may even blame, her or him for getting into or remaining in an abusive relationship.

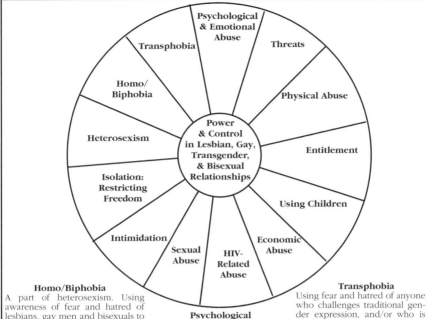

Homo/Biphobia

A part of heterosexism. Using awareness of fear and hatred of lesbians, gay men and bisexuals to convince partner of danger in reaching out to others. Controlling expression of sexual identity and connections to community. Outing sexual identity. Shaming. Questioning status as a "real" lesbian, gay man, bisexual.

Heterosexism

Perpetuating and utilizing invisibility of LGB relationships to define relationship norms. Using heterosexual roles to normalize abuse and shame partner for same sex and bisexual desires. Using cultural invisibility to isolate partner and reinforce control. Limiting connection to community.

Intimidation

Creating fear by using looks, actions, gestures and destroying personal items, mementos or photos. Breaking windows or furniture. Throwing or smashing objects. Trashing clothes, hurting or killing pets.

Using Children

Threats or actions to take children away or have them removed. Using children to relay messages. Threats to or actual harm to children. Threats to or revealing of sexual or gender orientation to children or others to jeopardize parent-child relationship, custody or relationships with family, friends, school or others.

Psychological & Emotional Abuse

Criticizing constantly. Using verbal abuse, insults and ridicule. Undermining self-esteem. Trying to humiliate or degrade in private or public. Manipulating with lies and false promises. Denying partner's reality.

Threats

Making physical, emotional, economic or sexual threats. Threatening to harm family or friends. Threatening to make a report to city, state or federal authorities that would jeopardize custody, economic situation, immigration, or legal status. Threatening suicide.

HIV-Related Abuse

Threatening to reveal HIV status to others. Blaming partner for having HIV. Withholding medical or social services. Telling the partner she or he is "dirty." Using illness to justify abuse.

Sexual Abuse

Forcing sex. Forcing specific sex acts or sex with others. Physical assaults to "sexual" body areas. Refusing to practice safer sex. In S&M refusing to negotiate or not respecting contract/scene limits or safe words.

Physical Abuse

Slapping, hitting, shoving, biting, choking, pushing, punching, beating, kicking, stabbing, shooting or killing. Using weapons.

Transphobia

Using fear and hatred of anyone who challenges traditional gender expression, and/or who is transsexual, to convince partner of danger in reaching out to others. Controlling expression of gender identity and connections to community. Outing gender identity. Shaming. Questioning validity of one's gender.

Isolation: Restricting Freedom

Controlling personal social contacts, access to information and participation in groups or organizations. Limiting the who, what, where and when of daily life. Restraining movement, locking partner in or out.

Entitlement

Treating partner as inferior; race, education, wealth, politics, class privilege or lack of, physical ability, and anti-Semitism. Demanding that needs always come first. Interfering with partner's job, personal needs and family obligations.

Economic Abuse

Controlling economic resources and how they are used. Stealing money, credit cards or checks. Running up debt. Fostering total economic dependency. Using economic status to determine relationship roles/norms, including purchase of clothes, food, etc.

Figure 10-1   Power and Control in Lesbian, Gay, Transgender, and Bisexual Relationships

Sexual Assault

Data from the National Violence Against Women Survey (NVAWS) reveal that sexual assault and rape are reported to affect approximately 17.6% of women and 3% of men over the life span.[13] These prevalence figures, despite being the most recent national surveillance data available, are over a decade old. They are acknowledged to be underestimates, as they were obtained by a random digit-dial telephone survey that queried adults only (18 years old or older). In addition, data could not be obtained from individuals who were not willing, or did not feel safe, to answer a lengthy phone interview in their homes; who elected not to disclose a history of rape or sexual assault to the interviewer; were homeless or living in an institutional setting; who did not speak English or Spanish; or who did not have a residential phone. Still, NVAWS represents the most accurate figures available, using accepted surveillance methodology.

The proportion of victims within the NVAWS cohort who self-identify as LGBT is unknown. Reliable estimates of rates of sexual victimization in the LGBT community are not available. However, it is thought that men, and gay men in particular, may experience sexual assault at a much higher rate than reported. Underreporting by gay men may be due to fears that their victimization will not be believed because they are gay, shame associated with having been victimized, or uncertainty of their own victimization because of assumptions that sexual assault only happens to women. A previous study conducted 20 years ago noted that 10.5% of men experienced rape or sexual assault over the life span.[14]

Legal definitions of sexual assault vary from state to state and cover a range of unwanted sexual contact behaviors. In contrast, the legal definition of rape is fairly consistent nationwide, and encompasses three required elements: penetration of a person's vagina, anus, or mouth by another, using an object or body part; the use of force; and lack of consent.

While rape of any individual typically results in both physical and psychological trauma, male victims may be at a distinct disadvantage due to the lack of available resources, a societal lack of understanding of male-on-male rape, and gender issues that often lead to increased shame and isolation for male victims.[15] Virtually all rape survivors fear that they will not be believed, that they will be blamed for the assault, and/or that communities and systems will not effectively hold perpetrators responsible.

Dating violence: Rape or sexual assault that occurs within the context of dating or in the course of an acquaintance relationship can happen to LGBT individuals in the same way that it can happen to heterosexual women. For LGBT survivors of this type of violence, there is the added burden of knowing that, in order to obtain medical care following an assault, the patient will have to disclose his or her sexual orientation to the provider. For women who are raped by other women, there is the added concern of not being believed because many providers are not aware that women can perpetrate sexual violence.

Typical concerns of victims: Survivors of rape and sexual assault are likely to express a range of concerns when discussing the incident with a medical provider. For lesbian victims, concerns about pregnancy and STIs may be enhanced because these are not issues that they typically need to deal with—women whose only sexual contact is with other women do not need to worry about pregnancy, and many mistakenly believe that they also do not need to be concerned about STIs. In some cases, these women may not receive regular gynecological care, and a pelvic exam after a rape may be experienced as repeat victimization.

It is also important for the provider to understand the sense of loss that can accompany being a victim of rape or sexual assault, as well as trauma symptoms that can emerge either acutely or months or even years after such an incident.

Rape kits or evidence collection: Most states have legislation and/or standard procedures guiding the collection of evidence after a rape. Typically evidence is collected by a certified Sexual Assault Nurse Examiner (SANE) if one is available in the emergency setting. Forensic evidence is collected in a standardized manner using a specially designed sexual assault evidence collection kit, or "rape kit," for evidence collection. These kits are completed at the time of the medical exam following a sexual assault. Some evidence, for example oral swabs, can only be collected within the first 24 hours following an assault, while it is possible to obtain valid samples of selected material including vaginal secretions up to 120 hours after the assault. Specific procedures are specified by various state statutes, and procedures must be followed exactly to ensure that the chain of evidence is preserved, so that evidence will be usable in court proceedings that may ensue. Because of the invasive nature of these exams and the difficulty most survivors have in enduring an invasive procedure after being traumatized by a sexual assault, it is important that providers understand the importance of allowing the patient to have a medical advocate from a rape crisis center or other support person with them during the exam. In most states, significant portions of the rape evidence collection kit can be completed on male victims as well. Thus, the opportunity for both standardized evidence collection and psychological support must be offered to male victims in the same way that it is offered to female victims.

Evaluation

General Considerations

Patients should be interviewed in private, without the partner, children, other relatives, roommates, or friends present. A history of previous trauma, chronic pain complaints, or psychological distress should be sought from direct history or from the medical record.

All patients, heterosexual and LGBT alike, should be queried periodically as a matter of routine standard practice about a life span history of trauma, including domestic violence and sexual assault. LGBT patients can be queried about direct or indirect exposure to hate crimes.

Hate Crimes

Direct victims of homophobic hate crimes most often present to emergency services with physical injuries resulting from the crime itself. Evaluation and management should proceed according to accepted trauma evaluation and treatment protocols, with particular attention to the possibility of sexual victimization occurring in the course of hate crime perpetration. Particular sensitivity should be used when interviewing patients who have been victims of suspected hate crimes, as the physical injuries sustained in an attack may be compounded by feelings of humiliation and fear of revictimization by the perpetrator and even police, healthcare providers, family, and others in positions of authority or importance.

Bystanders and other witnesses to hate crimes, as well as family, friends, and others connected to the LGBT community, can present to the healthcare system with symptoms that arise from secondary traumatization due to indirect victimization. Because of the global sense of vulnerability engendered by hate crimes, patients, even if not directly victimized themselves, may not volunteer that they have been witnesses to a hate crime or that they are close to someone who has been victimized. Indeed, patients who present with physical or psychological complaints resulting from being an indirect victim of a hate crime may not even be aware of the relationship between hate crime occurrence in their community and their own symptoms. For these reasons, careful, sensitive, nonjudgmental, and open-minded inquiry should be undertaken routinely in all patients who may be at risk from hate crimes.

Familiarity with local statutes regarding hate crime laws will help providers to direct patients toward appropriate resources and will assist the provider in understanding any mandatory reporting requirements. Particularly if the patient is elderly, disabled, or a minor child, mandatory reporting may be required. Special consideration should be given to the possibility that the patient may not be "out" (ie, others may not be aware that the patient is LGB or T). In addition, especially if the patient is a minor, an evaluation of the patient's physical and psychological safety at home should also be considered, since mandatory reporting may alert the patient's parents to the patient's previously closeted sexual orientation.

Domestic Violence

Victims of violence in relationships often do not "look battered." In fact, there may be no physical evidence of abuse at the time of the clinician's encounter with the patient. Because of this, routine inquiry about current and past domestic violence should be undertaken with all patients, including those who self-identify as LGBT, regardless of the presence or absence of "red flag" indicators of abuse. Because some gay, lesbian, or bisexual patients have not disclosed their sexual orientation to their clinicians, questions about abuse should be asked in gender-neutral language, so that the provider does not assume that a given patient is heterosexual and so that the provider can be alerted to the true nature of the injury (ie, abuse in the context of a relationship rather than from a random assault). Additionally, asking questions in gender-neutral language allows the patient to answer questions honestly and is more likely to engender trust in the clinician and in other members of the healthcare team.

Abusive relationships are characterized more by controlling patterns of behavior than by single violent incidents. In fact, physical violence is by no means universal in domestic violence and is almost never the first manifestation of abuse. When physical abuse does occur, it tends to become recurrent and progressive, increasing in frequency and severity over time. Although battered individuals may sustain life-threatening physical injuries, they also can suffer less obvious effects that can be just as debilitating, if not more so. In addition to physical trauma, victims may present with a variety of other medical problems, including chronic pain syndromes, somatization disorders, posttraumatic stress disorder, anxiety, depression, and alcoholism or other substance abuse. The LGBT community experiences the same spectrum of physical and psychological effects and reactions to abuse as does the heterosexual community.

Although victims of domestic violence access medical services more frequently than do non-abused individuals, most—especially those who are LGBT—do not volunteer a history of abuse even to their primary care clinicians. Abused patients are more likely to disclose a history of victimization if the clinician is perceived to be knowledgeable, nonjudgmental, accepting of LGBT identity, respectful, and supportive, as well as one who practices trauma-aware care.

Sexual Assault

LGBT patients who have been raped or sexually assaulted may be seen in the healthcare setting acutely, often within hours of an attack. Rape and sexual assault in the LGBT population may occur in the context of domestic violence in ongoing or concluded relationships, as a "date rape" in new or even incipient relationships, or in the context of hate crimes, the latter most often committed by strangers.

LGBT patients can also present with long-term sequelae from assaults that have taken place months to years prior—including during childhood. The most frequent perpetrators of sexual violence in childhood include family members, trusted acquaintances, and romantic partners. Many LGBT survivors of childhood sexual abuse may have been told at some point that their LGBT identity formed because of the abuse, or that they were "chosen" for sexual activities during childhood because they were LGBT. Both perceptions are incorrect and are blatant manifestations of the array of manipulative behaviors perpetrated on children for the sexual gratification of trusted adults. It is critical to convey to patients that sexual abuse during childhood does not cause someone to become gay or lesbian and that same-sex attraction is neither the cause nor the result of rape.

Disclosure of sexual assault victimization can be exceedingly difficult for members of the LGBT community. Patients may fear being stigmatized by the healthcare provider if the gender of the perpetrator and the nature of the assault is disclosed during the course of medical assessment.

As in the case of hate crime victimization and domestic violence, the clinician should assure the patient that he or she is believed, respected, and valued. A trauma-aware, respectful clinical encounter not only will place the patient at ease to the extent possible, but also will facilitate healing and reintegration from the trauma of sexual assault.

Routine Inquiry and Assessment

Use your RADAR: The acronym "**RADAR**," developed in 1992 by Elaine Alpert for the Massachusetts Medical Society's Campaign Against Violence, summarizes steps clinicians should take in recognizing and treating victims of hate crimes, domestic violence, and sexual assault.

Remember to ask routinely about violence and victimization in your own practice.

Ask directly about violence with such questions as "At any time, has anyone hit, kicked, or otherwise hurt or frightened you?" Interview your patient in private at all times.

Document information about "suspected hate crimes, domestic violence, or sexual assault" in the patient's chart.

Assess your patient's safety. Is it safe to return home? Find out if any weapons are kept in the house, if the children are in danger, and if the violence is escalating.

Review options with your patient. Know about the types of referral options (eg, LGBT advocacy services, domestic violence shelters, support groups, legal advocates).

Patients voice clear preferences in favor of their clinicians taking the initiative to inquire, as a matter of standard practice, about violence and abuse during the course of both routine and emergency clinical encounters. Again, the importance of using gender-neutral language cannot be understated. Lesbians who are asked whether or not they were abused by a boyfriend may be much less likely to disclose than lesbians who are asked whether they were abused by a partner, spouse, "someone you live with," or "girlfriend or boyfriend".

A single question, asked routinely and nonjudgmentally in the course of the social history, can significantly increase the detection rate of current or prior trauma and can allow your patient to feel more comfortable disclosing a history of abuse. This sample question can be adapted as needed to individual practices and can be used as an initial screening question for exposure to domestic violence, sexual assault, and hate crimes:

> "At any time, has anyone hit, kicked, choked, threatened, forced him or herself on you sexually, touched you in a sexual way that was unwanted, or otherwise hurt or frightened you?"

Should your patient disclose that she or he has been victimized, or if you suspect domestic violence, sexual assault, or hate crime victimization in the absence of direct disclosure, asking the following specific questions in a safe and confidential setting can help to determine the extent of abuse and the possible risk to your patient:

- How were you hurt?
- Has this happened before?
- When did it first happen?
- How badly have you been hurt in the past?
- Have you needed to go to an emergency room for treatment in the past?
- Have you ever been threatened with a weapon, or has a weapon ever been used on you?
- Have you ever tried to get a restraining order against a partner?
- Have your children (if the patient is a parent or caregiver) ever seen or heard you being threatened or hurt?
- Have your children ever been threatened or hurt by your partner?
- Do you know how you can get help for yourself if you were hurt or afraid?

It is helpful to ask adolescent patients questions such as these:

- Have you begun to date?
- Has your boyfriend or girlfriend ever threatened to hurt you, or have you ever threatened to hurt him or her?
- Have you ever been afraid of your boyfriend or girlfriend?
- Have you ever had a pushing or shoving fight with a boyfriend or girlfriend?
- Have you ever gotten hurt from a fight with a boyfriend or girlfriend?
- Have you begun to have sex?
- Has anyone ever made you have sex when you didn't want to?
- Have you talked to anyone else about this?

As important as it is to ask the right questions, it is equally important to refrain from asking questions in a manner that might frighten or intimidate your patient, increase your patient's sense of humiliation and shame about the violence, or be interpreted as blaming the victim for the situation.

One should never ask the patient what she or he did to bring on the violence, why she or he has remained in the relationship, or why she or he has returned once having left. In addition, it is critical that the clinician not break patient confidentiality by disclosing any information or discussing the case or any concerns with the patient's partner, a family member, or with anyone else.

Physical Examination and Documentation

Be highly suspicious of victimization with these physical findings:

- any evidence of injury, especially to the face, torso, breasts, or genitals
- bilateral or multiple injuries
- delay between onset of injury and presentation for care
- patient's explanation inconsistent with type of injury
- prior use of emergency services for trauma or other care
- chronic pain symptoms where no etiology is apparent
- psychological distress (ie, anxiety, depression, sleep disorder, or suicidal ideation)
- evidence of rape or sexual assault.

Document all findings carefully in the medical record. You may wish to draw a picture freehand, or include a labeled photograph to supplement your written description. It is important to describe the patient's symptoms and signs accurately and to indicate "domestic violence" or "suspect violence due to hate crime" as a diagnosis or problem when appropriate. The clinician should obtain written consent for photographic documentation from the patient prior to taking photographs, should initial (or sign) and date each photograph, and should append a statement with language similar to the following:

These photographs were taken of (name of patient) on (date) by me and are accurate, unedited and unaltered.

Digital photographs, if accompanied by the above statement, are perfectly acceptable for medical and medico-legal documentation.

Documentary evidence of a completed rape can be collected up to five days after the crime occurs. Physical evidence that can be used for medical assessment and possible criminal prosecution should be obtained using an accepted sexual assault evidence kit ("rape kit"), which can be found in most hospital emergency departments. Unless the patient is unwilling or unable to present to the emergency department, the examination and evidence collection should be conducted in the emergency setting. An increasing number of hospital emergency departments utilize the services of Sexual Assault Nurse Examiners (SANE) who have specific training in forensic nursing, evidence collection, and crisis counseling. Should a patient call your office before presenting to the emergency department, she or he should be told to refrain from showering, bathing, or douching before arriving at the hospital. Victims should be instructed to put all clothes worn during the assault in a paper bag to bring to the hospital as additional evidence.

Risk Assessment

Once a patient has disclosed being the victim of a hate crime or being in a threatening or violent relationship, the clinician can play an invaluable role in helping the patient assess the level of risk, initiating discussion of the need for a safety plan, and making referrals to appropriate services, including law enforcement as indicated. The most important determinants in assessing risk are the patient's level of fear and her or his own appraisal of both immediate and future safety needs. However, since patients may minimize or deny the danger of their situations, the following indicators of escalating risk should be explored with the patient:

- an increase in the frequency or severity of assaults (if the abuse is recurrent or chronic, such as in domestic violence)
- increasing or new threats of homicide or suicide by a partner
- the use or availability of a firearm
- new or increasingly violent behavior by the perpetrator outside the relationship

Time Management

Clinicians may be reluctant to engage in inquiry and assessment regarding hate crimes, domestic violence, and sexual assault because of concerns that they have insufficient time to screen and respond, given the multiple responsibilities and time pressures that they face in daily practice. Judicious time management, however, will allow for both universal inquiry and for targeted follow-up. Inquiry about violence and abuse (usually undertaken as the presenting issue in emergency presentations for trauma or in the primary care setting as part of the social history) should take no more than ten seconds yet should have a dual beneficial effect: the clinician will be reassured that the patient is not currently victimized or at risk, and the patient will be made aware that the clinician is concerned, knowledgeable, and able to respond should violence become an issue at any time in the future.

It bears keeping in mind that most patients who disclose prior or ongoing victimization, despite dealing with a difficult medical and social issues, are not in acute danger at the time of the visit. Should the patient disclose victimization, the clinician should conduct a brief danger assessment, offer information and hotline numbers, convey concern and support for the patient, and arrange to see the patient in follow-up to discuss the abuse in greater detail, as well as resource and referral options. Such an encounter should encompass approximately two to three minutes. Only rarely will the clinician be confronted with a patient in extreme danger or who has acute needs. In this situation, a true medical emergency exists, and urgent action will need to be taken.

Screening for violence and victimization, therefore, should not add substantially to the clinician's schedule and may ultimately save time by allowing the clinician to budget time prospectively.

Intervention

Guiding Principles of Intervention

Clinicians and other health professionals should bear in mind four guiding principles of intervention when addressing violence with their patients: (1) victim safety, (2) victim empowerment, (3) perpetrator accountability, and (4) advocacy for social change.[16]

Victim safety: Patient assessment, documentation, safety planning, communication, intervention, and follow-up must be conducted with utmost concern for the immediate and long-term safety of the victim and her or his dependent children. The clinician should ask, "Is what I am asking, doing, or recommending going to help my patient become safer, or at least not place the patient at risk for further harm?"

Victim empowerment: Abused individuals have had their freedom to make informed, independent choices about their (and their children's) lives restricted by the perpetrator's controlling and intimidating behavior. Facilitating the patient's ability to make her or his own choices is key to restoring a sense of purpose and well-being for victims of hate crimes, domestic violence, and sexual assault and can facilitate a patient's readiness to take proactive steps toward safety and healing. Letting the patient know that his or her sexual orientation or gender identity will not become the focus of treatment is also important. Many patients fear that they will be pathologized because they are LGBT, which would disempower the patient and would not contribute towards healing.

Perpetrator accountability: It is important to reframe the violence as occurring because of the perpetrator's behavior and actions, not the victim's. It thus follows that the need to take definitive steps to end the violence is the perpetrator's responsibility. This guiding principle assumes the importance of victim safety but rejects victim-blaming and other excuses offered by offenders as "explanations" for the violence.

Advocacy for social change: Clinicians acting alone simply cannot meet all the needs of LGBT victims of violence. As healthcare professionals and systems grapple with the complex issues involved in understanding and responding to hate crimes, domestic violence, and sexual assault, the need to collaborate with others in healthcare, as well as those in law enforcement, the faith community, and society-at-large, becomes apparent. Clinicians can be important catalysts for change so that violence in all of its forms can be more effectively identified, and ultimately prevented, and so that LGBT patients can receive the same level of care that is provided to heterosexual patients.

Trauma-informed Care

Medical providers should employ principles of trauma-informed care (also known as "trauma-aware care") when evaluating and caring for patients who have been victims of hate crimes, domestic violence, or sexual assault. Without understanding the sequelae of trauma and the range of short-term and long-term adaptive coping responses employed by survivors, clinicians run the risk of misdiagnosing the patient's condition and therefore being unable to assess and treat the patient appropriately.[17] For example, a male patient who frequently presents to the emergency department with facial contusions and broken ribs may be treated for his physical injuries, assuming the cause of the injuries is a street fight or bar brawl. Unless, however, the attending clinician understands that it is his boyfriend who is inflicting these injuries, the problem will never be fully addressed, and the patient will not be offered appropriate intervention and resources. The patient may continue to present with additional physical and psychological injuries unless and until appropriate interventions can be made.

Specific Interventions

Specific interventions by the clinician should include the following:

- communicating concern for the patient's safety
- evaluating the need to file a mandated report to the appropriate agency for children, elderly, or disabled patients, and in most states, for attacks involving deadly force (firearms, knives, and other lethal weapons)
- diagnosing and treating specific injuries and other medical problems related to ongoing or past victimization
- diagnosing and treating psychological and behavioral problems in victims

- discussing safer sex practices and protection against sexually transmitted infections (STIs) and pregnancy, especially for patients who have been raped or who have experienced coercive sexual activity
- prescribing, only when clearly indicated, tranquilizers or other sedating psychoactive medications, keeping in mind that they could impair the victim's ability to respond appropriately should she or he need to flee
- informing the patient that domestic violence does occur in LGBT relationships, that men can be victims of sexual assault and rape, and that the symptoms experienced after a hate crime are valid and deserving of treatment
- referring as appropriate to experts in the community who provide direct service to LGBT survivors of hate crimes, domestic violence, or sexual assault (local or national hotlines and domestic violence programs may be used as sources for referrals; see Appendix A for resources)
- reframing the violent behavior as unacceptable and criminal
- placing responsibility for the violence unequivocally on the perpetrator
- assuring follow-up both for the presenting complaint and for comprehensive primary care

Treatment and Follow-up

Appropriate medical treatment delivered in a manner that is nonjudgmental, compassionate, sensitive, and trauma-aware is critically important in fostering a sense of dignity and fostering healing in patients who have been victimized. Referrals to community-based experts in LGBT counseling and advocacy is key in addressing the profound isolation that many patients feel. Follow-up care with referral to comprehensive prevention-focused primary care is encouraged for all patients who do not have primary care clinicians.

Information about how to prevent pregnancy might be new to lesbians who have never been sexually active with men, and thus care must be taken by the provider to provide this information in a sensitive and caring manner. Further, information about screening for STIs needs to be given in a similarly sensitive manner, and this also might be an opportunity for the provider to educate the patient about the transmission of STIs.

Safety Planning

Every person who has suffered victimization resulting from hate crimes, domestic violence, or sexual assault should have a safety plan developed with an advocate or other trusted person. To develop a safety plan, the patient's level of danger and the resources needed to flee suddenly must be addressed. The plan should include a place to go (friends, family, or shelter) and other resources for daily living such as money, personal papers, car keys, and a change of clothing for the patient and her or his children. If an order of protection (restraining order) has been issued, your patient should carry a copy with him or her at all times. Inform your patient that local LGBT advocacy organizations, as well as domestic violence programs and rape crisis centers, provide free and confidential services, and that trained advocates from these programs can provide information regarding the following:

- legal rights
- police and court procedures for protective orders
- shelter availability and
- support groups and other support resources

Encourage your patient to call a local, statewide, or national hotline for further information and support. Provide a private, safe space for your patient to make those calls if at all possible. Such a call in no way commits the patient to a course of action, but it can better inform and empower individuals to make informed decisions. Quite often, the same information needs to be provided more than once. A list of resources can be found in Appendix A.

Prevention

Primary Prevention in the Office Setting

Clinicians and other healthcare providers should communicate a strong message that violence against LGBT individuals—particularly presenting as hate crimes, domestic violence, or sexual assault—is a legitimate healthcare and public health issue. There are many ways to bring effective primary and secondary prevention into the office setting. Posters and brochures should be displayed prominently in waiting and examination rooms, and in private areas such as bathrooms. Office staff should receive periodic in-service training about hate crimes, domestic violence, or sexual assault, referral resources, protocols, and office safety procedures. Frank discussion with all patients about healthy relationships, respect for the autonomy of others, and nonviolent means to address conflict should be encouraged.

When clinicians take a stand against violence, they join with the efforts of others who work to deliver the important cultural message that it is wrong, and against the law, to use intimidation and violence for any reason against an individual or a group. Clinicians can communicate this message effectively in the course of routine office practice. When clinicians and office staff model competence and concern about hate crimes, domestic

violence, and sexual assault, patients can more effectively face these difficult issues.

Help for Clinicians and Colleagues

Individual clinicians and other healthcare professionals may themselves be
LGBT and may not yet have come out to others in the work setting. In addition, some may have been victimized as children or as adults, or may currently be in an abusive relationship as a victim or a perpetrator. Those
whose lives have been affected by abuse in any form are urged to seek
help from a hotline or direct service organization or from a trusted colleague, therapist, family member, or other source of support.

Clinicians as Agents of Community Change

The clinician's role should not be restricted to the examining room or hospital ward. Clinicians are respected in the community; their opinions are
sought out and given great credence, and their influence as role models
and community leaders is clear. Thus, it is crucial that clinicians use their
positions of leadership and respect in joining in community coalitions;
advocating for improved services, laws, and practices; and modeling
respectful, nonviolent behavior. In short, clinicians can very effectively
"teach peace" in the course of their professional and personal activities.[18]
The "public health" role of the clinician as leader, advocate, and change
agent is perhaps as important as the "private health" job of providing expert
care for individual patients.

Summary Points

- Traumatic events cause disruptions in arousal, attention, perception,
  and emotion. Trauma caused by hate crimes, domestic violence, and
  sexual assault is of particular concern for LGBT individuals.
- Anti-LGBT hate crimes that include physical violence are often severe
  and can lead to a loss of trust in service providers, feelings of shame,
  and internalized homophobia, as well as long-lasting depression and
  anxiety. Hate crimes can also affect other community members who,
  upon hearing about the occurrence of a hate crime, experience symptoms of trauma.
- Victims of hate crimes and sexual assault often present acutely to
  emergency rooms or other healthcare settings. Evaluation and management should proceed according to accepted trauma evaluation
  and treatment protocols, with particular sensitivity to the needs of
  LGBT patients.

- Routine inquiry about domestic violence should be undertaken with all patients, regardless of the presence or absence of physical indicators of abuse. LGBT victims of domestic violence often feel uncomfortable disclosing the full extent of the threat they are experiencing from partners and may believe that clinicians do not understand or take seriously domestic violence in LGBT relationships. Male victims in particular may feel an increased sense of shame about their fear of an intimate partner.
- The acronym "**RADAR**" summarizes steps clinicians should take in recognizing and treating victims of hate crimes, domestic violence, and sexual assault:
  - **R**emember to ask routinely about violence and victimization in your own practice.
  - **A**sk directly about violence with such questions as "At any time, has anyone hit, kicked, or otherwise hurt or frightened you?" Interview your patient in private at all times.
  - **D**ocument information about "suspected hate crimes, domestic violence, or sexual assault" in the patient's chart.
  - **A**ssess your patient's safety. Is it safe to return home? Find out if any weapons are kept in the house, if the children are in danger, and if the violence is escalating.
  - **R**eview options with your patient. Know about the types of referral options (eg, LGBT advocacy services, domestic violence shelters, support groups, legal advocates). Referrals to community-based experts in LGBT counseling and advocacy is key in addressing the profound isolation that many patients feel.
- The clinician should assure the victim of violence that he or she is believed, respected, valued, and not responsible or to blame for the abuse or assault.
- The clinician can help the patient to assess the level of risk of future victimization. The most important determinants in assessing risk are the patient's level of fear and her or his own appraisal of safety needs.
- The clinician can also initiate discussion of the need for a safety plan and make referrals to appropriate services, including organizations that specialize in serving LGBT people.

References

1. **National Library of Medicine and National Institutes of Health**, with Merriam-Webster online. Medline Plus Medical Dictionary; 2005. Available at http://www.nlm.nih.gov/medlineplus/mplusdictionary.html.
2. **Herman J**. Trauma and Recovery. Basic Books; 1992:34.
3. **Van der Kolk BA, Roth S, Pelcovitz D, et al**. Disorders of extreme stress: the empirical foundation to a complex adaptation to trauma. Journal of Traumatic Stress. 2005;18:389-99.

4. **Van der Kolk BA**. The body keeps the score: approaches to the psychobiology of post-traumatic stress disorder. In: Van der Kolk BA, McFarland AC, Weisaeth L, eds. Traumatic Stress: The Effects of Overwhelming Experience on Mind, Body, and Society. Guilford Press; 1996:214-41.

5. **Noelle M**. The Psychological Effects of Hate-crime Victimization Based on Sexual Orientation Bias: 10 Case Studies [dissertation]. Clinical Psychology Program, University of Massachusetts Amherst; 2003.

6. **Fenway Community Health Center**. Fact Sheet: Survivors of Anti-LGBT Violence. Common Reactions; 2001.

7. **Berrill K**. Antigay violence and victimization in the United States: An overview. In: Herrick GM, Berrill K, eds. Hate Crimes. Sage; 1992:19-45.

8. **Herek GM, Gillis R, Cogan JC, et al**. Hate crime victimization among lesbian, gay, and bisexual adults: prevalence, psychological correlates, and methodological issues. J Interpers Violence. 1997;12:195-215.

9. **Federal Bureau of Investigation**. Hate crime statistics 2005. Available at http://www.fbi.gov/ucr/hc2005/index.html.

10. **National Coalition of Anti-Violence Programs**. Anti-lesbian, gay, bisexual and transgender violence in 2005. Available at http://www.ncavp.org/publications/National Pubs.aspx.

11. **Briere J, Spinazzola J**. Phenomenology and psychological assessment of complex post-traumatic states. Journal of Traumatic Stress. 2005;18:401-12.

12. **Walker L**. The Battered Woman. Harper & Row; 1979.

13. **US Department of Justice, Office of Justice Programs**. Special Report: Extent, Nature and Consequences of Rape Victimization: Findings from the National Violence Against Women Survey. Report NCJ 210346. US Department of Justice; January 2006.

14. **Sorenson SB, Stein JA, Siegel JM, et al**. The prevalence of adult sexual assault. American Journal of Epidemiology. 1987;126:1154-64.

15. **Munro K**. The treatment needs of sexually abused men, 2000. Available at http://www.kalimunro.com.

16. **Warshaw C, Ganley AL**. Improving the Health Care Response to Domestic Violence: A Resource Manual for Health Care Providers. Family Violence Prevention Fund; 1995.

17. **Clardie S**. Post-traumatic stress disorder within a primary care setting: effectively and sensitively responding to sexual trauma survivors. Wisconsin Medical Journal. 2004;103: 73-7.

18. **Glidden D**. Personal communication. 1996.

Chapter 11

Sexual Health

DEMETRE C. DASKALAKIS, MD
RAPHAEL LANDOVITZ, MD
MICHELLE CESPEDES, MD

Introduction

Sexual health is a crucial aspect of primary care. Caring for the whole patient, regardless of gender, sexual orientation, or sexual expression, should include a frank and open discussion about sexual activity, desire, function, and satisfaction. The first principle of promoting sexual health is to provide an open and nonjudgmental environment where patients feel safe enough to discuss their sexual health with a clinician. This is particularly important for lesbian, gay, bisexual, and transgender (LGBT) patients, who may experience shame or stigma associated with their sexual or gender identities. The second and equally important principle for optimizing sexual health is to obtain a thorough sexual history. The sexual history is no different than any other part of a complete medical evaluation and should be a routine and normalized part of the patient-provider interaction. Through the use of nonjudgmental questions, such as "Do you have sex with men, with women, or both?" the clinician avoids incorrect assumptions about sexual behavior and opens a dialogue that provides data important to counseling, management, and prevention. Following up with more specific questions on types of sexual activity, types of partners (eg, casual, monogamous), and use and type of protection, will guide the clinician's approach to screening, sexually transmitted infection (STI) diagnostics, and therapeutics. In assessing disease risk, the focus of the sexual history should be on behavior, rather than the sexual identity of the patient, particularly since behavior and identity do not always align. Men who have sex with men (MSM) may have sex with women and may not identify as gay or bisexual. Women who have sex with women (WSW) may have sex with men and may not identify as lesbian or bisexual. Transgender people may have sex with men, with women, or with both and may not identify themselves as gay, lesbian, or bisexual. At the same time, clarifying sexual self-identity is important for treating the whole patient and for building rapport; in particular, it is important when counseling patients about sexual satisfaction, when identifying any identity-related issues, or when helping reduce institutional barriers to care.

Other chapters in this book provide detailed suggestions on how to create a welcoming environment for LGBT patients (see Chapter 1), how to talk with patients about sexual self-identity (see Chapter 3), and how to take a sexual history and provide risk-reduction counseling (see Chapter 15). The following chapter goes into greater depth on sexual risk-taking behaviors, principles of safer sex, and the identification and treatment of sexual dysfunction and sexually transmitted diseases. Together, these chapters aim to provide clinicians with the tools and knowledge necessary to optimize the sexual health of their LGBT patients.

Optimizing Sexual Health and Satisfaction

Elements of both sexual identity and the specifics of sexual activity are critical in assessing the emotional and physical intactness of a patient's sexual life. Gay, lesbian, bisexual, and transgender individuals face many of the same issues regarding sexual dysfunction as heterosexuals but also have some unique challenges that an informed provider can address. From the provider perspective, the first step in optimizing the sexual health of these populations is to address one's own assumptions and limits. A provider uncomfortable with same-sex behaviors and gender issues is limited in their ability to care for this population and should have a low threshold to refer such patients to other care givers.[1,2] In some surveys, 3%-6% of patients seen by physicians are gay or lesbian.[3] Many more may not disclose their status in an often unwelcoming healthcare system. Increasing data indicate that sexual minorities may represent a significantly underserved group of patients. These patients often experience psychological and substance abuse issues which must be addressed as part of their overall treament in order to optimize outcomes, making the creation of a safe space for open discussions of sexual identity mandatory for optimal primary care and risk reduction/preventive counseling.[3,4]

Approaching sexual function and contentment among LGBT patients requires an open-ended approach free of assumptions and judgments of how desire and sexuality can or should be expressed. Sexuality, desire, and intimacy should be approached on the patient's terms to optimize their sexual health. Vocabulary should match that used by the patient. Beyond identifying what kind of sex a patient has, their level of satisfaction with how they express themselves sexually should be explored.

Sexual dysfunction limits the quality of life and may be a sign of psychiatric or medical illness or other social factors in both men and women. Clinical evaluation of sexual function begins with open-ended and frank history-taking fostered by a shame-free environment. Erectile dysfunction, ejaculatory issues, anal fissures, and hemorrhoids are all noninfectious issues that may impact the sexual health of MSM. WSW are prone to many of the same problems that impact heterosexual women, such as hypoactive sexual desire, sexual pain, and vaginal dryness.

Medical Evaluation of Men with Sexual Dysfunction

Erectile dysfunction (ED) is a common complaint among men and may be cause by both psychogenic issues, medical disease, medications, or a combination of the two. Certain aspects of history are necessary to better characterize the nature of erectile difficulties. Medical ED is usually gradual in onset. Most rapid-onset ED is associated with a psychogenic etiology or obvious surgery or trauma. Organic causes of ED are often associated with the lack of spontaneous erections such as those experienced in the morning upon waking. A complete review of prescription, recreational, and over-the-counter drug use, as well as alcohol use, should be performed to identify an easily reversible pharmacologic cause of ED.

The physical exam should focus on the etiologies of ED: endocrine, vascular, and neurologic. The testicular exam should focus on atrophy, masses, and symmetry, and the thyroid should be examined for any abnormality. Visual fields should be tested to identify any defects that may be caused by a pituitary adenoma, and the chest should be examined for gynecomastia. Peripheral pulses should be assessed for any evidence of vascular insufficiency. The cremasteric reflex should be elicited to check the integrity of central erection function. Laboratory evaluation should include thyroid function tests, glucose tolerance testing, lipid testing, prolactin testing, and testosterone level tests. Nocturnal penile tumescence testing may be necessary if no obvious cause is identified as a gateway to more complex tests of penile vasculature.

Several treatment modalities are available to address ED beyond treating underlying organic and psychogenic causes. These include prostaglandin injections, vacuum devices, and implants. In the last several years these have been eclipsed by the phosphodicsterase-5 (PDE-5) inhibitors such as sildanefil, tadalafil, and vardenafil. These drugs have shown efficacy in treating ED or multiple etiologies and are frequently prescribed and used by MSM.[5] Special attention should be paid to concurrent medications like protease inhibitors and nitrates (including amyl nitrate poppers) given known severe drug-to-drug interactions. Additionally these drugs may be associated with increased sexual risk-taking and the transmission of HIV and other sexual infections, so men should be reminded about safer sex and risk-reduction behaviors.[6] ED in the context of condom use may also be a reason that some MSM, specifically those with HIV, may engage in unprotected sex.[7,8]

Ejaculatory complaints may include premature ejaculation, retrograde ejaculation, decreased volume of ejaculate, and retarded ejaculation. The most common complaint, premature ejaculation, is not associated with any organic cause and may be treated with exercises to train the patient to better delay ejaculation or with medications such as selective seritonin reuptake inhibitors (SSRI).[9] These antidepressants are not surprisingly among the drugs that cause retrograde and retarded ejaculation. Retarded and retrograde ejaculation may be associated with HIV or antiretroviral-associated neuropathy.[8]

Anal complaints include hemorrhoids and fissures that may interfere with receptive anal sex. Topical therapies for treating hemorrhoids, stool softeners, sitz baths, and topical anesthetic creams may help with these often uncomfortable conditions. The role of anal sex among MSM is fairly complex, and it is wrong to assume that all MSM engage in this activity. Some MSM may complain about physically tolerating anal sex or about feelings of coercion by a partner to engage in this activity. Relaxation techniques and anal dilators may be indicated, based on specific complaints regarding tolerance of anal sex.

Medical Evaluation of Women with Sexual Dysfunction

Sexual dysfunction among women is more complex than among men. Decreased sexual desire, sexual pain, and anorgasmia are common presenting complaints. Some of these are associated with advancing age and hormonal changes associated with menopause, but other organic and psychogenic conditions may be involved in these syndromes.

Changes associated with hormones occur as a women enters her midlife. Declines in estrogen are associated with urogenital atrophy, vaginal dryness, and urinary incontinence. Over time vascular changes lead to changes in vaginal and clitoral tissues that decrease sensation, elasticity, and the ability to self-lubricate. These in combination may cause genital pain with sexual activity (dyspareunia) and create a cycle of anxiety and fear that makes sexual activity physically and mentally unpleasant. Although typically thought of as "male hormones," androgens play a role in desire and the physiologic sexual response. Routine clinical testosterone levels may or may not be sensitive enough to identify deficiency. Beyond midlife changes, premature ovarian failure, oopherectomy, adrenal insufficiency, and other hormonal therapeutics may also cause androgen deficiency. Other hormonal causes that merit evaluation are pituitary tumors, hyperprolactinemia, and thyroid disease. Hormonal replacement therapies are often recommended when deficiencies are identified. Physical examination should include a complete gynecologic exam focusing on evidence of atrophy and obvious causes of genital pain.

Loss of desire may be related to hormonal changes but like ED may be related to a whole host of medical conditions including vascular disorders, activity-limiting conditions, diabetes, and neurological disease. Physical examination should focus on neurologic evaluation, assessment of visual fields, and a vascular assessment. Historical evaluation should focus on a complete review of prescription, over-the-counter, and recreational drug use. A thorough psychiatric exam and screening for domestic abuse should also be conducted.[10] Often issues of sexual pain may impact on desire, so causes of dyspareunia should be pursued.[11]

Sexual pain syndromes include dyspareunia and vaginismus. These interrelated phenomena are often difficult to diagnose and treat. Causes as diverse as herpes simplex infection, atrophic vulvitis, topical irritants, and vaginal dryness may be etiologies of superficial dyspareunia. Deeper genital pain may be caused by pelvic inflammatory disease, endometriosis, ovarian cysts, and bowel disease. Treatment relies on the underlying diagnosis. Vaginismus is a conditioned response to genital pain that manifests itself as involuntary contraction of the perivaginal muscles, preventing penetration by a partner. Both physical and psychological etiologies may contribute to vaginismus. Counseling and vaginal dilators alone or in combination may be used to address this issue. Addressing dyspareunia will also help vaginismus.[11]

Anorgasmia is a very complex condition that is categorized by the inability to achieve an orgasm. This problem may be situational or absolute. Women may have never experienced an orgasm or may have had orgasms successfully in the past. Although not formally studied in WSW, anorgasmia is often associated with sexual repression of sensations and emotions, a phenomenon that may accompany issues surrounding sexual identity. Treatment involves a complex combination of therapy, self-exploration, and couples' counseling.[11] Limited and conflicting data exist regarding the use of PDE-5 inhibitors to enhance female sexual desire and response.[12]

LBGT patients should be encouraged to explore sexuality in a way that enhances their quality of life. Healthcare providers should address issues that limit such exploration while providing sex-positive advice regarding harm reduction to avoid the risk of sexually transmitted infections. The clinician's role in optimizing sexual health is to provide patients with the tools and knowledge necessary to engage in physically and emotionally gratifying safer sex.

Optimizing the Sexual Health of Transgender Patients

Very little has been written in the medical literature about the sexual satisfaction and happiness of transgender patients. The range of sexual expression and gender identities within this group is vast. The issue of sexual satisfaction is often intimately tied to satisfaction with gender, gender role, and perception of self. Although beyond the scope of this chapter, it is important that primary care providers maintain open communication with all patients to allow them the opportunity to express any transgender feelings or questions. Many guidelines exist to assist in the assessment of the trans-seeking or transgender patient. The therapeutic approach to a transgender patient includes an openness to fluidity in guidelines to match individual gender needs. Societies like the Harry Benjamin International Gender Dysphoria Association (HBIGDA) provide a structure to assist in optimizing the gender identity of transgender patients, including recommendations for psychotherapy in association with "triadic therapy"—real-life experience in the desired gender role, hormonal therapy, and surgery to achieve the desired anatomical gender. Transgender patients exist on a broad spectrum of gender needs and identities. Many have goals that do not include all aspects of the triad, an observation that providers should respect and understand.[13]

Sexual satisfaction and dysfunction among this population has not been studied, and much of the research on this population has focused on transgender individuals involved in high-risk behaviors such as commercial sex work. History and physical examination should focus on the organ systems present and not the perceived gender of the patient. It is also important for the primary care providers to avoid assumptions about sexual identity, the specifics of sexual activity, and the gender of client's partners. (More on providing healthcare to transgender patients can be found in Chapters 12 and 13.)

Principles of Safer Sex

Many sexually transmitted infections (STIs) are bodily-fluid borne, and transmission requires contact with fluids such as semen, blood, and vaginal secretions. Transmission can usually be prevented with use of "safer sex" techniques that limit the exchange of fluids. Like universal precautions in a healthcare setting, all sex partners should be approached as if they are potentially able to transmit sexual infections, and efforts should be made to avoid contact of mucous membranes like the mouth, rectum, and vaginal and urethral meatus with blood or anogenital secretions. Other infections such as hepatitis B are similarly transmitted, though this can be prevented through immunization.

Certain sexual activities are higher risk than others, and special attention should be paid to reduce harm when engaging in these activities. Because of ethics and logistics, precise measurements of the efficiency of HIV transmission for specific acts are not feasible. For MSM, the highest risk activity for acquiring HIV infection is receptive anal intercourse (approximately 50/10 000 exposures), followed by insertive anal intercourse (6.5/10 000 exposures), and followed distantly by oral sex (.5-1/10 000 exposures).

Activities such as mutual masturbation, body-to-body contact without fluid exchange, and role-play activities without fluid exchange do not transmit HIV. Transmission of syphilis, human papillomavirus (HPV), *Herpes simplex* virus (HSV), Molluscum contagiosum, and ectoparasites is still possible with these activities. "Rimming" (oral-anal contact), "water sports" (urine play), and "scat" (fecal play) are lower risk for HIV, although blood contamination is possible, increasing the chance for transmission of HIV and viral hepatitis. Though low risk for HIV, fecal-oral contact may, however, put individuals at risk for hepatitis A, bacterial STI, enteric infections, and intestinal parasites.[14] Sex toys, such as dildos that are inserted in mucous membranes and shared between partners can transmit HIV, hepatitis A or B, and other STIs if not properly sterilized. It is recommended that dildos and other toys not be shared or be cleaned with bleach between partners and used with condoms. Needles for piercing or other play should not be shared or should be sterilized between uses.[15]

Interventions aimed at preventing STIs in WSW should focus on minimizing the sexual transfer of vaginal fluids and menstrual blood between sexual partners. Interventions include the use of latex gloves and other latex barriers such as dental dams for vaginal-digital insertion, anal-digital insertion, and oral sex. Use of lubricants should be encouraged to decrease mucosal irritation and tearing, a potential portal of entry for HIV and other viral infections. Condoms used with insertive objects should be changed between partners, and efforts should be made to avoid the introduction of fecal flora into the vagina. As noted above, patients should be encouraged to clean dildos and other sex toys with bleach before using or storing them.

The first general principle of safer sex is making clear assessment of risk and risk-taking behaviors. Safer sex is a continuum and should be approached using a harm reduction model. Some individuals are more willing to accept risk than others, and counseling should focus on optimizing individual risk rather than forcing an individual's sexuality into a series of guidelines or recommendations. Abstinence may be the correct approach for some individuals, while reducing unsafe behavior by a fraction may be the best intervention for others. Individuals should be advised to have a preemptive plan rather than just reacting to certain situations that may occur. Individuals should be advised to contemplate what risk they are willing to accept prior to an encounter, as well as what preventive intentions they will operationalize in those settings. Rational decision-making, however, is less effective while under the influence of drugs and alcohol, so minimizing substance use and abuse when possible is critical to realizing the intention of safer sex.[15]

The second principle of safer sex is barrier protection. Latex barrier use during activities where fluids may be exchanged is central to safer sex. Counseling regarding barrier protection should focus on correct use of a condom, avoidance of contamination of barriers with body fluids, and the use of adequate *water-based* lubrication to avoid condom malfunction, breakage, and minimize mucosal trauma. Both male condoms and female condoms, though less studied, may have a role in reducing HIV and STI transmission among MSM.[16] Men who have sex with men should be advised to avoid even brief unprotected anal penetration, termed "dipping," given the presence of HIV in pre-ejaculate (pre-cum).[17] The phenomenon of "barebacking," or purposeful unprotected anal intercourse (UAI), is psychologically complex and often linked to drug-using behaviors.[18] This behavior continues to be an important target for preventive interventions to reduce the risk of HIV and other STIs among MSM. Additionally, barriers should be encouraged even if both partners are HIV-infected to prevent transmission of STIs, as well as to avoid the possibility of HIV superinfection with multiple strains of HIV of varying virulence and susceptibility to HIV medications. Patient materials on correct condom usage can be found in Appendices C, D, and E.

For oral sex, unlubricated condoms should be recommended and can be cut open to create a makeshift dental dam (as can plastic wrap). Counseling should be tailored to the individual's self-negotiated risk level. Although reports of HIV infection through exclusively oral-genital contact have been reported, this activity carries a lower risk than others exposures. Breaches in the oral mucosa, gingival inflammation, ejaculation in the mouth, sexually transmitted infections, trauma, and other oral infections appear to increase risk of oral transmission of HIV.

Magnitude of Risk of Various Sexual Practices

Many patients and physicians alike struggle to quantitate the relative risks of various sexual practices for the transmission of specific sexually transmitted diseases. Most attention focuses on HIV, although other STIs transmit much more efficiently. Some patients may prefer a risk/benefit analysis in order to help them evaluate their sexual practices, but making such quantitative assessments can be challenging, given the paucity of data. While 100% barrier use (most often latex condoms with water-based lubricant) for all potentially infectious secretion exposures to mucous membranes is the most conservative and effective approach to decrease STI transmission, often patients choose less complete protection, or no protection at all—for a multitude of reasons.

While the relative risk of various exposure types have been quantitated with varying degrees of precision, these all presuppose that the potential source of infection is an HIV-infected person and that all sources have the same degree of infectiousness. It is likely that the source's degree of infectiousness may contribute to the relative risk of any given exposure, in a "dose-dependent" manner. That is to say, the higher the source's plasma viral load, the greater the risk of HIV transmission from any given exposure. Other cofactors may influence the likelihood of HIV transmission per unprotected sex act, such as the presence of a concomitant STI. Therefore, when assessing a patient's risk of acquiring HIV, it is of paramount importance to elicit as much information regarding the source person as possible, in addition to the details of the exposure itself (see Table 11-1).

Patients may ask if risk of HIV transmission can be decreased if the partner withdraws before ejaculation, but this has not been studied in a controlled fashion, and definitive data is unlikely to be forthcoming. It is, however, worth noting that in some series, pre-ejaculate of HIV-infected men carried detectable and replication-competent virus in as many as 15% or more of such patients.[19]

Ulcerative and non-ulcerative STIs have been found to be independent risk factors for HIV transmission in most studies. There is some additional evidence that treatment of intercurrent STIs can lower shedding of infectious viral particles.[20] Lack of circumcision has been found to be a strong predictor of both HIV transmission and susceptibility to HIV acquisition.[21] These observations have made both treatment of STIs and circumcision attractive targets for prevention studies.

HIV Risk-taking Behaviors among MSM

The advent of highly active antiretroviral therapy (HAART), while having profound benefits for people living with HIV, has been coincident with a resurgence of unsafe sexual practices among MSM in an era of therapeutic optimism. Perceptions of HIV as a treatable, chronic, and therefore less lethal disease have been associated with contributing to a laxity in MSM's adherence to safer sexual practices.

Unprotected anal intercourse (UAI) is most highly associated with HIV transmission. Evidence of an increase in other rectal STIs, including rectal gonorrhea, HSV, and HPV,[22] can been taken as a surrogate marker for UAI.

Table 11-1   Estimated Per-Act Risk for Acquisition of HIV[40]

Exposure Route	Risk per 10 000 Exposures to an Infected Source
Blood transfusion	9000
Needle-sharing-drug use	67
Receptive anal intercourse	50
Occupational Needle stick	30
Receptive penile-vaginal sex	10
Insertive anal sex	6.5
Insertive penile-vaginal sex	5
Receptive oral intercourse on a man	1
Insertive oral intercourse on a man	0.5

A prospective analysis of Canadian MSM in Montreal from 1997 to 2003 recently demonstrated a small but significant increase in rates of UAI among HIV-uninfected MSM having sex with both casual partners of unknown HIV serostatus (8.2% to 12.2%), and known serodiscordant partners (15.7% to 18.8%).[23] Similar findings have been seen in other cities.

While some evidence exists that HIV-infected patients with decreased levels of plasma HIV RNA may be less likely to transmit HIV to their partners, this may generate a false sense of security that may lead to increased unsafe sexual practices. A recent meta-analysis tried to assess the impact of HAART treatment on unsafe behavior practices. In this study, HIV-infected persons taking HAART were no more likely to engage in high-risk behavior than untreated HIV-infected persons. They also found that HIV-infected persons taking HAART were not more likely to engage in high-risk behavior if their HIV RNA levels were below the limit of detection than if their HIV RNA levels were detectable; however, HIV-infected persons were more likely to engage in high-risk sexual behavior if they believed that HAART reduces HIV transmission.[24] Other studies have not found that beliefs regarding transmissibility and HAART are correlated with risk-taking behavior. Among heterosexual couples who were not on HAART, a ten-fold increase in HIV RNA in serum has been shown to roughly correlate with a 2.5-fold increase in risk of HIV transmission.[21] The relationship between plasma and genital secretion viral load is, however, not absolute. It is important for patients and physicians to remember that there is no HIV RNA level below which transmission of HIV absolutely does not occur.

Studies have repeatedly found correlations between UAI and multiple different recreational drugs. Methamphetamine and inhaled nitrates ("poppers") have been most often associated with unprotected intercourse, but marijuana and alcohol abuse have also been associated with risky sexual practices, and drugs used to treat erectile dysfunction have been abused and associated with risky sex among MSM. The use of the Internet for solicitation of sex partners also appears to be associated with UAI.[25] A 2001 survey of "circuit party" attendees in the San Francisco area found increased UAI during the circuit party among those that used drugs.[26] Many health departments are utilizing observational research to target individuals at high risk and settings associated with high-risk behavior such as commercial sex venues like bathhouses, gyms, sex clubs, and circuit parties, as well as Internet chat sites.

HIV Risk Behavior among WSW

Surveys of behavioral risk factors of WSW are not standardized and differ in their inclusion criteria, location for recruitment (eg, STI clinic, shelters, Internet surveys), and definition of WSW. As a result, the findings of these surveys cannot be generalized to all WSW. Reports consistently show that women who report having sex with at least one female partner in their lifetime have an increased risk of STI acquisition than women who exclusively have sex with men.[27] In a study of STI clinic clients, women who had sex with both men and women were at greater risk of HIV infection as compared to women who exclusively had sex with women or heterosexual women.[28] The risk correlated to risk-taking behavior, substance abuse, and number of partners over the past year.

Women who have sex with women and self-reported bisexual women are more likely to have sex with MSM and may be exposed to STIs more traditionally considered in MSM. Compared to WSM they also self-report increased risk-taking sexual behavior under the influence of alcohol or illicit drug use. Risk for transmission of STIs in WSW can also be categorized into the categories of penetrative practices and non-penetrative practices (see Table 11-2).

A small survey of WSW found that participants rarely cleaned sex toys between vaginal penetrative sex for the purpose of reducing STI transmission.[29] Insertive practices in the presence of menstrual blood increase the risk of transmission of blood-borne STIs including HIV and hepatitis B. To date there is no data that reliably quantifies the risk of transmission of STIs in WSW per sex act for practices that are common in this population.

HIV Risk Behavior among Transgender Patients

HIV infection is a major issue in the transgender community. Much of the literature reporting on this population focuses on individuals who engage in sex work, so estimates of prevalence are increased due to the population being evaluated. Estimates of prevalence of HIV infection in published studies range from 11%-68 percent.[30-34] Two studies focused on transgender participants who did not work in the sex industry and found a higher

Table 11-2   Stratified Risk of Sexual Practices of Women Who Have Sex with Women.

Level of Risk	Activity
Low risk	clothed genital stimulation
	nipple stimulation
	condom use with sex toys
Risky	cunnilingus without barrier protection (dental dam)
	vaginal or anal-digital insertion without condom
	vaginal or anal fisting without gloves
High-risk	cunnilingus during menses without barrier protection
	unprotected anal rimming
	shared sex toys without changing condoms between sex partners

prevalence of HIV risk behaviors than in non-transgender participants.[35,36] Some studies have demonstrated that transgender persons of African-American descent, those in a lower socioeconomic stratum, and those with less education may be at enhanced risk for HIV infection.

Beyond traditional sexually risky behavior, substance use, specifically hormonal and nonhormonal injection drug use, appears to be more frequent in this population and may be tied to higher risk sexual behavior. Issues of identity, domestic abuse, commercial sex work, and sexual violence are critical to address in a HIV-risk assessment of a transgender patient.[37] The social stigma of transgender identity often results in significant employment discrimination, forcing many of these individuals into sex work and social networks that may be associated with higher risk activities. Although not well studied, risk-taking among female to male transgender persons may be significant and should be investigated further. More research is necessary to develop effective sexual and drug harm reduction approaches to address this diverse and susceptible population. Specific behaviors likely carry the same risk in this population as in MSM and WSW as discussed above; specific research in this population regarding magnitude of risk of certain behaviors is unavailable.

Strategies to Reduce HIV Transmission

While abstinence and sexual intercourse with one mutually faithful uninfected partner are the only totally effective prevention strategies, these strategies are often either impractical, unacceptable, or unrealistic. Several proven and a few experimental strategies provide risk reduction in the setting of higher risk activities.

Condoms

Condom use cannot completely eliminate the risk of transmission of HIV, but laboratory and epidemiologic data has provided some information about the efficacy of condom use. In vitro data have shown latex condoms to be effective barriers to HIV, hepatitis B virus (HBV), and a number of STIs such as syphilis, gonorrhea, and chlamydia. Several studies strongly suggest the efficacy of condom use in people at risk for HIV.[38] However, many of these studies do not distinguish between "consistent" condom use (ie, condom use for all episodes of sexual intercourse) and "inconsistent" condom use (ie, anything less than use for all episodes)—therefore estimates of 70% protection likely represent the worst case scenario for the protection afforded by inconsistent, but frequent, condom use. Meta-analysis of available data suggest the true protection of appropriate condom use is approximately 95%.[38]

Circumcision

Circumcision is also being explored as a preventive intervention. In one noninterventional study of heterosexual serodiscordant couples, male circumcision was associated with a decreased risk of transmitting and acquiring HIV. A subsequent meta-analysis of multiple studies has found the protective effect of circumcision to be as high as 70%. This observation has led to the design of three large, randomized controlled trials of circumcision in heterosexual men in Africa. The results of the South African trial showed a 61% reduction in transmission in the circumcised cohort, as have two other randomized controlled trials.[39] Further research is needed to evaluate the role of circumcision and HIV transmission among MSM.

Bioprophylaxis

Bioprophylaxis refers largely to the use of biologically active therapeutic agents to prevent HIV infection. This burgeoning field at the interface between prevention and treatment draws on expertise from both fields and holds both exciting promise and new challenges. It is certain that any biomedical intervention will have to be intimately tied to behavioral modification to be effective at reducing risk over the long term.

Postexposure Prophylaxis (PEP) is broadly defined as the administration of antiretroviral agents to a patient after an exposure or potential exposure to HIV. Animal studies, a healthcare worker case control study, and observational studies all point to the efficacy of promptly administered antiretrovirals in preventing HIV transmission after an exposure. PEP has been recommended by the US Public Health Service (PHS) for occupational exposures to HIV since 1996. More recent observational and anecdotal data has prompted the US PHS to publish guidelines regarding non-Occupational Postexposure Prophylaxis (nPEP).[40] These guidelines extend PEP to sexual and nonoccupational percutaneous exposures using a decision tree similar to that used in occupational exposures. nPEP is recommended to be initiated within 72 hours after a high-risk sexual or percutaneous exposure to a potentially or known HIV-infected source.[40] nPEP has demonstrated cost effectiveness for receptive anal sex partners of HIV-infected men. Cost effectiveness data in other exposures have been conflicting.

Pre-Exposure Prophylaxis (PrEP) is a novel strategy currently under investigation, in which antiretroviral agents are used *in anticipation* of an exposure to HIV in high-risk individuals. Preclinical data has suggested that this strategy may be viable. Significant coverage in the lay media of PrEP use in combination with recreational drugs has led to concerns among clinicians and public health professionals. Large efficacy studies are ongoing in a variety of populations. Concerns about such strategies have focused on the selection for drug-resistant HIV while high-risk individuals are taking PrEP, adherence issues, long-term toxicity of chronic ARV administration in uninfected individuals, access to medications in underserved populations, and behavioral disinhibition which may accompany perceived protection against infection. Currently, this prevention strategy should not be recommended outside a study context. Behavioral interventions are likely to be a critical element to any successful PrEP effort.

Genital HSV has been shown to increase the risk of acquiring or transmitting HIV sexually.[41] A small study recently demonstrated a decrease in plasma and genital secretion HIV in West African women during suppressive therapy with valacyclovir over a 3-month period.[41] Larger trials are now underway which are evaluating the impact of prophylactic acyclovir in reducing HIV transmission and acquisition in HSV-2-infected persons. Data suggest that suppressing HSV-2 shedding may impact HIV transmission and acquisition.

Preventive vaccination against HIV would be an ideal bioprophylactic. Despite initial excitement regarding the field of HIV vaccinology, a completely protective therapeutic vaccine has remained elusive, and traditional methods of vaccine development have not yielded effective, durable protection. The genetic diversity of the virus, infidelity associated with the viral replication process, and the persistence of replication despite the presence of both humoral and cell-mediated immune responses all contribute to the complexity of vaccine development. Protective vaccination has proven a challenging goal but is an ongoing focus of significant research.

Microbicides are topically applied preparations that are currently in clinical development. These agents are being designed to have activity against HIV and other STIs and could be applied in anticipation of sexual intercourse. If proven effective and safe, microbicides will be available in gel, cream, film, or suppository form. Both "nonspecific" microbicides (detergents, surfactants, pH modifiers, and polyanions) and "specific" entry inhibitors are under investigation. Currently, 14 agents are in varying stages of clinical development in humans, with five of these agents in Phase 3 trials. While all of these agents are currently in development for vaginal use, trials planned for rectal use of these agents as well: it is not a foregone conclusion that efficacy vaginally will correspond to efficacy rectally for reasons of microenvironment, pH, closed vs. open space, and inherent mucosal differences. Microbicides for rectal use would likely be combined with a lubricant preparation.

The microbicide field experienced a setback in development when the topical contraceptive, nonoxynol-9 (N-9), despite potent in vitro activity against HIV, was shown to increase mucosal inflammation and actually increase HIV transmission when used by African female sex workers. This finding underscored the need for extreme caution in the safety considerations of microbicide development.[42]

HIV Testing: Counseling and Technologies

The Centers for Disease Control and Prevention (CDC) has established guidelines for HIV counseling that were revised in 2006 to make HIV testing a more routine part of clinical care and to reflect the availability of rapid, point-of-care HIV testing.[43] Many of the elements traditionally associated with HIV testing, such as separate written consent and pretest and posttest counseling, have been abandoned to streamline the testing process. Although these new guidelines have removed many administrative hurdles, individual jurisdictions will need to address these updated guidelines with changes in laws governing HIV testing. It is important during this time of transition that primary care providers keep regional regulations in mind as they evolve with CDC guidelines. For now, separate written consents and test-related counseling are still legal requirements in many jurisdictions. Changes in CDC guidelines include the following:

- HIV screening is recommended for patients in all healthcare settings after the patient is notified that testing will be performed unless the patient declines (opt-out screening).
- Persons at high risk for HIV infection should be screened for HIV at least annually. The CDC's *Sexually Transmitted Infection Guidelines*, also published in 2006, recommend that some MSM be tested every three to six months.[44]
- Separate written consent for HIV testing should not be required; general consent for medical care should be considered sufficient to encompass consent for HIV testing.
- Prevention counseling should not be required with HIV diagnostic testing or as part of HIV screening programs in healthcare settings.[43]

The first serologic test for HIV was approved by the Food and Drug Administration (FDA) in 1985. Although many new versions of this test exist, serologic testing remains the primary modality used to screen for and diagnose HIV infection. Serologic tests to detect antibodies against HIV are effective in diagnosing most established infections. These HIV-antibody tests have a window period during the acute and early phase of infection that may result in a false negative antibody test for HIV. Both serologic tests that recognize the HIV p24 antigen and molecular tests that detect HIV RNA by nucleic acid amplification are often used to supplement standard antibody tests when it is suspected that individuals have been very recently exposed to HIV infection (see Figure 11-1).

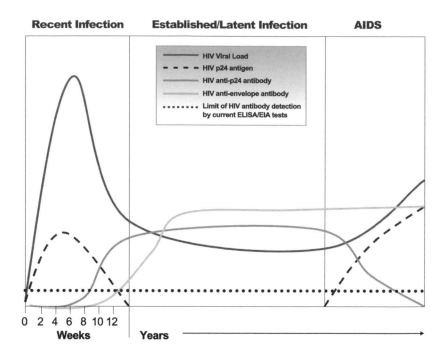

Figure 11-1   Laboratory testing in HIV and AIDS.
Created by Demetre C. Daskalakis, MD, used with permission.

Serologic Tests for HIV Infection

HIV Antibody Tests: Enzyme-Linked Imunosorbant Assays (ELISA) were the first FDA-approved HIV diagnostic. Subsequent generations of ELISA tests that detect antibodies against HIV are increasingly sensitive (> 99.9%) and work on a fundamental principle similar to the original HIV test. Positive HIV antibody ELISA tests require confirmation with more specific tests such as a Western Blot, covered below. The available rapid HIV tests that provide point of care results are variations of the standard HIV antibody-detecting ELISA. Antibody-detection tests may miss early stages of HIV infection before adequate titers of antibody are formed to reach the threshold of test detection. This is often called the "window period" of the ELISA.

HIV Antigen Tests: p24 is the protein that makes up the structural core of the HIV virus. It becomes detectable by serologic tests within two to three weeks of infection. The test shortens the window period of HIV antibody-detecting ELISA tests but has limited use in diagnosing later stages of infection. As graphically demonstrated in Figure 11-1, p24 levels in the blood decrease as antibodies against p24 neutralize and clear this antigen from the blood. Immune complex disassociation procedures may be used to free bound antigens and enhance the sensitivity of this test during later infection. These antigen-detecting tests can be used to monitor therapy and diagnose early or acute HIV infection, but they have essentially been replaced by nucleic acid amplification testing.

Newer Generation HIV Serologic and Rapid Tests: Several variations of HIV screening serology tests are in use, including fourth generation ELISA and rapid HIV tests. Both of these variations of the standard ELISA provide added clinical functionality to serologic tests traditionally used to diagnose. The fourth generation ELISA couples p24 antigen detection with standard HIV-antibody detection further decreasing the "window period" of serologic testing. Rapid HIV tests adapt the standard ELISA to an easy-to-administer and interpret point-of-care test using oral fluids or finger stick blood. Like a standard ELISA, positive results are preliminary until a more specific test confirms infection. Results are often available within 20-40 minutes, allowing for more successful measures to link patients with preliminarily positive results to care. Initial proceedings at the FDA have been initiated to consider home access to rapid HIV tests.

The HIV Western Blot: Screening ELISA tests for HIV require confirmation using more specific tests since false positive tests are possible. Causes of false positive HIV screening tests include multiple pregnancies, rheumatologic conditions, and other medical conditions, as well as involvement in HIV vaccine studies. The most commonly used confirmatory test in the United States is the HIV Western Blot, which is considered the "gold standard" for validation of screening results. Like ELISA tests, the Western Blot detects antibodies against HIV but in a more specific manner. There are no universal criteria for interpreting the Western Blot Test, and criteria vary from country to country. When combined with ELISA screening tests, the specificity of this algorithm approaches 99%. Newer rapid technologies are emerging based on the Western Blot that may allow for point-of-care confirmatory testing to supplement the benefits of rapid HIV testing for follow-up and connection to clinical care.

Molecular Diagnostics

Nucleic Acid Amplification Testing (NAAT): Although not approved by the FDA as a diagnostic test, many centers of excellence are utilizing HIV NAAT to diagnose individuals with "acute" HIV infection. NAAT uses several technologies but is colloquially referred to as "HIV viral loads." As graphically illustrated in Figure 11-1, high levels of virus are present as early as five to seven days after infection with HIV, several weeks before antibody is detectable. False positive tests are possible given the high specificity of NAAT in detecting HIV infection. False positives are possible but are not reproducible and are characterized by low-level viral detection (1000-3000 copies/mL).

Primary HIV Infection

Primary HIV infection is perhaps one of the most important and least recognized presentations of a sexually transmitted infection. Although no consensus definition exists, primary HIV infection includes preseroconversion and recent (< six months) infection. In as early as one week after exposure to HIV, an individual may present with nonspecific symptoms that are often interpreted to represent other, often less clinically significant, disease presentations. These symptoms are often associated with explosive levels of viremia with an occasionally precipitous, but usually temporary, drop in total T helper cell count (see Figure 11-2). Despite high HIV viral loads, acute infection is associated with antibody levels below the level of detection of standard HIV serologic testing. This "window period" is characterized by negative HIV antibody tests with detectable viremia using molecular techniques.

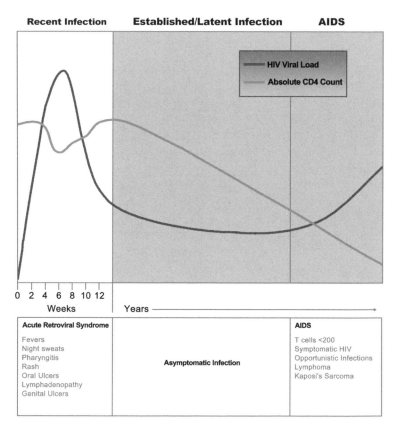

Figure 11-2   Primary HIV infection in the context of AIDS natural history. Primary HIV infection occurs within the first few weeks after exposure (see unshaded area of graph). It is associated with very high viral loads (darker line) and often temporary declines in total CD4 counts (lighter line). The early phase of HIV infection is often associated with clinical symptoms called Acute Retroviral Syndrome.

Created by Demetre C. Daskalakis, MD, used with permission.

The early phase of HIV infection may be important to recognize for both the public and the individual's health. Several studies have modeled and demonstrated that acutely infected individuals may be "hyper-infectious" and may disproportionately contribute to the ongoing transmission of HIV.[45] Diagnosing individuals during this phase of infection may allow for an opportunity to identify and modify behaviors that facilitate transmission within sexual networks. Although more controversial, there is some data that treating individuals with acute HIV infection may impact their future immunologic and virologic parameters. This continues to be an area of intense study.

Clinical Features

The syndrome associated with primary HIV infection is called Acute Retroviral Syndrome (ARS). In some series, up to 92% of patients may demonstrate the symptoms of acute infection, but the diagnosis is missed up to 80% of the time. ARS is often associated with a mononucleosis-like illness with fever, fatigue, lymphadenopathy, and pharyngitis. It may additionally present with a disseminated rash that does not spare the palms and soles. It is often mistaken for the rash of secondary syphilis or other viral, bacterial, and ricketsial exanthems. Oral and genital ulcers may also occur that may or may not be associated with pain. In addition to the mucocutaneous manifestations, patients with ARS may also present with aseptic meningitis, mimicking the presentation of primary HSV and other infections. Laboratory findings include elevated liver function tests, atypical lymphocytes, thrombocytopenia, and leucopenia. Acute viral hepatitis, cytomegalovirus disease, Epstein-Barr virus disease, and a host of other conditions may present in a similar fashion, posing a significant diagnostic challenge (see Table 11-3). Although rare, individuals with primary HIV infection may also present with opportunistic conditions such as Pneumocystis pneumonia and oral candidiasis.

Diagnostics/Therapy

The acute retroviral syndrome of recent HIV infection often occurs during the window phase of standard HIV antibody tests. If acute HIV infection is suspected, then serologic testing should be supplemented by HIV viral load testing. Standard consent and pretest and posttest counseling rules are applicable to viral load testing as per jurisdiction standards. Treatment remains controversial, with some experts advocating initiation of HAART for immunologic and public health purposes.

Table 11-3   Signs and Symptoms of Acute HIV Infection[101]

Signs, symptoms, and findings	Frequency
Fever	80%-90%
Pharyngitis	70%-90%
Lymphadenopathy	40%-70%
Headache	32%-70%
Arthralgia/Myalgia	50%-70%
Lethargy/Malaise	70%-90%
Gastrointestinal Complaints	30%-60%
Meningitis	24%
Encephalitis	rare
Peripheral Neuropathy	rare
Maculopapular Rash	40%-80%
Mucocutaneous Ulcers	5%-20%
Thrombocytopenia	45%
Leukopenia	40%
Elevated Liver Function Test	21%

Preventive Sexual Healthcare Screening

In the 2006 *Sexually Transmitted Infection Guidelines*, the CDC has made recommendations about appropriate screening of asymptomatic MSM who are sexually active. STI screening should include a review of symptoms associated with common sexually transmitted infections, and specific laboratory testing which is guided by exposure history. Most evaluations should be performed yearly unless the patient confirms that he has multiple or anonymous partners, has sex in relation to illicit drug use, or has partners that participate in such activities. In such individuals, testing every three to six months may be more appropriate.[44] Annual testing should include HIV serology, syphilis serology, screening for urethral *N. gonorrheae* (GC) and *C. trachomatis* (CT) infection in men who have participated in insertive anal intercourse within the prior year, screening for rectal GC and CT in men who have been the receptive anal intercourse partner in the preceding year, and screening for pharyngeal GC infection in men who participated in receptive oral intercourse within the prior year. Additionally, a low threshold should be used to test MSM for STI and HIV if presenting with any suspicious symptoms.[44]

For WSW, prevention must include education and improving perceptions of risk for STI and HIV. Decreasing the marginalization of this population in the medical community is essential. Practitioners should facilitate open discussions about sexual preferences and practices. Patients should be offered routine Pap and cervical GC and CT screening, as is the standard of care, regardless of their current sexual behavior with women or men. WSW, similar to all sexually active adults, should be encouraged to be HIV tested and to know the HIV status of their partners. Vaccination against hepatitis A and B should be offered to sexually active WSW. Syphilis screening should also be done routinely since oral transmission has been documented between women. Adequate mental health and substance abuse screening and referrals for harm reduction should be performed as intravenous drug use continues to be a significant risk factor for HIV and blood-borne virus transmission in this population.

Although the CDC provides no specific guidelines for transgender individuals, Chapter 13 discusses appropriate preventive screening for members of this community. If identified to be at high risk for HIV, transgender clients should be screened once every three to 12 months depending on specific behaviors. Screening for STI should be a routine part of care and should be performed at minimum yearly. Specific interventions and screening tests should be based on the organs present.[46]

Management of Sexually Transmitted Infections in MSM and WSW

MSM may present with several syndromes typical of sexually transmitted infections. It is important to think broadly and generate adequate differential diagnoses to ensure appropriate diagnostic and therapeutic considerations based on clinical presentations (see Table 11-4).

Table 11-4   Differential Diagnosis of Common STI Presentations in MSM

Genital Ulcer Disease	Urethritis	Disseminated Rash	Proctitis
Syphilis	Chlamydia	Secondary syphilis	Gonorrhea
Herpes Simplex	Gonorrhea	Primary HIV infection	Herpes Simplex
Chancroid	Ureaplasma	Erythema multiforme	Chlamydia
Primary HIV infection	Trichomonas	Pityriasis rosea	Lymphogranuloma venereum
Lymphogranuloma venereum	Mycoplasma	Other viral exanthem	Syphilis
Granuloma Inguinale	Herpes Simplex	Steptococcal-associated	Inflammatory bowel disease
Trauma	Adenovirus	Drug rash	Trauma
Neoplasm	Hypersensitivity to topical agents	Disseminated Gonorrhea	Enteric bacteria
Behcet's disease	Reiter's syndrome	Lichen planus	Enteric parasites
Reiter's syndrome	Urethro-meatal wart	Scabies	Retained foreign body
Fixed Drug Eruption	Other less common bacteria	Rickettsial Infection	

Chlamydia Species Including Lymphogranuloma Venereum

Chlamydia trachomatis (CT) is a gram-negative obligate intracellular organism that is the most common cause of sexually transmitted infections in both men and women.[47] In 2004, more than 900 000 cases of CT were reported to the CDC, compared to 300 000 cases of gonorrhea.[48] The prevalence of CT among MSM was thought to be low, but with increasing concern that inflammatory genital tract diseases may increase risk for HIV transmission, renewed interest has emerged in screening and preventing CT infection among MSM.[20] In a recent study of men presenting to San Francisco STI clinics, 15.2% of MSM with gonococcal urethritis were also infected with CT. Of those with nongonococcal urethritis (NGU), 18% had CT infection.[49] Chlamydia cervicitis appears to be rare among WSW who do not have sex with men.

The most common strains causing human infection are serovars A through K. These strains have a tropism for the epithelium of the eye and genital tract and are responsible for classic presentations such as trachoma and urethritis. Serovars L1, L2, and L3, which are responsible for Lymphogranuloma venereum (LGV) infection, infect epithelial cells as well, but have enhanced tropism toward monocytes and macrophages and lead to more systemic disease manifestations. Previously a disease of the developing world, LGV has re-emerged among highly sexually active MSM.[50]

Spectrum of Disease

Urethritis is the most common presentation of CT infection in men and is characterized by penile discharge and/or dysuria. It is important to remember that chlamydia is only one of several pathogens that can present with urethritis. The discharge associated with chlamydia urethritis is often described as mucoid or watery. In one study, however, eleven percent of men with confirmed CT and NGU had purulent-appearing discharge more classic for gonococcal urethritis. It is not possible to differentiate causes of urethritis by discharge character alone. A recent study of men presenting with NGU to STI clinics in Australia raised the possibility that absence of > five WBC/high power field (HPF) may not be a sensitive enough finding to rule out urethritis among symptomatic men.[51]

Procititis may also be a manifestation of CT in MSM. In one retrospective study, eleven percent of cases were attributed to chlamydia alone, while an additional seven percent were attributed to gonorrhea and chlamydia coinfection.[52] The diagnosis of rectal chlamydia infection poses a significant challenge given the lack of an easy way to culture the organism. Some research indicates that nucleic acid amplification tests (NAAT) using swabs approved for urethral specimens may have a role in diagnosing chlamydia proctitis. Some independent laboratories have therefore initiated nucleic acid testing on rectal specimens acquired on a rectal swab.[44,52] Empiric therapy for proctitis should include coverage for chlamydia when these diagnostic technologies are unavailable.

In 2003, an outbreak of Lympogranuloma venereum (LGV) caused by the L2 serovar of chlamydia occurred among MSM in the Netherlands presenting with proctitis.[50] Subsequently cases were identified in other western countries including the United States. Risk factors for the incident cases included involvement in "leather scene" parties (parties where extreme sexual practices, such as bondage, sadism, and masochism take place), unprotected anal intercourse (receptive or insertive), and non-genital anal penetration (fisting and sex toys).[50] Classically, LGV is on the differential diagnosis of ulcerative genital disease and has a 3-30 day incubation period. Generally after a subtle, non-painful papule resolves, unilateral inguinal lymphadenopathy develops. Secondary LGV presents very differently in men inoculated rectally and in women inoculated vaginally. Since rectal and cervical lymphatics drain to retroperitoneal lymph nodes, MSM who engage in anal intercourse and women may not present with inguinal lymphadenopathy but rather proctitis due to retroperitoneal lymphatic congestion. After this second stage, untreated LGV can lead to lymphatic obstruction, genital lymphedema, rectal strictures, and fistulae.

Along with GC, chlamydia is a very common cause of epididymitis among men 35 years of age and younger. In one study, nine of eleven men with epididymitis had chlamydia detected in their genital tract.[53] Additionally, gonorrhea is often a copathogen involved in epididymitis, as are many enteric gram-negatives in MSM who engage in insertive anal sex.

Chlamydia prostatitis remains a topic of intense speculation. Prostatic secretions need to pass through the urethra, so chlamydia detected may be of urethral rather than prostatic origin. Although limited by the possibility of urethral contamination of specimens, small series of patients demonstrate the possibility of an association between chlamydia and chronic prostatitis.

Mucopurulent cervicitis may occur in WSW and is usually found in women who also have sex with men.

Chlamydia Diagnostics

Tissue culture of *Chlamydia trachomatis* is expensive and work-intensive, and it requires specialized specimen-handling. Culture has therefore been rendered obsolete by nonculture methods to detect chlamydia.

Non-culture, non-nucleic acid methods: Direct fluorescent antibodies (DFA) against the major outer membrane protein (MOMP) found on elementary bodies of CT may be used to detect chlamydia. DFA may be less sensitive in male urethral samples (< 70%) than in cervical samples.[54] Enzyme-linked antibodies against the lipopolysaccharide (LPS) of chlamydia can also be used to detect chlamydia. Sensitivity ranges from 43%-92% with a specificity of 97% for male urethral specimens. Sensitivity decreases with urine samples.[54]

Nucleic Acid-based Tests: These tests are the most frequently used for asymptomatic screening and symptomatic testing for chlamydia genital infection. Currently approved DNA probe tests can be used on urethral and endocervical specimens, although emerging data indicates they may also be used on rectal specimens. Reported test characteristics for chlamydia include a sensitivity of 92.6%, specificity of 99.8% with associated positive predictive value in a background of 5% prevalence of 96.1% and a negative predictive value of 97.9% in a background of 10% prevalence. Nucleic acid amplification tests (NAAT) utilize molecular techniques that can amplify even small amounts of chlamydia nucleic acid to detect infection. A meta-analysis of 29 studies evaluated the sensitivity and specificity of CT-NAAT techniques in identifying chlamydia infection. Sensitivities and specificities for urethral specimens ranged from 88%-96% and 96%-99%, respectively. NAATs performed similarly in non-invasively acquired urine samples with sensitivities and specificities of 84%-93% and 94%-99% respectively.

LGV Diagnostics

LGV infection of the rectum poses a more significant diagnostic challenge given the need for longer therapy to eradicate infection. Molecular techniques are emerging to test for this rectal infection by LGV serovars of chlamydia.[54] For now, LGV diagnosis relies on clinical suspicion and serologic tests. A titer of 1:256 or greater using the complement fixation chlamydia serology or an IgG titer of > 1:128 using the microimmunofluorescenence test in the correct clinical setting is suggestive of LGV infection. These tests do not differentiate between different serovars of chlamydia, but the more invasive strains of LGV tend to generate much higher antibody titers than the less invasive D through K serovars.

Therapeutics[44,55,56]

Azithromycin and doxycycline are the main drugs used for treating chlamydial infections. Given the high risk of gonococcal coinfection, all treatment regimens should include empiric therapy for gonorrhea. Lymphogranuloma venereum requires a longer duration of therapy (usually three weeks). Partners of patients with chlamydial infection should be evaluated and treated even if their last contact was greater than 60 days prior to the onset of symptoms in the index patient. Abstinence should be encouraged until seven days after a single-dose regimen or at the end of a standard seven-day regimen of therapy. Asymptomatic partners of LGV cases who have had sexual contact within 30 days prior to symptom onset in the index patient should be examined and treated for urethral or cervical infection with standard single dose or seven-day regimens used to treat chlamydia infection (see Table 11-5).

Table 11-5   Chlamydia Treatment

Type of chlamydia	Treatment*	Special Considerations
Standard Chlamydia	Azithromycin 1 gram PO x 1 dose	Treat for gonorrhea as well
	Doxycycline 100 mg PO every 12 hrs x 7 days	Treat for gonorrhea as well
	Erythromycin base 500 mg QID x 7 days	Treat for gonorrhea as well. Consider test of cure 3 weeks after therapy is complete.
	Erythromycin ethylsuccinate 800 mg QID x 7 days	Treat for gonorrhea as well. Consider test of cure 3 weeks after therapy is complete.
	Ofloxacin 300 mg every 12 hrs x 7 days	Treat for gonorrhea as well
	Levofloxacin 500 mg PO QD x 7 days	Treat for gonorrhea as well
Lymphogranuloma Venereum (LGV)	Doxycycline 100 mg PO every 12 hrs x 21 days	Treat for gonorrhea as well
	Erythromycin base 500 mg QID x 21 days	Treat for gonorrhea as well
	Azithromycin one gram PO q Week x 3 weeks	Less data, some experts think this regimen may be equivalent. Treat for gonorrhea as well.

*Treatment of gonorrhea if not ruled out. Some favor empiric therapy in all cases.

Other Causes of Nongonococcal Urethritis in MSM

Traditionally, chlamydia was thought to be the cause of the majority of NGU, but several other pathogens may play a significant role in urethritis.[51] Other bacteria implicated in NGU include organisms treated by regimens recommended for treating chlamydia such as *Mycoplasma genitalium* and *Ureaplasma urealyticum* and *parvum,* as well as bacteria not treated by these regimens such as *Gardnerella vaginalis.*[57] Direct causality is difficult to establish since these organisms may also be commensals of the genital tract.

In addition to bacteria, both protozoa and viruses have been implicated in NGU. *Trichomonas vaginalis,* a protozoan parasite, has been identified as a cause of persistent urethritis. In one study, this protozoan was isolated in 15% of men with persistent urethritis after appropriate treatment.[58] Less data is available about *T. vaginalis* among MSM as a cause for NGU. There is also some evidence that adenoviruses and herpes simplex-1 and -2 may be the cause of some NGU without identified causality, specifically in MSM.[51]

Standard therapy for chlamydial urethritis should be employed as first line for NGU (see Table 11-5). If patients return with persistent urethritis and re-exposure/treatment noncompliance are not the cause of failure, culture for *T. vaginalis* should be obtained and the patient treated for this parasite with metronidazole (single oral 2-gram dose) or tinidazole (single oral two-gram dose) along with another dose of azithromycin (single oral one-gram dose). Up to one percent of men with NGU may go on to develop reactive arthritis; three go on to develop further rheumatologic manifestations like uveitis. Use of antimicrobials in the management of these late sequels continues to be controversial.

Gonorrhea

Infection with *Neisseria gonorrheae* (GC), a gram-negative diplococcus, is the second most common reported sexually transmitted disease in the United States. Although GC rates appear to be decreasing, some estimate that twice as many new infections with gonorrhea occur than are reported. Although women represent an increasing number of new gonorrhea infections, MSM represent between 20%-36% of cases of new gonorrhea infections reported every year.[59-60] In addition to high rates of infection, MSM activity is also associated with increasing rates of GC resistance to agents routinely used to treat this STI.

Spectrum of Disease

Gonorrhea most commonly presents as a localized infection and can cause disease in any part of the male or female genital tract. Additionally, infection of the oropharynx, or the rectum through anal and oral sex, respectively, occurs more commonly among MSM than men who have sex with women exclusively. Untreated infections can lead to both local complications and dissemination of disease (disseminated gonococcal infection or DGI). Incubation can be as short as three days and as long as three weeks. In one study of 1749 cases of gonorrhea in men, 86% of patients were symptomatic within 14 days of their postulated exposure.[61] In that same study, 1615 men had urethral infection and most commonly complained of discharge (82%) or pain with urination (53%). Ten percent of men with urethral infection had no symptoms of gonorrhea.[61] Long-term complications of gonorrhea can include chronic prostatitis and infection of deeper structures of the genital tract like seminal vesicles and associated glands.

Urethritis is the most common presentation of gonorrhea infection in men. It is important to remember that gonorrhea is only one of several pathogens that can present with urethritis. The discharge associated with gonorrhea is often described as mucopurulent, but it is not possible to differentiate discharge associated with gonorrhea from other causes of urethritis by appearance alone. Incubation time for development of symptoms after gonorrhea exposure tends to be shorter than for chlamydia, two to seven days compared to five to ten days. *Epididymitis* can also be caused by GC, but chlamydia and gonorrhea coinfection is more likely to cause this presentation than is GC alone.[62]

Proctitis is frequently caused by gonorrhea; 30% of cases in one retrospective analysis of MSM were attributed to gonorrhea.[52] Many other infections may present with similar symptoms, as may inflammatory bowel disease. Additionally, many men present with symptoms of proctitis without evidence of urethritis. Many men with culture-proven proctitis did not report any of the classic symptoms associated with this manifestation of gonorrhea. This finding is particularly worrisome given the association between proctitis and incident HIV infection.

Mucopurulent Cervicitis caused by gonorrhea can occur in WSW but is more commonly reported in WSW who have sex with men.

Gonococcal pharyngitis is on the differential of acute, exudative infections of the oropharynx. These infections may present without symptoms or like group A streptococcal pharyngitis with exudates and cervical lymphadenitis. Pharyngeal infections may occur in up to ten percent of MSM presenting with gonorrhea.

Disseminated gonorrheal infection (DGI) occurs in 0.5%-3% of individuals with gonorrhea infection. DGI may present with the classic triad of tenosynovitis, dermatitis, and polyarthralgias without purulent arthritis or with purulent arthritis without associated skin lesions.[63] The majority of patients with purulent arthritis have involvement of only one joint, although multiple joints may be involved; knees, wrists, and ankles are the most frequently involved joints. DGI is often associated with asymptomatic mucosal infection with few patients complaining of genital symptoms before their disseminated disease is manifest.[63] Some autoimmune diseases and congenital or acquired defects in the complement system are associated with DGI, prompting most to screen individuals for lupus and complement deficiency during the convalescence of disseminated gonorrhea.[63] There does not appear to be an increased incidence of DGI among people living with HIV.

Diagnostics

Gram stain continues to be a simple and cost-effective approach to diagnosing urethritis caused by gonorrhea. Cervical or urethral sample obtained with a cotton swab can be gram stained for evaluation under a light microscope. This technique yields a cell count per high-powered field that aids in the diagnosis of urethritis or cervicitis, as well as bacteriologic data. The presence of gram-negative diplococci within cells or in the extracellular area is diagnostic of gonorrheal urethritis. The swab used to obtain the microscopy specimen can also be used for gonorrhea culture. Historically, gram stain performs about the same as culture in most studies. One more recent study revealed that gram stain may be less sensitive in asymptomatic men (81%) while still excellent in those with symptoms (94%).[61] The gold standard diagnostic for gonorrhea remains culture on Thayer-Martin media.

Culture remains important in diagnosing gonorrhea in nongenital areas and is the only currently available way to define antibiotic susceptibilities for *N. gonorrheae*, an issue that may be important with emerging fluoroquinolone (FQ) resistance among isolates from MSM.

Molecular tests are available for diagnosing GC infections. The two most readily available are DNA probe tests and nucleic acid amplification tests (NAAT). The DNA probe tests that are currently approved by the FDA can be used on urethral and endocervical specimens. Reported test characteristics for gonorrhea include a sensitivity of 95.4%, specificity of 99.8% with associated positive predictive value in a background of 5% prevalence of 96.2% and a negative predictive value of 97.9% in a background of 10% prevalence. Although not approved for such testing, the DNA probe tests may play a role in diagnosing extragenital gonorrhea in the oropharynx and anorectum. Nucleic acid amplification tests (NAAT) utilize molecular techniques that can amplify even small amounts of gonorrhea nucleic acid to detect infection. These tests appear to be more sensitive than culture in most studies, with sensitivities > 98%. Additionally, these assays can be used to test urine as well as urethral and cervical swabs, increasing patient acceptability and with similar performance parameters to invasive testing.

Therapeutics

Knowledge of a patient's sexual behaviors and travel history is central in selecting a treatment regimen for gonorrhea. Geographic locale at time of infection, MSM behaviors, and anatomic site of infection all influence provider choices from treatment guidelines given emerging resistance patterns. Ideally, patients who engage in MSM activity should be treated for gonorrhea with either ceftriaxone or cefixime as first-line therapy (see Table 11-6).[44,55] Many providers, however, have used fluoroquinolones (FQ) in the past because of their ease of administration and as a first-line choice for penicillin allergic patients. Most recently an increase in FQ resistance among MSM and people visiting Hawaii, California, Asia, and Wales has prompted a change in treatment guidelines in such scenarios.[64] This resistance has spread throughout many communities in the United States, so clinicians should use extended spectrum cephalosporins to treat GC in MSM. If FQ use cannot be avoided in a particular scenario, providers are advised to have vigilance for treatment failures and to consider use of culture-based diagnostics to allow susceptibility testing of isolates.[64] Few options are available for treatment of penicillin allergic patients with the discontinuation of distribution of spectinomycin in the United States. It is important to either avoid FQ or have increased vigilance for treatment failure.[55] Patients should return for a test of cure only if symptoms persist. Additionally, all regimens should include empiric therapy for chlamydia if CT infection is not ruled out. Sex partners should be treated for gonorrhea if their last encounter was > 60 days from index case symptom onset or diagnosis.

Table 11-6 Treatment Regimens for Gonorrhea[44,55]

Anatomic Site	Treatment*	Special Considerations
Urethra, Cervix or Rectum	Cefixime 400 mg PO x 1 dose Ceftriaxone 125 mg IM x 1 dose	Only recently available again
	Ciprofolxacin 500 mg PO x 1 dose	Avoid in MSM and select geographic acquisition because of resistance
	Ofloxacin 400 mg PO x 1 dose	Avoid in MSM and select geographic acquisition because of resistance
	Levofloxacin 250 mg PO x 1 dose	Avoid in MSM and select geographic acquisition because of resistance
	Spectinomycin 2 g IM x 1 dose	Discontinued
	Azithromycin 2 g PO x 1 dose	Expensive, GI distress, Use in penicillin allergic patients, treats chlamydia
Pharynx	Ceftriaxone 125 mg IM x 1 dose	
	Ciprofolxacin 500 mg PO x 1 dose	Avoid in MSM and select geographic acquisition because of resistance
	Azithromycin 2 g PO x 1 dose	Expensive, GI distress, Use in penicillin allergic patients, treats chlamydia
Disseminated (induction)	Ceftriaxone 1 g IM/IV every 24 hrs Cefotaxime 1 g IV every 8 hrs	
Continue until 24-28 hrs of improvement before switching to continuation	Ceftizoxime 1 g IV every 8 hrs Ciprofolxacin 400 mg IV every 12 hrs	Avoid in MSM and select geographic acquisition because of resistance
	Ofloxacin 400 mg IV every 12 hrs	Avoid in MSM and select geographic acquisition because of resistance
	Spectinomycin 2 g IM every 12 hrs	Discontinued
Disseminated (continuation)	Cefixime 400 mg PO every 12 hrs Ciprofloxacin 500 mg PO every 12 hrs	Avoid in MSM and select geographic acquisition because of resistance
Treat for an additional week after completion of IV/IM induction	Ofloxacin 400 mg PO every 12 hrs	Avoid in MSM and select geographic acquisition because of resistance
	Levofloxacin 500 mg PO every 24 hrs	Avoid in MSM and select geographic acquisition because of resistance

*Treatment of chlamydia if chlamydia not ruled out. Some favor empiric therapy in all cases

Partners within the previous 60 days should be tested and treated as indicated. Additionally, safer sex should be encouraged and unprotected sex avoided entirely until treatment is complete and symptoms have resolved.

Syphilis

Syphilis is caused by *Treponema pallidum*. Disease manifestations are protean and often difficult to diagnose in the asymptomatic early stages and clinically variable later stages of infection. This infection can have long-term consequences that make it an important public health threat. In 2000, the CDC targeted *T. pallidum* for eradication. But, in 2001, the rates of syphilis began to increase, and the majority of the cases were disproportionately among men. In 2004, the CDC estimated that 64% of all primary and secondary syphilis cases were among MSM based on this gender disparity; non-Caucasian MSM appear to be disproportionately affected. Oral sex, traditionally thought of as a safer activity, has been implicated in the ongoing MSM syphilis epidemic. Non-gay-identified MSM and increasing evidence of transmission through sexual partnerships initiated through the Internet are areas that are being explored as targets for preventive interventions. Although the burden of disease appears to be less in WSW, oral-genital transmission of syphilis has been reported between women and due vigilance should be paid for diagnostics and screening of this population.

Spectrum of Disease

Treponema pallidum infection has been referred to historically as the "great imitator." No discussion of clinical manifestations of this disease could cover the complete spectrum of illness attributed to syphilis. Transmission of syphilis is through contact with infectious lesions on the skin or mucous membranes and through body fluids.[65] One half to two thirds of individuals exposed to a patient with syphilis in its early, infectious stages will go on to display clinical or serologic evidence of infection. Many infected people may have no manifestations or such mild manifestations of early disease that they do not come to clinical attention. Retrospective trials and case reports during the early days of the HIV epidemic raised the possibility that syphilis may present atypically among this population of patients, so special attention and screening is necessary among HIV-infected people. Syphilis is divided clinically into three stages: primary, secondary, and tertiary.

Primary syphilis is associated with a painless skin lesion, termed a chancre. This lesion appears within about 21 days of exposure and is often not detected. These lesions are described as non-tender, non-purulent ulcers with indurated borders. They are usually solitary, although multiple chancres have been reported in people with HIV. A minority of chancres in men with genital ulcer disease display the classic characteristics attributed to the lesion of primary syphilis, so a low threshold should be maintained for testing people with atypical lesions.[66] This stage is infectious via sexual contact.

Secondary syphilis may become manifest four to ten weeks after the appearance of the chancre, patients may present with symptoms of the secondary phase of syphilis. The most common presenting complaint is a rash. The rash can take many forms but is most commonly described as erythematous or copper-colored macules with a distribution that may not spare the palms or soles. Lesions may have other morphologies, but they are usually not vesicular.[65] Condyloma lata and mucous patches are other dermatologic manifestations of secondary syphilis. Although rash is the most common manifestation, other symptoms and signs may be appreciated in secondary syphilis. Secondary syphilis may present with fever, malaise, sore throat, and lymphadenopathy. Aseptic meningitis, cranial nerve involvement, and ocular involvement in the form of uveitis may also occur and represent the earliest stages of neurosyphilis. Syphilis is also a cause of proctitis, though often less symptomatic than other causes. Patients in this stage of disease can transmit syphilis through sexual contact.

Most people with secondary syphilis will enter an asymptomatic period called *latent syphilis* that is characterized by serologic evidence of infection in the absence of symptoms. This phase is less infectious, but up to 24% of latently infected individuals may have recurrence of secondary syphilis. The latent period is further divided into *early* and *late latent* infection. This distinction is based on previous negative tests or exposure within the previous year, as well as symptoms consistent with syphilis within that same time frame. Syphilis is transmitted from mother-to-child during latency but not through sexual activity.

One third of individuals untreated during earlier phases of syphilis will go on to have late sequelae, termed *tertiary syphilis.* Individuals diagnosed during this phase of infection are noninfectious. These manifestations include cardiovascular disease, gummatous disease, and late neurosyphilis. Incubation times for this stage of disease are in the order of 2-50 years after initial infection.[65] HIV-infected individuals may progress more rapidly, be more prone to CNS and ocular involvement, and have more significant gummatous disease manifestations than their HIV-uninfected counterparts.

Diagnostics[65]

Treponema pallidum cannot be cultured, so indirect diagnostics are the mainstay of diagnosing syphilis. Although examination of fluids from genital and mucosal lesions using darkfield microscopy may allow identification of treponemes, this technology is not sensitive and often unavailable. Serologic testing algorithms are standard screening and diagnostic tests for syphilis. Non-treponemal tests (Venerial Disease Research Laboratory [VDRL] and Rapid Plasma Reagin [RPR]) are initially sent with positive confirmed using treponemal tests (*T. pallidum* particle agglutination [TPPA] or fluorescent treponemal antibodies [FTA-abs]). The VDRL and RPR are 78%–86% sensitive in primary infection, 100% in secondary infection, and 95%–98% in latent infection. False positive non-treponemal tests may occur and need confirmation with more specific treponemal testing. The RPR and VDRL are also important in assessing treatment response as is described in the section below.

A diagnostic question that causes significant confusion is when to perform a lumbar puncture to evaluate a patient for CNS involvement with syphilis. The CDC recommends lumbar puncture of individuals with syphilis if there are neurologic or ocular signs or symptoms, in late latent or syphilis of unknown duration in HIV-infected individuals, in active tertiary syphilis, and in treatment failure of regimens that do not treat CNS involvement. Cerebrospinal fluid (CSF) should be tested for cell count, protein, and CSF VDRL and/or CSF FTA. There are no standardized guidelines to define a positive CSF result. A positive CSF VDRL or FTA is an absolute indication to treat for neurosyphilis. Five or more white cells on cell count and/or elevated protein > 45 mg/dL are also considered evidence of CNS involvement.[55]

Therapeutics

Resistance to penicillin has not emerged in *T. pallidum* given the ongoing clinical success noted among treated individuals. Therapeutic decisions require a clear perspective of disease stage, timing, and symptoms. Follow-up of non-treponemal test titers are necessary after therapy to guide further diagnostics and treatment strategies. Patients being treated for syphilis should be warned about the Jarisch-Herxheimer reaction, a not uncommon febrile response to therapy that is often flu-like. It can occur as early as two hours after treatment and usually resolves within 12–24 hours. All that is required is symptomatic therapy with antipyretics and analgesics (see Table 11-7).

Table 11-7   Treatment of Syphilis[55]

Stage	Treatment	Penicillin Allergy
Primary, Secondary, or	Benzathine Penicillin G	Doxycycline 100 mg PO two x day for 14 days
Early Latent Syphilis*	2.4 million units IM x one time	
Late Latent Syphilis**	Benzathine Penicillin G	Doxycycline 100mg PO two x day for 28 days
Syphilis of Unknown Duration	2.4 million units IM weekly	
Tertiary Syphilis	x three weeks	
Neurosyphilis	Aqueous crystalline penicillin G	Desensitize penicillin allergic
Ocular syphilis	three to four million units every four hrs for	patients. Ceftriaxone 2 grams IV x 14 d
Auditory syphilis	ten to 14 days	is an alternative option. CONSULT ID.
	or	procaine penicillin Avoid probenecid in
	2.4 million units IM once daily	sulfonamide allergic patients with probenecid 500 mg four x day for ten to 14 days

Follow-up non-treponemal tests should be checked in all patients treated for syphilis at six and 12 months after therapy. HIV-infected patients should also be tested at three, nine, and 24 months given some evidence that treatment failure may be more common in this population. Between five and eleven percent of patients may require re-treatment or, treatment intensification because of inadequate serologic response to therapy. An appropriate response to therapy is defined as resolution of symptoms and a four-fold absolute drop (or, two-fold serial dilutions) drop in VDRL or RPR titer at six months after treatment. The presence of clinical symptoms, less than a four-fold dilution in non-treponemal test titer within six months of treatment or persistent four-fold increase at six months after therapy is considered a failure. Those failed by treatment should have their CSF evaluated and either be treated for neurosyphilis or late latent disease, guided by these CSF results. Patients with neurosyphilis should have repeat lumbar punctures three to six months after therapy and every six months for three years or until CSF findings normalize.

All individuals diagnosed with syphilis should be offered HIV testing. Sexual contacts of individuals treated for primary, secondary, early latent syphilis, or syphilis of unknown duration with non-treponemal titers > 1:32 should be contacted for testing and potentially empiric treatment of early disease. Sex partners of patients who have latent syphilis should be evaluated clinically and serologically for syphilis and treated based on these findings.[55]

Herpes Simplex Virus Infection

Herpes simplex type-1 and type-2 (HSV-1 and HSV-2) are transmitted by skin-to-skin contact or contact with a mucus membrane and are the most common cause of genital ulcers. These viruses have the ability to generate latent infection in peripheral nerves after primary exposure and can lead to recurrent vesicular and ulcerative disease. Shedding of this virus occurs with or without the presence of ulcerative or vesicular lesions and can be transmitted through intimate or sexual contact with a completely asymptomatic carrier.

The seroprevalence of HSV is on the rise, with seroepidemiologic surveys estimating that more than 30 million people have genital HSV infection.[67] Traditionally, HSV-1 was thought to be restricted to orolabial herpes with HSV-2 causing the preponderance of genital infections. More recently, increasing rates of HSV-1 genital infection have been detected among sexually active adults. MSM are one of the groups with the highest rates HSV seroprevalence in the United States. Beyond being a clinical annoyance with recurrent and painful lesions, HSV disease may represent a significant risk factor for HIV transmission among MSM whether or not the HSV infection is symptomatic.

To date, the transmission of Herpes simplex virus between WSW has not been confirmed as an STI in this population. Marrazzo and colleagues found that the prevalence of antibodies to HSV type-2, the type associated with genital outbreaks, in a cohort of WSW is comparable to heterosexual women and is associated with history of having a male sexual partner with herpes. The prevalence of antibodies to HSV-1 associated with oral lesions was higher in WSW than in their heterosexual counterparts and was proportional to the number of lifetime female sexual partners. There was no relationship of the detection of antibodies to a history of an HSV outbreak in WSW. Since HSV can be transmitted in the absence of a detectable outbreak and the presence of open lesions facilitates transmission of other STIs, WSW should be counseled on the possible increased asymptomatic carriage of the oral HSV type and encouraged to engage in protected sex.

Spectrum of Disease

Clinical manifestations of herpes infection are complicated by the ability of HSV to remain latent in infected individuals, many of whom do not recall their first episode of infection. *Primary Infection* is defined as a new HSV infection in someone without serologic evidence of prior exposure. *Non-Primary First Episode Infection* is defined as a genital infection with HSV in someone previously exposed to the other type. An example of this would be a new genital HSV-1 infection in someone with preexisting serologic evidence of HSV-2 but not HSV-1 exposure. Dual genital infection with HSV-1 and -2 is possible and may be associated with more frequent recurrences. *Recurrent Infection* is reactivation of latent genital HSV. The cultured virus from these lesions should be congruent with the type of antibodies detected in serologic testing. An example would be isolation of HSV-2 from a genital lesion in an individual with detectable antibodies to HSV-2 in their blood. Generally speaking, the most significant, and often systemic, manifestations of HSV disease occur with primary infection. Recurrent infection tends to be milder, as does non-primary first episodes of genital HSV because of preexisting immunity and partial cross-type immunity, respectively.

The classic skin lesions of HSV begin as papules that evolve into vesicles and pustules. Rupture of these vesiculopustular lesions result in ulcers that crust over and heal without scar. The local disease manifestations of herpes simplex in MSM include genital ulcers, urethritis, and proctitis. Although often more severe in women, primary HSV infection in men may present with systemic symptoms 2-12 days after exposure. These symptoms may include painful vesiculopustular lesions that ulcerate (genital, perianal, or rectal), fever, painful and tender regional lymph nodes, fever, mucopurulent anal discharge, tenesmus, anal pain, dysuria, and watery urethral discharge. Primarily infected individuals may have multiple bilateral lesions that usually resolve within three weeks. HSV proctitis is most frequently described among MSM, and the other causes of proctitis, as described above, should be entertained and treated. Anoscopy may reveal mucosal ulceration. In one series of 101 MSM with proctitis, 13% of cases were caused by HSV alone. An additional 3% of cases were caused by mixed infections including HSV.[52] Other HSV presenting complaints include dysuria, pain and itching, painful regional lymph nodes, and systemic symptoms (fevers, headache, malaise, fatigue).

Recurrent disease is more common with HSV-2 infection (60%) than with HSV-1 (14%).[68] Systemic manifestations are uncommon, but about 50% of these recurrences are heralded by a local prodrome of localized pain or tingling 12–24 hours before visible lesions. There are usually fewer lesions so that the distribution tends to be unilateral. Recurrences may be more frequent among men than women. Lesions are shorter lived in recurrences than in primary infection. It is important to remember and teach patients that virus may be shed even in the absence of recurrent genital disease.

Other than dermatologic manifestations, neurological manifestations may also occur in the primary phases of genital HSV infection. 8%-25% of individuals with primary HSV infection may present with an aseptic meningitis syndrome with headache, photophobia, and neck stiffness. The cerebrospinal fluid formula includes a pleocytosis with 300-400 cells/mm3 with a lymphocyte predominance and normal chemistries, although hypoglycorrhachia may occur.[69] Recurrent aseptic meninigitis referred to as Mollaret's meningitis may be associated with HSV-2.[70] 2%-15% of individuals may present with this symptom as a reflection of sacral autonomic involvement. Again this appears to be more common in women. Sudden onset of impotence may also occur in the setting of sacral nerve involvement. Transverse myelitis is a very rare manifestation of HSV infection; symptoms include leg weakness, sensory disturbances, and bowel/bladder disturbances.

Diagnostics

Herpes is one of the possible etiologies of genital ulcer disease. It is difficult to ascertain the pathogen responsible for ulcerative disease by history and physical examination alone. Generally, the dermatologic manifestation of herpes is that of multiple shallow but painful ulcers that start as vesiculopustular lesions. Recurrence is a characteristic of herpes that may help differentiate it from other genital ulcer disease. It is often necessary to supplement clinical intuition with diagnostic tests.

Culture of a freshly unroofed vesicular lesion is the most specific diagnostic for herpes but suffers from having a sensitivity of around 50%. The yield is better in primary infection compared to the lower viral burden associated with recurrences. Standard viral media should be used and the sample should be collected with a Dacron swab. Culture may take up to ten days to demonstrate the presence of HSV.

Cytology (Tzanck smear) is done by smearing cells taken from a fresh blister or ulcer onto a microscope slide. The cells are stained with a stain, such as Wright's stain, and then examined under a microscope. The characteristic findings associated with herpes virus infection are multinucleated giant cells. These nuclei appear to be molded to fit tightly together. Dark inclusion bodies may be visible in the cytosol of these cells. The Tzanck smear allows for rapid diagnosis, but it does not help differentiate between HSV-1, HSV-2, and varicella virus.

Direct fluorescent antibodies (DFA) against HSV-1 and HSV-2 can be used to enhance detection of infected cells using microscopy. A scalpel is used to scrape (not cut) the base of ulcerative lesions or an unroofed vesicle. Antibodies directed against type-specific antigens are then used, to fluorescently stain the specimen. This test is quick, relatively inexpensive, and specific. It is less useful in later-stage HSV lesions and during secondary episodes.

Serologically confirmed presence of antibodies against HSV-1 or HSV-2 does not rule out other infections as a cause of genital ulcer disease. Over the past few years, the diagnostic tests have become much improved in terms of sensitivity and specificity. Serologic screening for asymptomatic individuals is not currently recommended, but if current studies show that acyclovir suppression prevents HIV transmission for HSV-2 seropositive individuals, then recommendations may change. HSV-2 serological testing for HIV-infected patients, people with recurrent genital ulcerations, and pregnant women may be considered. Real-time PCR performs very well as an HSV diagnostic but is limited by availability and cost.

Therapeutics
The first-line agents for treatment of HSV genital infections are acyclovir, valacyclovir (pro-drug of acyclovir), and famcilovir (a pro-drug of penciclovir). Several considerations come into play when designing a regimen to address HSV infection. Acyclovir is limited by poor bioavailability, high pill burden, and frequent dosing. Nevertheless, it is the standard of care for HSV therapy and is very cheap. Treatment during the primary HSV outbreak decreases pain, shortens time to healing, and decreases viral shedding.[44] More severe manifestations of primary infection like aseptic meningitis or severe host immunocompromise may prompt initial therapy with IV acyclovir at a dose of 5-10mg/kg every 8 hours, but most can be treated with oral medications. Therapy may be extended for immunocompromised

Table 11-8   Treatment of Primary HSV Outbreak

Drug	Dose and Duration	Comments
Acyclovir	400 mg PO TID for 7–10 days	Increased compliance with TID dosing
	200 mg PO five x day for 7–10 days	
	5-10 mg/kg IV Q8 hours for 7–10 days	For more severe manifestations
Famciclovir	250 mg PO TID for 7-10 days	
Valacyclovir	1 gram PO BID for 7-10 days	Caution in severe immunocompromise due to possible risk of TTP/HUS

patients or those who are slow to respond. Treatment does not reduce the frequency of recurrent outbreaks (see Table 11-8).

Episodic treatment of recurrences should be initiated within one day of outbreak, so patients should be given a supply or refills of the selected antivirals to allow them to initiate therapy expediently (see Table 11-9).

Another option for addressing HSV recurrences is chronic suppressive therapy. While on therapy, this strategy decreases the number of outbreaks (up to 70%-80%), decreases asymptomatic shedding, and reduces transmission rates to uninfected partners.[71] The data implicating the role of HSV infection in transmission and acquisition of HIV may portend a future role for HSV suppression as a HIV preventive technique. Most guidelines recommend reserving suppressive therapy for individuals with greater than six outbreaks per year and discontinuing every 12 months to readdress the need for chronic suppression. Many providers have a lower threshold to start suppression and many patients are unwilling to experiment with possible recurrence. There may also be a harm reduction benefit of therapy to avoid HSV recurrences by possibly decreasing HIV transmission between partners. There may be a role for longer chronic suppression in immunocompromised people who have had severe mucocutaneous HSV infection (see Table 11-10).

Resistant strains of HSV can occur in immunocompromised patients, some of whom may develop lesions while on suppressive therapy. Treatment failure in this population should prompt culture and susceptibility testing of lesions not improving on seven to ten days of therapy. Other

Table 11-9   Episodic Treatment of Recurrent Genital HSV

Drug	Dose and Duration (normal immune system)	Dose and Duration (compromised immune system)
Acyclovir	400 mg PO TID for 5 days	400 mg PO TID for 5-10 days
	200 mg PO five x day for 5 days	200 mg PO 5x day for 5-10 days
	800 mg PO BID for 5 days	
Famciclovir	125 mg PO TID for 7-10 days	500 mg PO BID for 5-10 days
Valacyclovir	500 mg PO BID for 3-5 days	1 gram PO BID for 5-10 days
	1 gram PO QD for 5 days	

Table 11-10   Suppressive Therapy for Recurrent Genital HSV

Drug	Dose (normal immune system)	Dose (compromised immune system)
Acyclovir	400 mg PO BID	400-800 mg PO BID-TID
Famciclovir	250 mg PO BID	500 mg PO BID
Valacyclovir	500 mg PO QD	500 mg PO BID
	1 gram PO QD for 5 days	

antivirals such as foscarnet or topical/systemic cidofovir may be necessary to address resistant infections.

Counseling

Patients diagnosed with herpes need to be educated on the natural history of disease, specifically that recurrences are possible and that these events can be addressed with episodic or suppressive antivirals. Disclosure to sex partners should be encouraged, and patients should be reminded that asymptomatic shedding may occur leading to disease transmission. Individuals with prodromal or active symptoms should avoid sexual activity. Condoms may prevent transmission if they cover the lesions. Partners should be evaluated for previous HSV outbreaks and taught to recognize the symptoms. HSV-2 type specific serology may have a role in informing asymptomatic partners about their exposure status.[55]

Other Infectious Causes of Genital Ulcer Disease

Genital herpes and syphilis are the most common causes of genital ulcer disease (GUD) in the United States. A distant third is chancroid, caused by *Haemophilus ducreyi*.[44] In addition to these three STI, other infectious causes of genital ulcers include acute HIV infection, lymphogranuloma venereum (caused by certain serovars of *Chlamydia trachomatis*), and granuloma inguinale (caused by *Klebsiella granulomatis* formerly *Calammatobacterium granulomatis*). Other noninfectious causes include fixed drug eruptions, Behçet's disease, traumatic injuries, and neoplasm. This section will focus on chancroid and granuloma inguinale since the other infectious causes have been dealt with elsewhere in this chapter. Treatment decisions are often made based on local epidemiology and clinical characteristics of the patient's presentation. It is often difficult to clinically diagnose the etiology of a genital ulcer, but certain characteristics of the ulcer and other clinical features may aid in diagnosis (see Table 11-11). Close follow-up is necessary to guarantee correct management decisions have been made. Multiplex PCR testing may become available that tests for HSV, *T. pallidum*, and *H. Ducreyi*; until then, workup of genital ulcers should include a complete history and physical, RPR or VDRL, HSV DFA, culture or Tzanck prep, gram stain of edge of the ulcer looking for *H. ducreyi* forms, and LGV PCR or serology if epidemiologically suspected.

Although rare in the United States, *chancroid* is an infection that has a worldwide distribution. H. Ducreyi is a difficult-to-culture etiologic agent of this GUD. It is seen most frequently in uncircumcised men who are non-Caucasian and is rarely identified in women. After exposure, symptoms develop within one to seven days, although incubation periods of several weeks have been reported. There is no specific association between chancroid and MSM.

Chancroid is classically described as painful, often multiple, ragged-appearing ulcers with surrounding erythema and an associated necrotic

Table 11-11   Characteristics of Sexually Transmitted Genital Ulcer Disease

Genital Ulcer Disease	Incubation	Pain*	Typical Ulcer**	Constitutional symptoms	Lymphadenopathy
Syphilis	7-90 days	No	Indurated borders, clean base. Heals spontaneously. Usually solitary	Rarely	Non-tender and may be bilateral
Herpes Simplex	2-7 days	Yes	Multiple. Ulcer with erythematous base. Start as vesicles. Spontaneous healing.	Yes in primary infection	Bilateral, may be tender
Chancroid	3-10 days	Yes	Sharp border, often described as ragged and undermined. Not indurated. Usually multiple.	No	Usually unilateral and suppurative
Lympho-granuloma Venereum	5-21 days	Not usually	Usually is not observed. Small and shallow with rapid spontaneous healing.	Yes	May be bilateral, tender, may be suppurative
Granuloma Inguinale	7-90 days	Rarely	Extensive beefy granulation-like tissue in ulcer.	Rarely	Pseudoadenopathy

* May be painful if secondarily infected.
**May present atypically.

exudate. Fifty percent of patients will have painful regional lymphaden-opathy. These lymph nodes may become suppurative and rupture, leading to sinus tract formation.

Gram stain from the edge of an ulcer or aspirate of an involved lymph node may reveal "tracking" gram-negative rods in a "school of fish" con-formation. Culture is difficult but should be performed if clinically indi-cated. All patients with suspected chancroid should be tested for syphilis and HIV in addition to other STIs.

Treatment of chancroid is often based on clinical features of the patient's presentation before other data is available. Regimens recom-mended for treatment include Azithromycin one gram PO x one dose, Ceftriaxone 250 mg IM x one dose, Ciprofloxacin 500 mg PO BID x three days, or Erythromycin base 500 mg PO TID x seven days. HIV-infected and uncircumcised men may not respond to therapy, so follow-up is of the essence 3-7 days after therapy is initiated. Improvement should be observed in the ulcers, although they may take weeks to heal and may still scar. Lymphadenopathy is slower to improve and may require surgical management.[44] All sexual contacts within ten days of symptom onset should be treated even in the absence of symptoms.

Granuloma inguinale, also called Donovanosis, is caused by intracellular gram-negative rod *Klebsiella granulomatis* (previously called *Calammatobacterium granulomatis*). These are intracellular organisms than infect mononuclear cells. The organism cannot be cultured, but microscopic evaluation may reveal characteristic Donovan bodies within mononuclear cells. This infection is rare in the United States but may be seen in travelers returning from parts of India, South America, Papua New Guinea, Australia, and Africa, where Granuloma inguinale is a more common cause of GUD.

Granuloma inguinale begins with a small, painless nodule or papule that appears 8-80 days after exposure. The nodule then progresses to a beefy red, friable, granulomatous ulcer. Multiple and coalescent ulcers may occur. Spontaneous healing with scar and deformity may occur. Lymphatic obstruction from keloid formation may result in elephantiasis of the genitals, and rectal infections may occur in MSM and others who engage in anal intercourse. Rare bone and joint involvement has been described. Granulomas may spread to the inguinal region and mimic lymphadenitis, a finding termed pseudobubos. Culture is not currently available. Identification of typical Donovan bodies on microscopy of crush preparation or biopsy is the only diagnostic aid beyond history and identification of the typical ulcer. The ideal regimen for granuloma inguinale has not been established. Relapse 6-18 months after therapy is not uncommon. Regimens recommended by the CDC include doxycycline 100 mg PO BID or Trimethoprim/Sulfamethoxazole one double strength tablet PO BID for at least three weeks. Cirpofloxacin, erythromycin, and azithromycin are other alternatives.

Follow-up again must be rigorous given the possibility of relapse and the lack of clear diagnostics. Therapy should be continued until lesions have completely healed. Aminoglycoside therapy may need to be added if improvement of lesions is not noted a few days after initiation or if the patient is HIV infected. Sexual partners should be evaluated for signs and symptoms of infection; the role for empiric therapy in the absence of symptoms is unclear.[44]

Non Ulcerative Genital Lesions

Although many genital ulcers begin as papules or vesicles, some sexually transmitted infections present with dermatologic manifestations in the genital and perianal areas with lesions that do not ulcerate. These include genital warts and Molluscum contagiousum. In addition to fixed dermatologic manifestations, ectoparasites such as crabs and scabies may also be transmitted through sexual contact.

Genital Warts

Genital warts are caused by human papillomavirus (HPV), a family of DNA viruses that infect epithelial cells. Beyond being responsible for genital warts, likely the most common sexually transmitted infection in the United States, HPV has also been linked to cervical cancer in women and precancerous anal dysplasia and anal neoplasia among MSM, as well as rare penile cancers. Over 50 serotypes of HPV exist, many of which cause routine warts, some of which demonstrate enhanced tropism toward the anogenital region, such as serotypes 6 and 11. In addition to genital tropism, some serotypes, such as serotypes 16, 18, 31, 33, and 35, are associated with increased risk of cervical and anal cancer.[72] In one study, PCR of anal cancers revealed that 84% of these tumors were positive for HPV-16.[73] Although the causal link between anal cancer and HPV is not definitive, some sources cite an increase in prevalence of this once rare tumor to 35 per 100 000 in MSM, a phenomenon that may be fueled by immunocompromise attributed to HIV infection.[74]

Beyond possible cancer risk among men who engage in receptive anal intercourse, an awareness of the specifics of sexual activity of MSM is necessary to diagnose more atypical manifestations of HPV infection such as intra-anal lesions, urethral lesions, and oral lesions.

Genital warts are usually diagnosed morphologically. Biopsy is rarely necessary unless there is uncertainty regarding the diagnosis, there has been failure of standard therapy, the patient is immunocompromised, or lesions are ulcerated, adherent, indurated, or otherwise atypical. Four morphologies of warts are observed. The first and most common are the cauliflower shaped structures of condyloma acuminata. These warts tend to occur on partially keratinized area of genitals such as the underside of the foreskin. Genital warts may also appear as flesh colored, dome-shaped papules that are one to four mm in diameter; as hyperkeratotic lesions with a thick, horny layer and tend to occur on fully keratinized areas of genital skin; or as flat warts that may not be visible without biopsy or trichloroacetic acid (TCA) application (a procedure with poor sensitivity that turns HPV lesions white).

Urethral-meatal warts may present with dysuria and are a less common cause of nongonococcal urethritis. These lesions are seen in 1%-25% of patients with genital warts, and urethral involvement without external manifestations is rare. Lesions may be visible with everion of the meatus or by using a pediatric nasal speculum, but may rarely be as deep as the prostatic urethra, requiring urologic evaluation.

Men who engage in receptive anal sex may develop external warts perianally; up to one third or one half of these men may also have internal lesions that are often asymptomatic. Some men, however, may present with anal itch, anal discharge or bleeding, anal pain, prolapsing lesions, as well as tenesmus or obstructive symptoms. Diagnosis depends on visualization by anoscopy with or without TCA. Oral warts may occur through orogenital contact and are usually asymptomatic. Inidividuals diagnosed with anogenital warts should be examined for oral lesions.

Several treatment options exist for genital warts. Choosing the appropriate intervention depends on location of the lesions, as well as accessibility for patient-directed therapy. The goal of therapy is to eradicate symptomatic warts. Untreated warts may regress but may be persistent in some individuals with normal or compromised immune systems. Treatment does not decrease infectivity.[44] Podofilox 0.5% topical solution or gel may be used in patient-applied therapy. Treatment cycles consist of three days of BID application podofilox followed by a four-day hiatus. This cycle may be performed up to four times. Alternatively, Imiquimod five percent cream may be applied by the patient to warts at bedtime, three times per week for up to 16 weeks. The cream should be washed off with soapy water 6-10 hours after application since local reactions are not uncommon. Some situations may call for provider-applied therapy. Options include ablation using cryotherapy every 1-2 weeks, podophyllin resin 10%-25% applied weekly, or trichloroacetic acid (TCA) applied to lesions weekly. In severe cases, surgical removal of interferon injections may be needed. External anal warts may be treated with cryotherapy, trichloroacetic acid/bicholoracetic acid (TCA/BCA), or surgery. Internal warts should be managed in consultation with a specialist. Internal warts may not always be treated but may trigger enhanced observation for oncogenic transformation by high-resolution anospcopy using TCA stain and biopsy. Treatment of urethral-meatal warts include standard cryotherapy of podophyllin. Oral warts are ablated with cryotherapy or surgery.

Persistence of high-risk subtypes of HPV (16, 18, 31, 33, 35, 45) causes cervical dysplasia and cancer. Types 16 and 18 account for the majority of cervical cancers, but one or more of these subtypes can be found in 90% of high-grade intraepithelial precursor lesions. Specific genital types of human papillomavirus are the causative agent of cervical cancer and genital warts. Worldwide, HPV causes significant morbidity and mortality that can be prevented with the use of routine Pap testing.

HPV is considered an STI and has been associated with age of first sexual intercourse and the number of male partners for heterosexual women. Routine Pap tests screen for the presence abnormal cells on the surface of the cervix and precancerous lesions. HPV has been detected in WSW, even in the absence of a history of sex with men.[75] Risk factors associated with HPV detection in WSW are an increased number of male partners and the use of insertive sex toys between female partners.

HPV appears to increase the risk for anal cancer and is thought to cause precancerous lesions called anal squamous intraepithelial lesions (ASIL). Some experts and centers of excellence in MSM healthcare offer screening for these lesions using anal Pap smears and referral of positive tests to specialists for high-resolution anoscopy. There are no official guidelines, so practice is center-dependent despite increasing evidence that HPV disease may pose a significant health threat to MSM, specifically those with HIV infection. Some experts recommend that HIV-infected MSM who engage in receptive anal intercourse be screened once a year and that HIV-uninfected MSM who engage in receptive anal sex be screened every three to five years. Screening should only be performed if a specialist able to perform a high-resolution anoscopy and a biopsy is available. It is unclear if identification of anal dysplasia impacts disease course, and surgical interventions for high-grade lesions are difficult and may not be definitive. There is some evidence that unlike other malignancies, HAART may have little impact in modifying progression of dysplasia from lower to higher grade lesions in HIV-infected individuals.

Protective immunity against HPV has been demonstrated by two vaccine products, one of which (Gardasil®), has been approved by the FDA for use in women between the ages of 9-26 years old. The other product (Cervarix®) is pending approval. Gardasil® is a quadrivalent vaccine that provides protection against HPV 6, 11, 16, and 18. HPV 16 and 18 are the strains responsible for the majority of cervical cancer (70%) and may be the dominant strains responsible for anal dysplasia in MSM. HPV 6 and 11 are responsible for 90% of genital warts. Cervarix® is a bivalent vaccine that targets only the more frequently oncogenic strains of HPV (16 and 18). The Merck FUTURE II trial compared Gardasil® to placebo in 12 167 women and demonstrated 97% efficacy in preventing high-grade cervical dysplasia and persistent HPV 16 and 18 infections. Similar data has been generated in trials of GlaxoSmithKline's Cervarix® vaccine. Studies of Garadsil® in men have demonstrated immunogenicity, but endpoints are more difficult to interpret given the low frequency of anal dysplasia in the US. Although approved for ages 9-26, the HPV vaccines will likely be more efficacious if given earlier in life due to the high rate of HPV acquisition soon after initiating sexual activity. Specific recommendations are pending.[76-78]

The implications for LBGT patients are significant. HPV vaccine joins hepatitis B vaccination as a preventive intervention that can prevent a sexually transmitted infection that can lead to cancer. Ongoing studies will be needed to evaluate specific efficacy and indications in this population. Given the reports of HPV transmission among WSW and the emerging literature about HPV-associated anal dysplasia among HIV-uninfected and HIV-infected MSM, preventive or therapeutic vaccination against HPV may make a significant impact on cervical and anal malignancy in LGBT populations.

Molluscum contagiousum

Molluscum contagiosum is classically described in children but may be sexually transmitted among adults, often with lesions in the genital area. Transmission of the pox virus responsible for this infection is by skin to skin contact. These lesions are usually of little consequence but may be more severe and diffuse in immunocompromised patients such as those with HIV infection.

Routine cases of molluscum come to clinical attention because of the presence of flesh-colored papules between 1-5 mm in diameter. In rare cases, these lesions can grow to about one cm and may be numerous and confluent in immunocompromised people. The classic molluscum lesion has a central dimple, or umbillication. Other lesions may have such an umbillication, such as disseminated fungal infections in immunocompromised individuals, and should be kept on the differential diagnosis of molluscum. Molluscum lesions are distributed over areas of contact around and on the genitals, as well as around the anus. Diagnosis is morphologic. Biopsy is rarely necessary but will demonstrate pox-virus inclusions. Molluscum is self-limited in most individuals, but treatment accelerates resolution and may impact transmissibility.[79]

The CDC does not offer formal guidelines for treating this non-ulcerative sexually transmitted infection. Most commonly, ablative therapies such as cryotherapy with liquid nitrogen, curettage, or light electrocautery are used to treat molluscum. There is limited evidence for the use of cidofovir in disseminated infection in immunocompromised individuals

Ectoparasites

Pediculosis Pubis (Crabs)

Itch tends to be the most prominent complaint of infestation with crabs, although some people recognize the parasite and its nits. Hairy individuals may have more disseminated infestations with the louse, only sparing the scalp. Direct visualization of the lice or nits makes the diagnosis. Medical treatment, hygienic interventions, and aggressive treatment of sex partners are all necessary to eradicate this infestation. The CDC recommends topical treatment regimens, including: permethrin 1% cream, lindane 1% shampoo, and pyethrins with piperonyl butoxide. Ivermectin 200 mcg/kg taken by mouth weekly for two consecutive weeks is a systemic option. Infested individuals should be directed to machine wash all bedding, clothing, and towels and to use a heated setting when drying the laundry. Alternatively, clothes and bedding may be dry cleaned or put in garbage bags for 72 hours to kill the parasites and nits. Sexual partners should be treated simultaneously to avoid re-infection. Patients with ongoing symptoms after one week should be re-treated.

Sarcoptes Scabies (Scabies)

The main symptom of scabies is persistent itch. Generally, these symptoms progress over two to three weeks prior to medical attention and can last indefinitely. Worsening of the itch at night is a common complaint of infested individuals. Serpiginous burrows may be seen on examination of affected areas, often the webs of the fingers, and are pathognomonic of this parasite. A more severe and infectious variety of scabies called Norwegian scabies may be seen in immunocompromised hosts such as those with AIDS. These lesions are more psoriatic-appearing and are also called crusted scabies.

Lesions may be scraped for microscopic exam to identify mites, eggs, or feces. Application of a washable marker to affected skin then washing off the excess may highlight the burrows, facilitating diagnosis. Many practitioners treat empirically in the correct clinical setting even in the absence of mite or burrow demonstration.

Medical treatment, hygienic interventions, and aggressive treatment of sex partners are all necessary to eradicate this infestation. Topical therapies include permethrin cream (five percent) and lindane (one percent). Ivermectin 200 mcg/kg weekly for two consecutive weeks is a systemic option for treating scabies. Norwegian scabies may require dual therapy with topical permethrin and systemic ivermectin. Lindane should be avoided since skin integrity may be compromised with crusted scabies, increasing the risk of neurologic side effects. Infested individuals should be directed to machine wash all bedding, clothing, and towels and to use a heated setting when drying the laundry. Alternatively, clothes and bedding may be dry cleaned or put in garbage bags for 72 hours to kill the parasites and nits. Sexual partners should be treated simultaneously to avoid re-infection. Symptoms may persist for up to two weeks since the itch is a manifestation of a hypersensitivity reaction to antigens that may be present despite the lack of living mites. Re-treatment should be considered in patients with ongoing symptoms after two weeks.

Other/Emerging STIs

Viral Hepatitis

Both hepatitis A and B are vaccine-preventable sexually transmitted infections that disproportionately affect MSM. Additionally, an increasing body of evidence indicates that hepatitis C infection may be more commonly transmitted through certain sexual activities practiced by some MSM. Hepatitis A, B, and C may all present with prodromal gastrointestinal and systemic symptoms and may go on to jaundice with very elevated liver function tests. Alternatively, infection may be mild or asymptomatic. All can be fulminant and may require liver transplantation in severe cases. Hepatitis A infection is generally self-limited and does not have a chronic phase of infection but can be quite severe. Hepatitis B and C, however, can go on to chronic infection with associated liver disease such as cirrhosis and hepatocellular carcinoma. Although a complete discussion of therapy of these infections is beyond the scope of this chapter, prevention of these infections is an important tenet of sexual health.

Hepatitis A is transmitted through fecal-oral routes and can be transmitted through sexual activities that include oral-anal contact (rimming). Rimming, however, is not the only sexual activity through which hepatitis A may be transmitted since inadvertent fecal contamination may occur with any sexual activity. Acute liver failure may occur and is more common in older people. Although hepatitis A virus clears, symptom relapse may occur in up to 15% of patients.

Serologic testing confirms hepatitis A infection, with hepatitis A virus (HAV) IgM being diagnostic for acute infection. Total HAV Ig positivity in the absence of a positive HAV IgM implies past infection and immunity. Total HAV Ig may or may not be positive after immunization. Treatment of individuals with acute HAV infection is supportive. MSM and WSW should be offered vaccination against Hepatitis A. These highly immunogenic vaccines are administered in a two-dose schedule at zero and six to 12 months. Given the insensitivity of serologic testing, no testing is recommended to demonstrate vaccine take. In the event of sexual exposure to an individual with hepatitis A, immunoglobulin may be used as postexposure prophylaxis. If hepatitis A vaccine had been administered greater than one month before contacts with a case, adequate protection is established so that immunoglobulin does not have to be administered. Vaccination is not adequate postexposure prophylaxis but may be administered at the same time, but at a different site, as the immunoglobulin.

Hepatitis B is a virus transmitted through exposure to blood or other body fluids. Unlike HAV infection, it is not transmitted through the fecal-oral route. Up to six percent of acutely infected adults go on to chronic infection with HBV and have a 15%-25% chance of dying from cirrhosis or hepatocellular carcinoma. The complete diagnosis of hepatitis B status relies on serologic testing that may be difficult to interpret, if the surface antigen or antibody are not detected. Serologic tests are used to diagnose HBV infection and to ascertain immunity to this virus or prior vaccination efficacy.

Hepatitis B vaccination is recommended for MSM and WSW given the risk of HBV transmission. Prevaccination testing is recommended to assess exposure status. The CDC recommends screening with anti-HB core antibody testing, although provider practice may include either hepatitis B surface antigen (HbsAg) and/or hepatitis B surface antibody (HbsAb) . Vaccine is generally administered in three doses to enhance immunogenicity. Several schedules exist, but most practitioners use the zero–one–six month schedule for vaccination. Postvaccination testing with a HBsAb is routine in the HIV-infected population six months after vaccination to demonstrate take of the vaccine.

Both vaccine and high-titer hepatitis B surface antibody immunoglobulin (HBsAb IgG) (HBIG) have a role in postexposure prophylaxis individuals who have had sexual contact with an acutely infected person. Both should be administered as soon as possible but within 14 days of last sexual contact. There is no role for HBV postexposure prophylaxis for an exposure to a chronically infected individual.

Hepatitis C virus (HCV) generally causes mildly symptomatic or asymptomatic acute hepatitis, but the majority of acutely infected individuals go on to chronic hepatitis with associated risk of cirrhosis and hepatocellular carcinoma. It is most efficiently transmitted through exposure to blood and blood products. Recent outbreaks have highlighted the possibility of more efficient sexual transmission among MSM than previously thought.[80] These cases appeared to be related to incident LGV infection, drug use, and sexual activities such as fisting that may cause more extensive mucosal damage to the rectum. HCV is diagnosed serologically. Some experts advocate use of molecular techniques to identify acutely infected individuals in certain clinical settings before serologies become positive. Chronic hepatitis C may be treated with a combination of interferon and ribavirin; additionally, although not standard of care, treatment of acute infection is being evaluated in clinical trials. No proven preexposure or postexposure prophylaxis is available for HCV infection.

Enteric Bacterial and Parasitic Infections

Several enteric bacteria and parasites may cause enteritis or colitis among MSM. Individuals may present with either bloody or nonbloody diarrhea, depending on the pathogen, as well as other symptoms like abdominal pain, cramping, and fever. Diagnostic considerations should include anoscopy, stool culture, stool ova and parasite exams, and stool antigen/immunoassay test to ascertain the infectious or noninfectious cause of these symptoms. Simple proctitis without symptoms of colitis or enteritis should be treated as rectal gonorrhea and chlamydia co-infection unless perianal and anal ulcers raise suspicion for HSV infection, in which case HSV therapy should be initiated. LGV and other causes may require further evaluation.

Several bacteria have been reported to cause infections among MSM. These include outbreaks of shigella, Salmonella enteritis, typhoid fever, and Campylobacter. Fecal oral transmission has been implicated in many of these cases, and most individuals present with bloody diarrhea with constitutional symptoms. Diagnosis is through stool culture, and treatment should be tailored to the isolate. Empiric therapy with ciprofloxacin 500 mg PO BID for 3-5 days is indicated in severe cases.

Parasites such as *Entamoeba histolyica* and *Giardia lamblia* may also cause enteritis and colitis. Generally *E. histolytica* causes bloody diarrhea while *G. lamblia* causes high-volume watery stools. Microscopic evaluation of stool may miss some cases of these parasites, so *Entamoeba* antigen testing and *Giardia* immunoassays are becoming more available and popular to diagnose these infections. *Giardia* is usually treated with metronidazole 250 mg PO TID for five days, although other agents are also available. *Entamoeba histolytica* is treated with metronidazole followed by a luminal agent to eradicate luminal cysts such as paromomycin.

Community-Associated Methicillin-Resistant
Staphylococcus Aureus (CA-MRSA) Infection

CA-MRSA has been recognized as an infection associated with hospitals since the mid-1960s. More recently outbreaks of MRSA skin and soft tissue infections have been noted among MSM, as well as other risk groups. Although not classically a sexually transmitted infection, there is some data that these infections may be associated with club drug use and recruitment of sexual partners at bathhouses and sex parties.[81] Although many of these infections have been among HIV-infected men, there is conflicting data about the association of CD4 count and colonization or infection.

MRSA infections present with furuncles, cellulites, deep folliculitis, abscesses, and cellulitis. Many people present complaining of an insect bite like lesion or sore. Given the frequency of MRSA infections in some MSM communities, it is important to send gram stain and culture of pus from these lesions to better direct therapy. These lesions tend to respond better to drainage than they do to antibiotics alone. The clone of MRSA causing the majority of these community infections (USA 300) has virulence factors that appear to make it more invasive and tenacious than standard strains of S. aureus. There is no accepted regimen, and therapy should be initiated for severe infections before culture data is available. The organism is always resistant to beta lactam antibiotics and variably susceptible to other oral antibiotics. In addition to drainage, several empiric oral regimens are possible based on presumed resistance. These include high dose trimethoprim-sulfamethoxazole, clindamycin (avoid this regimen if strain is erythromycin resistant or inducible clindamycin resistance is demonstrated in the microbiology laboratory), or linezolid 600 mg PO BID x 10-14 days. Close follow-up is necessary to make sure that antibiotic response is adequate and to decide if further drainage is needed. Some experts include rifampin in treatment regimens as well. Intravenous vancomycin still retains activity against all strains of CA-MRSA identified to date and should be used in severe infections. Individuals with recurrent infections and nasal carriage may benefit from mupirocin nasal eradication.

Special Considerations in Sexually Transmitted Infections among WSW

Both the medical community and WSW as a group hold the misconception that WSW have a lower risk of contracting STIs than their female heterosexual counterparts. This assumption is erroneous on two levels. First, many WSW have traditional risk factors for contracting STIs from men. Surveys of WSW have revealed that there is great variability in their sexual behavior, and many have had past or current sexual relationships with men.[82] In most self-report surveys, greater that 80% of women who self-identify as lesbians have had sex with men.[83] The prevalence of many STIs in WSW in comparable or exceeds that in heterosexual women (see Table 11-12).

Table 11-12   STI Prevalence in Studies of Women Who Have Sex with Women

STI	Bailey et al study[87]	Pinto et al study[102]	Diamant et al study[103]
Bacterial vaginosis	31.40%	33.80%	
Candida species	18.40%	25.60%	
Genital warts	1.60%		
Trichomonas	1.30%	3.50%	6%
Genital herpes	1.10%		3.30%
Chlamydia	0.60%	1.50%	4.60%
Gonorrhea	0.30%		3.30%
PID	0.30%		2%
Syphilis		0.70%	0.30%
HIV		2.90%	0.10%
Hepatitis B		7%	
Hepatitis C	0.00%	2.10%	
HPV infection		6.20%	4.80%
HPV cervical CIN		4.90%	

Secondly, STI transmission has been reported in the absence of a history of sexual contact with men. Cervical human papillomavirus has been reported to occur in 21% of lesbian women who report having no previous sexual contact with men.[84] Genital herpes is also prevalent in a significant number of WSW who never had previous sexual contact with men. Compared to their heterosexual counterparts, WSW are less likely to seek routine medical care including preventive screening.[27,85] Lesbians tend not to routinely disclose sexual behavior to their care providers.[86]

Bacterial Vaginosis

Bacterial vaginosis (BV), originally described in the late 1950s, is a common cause of vaginal complaints in women. Compared to age-matched heterosexual women, lesbians have a higher rate of bacterial vaginosis (BV). Lesbian couples tend to have concordant vaginal flora including the presence of BV. Studies have shown an increased risk associated with multiple sexual partners. There is evidence that supports the theory that in the lesbian population BV can be considered an STI. A Seattle cohort found a BV prevalence of 27% compared to the reported prevalence of 5%-20% in US women who have sex with men.

While vaginal irritation and pain on urination or after sexual activity is usually rare or mild, the condition is characterized by a copious gray-colored discharge and a distinct, foul-smelling "fishy" odor. The fishy vaginal odor can become more pronounced after sexual intercourse or during menses. Many women can be completely asymptomatic and are often diagnosed with BV during routine screening or in conjunction with another diagnosis.

The definitive bacterial agent of BV remains in dispute. The predominate bacteria of the normal vaginal flora is lactobacillus species. In BV lactobacillus is replaced by *Gardnerella vaginalis* and other species including *Prevotella bivia, Prevotella disiens, Peptostreptococcus,* and *Mobiluncus.* Some of the bacteria associated with BV are common colonizers of the rectum, and it may serve as a reservoir for BV-associated flora, similar to the pathogenesis of female urinary tract infections. BV has been associated with adverse outcomes in pregnancy including premature rupture of membranes, chorioamnionitis, postpartum endometritis, and fetal loss.[88,89]

The criteria for the diagnosis of BV in the presence of a vaginal discharge are a vaginal pH greater than 4.6, a positive whiff test with 10% potassium hydroxide (KOH), and the microscopic presence of clue cells. Clue cells represent the abundant coccobacilli bacteria adhering to vaginal epithelial cells. The treatment of BV is highly effective. The standard treatment is metronidazole 500 mg orally twice a day for seven days. The higher two-gram oral dose taken once has the advantage of witnessed compliance to treatment and coverage for trichomonas but is less effective and has an increased incidence of gastrointestinal side effects. Treatment can also be given intravaginally with preparations containing metronidazole or clindamycin.

While asymptomatic women found to have BV are usually not treated, special considerations should be taken into account with WSW patients. Given BV's association with adverse outcomes in pregnancy, all pregnant women and those actively trying to become pregnant should be treated. Since there is some evidence to support that BV may represent an STI in WSW, it can be concluded that treatment of an asymptomatic carrier may decrease transmission. This may be more relevant in the case of recurrent or refractory disease in a female partner in a monogamous lesbian couple. To date there is no clinical data to support treatment of asymptomatic partners.

Trichomonas Vaginalis

Trichomonas vaginalis is a protozoan parasite transmitted principally through vaginal intercourse. Trichomonads can also be spread through direct contact with infected material—underwear, wash cloths, or towels. Infection with the organism, while frequently asymptomatic, can cause vaginitis in women and urethritis in men. Symptoms include yellow-green, frothy, foul-smelling vaginal discharge, itching or tenderness in the vagina, pain during sex, or urinary frequency. Transmission of trichomonas has been reported among a lesbian couple. Unlike bacterial vaginosis, trichomonas has not been associated with adverse outcomes in pregnancy. Data from small studies in African women suggests that *Trichomonas* may play a role in facilitating HIV transmission. While there is definitive evidence that ulcerative STIs promote HIV acquisition, *T. vaginalis* may be an important cofactor. While expensive PCR-based diagnostic testing has been developed, the diagnosis can be made by visualization of the motile parasites on wet mount. Trichomonas vaginalis infections are usually treated with a one-time dose of metronidazole two gm orally. Studies have shown that at least five percent of clinical cases of trichomoniasis are caused by parasites resistant to the drug.

Vulvo-vaginal Candidiasis

Approximately 75% of all women will have at least one episode of vaginal candidiasis (VVC) in their lifetime. Symptoms include caceous vaginal discharge with accompanying vulvar puritis, irritation, and dysuria. Candida species can be normal colonizers of the female lower genital tract, and infection usually represents overgrowth. Based on heterosexual data, VCC is not normally acquired through sexual intercourse, although medical professionals sometimes offer treatment to male partners of women who have recurrent episode or more than four episodes a year. Frequent episodes of VCC should prompt an evaluation for an underlying cause of immunodeficiency, including diabetic screening and HIV testing.

PID and Mucopurulent Cervicitis

Pelvic inflammatory disease includes infections of the upper female genital tract, including endometritis, tubo-ovarian abscess, and salpingitis. *Neissera gonorrhea* and *Chlamydia trachomatis* are the most common implicated causative organisms. Empiric treatment for both gonorrhea and chlamydia should be initiated if adenexal or cervical motion tenderness is detected on manual exam. Infection with gonorrhea or chlamydia has been reported in WSW, but only in those with a history of sex with men. Asymptomatic male partners should be treated, but there are no established guidelines to recommend treatment to female partners of WSW.

HIV and Blood-borne Viruses

While there have been case reports of transmission of HIV between WSW who have no other risk factors, CDC data suggest that the absence of other risk factors is exceedingly rare.[90,91] In population-based survey data, HIV infection in WSW has mainly been through behaviors not associated with sex between women. Risk factors that have been consistently associated with HIV infection in WSW are a history of sex with MSM, intravenous drug use, the practice of needle sharing, and the exchange of sex for money.[92] There is a theoretical risk of transmission of HIV and other blood-borne STIs through mucous membrane exposure in the presence of infected vaginal fluids or menstrual blood. Hepatitis B and C share common routes of transmission with HIV. Surveys of sexual practices and STI prevalence in WSW rarely include infectious hepatitis. Prevention strategies implemented to reduce HIV infection should theoretically reduce the incidence of hepatitis B and C.

Special Considerations in Sexually Transmitted Infections among Transgender Persons

The sexual health of transgender individuals from the perspective of sexually transmitted infections is a particular challenge. Several barriers exist between patient and provider that require particular attention to optimize STI-related care. One common issue is the often overlooked close examination of the genitalia of transgender patients. It is important that screening, symptomatic testing, and syndrome identification be guided by a complete examination and understanding of the patient's sexual anatomy. Testing should be based on the specific anatomy and sexual organs present. Providers and patients are often of the erroneous belief that infections like gonorrhea do not affect surgically altered organs.[93–95] It is important to clarify symptoms experienced and their relation to specific sexual activity to guide diagnostics and therapeutics. Extraordinary sexual diversity exists among transgender patients, so enhanced efforts at obtaining a clear sexual and social history is critical. In the absence of guidelines, the provider needs to tailor their assessment to the transgender patient's unique risks and anatomy. Additionally, special emphasis should be given to assessing the transgender patient for domestic/partner violence and participation in sex work since these may be associated with incident STI and HIV.[96] Complete medical evaluation requires the knowledge of the transgender patient's hormonal status, as well as specific anatomy. For instance, female-to-male transgender people who are exposed to androgen therapy and who retain a cervix may demonstrate histologic changes consistent with dysplasia.[97]

Most studies of transgender patients and STI risk focus on sex workers. More effort should be made to enhance our knowledge about the behaviors and biology of individuals who do not engage in sex commerce. Although limited by the bias of studying sex workers, these studies demonstrate a high incidence of domestic violence and sex work-related violence among these individuals. When compared to MSM, transgender patients have an increased prevalence of syphilis, as well as a high rate of HSV, gonorrhea, and HPV infection.[96,98] STI interventions in this population should focus on routine harm reduction, as well as specialized counseling regarding injection drug use (both hormonal and nonhormonal) and social stigma with its significant effect on employability and access to services for this population.[99,100]

Conclusion

Sex, however or with whomever it is performed, should be a joyous part of life. Understanding a patient's sexuality and sexual activities allows for troubleshooting to maintain sexual satisfaction and preventive interventions to maintain sexual health. LGBT sex is not about pathology, HIV, or sexually transmitted infections; rather it is about satisfaction and good health. LGBT sex is normal sex. Omission of a sexual history from a medical assessment or minimization of sexual issues is not a neutral mistake. Not asking about sex implies a judgment that sex is not healthy or a part of healthcare. To marginalized communities that already doubt the validity of their sexual feelings, this tacit judgment is tantamount to invalidating the normalcy of their sexual selves. Asking about sexuality and sexual satisfaction affirms and validates your patient's sexual identity. Engaging your patient and partnering for their sexual health is equivalent to accepting and supporting a healthy sexual life without judgment or presumption.

Summary Points

- Asking about sexual identity and behavior are critical in providing appropriate healthcare to all patients.
- Sexual dysfunction is common among LGBT patients and should be discussed so appropriate interventions and therapies can be offered.
- Many patients do not know about the STI/HIV risks associated with certain behaviors. Educating them allows them to make informed decisions about the level of risk they are willing to accept.
- It is important to educate patients about safer sex, focusing on harm-reduction advice to minimize personal risk for HIV. It is also important to point out that safer sex techniques to prevent HIV do not always prevent other STIs.
- Routine screening for HIV and STIs should be a standard part of the healthcare of LGBT clients.
- Routine and streamlined HIV testing should be offered in all healthcare settings, following CDC guidelines and local laws.
- The signs and symptoms of STIs should guide the choice of diagnostic tests and therapies. Keep in mind special treatment considerations among LGBT patients such as the emergence of quinolone resistant gonorrhea among MSM.
- LGBT clients should be vaccinated against sexually transmitted pathogens like hepatitis A and B.
- Addressing the sexual health of LGBT patients should be a routine and normal part of their primary care.

References

1. **Bell R**. ABC of sexual health: homosexual men and women. BMJ. 1999;318:452–5.
2. **Potter JE**. Do ask, do tell. Ann Intern Med. 2002;137:341-3.
3. **Bonvicini KA, Perlin MJ**. The same but different: clinician-patient communication with gay and lesbian patients. Patient Education and Counseling. 2003;51:115-22.
4. **King M, Nazareth I**. The health of people classified as lesbian, gay and bisexual attending family practitioners in London: a controlled study. BMC Public Health. 2006;6:127.
5. **Briganti A, Salonia A, Deho F, et al**. Clinical update on phosphodiesterase type-5 inhibitors for erectile dysfunction. World J Urol. 2005;23:374-84.
6. **Swearingen SG, Klausner JD**. Sildenafil use, sexual risk behavior, and risk for sexually transmitted diseases, including HIV infection. Am J Med. 2005;118:571-7.
7. **Cove J, Petrak J**. Factors associated with sexual problems in HIV-positive gay men. Int J STD AIDS. 2004;15:732-6.
8. **Richardson D, Lamba H, Goldmeier D, Nalabanda A, Harris JR**. Factors associated with sexual dysfunction in men with HIV infection. Int J STD AIDS. 2006;17:764-7.
9. **Balon R**. Antidepressants in the treatment of premature ejaculation. J Sex Marital Ther. 1996;22:85-96.
10. **Butcher J**. ABC of sexual health: female sexual problems I: loss of desire-what about the fun? BMJ. 1999;318:41-3.
11. **Butcher J**. ABC of sexual health: female sexual problems II: sexual pain and sexual fears. BMJ. 1999;318:110-2.
12. **Mayor S**. Pfizer will not apply for a licence for sildenafil for women. BMJ. 2004;328:542.
13. **Harry Benjamin International Gender Dysphoria Association**. Standards of Care for Gender Identity Disorders [publication online]. 6th ed. 2001. Available at http://www.wpath.org.
14. **Gill SK, Loveday C, Gilson RJ**. Transmission of HIV-1 infection by oroanal intercourse. Genitourinary medicine. 1992;68:254-7.
15. **AIDS InfoNet. Safer Sex Guidelines**. The Body: The Complete HIV/AIDS Resource. 2005. Available at http://www.thebody.com/content/art6098.html.
16. **Wolitski RJ, Halkitis PN, Parsons JT, Gomez CA**. Awareness and use of untested barrier methods by HIV-seropositive gay and bisexual men. AIDS Educ Prev. 2001;13:291-301.
17. **Pudney J, Oneta M, Mayer K, Seage G III, Anderson D**. Pre-ejaculatory fluid as potential vector for sexual transmission of HIV-1. Lancet. 1992;340:1470.
18. **Halkitis PN, Parsons JT and Wilton L**. Barebacking among gay and bisexual men in New York City: explanations for the emergence of intentional unsafe behavior. Arch Sex Behav. 2003;32:351-7.
19. **Ilaria G, Jacobs JL, Polsky B, et al**. Detection of HIV-1 DNA sequences in pre-ejaculatory fluid. Lancet. 1992;340:1469.
20. **Cohen MS, Hoffman IF, Royce RA, et al**. Reduction of concentration of HIV-1 in semen after treatment of urethritis: implications for prevention of sexual transmission of HIV-1. AIDSCAP Malawi Research Group. Lancet. 1997;349:1868-73.
21. **Quinn TC, Wawer MJ, Sewankambo N, et al**. Viral load and heterosexual transmission of human immunodeficiency virus type 1. Rakai Project Study Group. N Engl J Med. 2000;342:921-9.
22. **Rietmeijer CA, Patnaik JL, Judson FN, Douglas JM Jr**. Increases in gonorrhea and sexual risk behaviors among men who have sex with men: a 12-year trend analysis at the Denver Metro Health Clinic. Sex Transm Dis. 2003;30:562-7.
23. **George C, Alary M, Otis J, et al**. Nonnegligible increasing temporal trends in unprotected anal intercourse among men who have sexual relations with other men in Montreal. J Acquir Immune Defic Syndr. 2006;42:207-12.

24. **Crepaz N, Hart TA, Marks G**. Highly active antiretroviral therapy and sexual risk behavior: a meta-analytic review. JAMA. 2004;292:224-36.

25. **Elford J, Bolding G, Sherr L**. Seeking sex on the Internet and sexual risk behaviour among gay men using London gyms. AIDS. 2001;15:1409-15.

26. **Mansergh G, Colfax GN, Marks G, Rader M, Guzman R, Buchbinder S**. The Circuit Party Men's Health Survey: findings and implications for gay and bisexual men. Am J Public Health. 2001;91:953-8.

27. **Fethers K, Marks C, Mindel A, Estcourt CS**. Sexually transmitted infections and risk behaviours in women who have sex with women. Sexually Transmitted Infections. 2000; 76:345-9.

28. **Marrazzo JM, Koutsky LA, Handsfield HH**. Characteristics of female sexually transmitted disease clinic clients who report same-sex behaviour. International Journal of STD & AIDS. 2001;12:41-6.

29. **Marrazzo JM, Coffey P, Elliott MN**. Sexual practices, risk perception and knowledge of sexually transmitted disease risk among lesbian and bisexual women. Perspectives on Sexual & Reproductive Health. 2005;37:6-12.

30. **Elifson KW, Boles J, Posey E, Sweat M, Darrow W, Elsea W**. Male transvestite prostitutes and HIV risk. Am J Public Health. 1993;83:260-2.

31. **Galli M, Esposito R, Antinori S, et al**. HIV-1 infection, tuberculosis, and syphilis in male transsexual prostitutes in Milan, Italy. J Acquir Immune Defic Syndr. 1991;4:1006-7.

32. **Modan B, Goldschmidt R, Rubinstein E, et al**. Prevalence of HIV antibodies in transsexual and female prostitutes. Am J Public Health. 1992;82:590-2.

33. **Spizzichino L, Casella P, Zaccarelli M, Rezza G, Venezia S, Gattari P**. HIV infection among foreign people involved in HIV-related risk activities and attending an HIV reference centre in Rome: the possible role of counselling in reducing risk behaviour. AIDS Care. 1998;10:473-80.

34. **Tirelli U, Vaccher E, Bullian P, et al**. HIV-1 seroprevalence in male prostitutes in northeast Italy. J Acquir Immune Defic Syndr. 1988;1:414-5.

35. **Nemoto T, Luke D, Mamo L, Ching A, Patria J**. HIV risk behaviours among male-to-female transgenders in comparison with homosexual or bisexual males and heterosexual females. AIDS Care. 1999;11:297-312.

36. **Stephens T, Cozza S, Braithwaite RL**. Transsexual orientation in HIV risk behaviours in an adult male prison. Int J STD AIDS. 1999;10:28-31.

37. **Clements-Nolle K, Marx R, Guzman R, Katz M**. HIV prevalence, risk behaviors, health care use, and mental health status of transgender persons: implications for public health intervention. Am J Public Health. 2001;91:915-21.

38. **Pinkerton SD, Abramson PR**. Effectiveness of condoms in preventing HIV transmission. Soc Sci Med. 1997;44:1303-12.

39. **Quinn TC**. Circumcision and HIV transmission: the cutting edge [Abstract 120]. Presented at the Conference on Retroviruses and Opportunistic Infections (CROI). Denver, CO; 2006.

40. **Smith DK, Grohskopf LA, Black RJ, et al**. Antiretroviral postexposure prophylaxis after sexual, injection-drug use, or other nonoccupational exposure to HIV in the United States: recommendations from the US Department of Health and Human Services. MMWR Recomm Rep. 2005;54:1-20.

41. **Renzi C, Douglas JM, Jr., Foster M, et al**. Herpes Simplex Virus Type 2 Infection as a Risk Factor for Human Immunodeficiency Virus Acquisition in Men Who Have Sex with Men. The Journal of Infectious Diseases. 2003;187:19-25.

41. **Nagot N, Foulongne V, Becquart P, et al**. Longitudinal assessment of HIV-1 and HSV-2 shedding in the genital tract of West African women. J Acquir Immune Defic Syndr. 2005;39:632-4.

42. **Dhawan D, Keller M, Klotman ME**. Topical microbicides: the time has come. AIDS Read. 2006;16:144-8, 155-8, 161; discussion 148, 156-7.

43. **Branson BM, Handsfield HH, Lampe MA, et al**. Revised recommendations for HIV testing of adults, adolescents, and pregnant women in health-care settings. MMWR Recomm Rep. 2006;55:1-17; quiz CE1-4.

44. **Centers for Disease Control and Prevention**. Sexually Transmitted Diseases Treatment Guidelines 2006. MMWR Morb Mortal Wkly Rep. 2006;55:1-100.

45. **Wawer MJ, Gray RH, Sewankambo NK, et al**. Rates of HIV-1 transmission per coital act, by stage of HIV-1 infection, in Rakai, Uganda. J Infect Dis. 2005;191:1403-9.

46. **Feldman J, Bockting W**. Transgender health. Minn Med. 2003;86:25-32.

47. **Mandell GL, Bennett JE, Dolin R**. Principles and Practice of Infectious Diseases. Vol. 2. 5th ed. Churchill Livingstone; 2000.

48. **Centers for Disease Control and Prevention**. Sexually Transmitted Disease Surveillance 2004 Supplement, Chlamydia Prevalence Monitoring Project Annual Report. U.S. Department of Health and Human Services, Centers for Disease Control and Prevention; 2005.

49. **Ciemins EL, Flood J, Kent CK, et al**. Reexamining the prevalence of Chlamydia trachomatis infection among gay men with urethritis: implications for STD policy and HIV prevention activities. Sex Transm Dis. 2000;27:249-51.

50. **Nieuwenhuis RF, Ossewaarde JM, Gotz HM, et al**. Resurgence of lymphogranuloma venereum in Western Europe: an outbreak of Chlamydia trachomatis serovar l2 proctitis in The Netherlands among men who have sex with men. Clin Infect Dis. 2004;39:996-1003.

51. **Bradshaw CS, Tabrizi SN, Read TR, et al**. Etiologies of nongonococcal urethritis: bacteria, viruses, and the association with orogenital exposure. J Infect Dis. 2006;193:336-45.

52. **Klausner JD, Kohn R, Kent C**. Etiology of clinical proctitis among men who have sex with men. Clin Infect Dis. 2004;38:300-2.

53. **Eley A, Oxley KM, Spencer RC, Kinghorn GR, Ben-Ahmeida ET, Potter CW**. Detection of Chlamydia trachomatis by the polymerase chain reaction in young patients with acute epididymitis. European Journal of Clinicial Microbiology & Infectious Diseases. 1992;11:620-3.

54. **Wagenlehner FM, Weidner W, Naber KG**. Chlamydial infections in urology. World J Urol. 2006;24:4-12.

55. **Centers for Disease Control and Prevention**. Sexually Transmitted Diseases Treatment Guidelines 2002. MMWR Recomm Rep. 2002; 51:1-84.

56. **Centers for Disease Control and Prevention**. Lymphogranuloma Venereum Among Men Who Have Sex With Men—Netherlands, 2003-2004. MMWR Morb Mortal Wkly Rep. 2004; 53:986-8.

57. **Burstein GR, Zenilman JM**. Nongonococcal urethritis—a new paradigm. Clin Infect Dis. 1999;28:S66-73.

58. **Hoosen AA, Coetzee KD, van den Ende J**. A microbiological study of failed penicillin therapy for gonococcal urethritis in Durban. S Afr Med J. 1990;78:189-91.

59. **Fox KK, del Rio C, Holmes KK, et al**. Gonorrhea in the HIV era: a reversal in trends among men who have sex with men. Am J Public Health. 2001;91:959-64.

60. **Mark KE, Gunn RA**. Gonorrhea surveillance: estimating epidemiologic and clinical characteristics of reported cases using a sample survey methodology. Sex Transm Dis. 2004;31:215-20.

61. **Sherrard J, Barlow D**. Gonorrhoea in men: clinical and diagnostic aspects. Genitourin Med. 1996;72:422-426.

62. **Holmes KK, Berger RE, Alexander ER**. Acute epididymitis: etiology and therapy. Arch Androl. 1979;3:309-16.

63. **O'Brien JP, Goldenberg DL, Rice PA**. Disseminated gonococcal infection: a prospective analysis of 49 patients and a review of pathophysiology and immune mechanisms. Medicine [Baltimore]. 1983;62:395-406.

64. **Centers for Disease Control and Prevention**. Increases in Fluoroquinolone-Resistant Neisseria gonorrhoeae Among Men who Have Sex with Men—United States, 2003, and Revised Recommendations for Gonorrhea Treatment, 2004. MMWR 2004; 53:335-8.

65. **Golden MR, Marra CM, Holmes KK**. Update on syphilis: resurgence of an old problem. JAMA. 2003;290:1510-4.

66. **DiCarlo RP, Martin DH**. The clinical diagnosis of genital ulcer disease in men. Clin Infect Dis. 1997;25:292-8.

67. **Benedetti J, Corey L, Ashley R**. Recurrence rates in genital herpes after symptomatic first-episode infection. Ann Intern Med. 1994;121:847-54.

68. **Reeves WC, Corey L, Adams HG, Vontver LA, Holmes KK**. Risk of recurrence after first episodes of genital herpes. Relation to HSV type and antibody response. N Engl J Med. 1981;305:315-9.

69. **Kimberlin DW, Rouse DJ**. Clinical practice. Genital herpes. N Engl J Med. 2004; 350:1970-7.

70. **Dylewski JS, Bekhor S**. Mollaret's meningitis caused by herpes simplex virus type 2: case report and literature review. Eur J Clin Microbiol Infect Dis. 2004;23:560-2.

71. **Corey L, Wald A, Patel R, et al**. Once-daily valacyclovir to reduce the risk of transmission of genital herpes. N Engl J Med. 2004;350:11-20.

72. **Palefsky JM, Cranston RD**. Virology of human papillomavirus infections and the link to cancer. UpToDate, Online Version 9.2. Available at http://63.240.11.74/topic.asp?file =tumorhiv/2277#3

73. **Frisch M, Glimelius B, van den Brule AJ, et al**. Sexually transmitted infection as a cause of anal cancer. N Engl J Med. 1997;337:1350-8.

74. **Daling JR, Weiss NS, Hislop TG, et al**. Sexual practices, sexually transmitted diseases, and the incidence of anal cancer. N Engl J Med. 1987;317:973-7.

75. **Marrazzo JM, Koutsky LA, Kiviat NB, Kuypers JM, Stine K**. Papanicolaou test screening and prevalence of genital human papillomavirus among women who have sex with women. Am J Public Health. 2001;91:947-52.

76. **Harper DM, Franco EL, Wheeler CM, et al**. Sustained efficacy up to 4.5 years of a bivalent L1 virus-like particle vaccine against human papillomavirus types 16 and 18: follow-up from a randomised control trial. Lancet. 2006;367:1247-55.

77. **Speck LM, Tyring SK**. Vaccines for the prevention of human papillomavirus infections. Skin Therapy Letter. 2006;11:1-3.

78. **Stanley MA**. Human papillomavirus vaccines. Reviews of Medical Virology. 2006;16:139-49.

79. **van der Wouden JC, Menke J, Gajadin S, et al**. Interventions for cutaneous molluscum contagiosum. Cochrane Database Syst Rev 2006:CD004767.

80. **Gotz HM, van Doornum G, Niesters HG, den Hollander JG, Thio HB, de Zwart O**. A cluster of acute hepatitis C virus infection among men who have sex with men—results from contact tracing and public health implications. AIDS. 2005;19:969-74.

81. **Lee NE, Taylor MM, Bancroft E, et al**. Risk factors for community-associated methicillin-resistant Staphylococcus aureus skin infections among HIV-positive men who have sex with men. Clin Infect Dis. 2005;40:1529-34.

82. **Makadon HJ**. Improving health care for the lesbian and gay communities. N Engl J Med. 2006;354:895-7.

83. **Diamant AL, Schuster MA, McGuigan K, Lever J**. Lesbians' sexual history with men: implications for taking a sexual history. Archives of Internal Medicine. 1999;159:2730-6.

84. **Marrazzo JM, Koutsky LA, Stine KL, et al**. Genital human papillomavirus infection in women who have sex with women. Journal of Infectious Diseases. 1998;178:1604-9.

85. **Fish J, Anthony D**. UK National Lesbians and Health Care Survey. Women Health. 2005;41:27-45.

86. **Roberts SJ, Sorensen L**. Health related behaviors and cancer screening of lesbians: results from the Boston Lesbian Health Project. Women Health. 1999;28:1-12.

87. **Bailey JV, Farquhar C, Owen C and Mangtani P**. Sexually transmitted infections in women who have sex with women. Sex Transm Infect. 2004;80:244-246.

88. **Hillier SL, Nugent RP, Eschenbach DA, et al**. Association between bacterial vaginosis and preterm delivery of a low-birth-weight infant. The Vaginal Infections and Prematurity Study Group. N Engl J Med. 1995;333:1737-42.

89. **Swedberg JA**. Bacterial vaginosis: etiology, association with preterm labor, diagnosis, and management. Compr Ther. 1989;15:47-53.

90. **Rich JD, Buck A, Tuomala RE, Kazanjian PH**. Transmission of human immunodeficiency virus infection presumed to have occurred via female homosexual contact. Clin Infect Dis. 1993;17:1003-5.

91. **Centers for Disease Control and Prevention**. HIV/AIDS and US women who have sex with women. Available at http://www.cdc.gov/hiv/pubs/facts/wsw.htm. Accessed July 31, 2006.

92. **White JC**. HIV risk assessment and prevention in lesbians and women who have sex with women: practical information for clinicians. Health Care for Women International. 1997;18:127-38.

93. **Fiumara NJ, Asvadi S**. Asymptomatic gonococcal urethritis in a male transsexual female. The British Journal of Venereal Diseases. 1978;54:130-1.

94. **Bodsworth NJ, Price R, Davies SC**. Gonococcal infection of the neovagina in a male-to-female transsexual. Sex Transm Dis. 1994;21:211-2.

95. **Haustein UF**. Pruritus of the artificial vagina of a transsexual patient caused by gonococcal infection. Hautarzt. 1995;46:858-9.

96. **Cohan D, Lutnick A, Davidson P, et al**. Sex worker health: San Francisco style. Sex Transm Infect. 2006;82:418-22.

97. **Miller N, Bedard YC, Cooter NB, Shaul DL**. Histological changes in the genital tract in transsexual women following androgen therapy. Histopathology. 1986;10:661-9.

98. **Pisani E, Girault P, Gultom M, et al**. HIV, syphilis infection, and sexual practices among transgenders, male sex workers, and other men who have sex with men in Jakarta, Indonesia. Sex Transm Infect. 2004;80:536-40.

99. **Lombardi E**. Enhancing transgender health care. Am J Public Health. 2001;91:869-72.

100. **Lombardi EL, Wilchins RA, Priesing D, Malouf D**. Gender violence: transgender experiences with violence and discrimination. J Homosex. 2001;42:89-101.

101. **Kahn JO, Walker BD**. Acute human immunodeficiency virus type 1 infection. N Engl J Med. 1998;339:33-9.

102. **Pinto VM, Tancredi MV, Tancredi NA, Buchalla CM**. Sexually transmitted disease/HIV risk behaviour among women who have sex with women. AIDS. 2005;19:S64-9.

103. **Diamant AL, Schuster MA, McGuigan K, Lever J**. Lesbians' sexual history with men: implications for taking a sexual history. Arch Intern Med. 1999;159:2730-6.

TRANSGENDER AND INTERSEX HEALTH

Chapter 12

Introduction to Transgender Identity and Health

RANDI KAUFMAN, PsyD

Introduction

The *Metamorphosis*, Franz Kafka's well-known story, opens with the preposterous plight of an ordinary man who has been transformed into a giant insect. Despite being an insect, Gregor Samsa continues to think and feel like a human being. However, as an insect he is unable to communicate with his family and is unable to solicit their help, their empathy, or even the ability to tell them who he is. Time passes in this bizarre, tortuous state of affairs, and Gregor slowly becomes aware that his situation is insurmountable, as he does not turn back into a human being. His will to survive persists for a time but eventually fades away. The turning point comes when his sister cries out that if this insect were in fact Gregor, he would have gone away willingly, as he would understand that his family could not live with "such a creature." Recognizing the agony his family feels, Gregor's wish to live is transformed into a wish to die. He dies in a state of meditation, suggesting that he wills himself into death, as a loving act toward his family.

The Metamorphosis is often read as a metaphor for spiritual disintegration, resulting from the impossibility of escaping one's circumstances. It suggests confusion, humiliation, ridicule, and utter isolation when others cannot see one for who one is. The story suggests that even despite being rejected, one may desire to sacrifice one's self in order to spare one's family, as the ultimate act of love.

In many ways, *The Metamorphosis* describes the predicament of a transgender person. In tandem with the realization that the relationship between their anatomical sex and gender identity is different from that of other people, transgender individuals quickly become aware that they are subject to rejection, ridicule, humiliation, and isolation. Like Gregor, some transgender individuals choose to sacrifice themselves in order to spare their loved ones. This sacrifice can be concrete and permanent, as in the case of suicide, or abstract, as when a person keeps this identity repressed, resulting in psychic death. Fortunately, many transgender people choose to come out, rather than to surrender.

Coming out as transgender is an act of courage that includes taking huge risks, being willing to test relationships, and trusting that peoples' caring and respect will supersede a negative outcome.

We are currently at a crossroads in our understanding and acceptance of gender identity development. On the one hand, the prevailing view of gender continues to be that a person is either a man or a woman and that their internal sense of being male or female is inextricably tied to their anatomy. This view is reflected by the fact that gender identity disorder is still listed as a diagnosis in the most recent *Diagnostic and Statistical Manual of Mental Disorders* (DSM-IV), thus labeling gender identity differences as mental illness. On the other hand, it is becoming increasingly clear that gender identity questioning is occurring more frequently, and current clinical thinking suggests that gender identity issues are not a sign of psychopathology.[1] The high incidence of mental health problems and substance abuse found in people with gender identity issues is now believed to result from cultural discrimination and intolerance, often coupled with a lack of social and financial supports needed to respond to these challenges. Understanding transgender issues within this larger psychosocial context, rather than as a mental disorder, has resulted in a movement toward taking gender identity disorder out of the DSM, similar to the way in which homosexuality was removed in 1973.

The purpose of this chapter is to provide a general context of transgender issues and experience so that healthcare providers may be more informed when working with the transgender population and thereby offer more sensitive, pertinent, and supportive care.

Definitions

Sex, Gender, and Gender Identity

The terms sex, gender, and gender identity tend to be used in different ways and can therefore be confusing. The two-sex, two-gender model that is most familiar to us today[2] uses the term "sex" to describe a person's body—that is, the objective biological (chromosomal) and anatomical (internal and external genital) characteristics that society recognizes as male or female. "Gender" is used variously to describe a person's gender identity (the internal sense of being male or female, regardless of biology), or gender role (the roles, behaviors and attributes—masculine or feminine—that a society considers appropriate for men and women). According to this binary model, every person is defined as either a man or a woman, gender is fixed and rooted in biological sex, and the accepted gender role is dictated by apparent gender. This model excludes intersex people, who are born with sex chromosomes, external genitalia, and/or internal reproductive organs that are not exclusively male or female. In addition, it fails to account for people who perceive themselves to be a gender that is different from the one they were assigned at birth, and it negates the experience of an emerging group of people who describe gender as other than just male or just female.

New models of sex and gender[3] are beginning to be described, moving us away from the familiar two-sex (male and female), two-gender (masculine and feminine) model where sex and gender are dichotomous constructs, toward models that might be described as "polysex" or "polygender." These models provide a more complete understanding of the diversity and complexity of sex and gender, and permit greater self-expression. The models further distinguish the differences between sex (the objective categorization of one's biology as male, female, or intersex), sexual orientation (whom one is attracted to), gender identity (a subjective sense of oneself as male, female, or other), gender role (cultural expectations that one follow a set of prescribed behavioral norms based on one's gender), gender presentation (how one looks),[4] gender performance (how one acts),[4] gender assignment (gender that is assigned at birth by a medical provider,[5] usually based on appearance of the external genitalia), and gender attribution (attribution of one person's gender by another, based on cultural interpretation of gender cues).[5]

What Does It Mean to Be "Transgender"?

Transgender people are individuals who transgress societally constructed gender norms in one manner or another. However, the language in the field is still evolving: the term "transgender" is used in so many ways that it is not possible to define precisely. Some use the word "transgender" as an umbrella term to refer to people whose feelings or behaviors do not match their assigned gender: examples include "cross-dressers" and people who identify as "MTF" (male-to-female) or "FTM" (female-to-male). Others use the word to describe a gender outside the constructs of male/female, to describe the experience of having no gender or multiple genders: examples include people who define themselves as "genderqueer," "androgyne," "gender bender," "beyond binary," and "polygender." Table 12-1 presents definitions of some common and less familiar terms that have been used to describe members of the transgender community.

Transgender people choose to present themselves to the world in a wide variety of ways. Some transgender individuals decide to alter their bodies through hormones or surgery in order to make their anatomy concordant with their gender identity. Others opt to express their gender in a less permanent fashion, by changing hairstyle or manner of dress. Still others

Table 12-1   Definitions of Transgender Terms

MTF: Male to Female (used with and without "transsexual")	A person born biologically male whose gender identity is female, who presents socially as a woman, and who often, but does not always, makes physical changes through hormones or surgery.
FTM: Female to Male (used with and without "transsexual")	A person born biologically female whose gender identity is male, who presents socially as a man, and who often, but does not always, makes physical changes through hormones or surgery.
Cross-dresser	Anyone who dresses in clothing not associated with their assigned sex; generally refers to a male who dresses as female, who may or may not want to change his gender; considered more politically correct than "transvestite."
Transvestite	Typically used to describe a biological male who dresses as a female, often for sexual gratification. This term tends to be viewed as disparaging and pathologizing.
Drag queen	A male who cross-dresses as a woman primarily for performance or show. Drag queens generally identify as males, often as gay males, and do not wish to change their gender.
Drag king	A female who cross-dresses as male and who may or may not want to change her gender.
Transwoman	Generally refers to someone who was born male and who identifies and portrays their gender as female. People will often use this term after taking some steps to portray their gender as female, or after fully transitioning; however, many who have fully transitioned prefer to be called women, rather than transwomen.
Transman	Generally refers to someone who was born female and who identifies and portrays their gender as male. People will often use this term after taking some steps to portray their gender as male, or after fully transitioning; however, many who have fully transitioned prefer to be called a man, rather than transman.
Intersex	A person born with genitalia that are neither exclusively male nor female, or that are inconsistent with chromosomal sex; sometimes not identified until puberty, when the person either fails to develop certain secondary sex characteristics, or develops characteristics that were not expected. Intersex is not considered a subcategory of transgender. However, people born with certain intersex conditions may be more likely than the general population to feel their gender assignment at birth was incorrect. The term "Disorders of Sexual Development" is recommended where the medical care of infants is considered.
Hermaphrodite	Previously used to describe intersex; now considered stigmatizing and outdated.
Passing	When someone is perceived as the gender they are presenting in their dress and mannerisms. For example: a male dressed as female is seen by others as female.
Getting Clocked/ Spooked	When a stranger sees through the gender someone is trying to portray. For example: a male who is dressed as female hears someone say, "that is a man in a dress."
Stealth	When a transgender person has transitioned into a different gender, lives as if born in that gender, and does not divulge that he/she is transgender.

Table 12-1   Definitions of Transgender Terms (continued)

Tranny	Short for transgender. Some people consider this term derogatory.
Tranny-chaser	Refers to someone who is attracted to and/or seeks out sex or relationships with transgender people. Some people consider this term derogatory.
Genderqueer	This new term is generally used in two ways: 1) as an umbrella term that includes all people whose gender varies from the norm, akin to the use of the word queer to refer to all sexual orientations different from the norm (heterosexual); or 2) to describe a subset of individuals who are born biologically female, but feel their gender identity is neither female or male. Clinical observation suggests that when seen in the binary of male/female, these individuals tend to feel more comfortable being seen as male and using male names and pronouns, but do not necessarily feel that their gender identity is male.
Boi/Tranny Boi	Another term for someone born female who feels that this is not an accurate or complete description of themselves. Other similar terms on the FTM spectrum include "Butch," "Boychick," "Shapeshifter," and "Boss Grrl."
Androgyne	Refers to someone whose gender identity is both male and female, or neither male nor female. An androgyne person might present as androgynous, and/or as sometimes male and sometimes female, and might choose to use an androgynous name. Pronoun preference typically varies, including alternately using male or female pronouns, using the pronoun that matches gender presentation at that time, or using newly developed gender-neutral pronouns.
Gender bender, beyond binary, polygender and gender outlaw	Similar to genderqueer and androgyne, these terms refer to gender variations other than the traditional, dichotomous view of male and female. People who self-refer with these terms may identify and present themselves as both or alternatively male and female, as no gender, or as a gender outside the male/female binary.

choose to do nothing at all. No matter how they choose to present themselves, most transgender individuals share one common desire: to be seen and respected for who they are.

Gender Identity versus Sexual Orientation

While gender identity and sexual orientation are distinct, they are closely intertwined; the process of exploring gender identity invariably includes exploring sexual orientation as well. The frequent misconception that transgender means gay may result from the tendency of some gay and lesbian people to present themselves in ways that depart from stereotypical gender norms or from the association of gay men with female impersonators. Gender identity and sexual orientation can be aptly distinguished by thinking about gender identity as the way a person feels inside about their gender (self) and thinking about sexual orientation as the gender(s) a person is attracted to (other).

A model developed by Grace Sterling Stowell, the executive director of the Boston Alliance of Gay, Lesbian, and Transgender Youth, depicts a triangle, with biological sex, gender, and sexual orientation being the three separate points.[6] Visually, this model describes both the ways in which these categories are separate, as well as the fact that they are related (see Figure 12-1).

Transgender people can have any sexual orientation; sexual orientation may change as they explore, and become more clear about, their gender identity. It is not helpful to use labels to describe a transgender person's sexual orientation, as labels can be confusing and misleading. Consider a biological male who has the gender identity of a female. For this person, being gay may mean feeling attracted to women; being heterosexual could mean feeling attracted to men. To further add to the confusion, sexual orientation labels may be used differently depending on whether someone is out about her or his gender identity. A biological male who identifies as female but who keeps her gender identity closeted may call herself "gay" to let others know that she likes men. On the other hand, a biological male who identifies as female and *is* out about her gender identity may call herself "straight" to let others know that she likes men. Clearly, if we want to know about someone's sexual orientation, we need to ask what gender(s) they are attracted to and refrain from making assumptions based on commonly used, but imprecise terminology.

Gender Identity Disorder and Gender Dysphoria

Gender identity disorder (GID) is a diagnosis defined by the *Diagnostic and Statistical Manual of Mental Disorders* (DSM-IV)[7] to aid in the identification of transgender individuals who might benefit from clinical intervention. On the positive side, inclusion of this category legitimizes gender issues as worthy of scientific investigation, which facilitates clinical research; it also validates the need for clinical care, which may in turn help facilitate change in medical insurance policies that currently exclude coverage for care related to gender identity issues. Criteria for establishing a

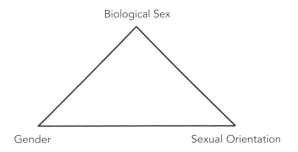

Biological Sex

Gender   Sexual Orientation

Figure 12-1   Stowell model, depicting relationships between sex, gender, and sexual orientation.

Adapted from an illustration by Grace Sterling Stowell. Used with permission.

diagnosis of GID are presented in Table 12-2. It should be noted that the diagnosis of GID only describes transsexuals—one subset of people who are transgender. The field of gender identity is still so new that the DSM description of GID has already become outdated.

On the negative side, the diagnosis of gender identity disorder has been criticized both as a diagnosis and in terms of its language. The word "disorder" indicates that a variation from gender norms is disordered or deficient, rather than simply different. It suggests that gender identities held by transgender people are not legitimate, but instead represent perversion, delusion, or immature development. Therefore, many people use the term "gender dysphoria," instead. Gender dysphoria describes persistent aversion toward some or all of one's physical characteristics and/or social roles that are ascribed according to biological sex. Often experienced as depression, anxiety, irritation, and/or agitation, gender dysphoria describes the sense that something is very wrong; rather than implying pathology, this term portrays a transgender person's emotional experience more aptly.[8]

How Does Gender Identity Develop?

Increasing knowledge suggests that gender identity development is much more complex than previously assumed, and there is no scientific consensus about a single pathway which leads to gender dysphoria.[9] Theories of causation tend to fall into two categories: nature/biology and nurture/socialization. The predominating biological theory suggests that a

---

Table 12-2   Definition of Gender Identity Disorder

Gender Identity Disorder in Adolescents and Adults, 302.85

Diagnostic Criteria:

A. A strong and persistent cross-gender identification (not merely a desire for any perceived cultural advantages of being the other sex). In adolescents and adults, the disturbance is manifested by symptoms such as a stated desire to be the other sex, frequent passing as the other sex, desire to live or be treated as the other sex, or the conviction that one has the typical feelings and reactions of the other sex.

B. Persistent discomfort with one's sex or sense of inappropriateness in the gender role of that sex. In adolescents and adults, the disturbance is manifested by symptoms such as preoccupation with getting rid of primary and secondary sex characteristics (e.g., request for hormones, surgery, or other procedures to physically alter sexual characteristics to simulate the other sex) or belief that one was born the wrong sex.

C. The disturbance is not concurrent with a physical intersex condition.

D. The disturbance causes clinically significant distress or impairment in social, occupational, or other important areas of functioning.

Specify if (for sexually mature individuals) Sexually Attracted to Males, . . . Females, . . . Both, . . . Neither.

neurohormonal disturbance takes place in the brain during embryological development. While the genitalia of the human embryo become differentiated as male or female during the 12th week of fetal development, the gender identity portion of the brain differentiates around the 16th week. If there is a hormonal imbalance during this four-week period, gender identity may not develop along the same lines as the genitalia.[10] It is hypothesized that the state of the mother's overall physical and mental health during pregnancy could cause such an imbalance. Severe emotional trauma or other stress or the ingestion of certain prescription or illegal drugs during pregnancy could interfere with fetal brain chemistry.

Theories of nurture claim that gender identity is taught through socialization. Early psychoanalytic theories suggested that gender identity disorder was due to disturbances such as difficulty separating and individuating from a parent,[11] an unresolved Oedipal complex, the physical or emotional absence of the primary caregiver during a child's early years, cross-gendered behaviors being reinforced, and the existence of a classically overbearing mother or a weak or absent father. These theories are inconsistent with clinical observation, which demonstrates that the psychosocial and familial experiences of transgender people, like those of everyone else, are extraordinarily diverse.

Failure of the nurture/socialization theories to account adequately for the complexity of gender identity is vividly illustrated by the case of Canadian twin boys.[12] In 1967, one of two identical male twins had his penis severely injured in a botched circumcision. After consulting John Money, a renowned expert in gender identity, the family decided to raise this twin as a girl. Female external genitalia were created surgically while he was an infant, and female sex hormones were administered. For twelve years, he participated in a program of "social, mental, and hormonal conditioning to make the transformation take hold in his psyche."[12] He was not told the truth about his history, however, and grew up believing he was born female. The case was presented as a success in the medical literature. The apparent outcome that gender was a result of socialization, rather than biology, gave credence to the women's movement in the 1970s, and was widely cited. The case brought fame to Dr. Money, who was called "one of the greatest sex researchers of the century."[10]

In 1997, the experiment was exposed as a failure. Dr. Milton Diamond, a biologist at the University of Hawaii, and Dr. Keith Sigmundson, a Canadian psychiatrist, documented how the twin rebelled against being socialized female. He resisted wearing dresses, insisted on standing up to urinate, and was bullied viciously at school.[13] When he was a teenager, he attempted suicide. His parents finally told him of his history at age 14; he then reverted back to male, taking male hormones. Although he lived the rest of his life as a man, David Reimer remained unhappy and said: "I'd give just about anything to go to a hypnotist to black out my whole past . . . Because it's torture. . . . What they did to (me) in the body is sometimes not near as bad as what they did to (me) in the mind."[13] Tragically, David Reimer killed himself in 2004, at age 38.

This anecdote demonstrates the importance of helping individuals who are questioning their gender identity to define themselves and supporting them as they gradually choose to reveal themselves to others. Attempts to force transgender persons to live in a gender that feels alien are not effective and can be extremely harmful.

Normal Developmental Questioning versus Gender Dysphoria

A certain amount of questioning gender and sexuality norms is a part of normal development, as discussed in the chapter on adolescence. It is important to note that questioning and/or exploring one's gender and/or gender identity does not necessarily indicate gender dysphoria or the diagnosis of GID. However, most transgender adults report knowing something was different about them at an early age. It is common to hear that by age four or five the person knew they were in the wrong body or learned that their gender was different from what they believed. To quote one client: "I thought I was a girl, and when we lined up in kindergarten I went to the girl's line. I was told 'go to the other line, you're a boy.' That's how I learned I was a boy."

Sometimes gender dysphoria can be avoided or tolerated in childhood, as the changes that come with puberty have not yet begun. Children may gravitate toward peers who mirror their gender identity or may choose to play stereotypical games associated with the gender they feel they are. However, children with gender dysphoria may show signs of distress very early. Biological girls may refuse to wear dresses, have long hair, or play with girls, and may try to stand up to urinate. Biological boys may want to dress up in their mother's (or sister's) clothing, play with girls, or sit down to urinate. Some children state or insist that they are the other gender or that they will become the other gender when they grow up. Diagnosing a child with GID can be tricky, as research shows that the majority of children with cross-gender behavior do not grow up to qualify for the diagnosis of GID in adulthood.[14]

Puberty is often a time that gender dysphoria becomes more apparent, both to the individual who is undergoing physical changes, and to others. Although many people are able to either ignore or bear their gender issues as children, the drastic changes associated with puberty create a harsh reality that no longer permits denial. Clients often describe puberty as a horrific time, during which they felt shocked, humiliated, and betrayed by their bodies. Not surprisingly, transgender adolescents often express dislike or even disgust about their bodies after secondary sex characteristics develop.[15] If these feelings of revulsion escalate, depression, suicidal feelings, and acts of self-harm may result.

Normal questioning crosses into gender dysphoria or gender identity disorder when a person develops persistent and preoccupying symptoms that become the main focus of their life. When this happens, there are usually concomitant difficulties in many other realms, including social, academic or occupational functioning. Normal development may be arrested or delayed. Many clients report a fear or avoidance of "growing up," and/or difficulty seeing the future: "I couldn't imagine a future, because I could never see myself as a female."

Consequences of Living in an Intolerant Society

The consequences of living in a intolerant society can be readily understood by considering the following questions: Have you ever seen someone whose gender was unclear? Did you stare? Did you feel uncomfortable? Did you want to figure it out? Why? How did you feel? Uncomfortable? Confused? Nervous? Intrigued? Why? Cultural norms dictate how we should behave based on how our sex, gender, and/or sexual orientation are perceived. For most people this is not problematic. However, people who do not conform to societal expectations often have these experiences:

- being stared at
- being ignored
- being engaged when otherwise they would have been left alone
- awkwardness in conversation
- discrimination
- violence

Gender identity impacts every aspect of a person's daily life: relationships with friends, family members, and romantic partners; work or school; and the ability to access healthcare. Consider the experience of a transgender person who needs to use a restroom, and discovers that rather than single-occupant (unisex) bathrooms, segregated facilities (male only or female only) are the only available options. How much time will a transgender person spend thinking about which restroom to use? How much will they worry about being hassled or harassed if they use the one that feels right? How uncomfortable will they feel if they have to use the one that does not feel right? What if someone calls the police while they are in the bathroom? This is just one example of the kinds of challenges transgender people encounter every day.

Lack of acceptance frequently leads to low self-esteem, shame, humiliation, and isolation. Transgender individuals are at extremely high risk for discrimination, lack of access to basic medical and mental healthcare, unemployment and underemployment, homelessness, substance abuse, HIV, depression, anxiety, suicidal feelings and/or attempts, sex work, and violent hate crimes. A problem in one area quickly leads to a problem in another. For example, financial problems resulting from unemployment can lead to loss of medical insurance (and subsequent poorer access to healthcare), as well as homelessness and reliance on sex work for income (with associated increased risk for various negative outcomes, including violence, substance abuse, and HIV). Once established, this vicious cycle can be hard to break.

Many medical and mental health providers lack knowledge about the specific health needs of the transgender population. The remainder of this section will review data regarding key areas of risk. The section in this chapter entitled "How Can We Help? Clinical Approach to Working with Transgender Patients" outlines standards of care and presents practical tips to help clinicians communicate sensitively and provide appropriate mental health and referral services. Specific information regarding hormonal and surgical management is presented in Chapter 13.

Depression

Depression is likely the most frequent symptom associated with gender dysphoria.[1] The depression is often chronic, as the majority of gender dysphoric people have been aware of their gender dysphoria from an early age, even as early as three or four. However, certain situations can increase the severity of the depression. These situations can easily be overlooked, however, as they are "ordinary" events to those who do not experience gender dysphoria. Without an understanding of gender dysphoria, these situations will not be recognized as possible precipitating events that can increase depression and/or suicidal feelings or attempts.

As noted previously, puberty is a particularly vulnerable time. As their bodies begin to show secondary sex characteristics of a gender that feels wrong, people with gender dysphoria often experience feelings of shock, confusion, horror, anger, upset, and betrayal, despite the fact that most understand puberty intellectually and anticipate the changes their bodies are likely to undergo. Before puberty, some transgender individuals believe that their bodies will change into the gender with which they identify, while others believe that their bodies will remain androgynous, without secondary sex characteristics. Once physical changes begin, it is no longer possible to hide in these fantasies.

Monthly menstrual periods and premenstrual symptoms in biological females who feel male, and erections, ejaculation, and nocturnal emissions in biological males who feel female can increase feelings of humiliation and depression acutely. For example, one client developed suicidal ideation every month when he had his period, but this resolved when he began taking testosterone and his menses ceased.

People with gender dysphoria often avoid masturbation and sexual activity with others, due to discomfort or even disgust with their genitalia. Those who are sexual often fantasize that their body matches their gender identity; in fact, many people are only able to be sexually aroused if they hold this fantasy. Biological male clients who identify as female say they imagine having a vagina while they are being penetrated anally; often their penis is tucked away, not to be seen or touched, increasing the believability of the fantasy. One client, a biological female who transitioned to male, became aware of his attraction to other men when gay men responded to him as a male. When he was perceived as female, however, sexual interest shown by men became repulsive and upsetting.

It is important to note, however, that feelings about one's body and with being sexual exist along a continuum of comfort. This range includes people who are only mildly unhappy with their bodies, to those who can hardly bear to wash themselves in the shower. There are also people who are not particularly uncomfortable with their bodies. Some clients say that if they were seen and treated as the gender they identify with, they would not feel the need to make any changes to their bodies. However, because gender identity is often perceived incorrectly, some of these individuals choose to change their bodies so they will be seen as the people they feel they are.

Depression can also arise in persons who do not necessarily qualify for the diagnosis of GID but do experience a certain amount of gender dysphoria. Such people may not identify as either male or female and therefore do not gain outside validation of a gender identity different from the male/female binary. For example, one client who was born biologically male and identified as androgyne sought to present her gender as androgynous, as this felt most genuine to her (the client is comfortable using both male and female pronouns). However, she found that although she could convincingly present as either male or female, she was not able to find a way to appear androgynous. Eventually she came to accept her gender identity as separate from her gender presentation. However, the client continues to experience depression, low self-esteem, and feelings of rejection and isolation due to the inability of others to recognize her as androgyne. Despite gender dysphoria, some people do not seek medical or mental healthcare and struggle with these issues without the benefit of professional help. Some manage to deal with their issues effectively; others continue to suffer the effects of being different, whether or not they come out about their gender variation.

Depression often requires psychopharmacological intervention. Some transgender people are leery of beginning medication, as they fear this will mean that their gender issues will not be fully addressed. Providers should appreciate that while medication can help alleviate depression, gender dysphoria will not resolve until underlying gender issues are addressed, using modalities such as individual psychotherapy and/or participation in a support group.

Hormone administration (generally female hormones) can also induce or increase depression. This type of depression can also be treated with medication. However, hormone administration often leads to a decrease in depression and brightening of mood, as the person sees tangible progress in resolving their gender dysphoria. Sudden withdrawal of hormones should generally be avoided, since this can precipitate mood swings and depression.

Anxiety

Some, but not all studies suggest that there may be a correlation between separation anxiety in childhood and later development of gender identity disorder.[16] However, consensus exists that anxiety disorders are common in people diagnosed with GID. Anxiety can be chronic, stemming from repression of gender dysphoria, as well as the fear that others will find out. Anxiety may also manifest more acutely, as is seen in situations that include being in public or anticipating being in public. In this case, the anxiety likely results from fear of or prior experience with public scrutiny, harassment, and/or violence. As with depression, management of anxiety disorders in this population often requires a multimodality approach that includes medications, psychobehavioral or cognitive behavioral therapy, and group support.

Self-harm

A review of the literature shows that populations who engage in self-mutilation include transsexuals,[17] people who self-mutilate for religious or cultural reasons,[18] people who suffer from psychosis, and individuals with severe personality disorders.[19] Among those with borderline personality disorder, self-mutilating behavior is an attempt to regulate affect.[20] Despite the abundance of information about self-mutilation in people with borderline personality disorder, reference to mutilation of the genitals in this population is virtually absent.

In the transgender population, however, self-harm to the body is usually directed specifically towards the genitalia.[21,22] When a person's physical self is discordant with their gender identity, the body feels alien. The purpose of genital mutilation is to remove the most offending parts,[23] with or without a plan to fashion new, more appropriate ones. Self-castration is rarely an impulsive act; rather, it usually occurs after long-standing conflict.[22] Depression and anxiety due to the wait for sex reassignment surgery can be triggering factors.[24]

Transgender people often have unrealistic expectations about what will happen after they harm their genitalia. Clients sometimes relate the belief that they will heal easily and be fine without any medical attention, ignoring the fact that castration or amputation of the breasts represent major physical trauma. Magical thinking is also quite common: for example, one client described repeatedly trying to slam her penis in a drawer to cut it off, with the belief that severing her penis would result in a vagina.

Suicide

The literature is replete with studies linking suicide with GID.[25,26,27] Studies of transgender populations in Philadelphia, Washington, Chicago, San Francisco, and Houston report suicidal ideation rates ranging from 16% up to 64%,[27] with most people attributing their suicidal thoughts to gender dysphoria. Clements-Nolle found that 62% of 392 MTF individuals were depressed, and 32% had attempted suicide.[28]

Recent studies have examined the relationship between gender role, sexual orientation, and suicide risk. Studies have found that cross-gender role is a unique predictor of suicidal symptoms, especially for boys, concluding that cross-gendered people, regardless of sexual orientation, appear to have a higher risk for suicidal symptoms.[26]

Substance Abuse

Substance abuse is also common. Transgender individuals are believed to be the most underserved group of substance abusers; however, few studies have been performed specifically in the transgender community.[29]

The Transgender Community Health Project in San Francisco surveyed 392 MTF and 123 FTM individuals in 1997. In addition to extremely high levels of HIV risk behaviors, 34% of the MTF group and 18% of the FTM group reported injection drug use.[30] Of this latter group, 91% shared syringes. Available studies also suggest that the use of tobacco is common in the transgender community.[31] Obtaining treatment for substance abuse is frequently a problem for transgender individuals. Many treatment programs segregate people by sex, which can lead transgender patients to feel humiliated or to decline treatment.[27] Also common is the view that taking hormones, or even psychotropic medication, represents drug use and that cessation of hormone use is therefore required prior to enrollment in a substance abuse treatment program.[27]

Unique features of substance abuse in the transgender community include the use of silicone to change the shape and appearance of the body and self-administration of illegally procured hormones. Since both may be injected, sharing works or failure to use a sterile technique can result in complications that include infections at the injection site, endocarditis, hepatitis, and HIV. The use of silicone, which has been condemned by the FDA and others,[25] is often of industrial-grade rather than medical-grade, which was once procured much more easily for breast implants. Undesired effects include respiratory stress, death, systemic illness, and disfiguration due to hardening and migration of the material.[25] Unsupervised use of hormones is also dangerous, as it is associated with increased risk for thromboembolism, abnormal liver function,[25] and adverse cardiac outcomes.

Sex Work

Sex work is common in the transgender community for a number of reasons. Sex work provides a means of financial support for transgender people who do not have other ways of supporting themselves. Transgender youth are at particular risk. Frequently banished from their homes when they come out, transgender youth often lack high school equivalency, and they may not even have reached the legal age of employment. Transgender adults who are fired because they come out at work often find it very difficult to get another job, either because they do not "pass," or because their previous employer will not give them a good recommendation.

In addition to being a means for survival, sex work may be viewed as a road to transition. Sex work can provide large amounts of money, often fairly quickly. This can be very tempting to a transgender individual who is desperate to transition but has no other ways to find the money to do so. The process and challenges of transition are described in more detail in the section entitled "Transition."

Besides providing financial help, sex work can be emotionally helpful. Transgender people often fear that no one will want to be romantic or sexual with them because of their gender identity. Being desired for one's body is incredibly powerful. It is something we all want, something we all seek. It is important for our self-esteem, for our need to be close to others, and our need to be loved. Sex work can provide the gratification and sense of normalcy a transgender person craves in being desired for their body and affirmed for their gender presentation.

Unfortunately, sex work is associated with significant risks. Prostituting often requires following the demands of the person paying for these services. This means that the sex worker is less likely to practice safe sex and is therefore vulnerable to infection with hepatitis C, HIV, and other STIs. Transgender sex workers are also at high risk for interpersonal violence.

HIV/AIDS

Recent studies report high rates of HIV in MTF populations: 21% in Chicago,[27] 22% in Los Angeles,[32] 21% to 30% in New York,[27] 27% in Houston,[27] 32% in Washington, DC,[27] and 26%, 35%, and 47% in San Francisco.[28,33] High levels of lifetime HIV-risk behaviors are observed among transgender women: in one study of 392 MTF individuals in San Francisco, 80% reported a history of sex work and 85% had participated in unprotected receptive anal sex.[30] The same study found that HIV prevalence was much lower in a second group of 123 FTM individuals (1.6%); however, this may not continue to be the case, as 28% of this group reported a history of unsafe receptive anal sex.

Information from eleven focus groups with 100 MTF and FTM people in San Francisco found that low self-esteem was the main reason for sexual risk taking.[31] Thus, it appears that for some transgender individuals, the risk of contracting HIV is considered less important than the gratification and sense of normalcy they experience in being desired for their body and affirmed for their gender presentation. The importance of addressing self-esteem issues with transgender clients cannot be overemphasized; clearly, clinicians also need to work hard on developing effective risk-reduction counseling techniques.

Violence and Safety Issues

Violence toward transgender individuals is common, both within and outside the home. Transgender people "can enrage others by their mere existence."[25] Looking androgynous, or having mixed gender characteristics, appear to be triggering factors for "trans-bashing."

Kenagy found that 53.8% of 78 transgender people had been forced to have sex, 56.3% of 80 transgender people had experienced violence in their home, and 51.3% of 80 transgender people had been physically abused.[34] In each case, MTF individuals were significantly more likely to have experienced this violence than FTMs. Transgender women of color are at highest risk.[27]

The murder rate of transgender people is extremely high. Statistics show that prior to 1999, a transgender murder occurred approximately once a month. Since then the number has increased to two murders per month.[35] According to transgender historian Candice "Kay" Brown, a murder rate of one MTF transsexual person each month computes to an average of 119 murders per 100 000 transsexuals, or six times greater than the national average.[35] This murder rate is more than three times that of African American men, who have the next highest recorded incidence.[35]

It should be noted that much of the violence experienced by transgender people is not reported, due to internalized transphobia, shame, and lack of confidence in authorities. In addition, violence against transgender people is often attributed incorrectly as gay bashing. Furthermore, transgender murders are often not reported in the news. In reaction, the Web site "Remembering Our Dead" (http://www.gender.org/remember/) was created to keep more accurate track of transgender murders.

Healthcare Access

Despite being at such high risk for adverse health effects, many transgender people are routinely refused care,[26,34] are unable to afford healthcare due to being unemployed or underemployed,[27] or do not seek care due to traumatic experiences in the past. There are documented cases of transgender deaths due to the delay, or even refusal, to provide urgent medical treatment.[31] Transgender youth, in particular, may not be able to access appropriate medical treatment for gender identity disorder, due to being underage. Ironically, failure to take proactive steps is a primary reason for the escalation of psychological problems, including suicide, alcohol and drug abuse, and homelessness,[26] creating a self-reinforcing cycle. Given such high risks, coupled with the incredible difficulty accessing medical and mental healthcare, the importance of developing programs that provide outreach services to the transgender community cannot be overemphasized. Outreach programs should take into account populations that are least likely to seek care, such as injection drug users, sex workers, youths, and the homeless. Example of model health access programs include: the Gay, Lesbian, Bisexual and Transgender Health Access Project in Boston, Mass (http://www.glbthealth.org/index.html), and the Transgender Healthcare Access Project at the Transgender Law Center in San Francisco, Calif (http://www.transgenderlawcenter.org/do/transform.html#health).

Reaching Self-Acceptance

As discussed in detail in Chapter 3, the process of reaching self-acceptance and developing a positive identity follows a very similar course for transgender individuals as it does for people who define themselves as lesbian, gay, or bisexual. The first step is to define oneself; subsequently, one must decide how much to reveal that identity to other people. Unlike LGB individuals, however, transgender people are often in the unique position of being less able to conceal their identities—that is, in living in a gender role that conflicts with their biological sex, they are frequently conspicuous to others. This lack of privacy poses particular challenges for transgender individuals who choose to undergo a "real life experience" on the road to making a more permanent physical transition toward a body that is in accord with their gender identity. This section reviews the three major important tasks transgender individuals must traverse on the path toward self-acceptance: self-exploration, coming out, and transitioning.

Self-exploration

A certain amount of questioning and experimentation around gender identity and sexual orientation is common in many adolescents and young adults as part of normal psychosexual development. For transgender people, the gradual realization that they are truly different from most of their peers, rather than merely experimenting, is often a daunting process. Some individuals, particularly those who have positive role models and strong supports, feel validated and euphoric when they discover that there are words to describe their experience and that they are not alone. For others, this time may be punctuated by feelings of confusion, anxiety, and depression. Not surprisingly, therefore, many transgender individuals find it helpful to consult a mental health professional during the process of questioning and clarifying their gender identity. The tasks of psychotherapy are reviewed below, in the section entitled "Mental Health Evaluation and Management."

Coming Out

When a transgender individual has reached a certain comfort level in exploring their gender issues, a frequent next step is to begin coming out to others. For transgender people, the coming out process strongly resembles that of LGB people. Coming out as transgender helps reinforce a person's identity, as well as making space to allow others to shift their perspective. Coming out is a life-long process. However, there is often a concentrated period of time during which a person first begins to come out to key people in their life.

Similar to coming out about sexuality, people make different choices about how, when, and to whom they choose to come out as transgender. Unlike sexual orientation, however, gender identity cannot be easily hidden if the person chooses to make physical changes to their body. Therefore, the person may need to come out to people they would not ordinarily choose to come out to if they could keep their identity private. Some transgender people feel their identity will be taken more seriously if they have already started the process of transition: "It would be hard for my family to see me as female if I still look completely male." They may therefore choose to begin hormone therapy first, so that their bodies will display the physical attributes of their gender.

The process of coming out may result in feelings of relief, euphoria, anxiety, or any combination of these and other emotions. Some transgender individuals report successful, easy experiences of coming out that go better than expected; others describe difficult, upsetting experiences that include being rejected, being challenged, and being misunderstood. A frequent occurrence is the need to educate people about what transgender is and is not: this can feel like a burden to a vulnerable person who longs for support and understanding. Some clients resent having to educate others: one person stated bluntly, "That's not my job." There is also a risk that the person coming out will take on, or be expected to adopt, the role of caretaker for friends and family who are having emotional difficulty handling the news. This, too, can cause resentment. As one client put it: "I'm the one who needs the support and understanding, but my family wants me to take care of them, because they're so upset about this. What about me?"

Some clients experience setbacks in their relationships in the short-term but are able to work through the issues with time, resulting in continued, sometimes better relationships in the long term. For example, one client's mother responded to her coming out in a judgmental and rejecting manner. They had no contact for two years, and the client believed that her mother was gone from her life forever. However, the two gradually began speaking again, and her mother eventually became more accepting. Another client's parents said they wished their child was "just gay," rather than transgender. Ironically, this statement shows the progress our culture has made in accepting different sexual norms, while at the same time demonstrating that we still have far to go to become more accepting of different gender norms.

Coming out at work presents particular challenges for transgender individuals. Fortunately, during recent years, many clients report being received well when they come out on the job, in large part because an increasing number of employers have already had experience with other transgender employees. Unfortunately, however, some clients continue to report being fired or let go. At times, their gender identity is explicitly cited as the reason for dismissal; more often, people are offered other explanations, but suspect that it was really about their gender. In addition, transgender people may have difficulty getting hired because they are visibly gender variant. There is often little recourse, since there is currently no uniform protection for transgender people.

Federal disability laws such as the Federal Rehabilitation Act and the Americans With Disabilities Act explicitly exclude protection for gender identity not resulting from a physical impairment. However, some state laws do not include this exception, and therefore in some states a transgender person may find protection. Title VII of the Civil Rights Act of 1964, which prohibits discrimination of employees on the basis of race, color, religion, sex, or national origin, fails to protect people based on sexual orientation or gender identity. In 1996 the Employee Non-Discrimination Act (ENDA) proposed protection for people based on sexual orientation, but this failed in the Senate by a 50-49 vote. In 2004, the Human Rights Campaign, an LGBT organization which is among the primary lobbyists for the bill, announced that it would only support the passage of the ENDA if it included transgender protections as well. As of April 2007, the most current proposed version of the ENDA includes protection based on gender identity, as well as sexual orientation. Currently [13] states, the District of Columbia, and [91] cities and counties across the country have now passed explicitly transgender-inclusive antidiscrimination laws. These laws currently cover [37%] of the US population. Participating states include Minnesota (passed in 1993), Rhode Island (2001), New Mexico (2003), California (2003), Illinois (2005), Maine (2005), and Washington (2006).

Transition

Transition is generally understood as a period of time during which a person makes life-altering decisions that frequently include making changes in their physical characteristics. However, not all transgender individuals choose to change their physical appearance. For people who do choose to make changes, the range of choices extends from temporarily altering their outward appearance to making permanent physical and/or anatomical changes.

There are a many ways people can alter their outward appearance to portray their gender differently. These include changing their gait, clothing, manner of speech, hairstyle, choice of makeup and jewelry, etc. For people who wish to portray their gender as male, other options include "binding" and "packing." Binding refers to hiding or minimizing the appearance of breasts through the use of constricting materials that include ace bandages, a sports ("frog") bra, duct tape, or an actual chest binder (compression vest). Binders are readily available through transgender and medical supply Web sites. It is also common to layer shirts, or wear shirts with a design that visually minimizes chest protrusion. "Packing" refers to visually creating the appearance of male genitalia in one's pants. Common items used for this purpose include a rolled up pair of socks, a strap-on dildo, or a "packer"—a soft male genital prosthesis that does not require the use of a harness. Some packers permit the wearer to urinate standing, which can enhance the person's feeling of having male genitalia, as well as increasing their safety when using a male restroom in public.

For people who wish to portray their gender as female, the creation of visible breasts without surgery is common. This often includes wearing "falsies"—prosthetic breasts made of silicone or foam that can be placed in a bra. However, many people find other creative, cheaper ways of fashioning breasts. One way is to knot a short length of pantyhose containing uncooked rice into a round shape, which allows for a very natural looking breast when inserted into a bra cup. Duct tape can also be used to pull the skin of the chest together to effect the look of cleavage. Another common technique to minimize male sex characteristics is "tucking"—that is, hiding the male genitalia from view. To tuck, one first slides the testicles up into the peritoneal cavity, then pulls the penis between the legs, securing it in place by wearing a tight pair of women's underwear.

Transgender individuals who want to change actual physical characteristics and anatomical features may elect to take hormones or to have surgery. For people who transition from male to female, surgery generally refers to sex reassignment surgery (SRS), but can also include breast augmentation and other forms of cosmetic surgery, such as facial feminization surgery (FFS). For people who transition from female to male, surgery may refer to "top" or "chest" surgery (mastectomy), or to "lower" surgery (eg, creation of a neophallus). Please refer to Chapter 13: Medical and Surgical Management of the Transgender Patient for further discussion.

When transitioning, transgender individuals often choose to change their first name to provide a gender cue. Frequently, there are clear, definitive reasons why specific names are chosen. Many people change their given name to the male or the female version (eg, Roberta transitions to Robert; Paul transitions to Paula), or to a different but similar name (eg, Melissa changes to Melvin; John changes to Joanne). Others adopt the name their parents would have chosen had they been born the opposite sex, thereby permitting important family members to share in this intimate journey. Finally, some people choose completely novel names for symbolic reasons. Examples include naming oneself after a close relative or person who has passed away, choosing a name in another language, or a term with religious or spiritual meaning, or deliberately selecting an androgynous name, such as Pat, Robin, or Chris. People who choose the latter option may do so because they reject the idea of gender as a binary system, or in order to avoid gender-specific names in an effort to help others accept their transition more easily.

Financial issues are often a big part of the transition process. Transition can be very expensive. Costs can include hormones, a new wardrobe, hair removal, hair replacement, a legal name change, surgery (cosmetic, chest, or sex reassignment surgery), and, almost invariably, psychotherapy. The inability to afford some or all of the things a person in transition feels are critical to accomplish interrupts the transition process and can trigger significant mental health sequelae, including depression, anxiety, and even suicide. Unfortunately, medical insurance pays for very little at this point in time: generally just psychotherapy, and sometimes hormones.

Transition includes a person's adjustment to their changing body. In addition to becoming accustomed to unfamiliar physical characteristics, this involves becoming increasingly aware of the different ways one is perceived by others as a result of those changes. For example, a biological male who successfully "passes" as female may suddenly encounter misogynous reactions. In addition, it is critical for transgender individuals who are transitioning to be aware that they are at particularly increased risk for physical violence during the transition period. The lack of clarity of a person's gender due to mixed gender cues is known to be a risk factor for violence.[25]

Importantly, the transgender person is not the only one who transitions. People in the transgender person's life also have to go through a process during which they gradually change their perception of the person's gender identity. It is understandable that people display a range of reactions, including curiosity, surprise, shock, and confusion. Learning that someone is transgender can precipitate feelings of hurt or betrayal. People may have shared confidences they would not have shared had they been aware of the transgender person's gender identity. Sometimes people feel a need to change how they interact with the transgender person based on their new understanding of their gender. To minimize negative impact, it is helpful to educate patients about what to anticipate and to encourage them to have supports in place before transitioning publicly. Health providers should also be aware that they, just like other people in transgender individuals' lives, may experience a sense of awkwardness in relating to their transgender patients for a period of time following transition.

How Can We Help? Clinical Approach to Working with Transgender Patients

One of the earliest practitioners to work with transgender clients was Harry Benjamin, a pioneering endocrinologist who worked with transsexuals in New York City in the 1950s. In response to the dearth of information available at the time, Dr. Benjamin wrote a set of clinical guidelines in 1979 to guide the treatment of patients with gender dysphoria. These guidelines, known as the *Harry Benjamin Standards of Care* (SOC),[36] have been revised six times by an international professional consensus group of medical practitioners, and remain in use currently. The organization responsible for the SOC is the World Professional Association for Transgender Health, Inc. (WPATH): formerly, WPATH was known as the Harry Benjamin International Gender Dysphoria Association. A brief summary of the SOC is presented in Table 12-3; the complete set of guidelines (a free 22-page PDF file) can be accessed at http://www.wpath.org.

In keeping with the SOC, the remainder of this section describes practical tips to help clinicians communicate more sensitively and effectively with transgender patients, lists useful educational resources for both clinicians and patients, and outlines a comprehensive approach to mental health evaluation and management. Medical and surgical management are also discussed briefly: for details, please refer to Chapter 13.

Table 12-3   Harry Benjamin Standards of Care, Version 6 (2001)

Summary of Contents

- Prevalence, natural history and cultural differences of gender identity variance throughout the world
- History of diagnostic nomenclature
- The role of the mental health professional
- Assessment and treatment of children and adolescents with gender dysphoria
- Goals and processes of psychotherapy for adults with GID
- Requirements for, and effects of hormone therapies
- Helping transgender patients adopt to their new gender role or presentation in every day life
- Surgical indications and ethics
- Basic guidelines for breast and genital surgery
- Recommendations for post-transition follow-up

Create a Nonjudgmental, Welcoming Environment

When working with transgender patients it is critical to provide an environment that is welcoming and nonjudgmental. Such an environment permits transgender patients to feel physically safe, accepted, and understood. In a meta-analysis of 221 studies that ranked the importance of various factors in determining satisfaction with care, transgender patients rated humane treatment as the number one factor; technical competence was rated second.[37] Clearly, as is true in caring effectively for all other patients, learning to treat transgender patients with compassion and respect is of paramount importance.

There are a number of ways in which this can be accomplished. It is important to speak frankly and to select appropriate language.[38] Clinicians who use incorrect or outdated language will fail to portray a sense of understanding and respect. The transgender person may conclude that the provider does not value their inner experience, leading to feelings of being misunderstood, overlooked, or rejected. For example, certain terms, such as "transvestite" and "hermaphrodite," have derogatory connotations and are best avoided. It is always best to ask how a patient self-identifies, rather than make assumptions based on their presentation, and to use the patient's own language during subsequent conversation. It is also useful to explicitly discuss how they and their friends and partner(s) wish to be addressed, in terms of what name and what pronouns they prefer. The use of available binary pronouns, such as "he" and "she" do not accurately reflect every person's sense of self.

Providers should take the responsibility for training office staff, since use of appropriate etiquette by all personnel promotes patients' confidence in the entire healthcare experience. Mistakes will happen and will likely be forgiven as long as it is clear that the person is making an effort to get it right; most transgender people are quite reasonable in understanding that changing language, or using unfamiliar language, takes time.[38]

Most healthcare providers receive little to no formal instruction regarding gender identity and the health needs of transgender patients. Given this truth, it is perfectly acceptable to admit ignorance. However, it is important for clinicians to seek out reliable information in order to increase their knowledge and skills. Transgender patients themselves are often excellent resources: most transgender people do not mind being asked pertinent questions that demonstrate concern and respect. A wide variety of educational resources is available, including books, movies and documentaries, articles in peer-reviewed journals, formal training programs, and continuing education conferences. In addition, clinicians should learn which specialists in their area routinely provide care to transgender patients, and consult with or refer to them when appropriate. A list of resources is presented in Appendix A.

Curiosity is normal; however, it is important to refrain from being voyeuristic. For example, if a transgender patient presents with an ear infection, treating the infection is the focus of care. Asking questions about gender reassignment surgery in this context is not appropriate, as it will not enhance care, and will quite likely feel intrusive to the patient.[38] However, it is also important not to avoid dealing with the person's gender when it is appropriate. Many transgender people are extremely sensitive about having their bodies looked at, touched, and prodded. It is common for transgender men to refuse breast and pelvic exams, and for transgender women to refuse testicular and prostate exams. It is critical to acknowledge the inherent sensitivity in participating in these exams and equally important to respect the patient's refusal of care. Taking the time to establish a solid alliance with the patient over a series of visits is often required before a patient will permit these exams.[38]

Last, but not least, it is important to be sure that the physical environment of the office is conducive to care. As noted in Chapter 15, visual cues that signal acceptance, such as a posted nondiscrimination policy that includes gender or medical brochures that address the health needs of diverse groups including transgender populations, are very helpful. In addition, it is critical to provide a restroom that is unisex. Having to choose which public restroom to use is something that most people never think about. For a transgender person, having to decide which gendered restroom to use can very easily cause anxiety, shame, and realistic safety concerns.[9] Although not an ideal solution, if unisex restrooms are not available, it may be possible to use a nongendered restroom provided for people with disabilities.

Help Patients Find Community Supports

While support is often an important component of care for people who are grappling with any medical or mental health issue, it is even more critical for the transgender population, given that our society remains largely uneducated, intolerant, and discriminatory. Discovering that they are not alone, finding and using appropriate supports, and developing a sense of community are critical factors that help transgender patients achieve self-acceptance. Therefore, health providers should be able to refer transgender clients to support groups, Web sites, and literature that will be useful and educational. A list of resources is presented in Appendix A.

Mental Health Evaluation and Management

Gender dysphoria is invariably associated with some level of psychological distress. Therefore, it is not surprising that many transgender individuals choose to seek help from a mental health professional at one time or another during the process of clarifying and consolidating their gender identity. In addition, the Harry Benjamin SOC strongly recommends that all transgender patients who desire hormones or surgery first undergo 12 weeks of psychological assessment and/or psychotherapy in order to protect against making impulsive decisions that have irreversible consequences. Most medical providers require a letter from a mental health professional that confirms the diagnosis of GID, states that the patient is mentally stable enough to make life-altering decisions, and asserts that they are psychologically ready to adapt to the numerous life changes physical transformation will bring.

During the initial evaluation, the mental health provider will ensure that the patient qualifies for the diagnosis of gender dysphoria or GID (see Table 12-2); assess for the presence of concomitant conditions such as depression, anxiety, or substance abuse; and recommend appropriate treatment as indicated. Table 12-4 lists a number of common mental health conditions that sometimes look like GID and must be ruled out.

Table 12-4   Mental Health Diagnoses That Can Present Like GID

Psychosis	• Rule out delusions of being the opposite sex.
Body Dysmorphic Disorder	• Distinguish between preoccupation with an imagined or slight defect in appearance versus a real aversion to one's genitalia.
Eating Disorders	• Distinguish between disordered eating behavior that results from disturbances in body perception associated with eating disorders versus disordered eating in an attempt to modify the body due to gender dysphoria.
Dissociative Identity Disorder / PTSD	• Evaluate for the presence of multiple personalities, which may include being a member of a different sex or gender. • Clarify that the patient's dissatisfaction with their body is based on identity, rather than a history of abuse, and a consequent desire to dis-identify from a certain gender.
Borderline Personality Disorder	• Distinguish between instability of self-image and relationships and acts of self-harm due to personality disturbance versus issues of gender identity.
Obsessive Compulsive Disorder (OCD)	• Repetitive, obsessive thoughts and/or compulsive behaviors in persons with OCD do not reduce anxiety, whereas thoughts/behaviors such as cross-dressing in persons with gender dysphoria afford relief.
Nonconformity to Stereotypical Sex Role	• Differentiate between gender dysphoria based on identity and anatomy versus dissatisfaction with sex role stereotypes.
Transvestic Fetishism	• Distinguish between the gender dysphoria that can emerge in heterosexual males who cross-dress for the purpose of sexual gratification and the strong and persistent cross-gender identification and discomfort with biological sex seen in GID.

Psychotherapy is intended to establish a safe and trusting environment where the patient can explore gender identity issues with assistance from an experienced professional. The goal of treatment is not to "correct" gender identity, nor is it to "correct" biological sex or gender presentation. Rather, the goal of treatment is to relieve the tension between gender identity, biological sex, and gender presentation, in order to increase psychological well-being and functioning. The patient, in collaboration with medical and mental health providers, largely determines the nature and degree of intervention necessary to accomplish this relief.

Psychotherapists who work with gender identity issues are often called "gender specialists." They may have a degree in psychology, social work, or psychiatry and have undergone training and supervision or consultation with another gender specialist. Because at this point in time very few, if any, training programs include specialization in gender identity issues, most practitioners have found ways to educate themselves through conferences, reading, workshops, and supervision. Names of knowledgeable mental health providers can be obtained from several of the resources listed in Appendix A.

Although beginning treatment can provide relief, the process of psychotherapy is often both frustrating and painful. Many of the issues a transgender person must face include the possibility of loss. Coming out as transgender means having the courage to risk the loss of one's family, friends, lover, job, financial stability, and sense of purpose. Discrimination, social intolerance, and facing an uncertain future can exacerbate or trigger a patient's depression, anxiety, substance use, or suicidal thoughts. Frequently, transgender people feel a sense of urgency to deal with their gender issues once they begin treatment. However, the mental health clinician may feel that other issues should be addressed first, such as stabilizing mood. For a transgender patient, having to postpone gender transition can result in immense frustration and anxiety. Given the current structure provided by the Harry Benjamin SOC, psychotherapists are in the position of being gatekeepers in the transgender person's process of transition: this can result in a tense therapy situation, which can be counterproductive.

Medical and Surgical Management

Details regarding hormone prescription, medical surveillance, and surgical management options can be found in Chapter 13. However, several areas deserve additional emphasis here. These include a general statement about the importance of sex reassignment surgery (SRS) in selected cases, description of the "real-life experience," and discussion of the literature that has examined outcomes following SRS.

Importance of Sex Reassignment Surgery

The Harry Benjamin SOC state that SRS, "when prescribed or recommended by qualified practitioners, is medically indicated and medically necessary. Sex reassignment is not 'experimental,' 'investigational,' 'elective,' 'cosmetic,' or optional in any meaningful sense. It constitutes very effective and appropriate treatment for transsexualism or profound GID."[36]

Real-life Experience

The SOC calls for a "Real Life Test" or "Real Life Experience" prior to SRS. This experience consists of fully adopting the gender role into which a patient is transitioning. It includes presenting oneself in the cross-gender role in all social interactions and adopting a gender-appropriate new name and pronouns. As noted in the SOC, "the real-life experience tests the person's resolve, the capacity to function in the preferred gender " and "assists both the patient and the mental health professional in their judgments about how to proceed."[36]

Outcomes Following Sex Reassignment Surgery

While many people transition successfully without surgery, there is a large body of literature about the success and positive consequences of SRS in people with GID.[39,40] For many transgender individuals, psychotherapy alone is unsuccessful in resolving gender dysphoria completely, while surgical reassignment is often effective. As noted by Morris et al: "No true transsexual has yet been persuaded, bullied, drugged, analyzed, shamed, ridiculed, or electrically shocked into an acceptance of his physique."[41]

The most comprehensive study of the effects of SRS examined over 70 studies, and eight previous reviews.[40] These data included more than 2000 patients in 13 countries over the course of 30 years (1961-1991). Results were satisfactory in more than 70% of MTF and in nearly 90% of FTM individuals. Specific positive outcomes of SRS include a decrease or disappearance of psychopathological features,[42] greater satisfaction with interpersonal relationships and social functioning,[43] a more positive physical self-image,[44] greater acceptance by family members,[45] an improvement in occupational functioning,[45] less difficulty finding sexual partners,[42] enhanced ability to achieve orgasm,[44] and/or greater sexual satisfaction.[43]

With regard to suicide, the literature cites a "marked decrease in suicidal tendencies postoperatively"[46] in MTF transsexuals. Most patients developed strong support systems and did well in other ways. Hunt and

Hampson found that patients no longer viewed themselves as "deviant" as they did before the surgery.[45] All 17 subjects in their study stated that despite the pain, expense, and delay involved in surgery, they would choose the same course again. Older studies describe a very small incidence of regret following SRS. The chief causes of regret include lack of family support,[47] failure to carry out the Real-Life Test, and disappointing surgical outcomes.[42] Regret is often temporary and dissipates within the first year.[39] A period of postoperative psychotherapy is recommended to facilitate adjustment.[38]

More recent studies show even higher rates of success, finding either that there were no regrets,[48] or less than 1% of people showing regret.[40] This increase in satisfaction is likely due to improved surgical technique, since recent studies suggest that "physical results of SRS may be more important than preoperative factors such as transsexual typology or compliance with established treatment regimens in predicting postoperative satisfaction or regret."[39] Difficulties experienced after surgery are usually temporary and disappear within one year.[49]

Success Stories

There are numerous examples of transgender individuals who have transitioned successfully and are leading full, satisfying lives. Some of these people are well-known, while others are known mostly in the transgender community.

The following people have transitioned from male to female:

- Christine Jorgensen, a famous pioneer, was one of the earliest people to transition. The *Daily News* broke the story on December 1, 1952, with headlines that read: "Ex-GI Becomes Blonde Bombshell," catapulting her into notoriety worldwide. Christine went to Scandinavia, began hormones in 1950, and underwent SRS in 1952-1954.
- Renee Richards, the famous tennis player, successfully sued the United States Tennis Association when it barred her from competing in the US Women's Open. This established an important precedent for the rights of transsexual athletes.
- Dana International (aka Sharon Cohen), who won the Eurovision Song Contest in 1998.
- Dr. Marci Bowers, a gynecologist, obstetrician, and SRS surgeon trained by Dr. Stanley Biber, the pioneering SRS surgeon in the US.

The following people have transitioned from female to male:

- Billie Tipton, a Jazz musician and early transgender pioneer, who lived successfully as a male, married a woman, and was discovered to be biologically female at the time of his death.
- Jamison Green, a writer and transgender activist, whose recently published a book entitled *Becoming a Visible Man.*
- Stephen Whittle, a senior law lecturer in the UK and vice president of Press for Change, who works to change laws in the UK that do not permit gender changes on birth certificates. Stephen transitioned at the young age of 19.

Conclusion

Gregor Samsa, the man who became an enormous insect, was a victim unable to escape his circumstances. He disintegrated psychically, spiritually, and eventually physically. Because he did not have a language to communicate with his family, there was no possibility for them to recognize or support him. He therefore remained isolated, humiliated, and miserable.

If we persist in using a binary model of gender, in which sex, gender, gender identity, and gender expression are viewed as either male or female, we will ensure that being transgender continues to be a fundamentally stigmatizing condition, accompanied by myriad psychosocial and medical problems. As health providers, it behooves us to practice in ways that promote the health and dignity of the people we serve. Providing sensitive and comprehensive care to transgender patients will work towards decreasing the prevalence of common secondary medical, mental health, and psychosocial problems and will promote the pledge of doing no harm.

It is also critical to remember that gender dysphoria is just one aspect of a person. As for any nontransgender individual, general healthcare for transgender people remains essential. Working with transgender patients challenges us to remain open minded, to consider gender, and identity in general, in a more complex way, and to appreciate the value of human diversity.

Summary Points

- Transgender people are individuals who do not conform to societally constructed gender norms for male or female. The broad category of transgender includes those who identify their gender as opposite their biological sex, those who cross-dress, those who identify as both male and female, those who identify as neither male nor female, and others who vary from cultural gender norms.

- New models and language are emerging that allow for a range of gender identity and expression beyond the binary concept of male and female.
- Gender identity disorder (GID) is a diagnosis defined by the *Diagnostic and Statistical Manual of Mental Disorders* (DSM-IV-TR) that describes those who have a strong and persistent cross-gender feelings. The diagnosis is used to aid in the identification of individuals who might benefit from clinical interventions to enhance adjustment.
- The term "gender dysphoria" describes the discomfort transgender people often feel about their body and about societal expectations regarding gender roles. Many transgender people prefer this term to GID. Gender dysphoria is generally experienced as a mix of depression, anxiety and agitation, and the sense that something is not right.
- Current clinical thinking suggests that gender dysphoria is not a sign of mental pathology. However, cultural intolerance can leave many transgender people with few social and financial supports needed to respond to the medical and emotional challenges of being gender variant; consequently, mental health issues often arise.
- Due to cultural misunderstanding and intolerance, transgender people face a great deal of discrimination; they often lack access to basic healthcare and support networks, and are at high risk for unemployment and underemployment, homelessness, substance abuse, HIV, depression, anxiety, suicide, self-harm, sex work, and hate crimes. Low self-esteem, shame, and humiliation are often part of the transgender person's daily experience.
- Gender identity and sexual orientation are closely intertwined, but are distinct. Gender identity describes a person's internal sense of being male or female regardless of biology; sexual orientation refers to the gender(s) a person finds attractive.
- Not every gender dysphoric person decides to change their physical appearance or transition to the other gender, and not every transgender person has gender dysphoria.
- Transitioning is very expensive and is not covered by most medical insurance plans. For those who choose surgery, sexual reassignment surgery has been shown to be highly effective in relieving gender dysphoria. There are numerous examples of transgender individuals who have transitioned successfully and are leading full, satisfying lives.
- Clinicians can provide sensitive and comprehensive care by creating nonjudgmental, welcoming environments, seeking reliable information, and helping patients find appropriate community supports.
- The Harry Benjamin Standards of Care (SOC) provides guidelines for the psychiatric, psychological, medical, and surgical management of gender dysphoric patients, including persons who wish to alter their physical appearance through hormone therapy and/or surgery (http://www.wpath.org).

References

1. **Israel GE, Tarver DE**. Transgender Care: Recommended Guidelines, Practical Information & Personal Accounts. Temple University Press; 1997.

2. **Laqueur T**. Making Sex: Body and Gender from the Greeks to Freud. Harvard University Press; 1990.

3. **Beemyn BG**. Trans on campus: measuring and improving the climate for transgender students. On Campus with Women [serial online]. 2005;34. Also available at http://www.ocww.org.

4. **Feldman S**. Components of Gender. Available at http://androgyne.0catch.com.

5. **Bornstein K**. My Gender Workbook. Routledge; 1998.

6. **Stowell GS**. Personal communication; 2001.

7. **Diagnostic and Statistical Manual of Mental Disorders**. 4th ed. American Psychiatric Association; 1994.

8. **Lev AI**. Transgender Emergence: Therapeutic Guidelines for Working with Gender-Variant People and Their Families. The Haworth Clinical Practice Press; 2004.

9. **Bockting WO, Coleman E**. A comprehensive approach to the treatment of gender dysphoria. In: Bockting WO, Coleman E, eds. Gender Dysphoria: Interdisciplinary Approaches in Clinical Management. The Haworth Press; 1992:131-55.

10. **Bradley SJ, Zucker KJ**. Gender Identity Disorder: A review of the past 10 years. Journal of the American Academy of Child and Adolescent Psychiatry. 1997;36:872-80.

11. **Lothstein LM**. Psychodynamics and sociodynamics of gender-dysphoric states. American Journal of Psychotherapy. 1979;33: 214-38.

12. **Colapinto J**. As Nature Made Him: The Boy Who Was Raised As a Girl. Harper Collins; 2000.

13. **Diamond M, Sigmundson HK**. Sex reassignment at birth. Long-term review and clinical implications. Arch Pediatr Adolesc Med. 1997;151:298-304.

14. **Green R**. Gender identity in childhood and later sexual orientation: follow-up of 78 males. American Journal of Psychiatry. 1985;142:339-41.

15. **Di Ceglie D, Freedman D, McPherson S, Richardson P**. Children and adolescents referred to a specialist gender identity development service: clinical features and demographic characteristics. International Journal of Transgenderism. 2002;6, Available at http://www.symposion.com/ijt/ijtvo06no01_01.htm.

16. **Coolidge FL, Thede LL, Young SE**. The heritability of Gender Identity Disorder in a child and adolescent twin sample. Behavior Genetics. 2002; 32:251-7.

17. **Alao A, Yolles JC, Huslander W**. Female genital self-mutilation. Psychiatric Services. 1999;50:971.

18. **Bhatia MS, Arora S**. Penile self-mutilation. The British Journal of Psychiatry. 2001;178: 86-7.

19. **McKay D, Gavigan CA, Kulchycky S**. Social skills and sex-role functioning in borderline personality disorder: relationship to self-mutilating behavior. Cognitive Behavioral Therapy. 2004;33:27-35.

20. **Paris J**. Understanding self-mutilation in borderline personality disorder. Harvard Review of Psychiatry. 2005;13:179-85.

21. **Master V, Santucci R**. An American hijra: a report of a case of genital self-mutilation to become India's "third sex." Urology. 2003;62:1121.

22. **Sirota P, Megged S, Stein D, et al**. Self-Castration. Harefuah. 1994;126:186-8,239,240.

23. **Haberman MA, Michael RP**. Autocastration in transsexualism. The American Journal of Psychiatry. 1979;136:347-48.

24. **Michel A, Mormont C**. Was Snow White a transsexual? Encephale. 2002;28:59-64.

25. **Denny D**. Transgendered youth at risk for exploitation, HIV, hate crimes. American Educational Gender Information Service, Inc.; 1995. Available at http://www.aidsinfonyc.org/Q-zone/youth.html.

26. **Van Wormer K, McKinney R**. What schools can do to help gay, lesbian, and bisexual youth: a harm reduction approach. Adolescence. 2003;38:409-20.
27. **Xavier J, Hitchcock D, Hollinshead S, et al**. An Overview of US Trans Health Priorities: A Report by the Eliminating Disparities Working Group. National Coalition for LGBT Health; August 2004.
28. **Clements-Nolle K, Marx R, Guzman R, et al**. HIV prevalence, risk behaviors, health care use, and mental health status of transgender persons: implications for public health intervention. American Journal of Public Health. 2001;91:915-21.
29. **Markowitz L**. Out of denial: an interview with Dana Finnegan and Emily McNally. 2002. National Association of Lesbian and Gay Addiction Professionals. Available at http://www.nalgap.org/news.htm.
30. **San Francisco Department of Public Health**. The Transgender Community Health Project: Descriptive Results. 1999. Available at http://hivinsite.ucsf.edu/InSite.jsp?doc=2098.461e.
31. **Bockting W, Knudson G, Goldberg J M**. Counseling and Mental Health Care of Transgender Adults and Loved Ones. 2006. Available at http://www.vch.ca/transhealth/resources/tcp.html.
32. **Simon TB, Reback C, Bemis C**. HIV prevalence and incidence among male-to-female transsexuals receiving HIV prevention services in Los Angeles County. AIDS. 2002; 14: 2953-2955.
33. **Nemoto T, Operario D, Keatley J, Han L, Soma T**. HIV risk behaviors among male-to-female transgender persons of color in San Francisco. American Journal of Public Health. 2004;94:1193-9.
34. **Kenagy, GP**. Transgender health: findings from two needs assessment studies in Philadelphia. Health and Social Work. 2005;30:19-26.
35. **Kolakowski V**. Another transgender murder: local TG group declares 'state of emergency and national crisis.' Bay Area Reporter. 1999;29:19.
36. **Harry Benjamin International Gender Dysphoria Association**. Standards of Care for Gender Identity Disorders [publication online]. 6th ed. 2001. Available at http://www.wpath.org.
37. **Hall JA, Dornan MC**. What patients like about their medical care and how often they are asked: a meta analysis of the satisfaction literature. Social Science and Medicine. 1988;27:935-9.
38. **Kaufman R**. Improving transgender healthcare. New Jersey AIDS Line. Summer 2006;29-30. Special LGBT Health Issue.
39. **Lawrence A**. Factors associated with satisfaction or regret following male-to-female sex reassignment surgery. Archives of Sexual Behavior. 2003;32:299-315.
40. **Pfafflin F, Junge A**. Sex Reassignment: 30 Years of International Follow-up Studies after SRS: A Comprehensive Review, 1961-1991 [publication online]. Translated from German into American English by Roberta B. Jacobson and Alf B. Meier. IJT Electronic Books; 1992. Available at http://www.symposion.com/ijt/pfaefflin/1000.htm.
41. **Morris J**. Conundrum. Harcourt Brace Jovanovich; 1974.
42. **Ross MW, Need JA**. Effects of adequacy of gender reassignment surgery on psychological adjustment: a follow-up of fourteen male-to-female patients. Archives of Sexual Behavior. 1989;18:145-53.
43. **Bodlund O, Kullgren G**. Transsexualism—general outcome and prognostic factors: a five-year follow-up study of nineteen transsexuals in the process of changing sex. Archives of Sexual Behavior. 1996;25:303-16.
44. **Rakic Z, Starcevic V, Maric J, et al**. The outcome of sex reassignment surgery in Belgrade: 32 patients of both sexes. Archives of Sexual Behavior. 1996;25:515-25.
45. **Hunt DD, Hampson JL**. Follow-up of 17 biologic male transsexuals after sex-reassignment surgery. The American Journal of Psychiatry. 1980;137:432-8.
46. **Stein M, Tiefer L, Melman A**. Follow-up observations of operated male-to-female transsexuals. Journal of Urology. 1990;143:1188-92.

47. **Landen M, Walinder J, Hambert G, et al**. Factors predictive of regret in sex reassignment. Acta Psychiatria Scandinavia. 1998;97:284-9.
48. **Krege S, Bex A, Lummen G, et al**. Male-to-female transsexualism: a technique, results and long-term follow-up in 66 patients. BJU International. 2001;88:396-402.
49. **Aude M, Ansseau M, Legros JJ, et al**. The transsexual: what about the future? European Psychiatry. 2002;17:353-62.

Chapter 13

Medical and Surgical Management of the Transgender Patient: What the Primary Care Clinician Needs to Know

JAMIE FELDMAN, MD, PhD

Introduction

Transgender persons represent an underserved community in need of sensitive, comprehensive healthcare. As discussed in Chapter 12, delivery of quality medical care to this population can be challenging for several reasons. Transgender identity and behavior are often socially stigmatized, leading many individuals to maintain a traditional male or female presentation and public role while keeping their transgender health concerns concealed. Lack of healthcare insurance, the experience of discrimination in the healthcare setting, lack of access to medical personnel competent in transsexual medicine, and possible discomfort with the body can lead transgender patients to avoid medical care altogether.[1] Thus, they often lack access to preventive health services and timely treatment of routine health problems.

In addition, most physicians and other healthcare professionals do not receive training in health issues specific to transgender patients and lack ready access to appropriate information or to a knowledgeable colleague. Long-term, prospective studies for most transgender-specific health issues are lacking, resulting in variable preventive care recommendations based primarily on expert opinion. However, by utilizing an increasing body of peer-reviewed, scientific research on transgender health, along with relevant data from the general population, one can develop an evidence-based approach to preventive care for transgender patients.

This chapter presents a general medical approach to transgender healthcare for the average primary care clinician who seeks to increase his or her skill in providing competent care to this population. Recommendations are made about what to include in the history and how to perform the physical exam, and suggestions for screening and prevention are presented as appropriate for individuals with varying physiological (hormonal) and anatomical (surgical) presentations. The nuances of hormone prescription are not discussed in detail here. For readers who seek this information, the following resources provide an excellent summary: *Transgender Primary Medical Care: Suggested Guidelines for Clinicians in British Columbia*[2] and "Preventive Care of the Transgendered Patient: An Evidence Based Approach," in *Principles of Transgender Medicine and Surgery*.[3]

General Guidelines

Patients explore transgender issues best in an environment of trust. Providers should refer to the transgender patient by their preferred name and pronoun, reassure the patient about confidentiality, educate clinic staff and colleagues regarding transgender issues, and respect the patient's wishes regarding potentially sensitive physical exams and tests (such as pelvic examinations or mammograms). Familiarity with commonly used terms and the diversity of identities within the transgender community is essential.

Hormonal and surgical treatment, discussed later in this chapter, can increase the quality of life for transgender individuals who desire to bring their bodies into greater congruence with their gender identity.[4] Efforts should be made to address health concerns that arise related to hormonal interventions or planned surgeries through behavior change, lifestyle change, or medication. Reduction or discontinuation of hormones should be a last rather than first resort and is not to be undertaken lightly as there can be serious psychological consequences.

The Transgender-Oriented Health History

As with any patient coming to establish care, providers should perform a comprehensive health history with their transgender patients. Please see Chapters 12 and 15 for specific suggestions regarding how to ask questions in a sensitive and respectful manner. The transgender-oriented health history should include the following elements:

The *general health history* should review current and past medical conditions, including all medications and the most recent physical exam (including Pap smear, and testicular and rectal exams, where appropriate). A thorough gynecologic and obstetric history is important in female-to-male patients, as there may be an increased incidence of polycystic ovarian syndrome (PCOS) in this population.[5]

In the *family history*, particular attention should be paid to any clotting disorders, cardiovascular disease, hypertension, diabetes, and mental illness. Any family history for breast, ovarian, uterine, or prostate cancer should also be noted, as these cancers are known to be influenced by exogenous hormones and may require different or more frequent screening if patients are taking feminizing or masculinizing hormones.

A *sexual health* history requires particular sensitivity for transgender patients. Discussion should be initiated gradually and pacing should depend on patient comfort. A screening sexual history should cover sexual orientation, risk behaviors related to sexually transmitted infections (STIs) and unintended pregnancy, and sexual function. If the screening history raises concerns, a more detailed sexual history is warranted.

The *psychosocial history* should include a review of a transgender patient's family, economic, and larger social environments, which can be sources of support or stress. Social isolation, rejection by family or community of origin, harassment, and discrimination can significantly impact a transgender individual's health. As a result of employment discrimination and family abandonment, many transgender people live in poverty in both rural and urban areas, and housing concerns are not uncommon.[6]

History of Feminizing or Masculinizing Interventions

Some transgender individuals utilize hormonal, surgical, or other interventions to bring their bodies into greater alignment with their gender identity. When establishing care with a transgender patient, a thorough history of these interventions is essential. For other patients, hormonal and surgical concerns are less prominent, and this part of the history is accordingly brief. Questions may include the following:

1. Has the patient ever taken cross-gender hormones?
Are there any complications or concerns regarding past
or current hormone use?
Feminizing and masculinizing medications have the potential for numerous drug interactions, and the primary care provider needs to be cognizant of these before prescribing anything new. Medically unsupervised use of hormones is common among transgender patients with limited access to care.[7] Patients may borrow hormones from friends or buy hormones illicitly. Increasingly, transgender persons are purchasing hormones over the Internet, usually from foreign suppliers and with little to no clinician involvement. The primary care provider should also inquire about "herbal hormones"—phytoestrogens or androgen-like compounds sold as dietary supplements such as red clover, black cohosh, and dehydroepiandrosterone (DHEA). Transgender patients with coexisting chronic medical problems will need closer follow-up once they begin hormones.

2. Has the patient undergone any feminizing or
masculinizing surgical procedures? Are there any
complications or concerns regarding past surgeries?

For individuals in the female-to-male (FTM) spectrum, surgeries may
include chest reconstruction, hysterectomy, salpingo-oophorectomy,
vaginectomy, metaidoioplasty or phalloplasty (penile construction), ure-
throplasty, scrotoplasty, and procedures to masculinize facial and body
contours. For individuals in the male-to-female (MTF) spectrum, surgery
may include orchiectomy, penectomy, vaginoplasty, breast augmentation,
facial feminization or tracheal shave and procedures to feminize body contours, and surgery to elevate voice pitch. Complications relating to genital
surgery (for both MTFs and FTMs) are not infrequent, particularly in
patients who underwent surgery many years ago when techniques were
less sophisticated and follow-up care less consistent. Surgical interventions
will be discussed in more detail later in this chapter.

3. Does the patient plan to pursue hormone therapy or
surgeries in the future? Are there any additional feminizing/
masculinizing interventions sought by the patient?

Awareness of future plans is useful in coordinating referrals and planning
relating to care for any coexisting medical, social, or psychological concerns. Nonmedical, peer-based resources are often useful for assistance
relating to appearance (clothing, hairstyle, makeup, footwear, etc), change
in legal name or sex designation, and gender-specific mannerisms. Referrals
may be sought for speech change therapy, hair removal, or hair transplant.

Transgender Physical Exam

Physical exams should be structured based on the organs present rather
than the perceived gender of the patient. For example, if there is any significant breast tissue, the patient needs routine breast/chest exams. The
prostate is not removed in vaginoplasty, and prostate exams should be performed for the MTF patient as indicated. If the uterus and cervix are present in FTMs, pelvic exams and Pap smears typically need to be done on a
regular basis, although these may be deferred for FTMs who have not had
penetrative vaginal intercourse.

Transgender patients may be uncomfortable with their bodies and may
find some elements of physical examination traumatic. Unless there is an
immediate medical need, sensitive elements of the exam (particularly
breast, genital, and rectal exam) should be delayed until strong clinician-
patient rapport has developed. Sensitive exams can be managed in a variety of ways, depending on patient preference; some patients prefer the
exam to be done as quickly as possible, while others require a slow pace
or even light sedation. It is important to discuss the purpose and specifics
of the exam (when, where, and how you will touch the patient) prior to

proceeding: when this is done clearly, most patients will understand. The physical exam provides an important opportunity to educate patients about their bodies and about the need for ongoing health maintenance.

A range of physical development is seen in patients undergoing hormone therapy. FTM patients may have beard growth, clitoromegaly, acne, and androgenic alopecia; those who have bound their breasts for numerous years may have rash or yeast infection of the skin under the breasts. MTF patients may have feminine breast shape and size, often with relatively underdeveloped nipples; breasts may appear fibrocystic if there have been silicone injections. Galactorrhea is sometimes seen in MTF patients with high prolactin levels, especially among those using breast pumps to stimulate development.[8] There may be minimal body hair and variable facial hair (depending on length of time on hormones and manual hair removal treatments such as electrolysis). Testicles may become small and soft; defects or hernias at the external inguinal ring may be present due to the practice of "tucking" the testicles up near (or into) the inguinal canal. Particularly in the absence of hormone therapy, findings suggestive of intersex conditions should be further evaluated.

Physical findings in postoperative patients will depend on the types of surgeries that have been done, the quality of the surgical work, the impact of postoperative complications, and any revisions that have been performed after the initial surgery. FTM patients after chest surgery will have scar tissue consistent with the type of procedure and may have large nipples or small grafted nipples. The FTM neophallus created from the release of an augmented clitoris (metaidoioplasty procedure) looks like a very small penis; a grafted penis constructed by phalloplasty will be adult-sized but more flaccid than in the natal male (erection is obtained through use of a stiffener or pump). MTF patients may have undergone breast augmentation with implants. MTF genital surgery typically involves simultaneous removal of the penis or testicles and creation of a neovagina; some patients may just have the testes removed, prior to or instead of vaginoplasty. There may be varying degrees of labial reconstruction and clitoral hooding, depending on the completion of surgical revisions. The neovagina typically appears less moist than in natal women, and may be stenosed internally if the patient does not dilate daily or is not sexually active.

Laboratory Requisition Forms

Most requisition forms for laboratory tests ask for the sex of the patient to provide the primary care provider with normal ranges for the results (which are often sex-dependent) and to flag abnormal results. Normal values for transgender persons who are undergoing or have completed gender transition have not been established for any laboratory test, and there is no consensus about how sex should be recorded on lab requests for the transgender patient. Clinicians must therefore balance consideration of the following issues in order to select the correct test in an appropriate manner: (a) the stress a patient experiences going into the lab with a sex on the form that conflicts with their name/appearance; (b) the need to obtain laboratory tests that are most appropriate to a patient's physiology; and (c) the need to minimize laboratory error.

Evidence-Based Decision-Making in Transgender Care

Currently, few prospective, large-scale studies exist regarding transgender healthcare. The best available evidence comes from a Netherlands historical cohort involving 816 male-to-female (MTF) and 293 female-to-male (FTM) transsexual patients, with hormone use ranging over two months to 41 years.[9] Morbidity and mortality were compared to age-gender specific statistics in the general Dutch population. As the study did not track a specific cohort over a long period of time, particularly into the over age 65 range, the long-term health effects of hormone therapy remain uncertain. Smaller scale studies on specific issues such as osteoporosis do exist, along with non-trans-specific evidence (ie, studies involving nontransgender men and women). In many areas, case reports or series are the major source of trans-specific data. Case studies suggest that certain conditions occur in the transgender setting; however, further research is needed to determine incidence and clinical significance.

In applying knowledge from the nontransgender setting to transgender patients, clinicians should look for rigorous studies that are highly relevant to the clinical context. For example, a large prospective study involving nontransgender women on postmenopausal hormone therapy may be relevant for MTFs over age 50 who are taking similar types of hormones for feminizing purposes. Evidence from nontransgender studies can be directly applied to similar transgender patients who have not had surgical or hormonal interventions, eg, studies involving nontransgender women are applicable to individuals in the FTM spectrum who have not taken testosterone or have not had masculinizing surgery.

Primary Prevention, Screening, and Management

Risks and recommendations for preventive care often depend on the patient's hormonal and surgical status and will be discussed according to these categories where applicable. The recommendations below are based on a systematic, evidence-based review of the transgender and appropriate nontransgender literature, supplemented by peer-reviewed expert opinion.

Vaccinations

Recommended vaccinations are the same for transgender and nontransgender patients. While vaccination of all children for Hepatitis B is now recommended, many transgender adults are not immune and could benefit from vaccination—particularly persons with more than one sexual partner in the last six months, patients with a recent STI, individuals who share needles to inject hormones or other substances, and those traveling to endemic areas.

Cancer Screening: Breast Cancer

MTF Patients, No Hormone Use
There is no evidence of increased risk of cancer compared to natal male patients, in the absence of other known risk factors (eg, Klinefelter syndrome). Routine screening, either in the form of regular breast exams or mammography, is not indicated.

MTF Patients, Past or Current Hormone Use
MTF patients who have taken feminizing hormones may be at increased risk of breast cancer compared to natal males, but they likely have significantly lower risk compared to natal females.[8] The length of feminizing hormone exposure, family history, BMI > 35, and use of progestins may further increase risk (by 37%-40%); however, screening mammography for MTF patients receiving hormone therapy is not currently supported by the evidence. Screening mammography is advisable in patients over age 50 with additional risk factors (eg, estrogen and progestin use > five years, positive family history, BMI > 35).[10] Annual clinical breast exam and periodic self-breast exam are not recommended for cancer screening but may serve an educational purpose. Breast augmentation, common among MTF patients, does not appear to increase risk of breast cancer, although it may impair the accuracy of screening mammography.[11]

FTM Patients, No Chest Surgery,
With or Without Testosterone Use
Breast exams and screening mammography are recommended as for natal females.

FTM, After Chest Surgery, With or Without Testosterone Use
Female-to-male patients who undergo breast reduction or mastectomy (chest reconstruction) retain some degree of underlying breast tissue for good cosmetic result. Case series do exist of breast cancer among female-to-male patients after chest surgery and on hormones.[12] The risk of breast cancer is reduced with chest surgery but appears higher in FTM patients than natal men, based on breast reduction studies in nontransgender

women. Risk is affected by age at chest surgery and the amount of breast tissue removed. Pre-chest surgery mammography is not recommended unless the patient meets usual natal female recommendations.[13] Yearly chest wall and axillary exams, along with education regarding the small but possible risk of breast cancer, are recommended.

Cancer Screening: Cervical Cancer

MTF, Following Vaginoplasty

If the glans penis has been used to create a neocervix, Pap smear should follow guidelines for natal females.[14] One can consider vaginal Pap smear for MTFs with history of genital warts.

FTM, Cervix Intact (Partial Hysterectomy or No Hysterectomy)

Pap smears can be traumatic for the FTM patient and should be kept to a minimum for patients at low risk of HPV transmission (ie, little sexual activity involving the genitals). Pap smears should follow recommended guidelines for natal females in patients with an intact cervix. There is no evidence that testosterone increases or reduces the risk of cervical cancer. As testosterone therapy can result in atrophic dysplasia-like changes to the cervical epithelium, the pathologist should be informed of the patient's hormonal status.[15] For patients otherwise at low risk of cervical cancer, atypical squamous cells of uncertain significance (ASCUS) and low-grade squamous intraepithelial lesion (SIL) Pap smears are unlikely to represent precancerous lesions. However, these changes are not well-characterized in the literature, and colposcopy may be indicated in patients at increased risk. Total hysterectomy should be considered in the presence of high-grade dysplasia or if the patient is unable to tolerate Pap smears.

FTM, After Total Hysterectomy (Cervix Completely Excised)

If there is no prior history of high-grade cervical dysplasia and/or cervical cancer, no future Pap smears are needed. If there is prior history of high-grade cervical dysplasia or cervical cancer, patients should have annual Pap smears of the vaginal cuff until three normal tests are documented, then continue Pap smears every two to three years (as recommended for natal females).

Cancer Screening: Ovarian or Uterine Cancer

FTM, Intact Ovaries and/or Uterus (No Hysterectomy), With or Without History of Hormones

Increased incidence of polycystic ovarian syndrome (PCOS) has been noted among FTMs even in the absence of testosterone use.[5] PCOS is a hormonal syndrome complex characterized by some or all of the following: failure to ovulate, absent or infrequent menstrual cycles, multiple cysts on the ovaries, hyperandrogenism, hirsuitism, acne, hidradenitis suppurativa, acanthosis nigricans, obesity, and glucose intolerance or diabetes. PCOS is associated with infertility, as well as increased risk of cardiac disease, high blood pressure, and endometrial cancer.[16] Screening for signs and symptoms of polycystic ovarian syndrome (PCOS) is therefore reasonable in all FTM patients. Some studies suggest an increased risk of ovarian cancer among female-to-male patients on testosterone therapy.[17] Pelvic exams should be performed every one to three years in patients over age 40 or with a family history of ovarian cancer, or yearly if PCOS is present. Given the risk of endometrial cancer among nontransgender women over 40 and all women with PCOS, providers should evaluate unexplained uterine bleeding, with transvaginal ultrasound, pelvic ultrasound, and/or endometrial biopsy. As pelvic exams may be distressing for female-to-male patients, a total hysterectomy should be considered if patients cannot tolerate ongoing pelvic exams, if fertility is not an issue, and if the patient's health will not be adversely affected by surgery.

Cancer Screening: Prostate Cancer

MTF, No Current/Past Hormones, No Surgery

Routine PSA screening in any usual risk population is not currently supported by evidence. The risks and possible benefits of PSA screening should be discussed with all patients, and routine screening considered in high-risk patients (African American, family history of prostate cancer) starting at age 45. Digital rectal exams should be performed as for natal males.

MTF, Past or Current Hormones, With or Without Surgery

The prostate is not removed in male-to-female genital surgery. Feminizing hormone therapy appears to decrease the risk of prostate cancer, but the degree of reduction is unknown. PSA screening is not recommended, as PSA levels may be falsely low in an androgen-deficient setting,[18] even in the presence of prostate cancer. A recent study demonstrated that 15% of nontransgender men with PSA levels less than four ng/mL (within the normal range) had prostate cancer.[19] Androgen antagonists may decrease serum levels of PSA, further complicating interpretation of PSA results in the MTF patient who is taking feminizing hormones.[20] Providers should consider screening in high-risk patients only, but digital rectal exams should be performed as per natal males, along with education regarding the small but possible risk of prostate cancer.

Cancer Screening: Other Cancers

Currently, there is no evidence that transgender persons are at either increased or decreased risk of other cancers. Screening recommendations for other cancers (including colon cancer, lung cancer, and anal cancer) should be followed as with nontransgender patients.

Cardiovascular Disease

All Transgender Patients

Assessing and treating cardiovascular risk factors is an essential primary care intervention for transgender patients. Regardless of hormone status, the transgender population as a whole has several risk factors for cardiovascular disease; feminizing or masculinizing hormone therapy further increases cardiovascular risks. Smoking is a concern for both FTM and MTF persons. MTF patients tend to present for transgender care at an older age (ie, early 40s)[21] with hypertension, diabetes, hyperlipidemia, or other conditions common in middle-aged male bodies. FTM patients who present with PCOS are at increased risk for hypertension, insulin resistance, and hyperlipidemia. Finally, cardiovascular risk factors are often undiagnosed or undertreated among transgender patients due to their relative lack of primary care. Prompt identification and management of cardiovascular risk factors may decrease the hazards associated with hormone therapy in these patients. Providers may consider performing a stress test before prescribing hormones to patients at very high risk or with any cardiovascular symptoms; as in nontransgender patients, daily aspirin therapy may be considered in patients at high risk for coronary artery disease (CAD).

MTF, Currently Taking Feminizing Hormones

The effects of feminizing hormones on CAD and cerebrovascular disease are not well characterized. There are several case reports of myocardial infarction and ischemic stroke among MTFs taking estrogen,[22] and increased risk has been noted among women on oral contraceptives. However, the retrospective 1997 Netherlands study found no increased incidence of CAD or cerebrovascular disease compared to rates in the general population.[9] Both the Heart and Estrogen/Progestin Replacement Study (HERS) and Women's Health Initiative (WHI) trials, prospective studies of hormone replacement among postmenopausal women, indicated no benefit and a probable increased risk for cardiovascular events with combined estrogen and progesterone therapy.[23,24] The estrogen-only arm of the WHI trial demonstrated an increase in cerebrovascular events but not cardiac events. The HERS and WHI trials were conducted using oral conjugated estrogen; it is unclear whether these effects extend to other oral or transdermal estrogens (which show reduced risk of venous thromboembolic events).[25] In both the HERS trial and the observational Nurses Health Study,[26] an increased number of cardiac events occurred in the first one to two years and decreased in subsequent years of hormone replacement. Therefore, close monitoring for cardiac events or symptoms is recommended for MTFs with risk factors, especially during the first one to two years of feminizing hormone therapy. In patients with preexisting CAD, there is increased risk of future events using estrogen and/or progestin. It may be possible to reduce risks by using transdermal estrogen, reducing the estrogen dose, and omitting progestin from the regimen.

FTM, Currently Taking Testosterone

The effect of testosterone on cardiovascular events in FTM patients is unclear. While both exogenous testosterone and hyperandrogen states (eg, PCOS) clearly increase cardiac risk factors as discussed, current evidence of increase in cardiac morbidity or mortality with PCOS is limited.[16] In FTMs with preexisting CAD who are using testosterone, there may be increased risk of future events. The extent of risk and resulting morbidity, and mortality are unclear, given the contradictory effects of testosterone replacement or increased androgens in nontransgender men and women.

Close monitoring for cardiac events or symptoms is recommended for FTMs at moderate to high risk for CAD. In FTMs with preexisting CAD, there may be an increased risk of future events. Individualized decision-making is key, but attention to published guidelines for secondary prevention is recommended.

Hypertension

MTF and FTM, Not Currently Taking Hormones

Hypertension screening and treatment should follow recommended guidelines for nontransgender patients. Ideally, blood pressure should be well controlled prior to initiating feminizing or masculinizing hormone therapy.

MTF, Currently Taking Estrogen

Exogenous estrogen can increase blood pressure, and transgender patients at risk may develop overt hypertension. While a significantly higher incidence compared to the nontransgender population was not noted in the Netherlands study,[9] the researchers defined hypertension as pressures greater than 160/95 mm Hg, considerably higher than current North American guidelines. Providers should monitor blood pressure every one to three months, and a systolic blood pressure goal of ≤ 130 mm Hg and a diastolic goal of ≤ 90 mm Hg is recommended. Use of the anti-androgen spironolactone may be considered as part of an antihypertensive regimen in FTM patients desiring feminizing therapy.

FTM, Currently Taking Testosterone

The risk of hypertension in FTMs is unclear. Exogenous testosterone can increase blood pressure,[27] and natal females with PCOS are at increased risk of hypertension. [16] However, a prospective study (N = 28) found no significant change in blood pressure after an average of 18 months of testosterone administration—even among subjects on double the normal dose of testosterone.[28] Providers should monitor blood pressure every 1-3 months, with recommended blood pressures goals of ≤ 130 mm Hg systolic and ≤ 90 mm Hg diastolic, especially in patients with PCOS.

Lipids

MTF, Not Currently Taking Estrogen
FTM, Not Currently Taking Testosterone
Screening for and treatment of hyperlipidemia should follow guidelines for nontransgender patients. Ideally, lipids should be well controlled prior to initiation of either feminizing or masculinizing hormones.

MTF, Currently Taking Estrogen
Studies in both nontransgender women and MTFs demonstrate increased high density lipoprotein (HDL) and decreased low density lipoprotein (LDL) cholesterol on estrogen therapy.[29,30] However, both the HERS and WHI trials, prospective studies of hormone replacement among post-menopausal women, indicated no benefit and a probable increased risk for cardiovascular events with combined estrogen and progesterone therapy.[23,24] Oral estrogen therapy, both in postmenopausal women and MTF patients, is known to increase triglycerides and has precipitated pancreatitis in several cases.[31] An annual fasting lipid profile is thus recommended for MTF patients taking estrogen. Transdermal estrogen is preferred for patients with hyperlipidemia, particularly hypertriglyceridemia. In order to incorporate the cardiovascular effects of feminizing hormone therapy into existing evidence-based guidelines, it can be considered as an additional cardiac risk factor. Target lipid levels for patients on treatment include an LDL of < 130 mg/dL for low-to-moderate risk patients and < 100 mg/dL for high-risk patients, consistent with current National Cholesterol Education Program Adult Treatment Panel (NCEP ATP) guidelines.[32]

FTM, Currently Taking Testosterone
Risk of atherosclerotic disease is increased in patients on masculinizing regimens because of increased LDL and decreased HDL cholesterol.[33] However, no extra cardiovascular morbidity was seen in the retrospective Netherlands study.[9] Both FTM patients and natal women with PCOS are at increased risk of dyslipidemias, although the effect on the risk of cardiac events is not yet determined.[16,34] An annual fasting lipid profile is recommended for patients on testosterone, and supraphysiologic testosterone levels should be avoided in patients with known hyperlipidemia. Daily topical or weekly intramuscular testosterone regimens are preferable to bi-weekly intramuscular injection. Target lipid levels for patients on treatment should follow NCEP ATP guidelines, as noted above. Exercise is recommended in all groups to treat low HDL levels.

Diabetes Mellitus

MTF, Not Currently Taking Estrogen
FTM, Not Currently Taking Testosterone

Providers should follow diabetes screening and management guidelines as for the nontransgender population. Additionally, providers should consider screening (by patient history) all FTM patients for PCOS and perform diabetes screening if PCOS is present.

MTF, Currently Taking Estrogen

Patients taking estrogen may be at increased risk for type 2 diabetes, particularly those with a family history of diabetes or other risk factors. Estrogen is known to impair glucose tolerance,[35] and there have been case reports of new onset type 2 diabetes among MTF transgender patients on estrogen.[36] A study of glucose tolerance among hyperandrogenic women on oral contraceptives demonstrated a significant reduction in glucose tolerance and the development of diabetes in two of the sixteen women,[37] suggesting that the presence of endogenous androgens plays a role in glucose metabolism as well. Finally, patients on feminizing hormones often gain weight and body fat, which may contribute to glucose intolerance. An annual fasting glucose test is recommended in patients with family history of diabetes and/or greater than five kg weight gain. Glucose tolerance testing (or A1c in patients unable to perform a GTT) may be considered in patients with evidence of impaired glucose tolerance without diabetes. Diabetes should be managed according to guidelines for nontransgender patients, but insulin-sensitizing agents are recommended if medications are indicated, given the underlying mechanism of insulin resistance associated with hormonal therapy. A decrease in estrogen dose may be indicated if glucose is difficult to control or the patient is unable to lose weight.

FTM, Currently Taking Testosterone

As noted above, there is limited evidence of a higher incidence of PCOS among FTM persons, who have an increased risk of glucose intolerance. However, there is no current evidence of an altered risk of type 2 diabetes in FTMs who are taking testosterone. Further research is needed to clarify how these findings affect the risk of diabetes in the FTM population. Providers should consider an annual fasting glucose test in patients with family history of diabetes and/or greater than five kg weight gain. Guidelines for managing diabetes mellitus are the same as for the nontransgender population.

Smoking

All Transgender Patients

Little is known about smoking prevalence or cessation patterns in the transgender population. Thirty-seven percent of transgender patients presenting to a Minnesota clinic for hormone therapy were current smokers, compared to 20% for the Minnesota population overall.[38] Among the transgender population, there are commonly multiple identified risk factors for smoking, including poverty, stressful living and work environments, and societal marginalization.

The trans-specific risks associated with smoking include an increased risk of venous thromboembolic events with estrogen therapy and reassignment surgery, possible increased risk of cardiovascular disease with both feminizing and masculinizing hormone therapy (especially over age 50), and delayed healing following surgery. Providers should screen all transgender patients for past and present tobacco use.

Inclusion of smoking cessation as part of comprehensive transgender care has been highly successful, particularly in association with hormone therapy. Buproprion, nicotine replacement, nicotinic receptor blockers, and behavioral modification techniques may be appropriate. A comprehensive approach involves consistent smoking cessation messages from all staff, frequent supportive follow-up of cessation efforts, and direct communication of the limitations and risks that smoking imposes on hormone therapy.[39]

Venous Thrombosis/Thromboembolism and Feminizing Hormones

MTF patients on any form of estrogen are at increased risk of venous thromboembolic events—potentially as high as a 20-fold increase.[9] Estrogen therapy is contraindicated in MTF patients with a history of venous thromboembolic events (VTE) or underlying thrombophilia (eg, anticardiolipin syndrome, Factor V Leiden). MTF patients over age 40, smokers, and highly sedentary patients are at particular risk of VTE and may benefit from lifestyle change, transdermal estrogen, and lower estrogen doses.[9,25] Providers should consider daily aspirin therapy in patients with risk factors for VTE who are taking estrogen. All MTF patients on or considering estrogen therapy should be warned regarding the risks of VTE, along with the signs and symptoms.

Osteoporosis

MTF and FTM, No Hormone Use, No Surgery

There is no evidence of increased or decreased risk among transgender persons. Providers should follow recommended guidelines for natal females in FTM patients; routine screening is not recommended for MTF patients, except as indicated by additional risk factors.

MTF, Past or Present Feminizing Hormones, Preorchiectomy

There is no current evidence that feminizing therapy increases risk of osteoporosis, but long-term prospective studies have not been done. Routine screening is not recommended except as indicated by additional risk factors. Calcium and vitamin D supplementation are recommended.

MTF, After Orchiectomy

The effect of feminizing hormones on bone density is controversial, particularly in the postsurgical patient. It is unclear how much estrogen is needed following gonadal removal to protect against bone loss, but studies in postmenopausal women suggest that very low dose estrogen (.025 mg transdermal estradiol or .3 mg conjugated equine estrogen [CEE]) may be sufficient.[40] Loss of bone density is most likely after orchiectomy in those patients with other risk factors (eg, Caucasian or Asian ethnicity, smoking, family history, high alcohol use, hyperthyroidism) and in those who are not fully adherent to hormone therapy. In general, estrogen therapy is advised to reduce the risk of osteoporosis. If there are contraindications to estrogen therapy, supplemental calcium (1200-1500 mg daily) and vitamin D (600-800 units daily) are recommended to limit bone loss, as has been recommended for postmenopausal women. Bone mineral density (BMD) screening is recommended for patients over age 60 who have been off estrogen therapy for longer than five years. If there are additional risk factors for bone loss in patients unable to take estrogen, weekly bisphosphonate therapy (with 35-70 mg alendronate or 35 mg risedronate) may be considered.

FTM, Past or Present Hormone Use, No Surgery

Opinion is mixed on the impact of testosterone on bone density prior to oophorectomy. Some studies demonstrate increased BMD or no change, while others report bone loss.[41,42] Some FTM patients may use Depo-Provera® to produce amenorrhea, which appears to result in bone loss with long-term use in nontransgender women.[43] Providers should consider BMD screening in FTMs over age 50 (or sooner in patients with additional risk factors for osteoporosis) who have been on testosterone therapy over five years. Supplemental calcium (1200-1500 mg daily) and vitamin D (600-800 units daily) are recommended to help maintain bone density.

FTM, Past or Present Hormone Use, Postoophorectomy (or Total Hysterectomy)

Although studies have found that exogenous testosterone maintains bone density to some degree, it may not be sufficient, especially after oophorectomy.[44] It is unclear how much testosterone is needed following gonadal removal to protect against bone loss. Bone loss is most likely in those patients with other risk factors (eg, Caucasian or Asian ethnicity, smoking, family history, high alcohol use, hyperthyroidism) and those who are not fully adherent to hormone therapy. Ongoing testosterone therapy is recommended in these situations. If there are contraindications to testosterone therapy, weekly bisphosphonate therapy (35-70 mg alendronate or 35 mg risedronate) can be considered. Providers should consider BMD screening in all FTMs over age 60, and in FTMs over age 50 (or sooner) in patients with additional risk factors for osteoporosis who have received testosterone therapy for greater than five years. Supplemental calcium (1200-1500 mg daily) and vitamin D (600-800 units daily) are recommended to help maintain bone density.

Sexual Health

Sexually Transmitted Infections (STIs)

Transgender individuals share many of the concerns regarding STIs, including hepatitis B and HIV, found in the lesbian, gay, and bisexual communities (see Chapter 11). There are a few transgender-specific considerations, however. If the category "men who have sex with men" (MSM) is extended to include transgender individuals (of any gender) who have sex with men (TSM), many transgender individuals would be considered in a population that is at increased risk for STIs. Sexual practices among transgender individuals vary greatly,[45,46] and assumptions should not be made about the gender of a patient's sexual partner(s), sexual activities, or individual risks. As discussed in Chapter 12, cofactors related to unsafe sex, such as depression, suicidal ideation, and physical or sexual abuse, are also increased among the transgender population: studies indicate that the need to affirm one's gender identity can drive high-risk sexual behaviors. Finally, because needle-sharing with injectable hormones (or silicone) is a trans-specific potential risk factor for transmission of HIV and hepatitis B/C, patients need to be educated regarding the risks as well as safe handling of needles and syringes.

STI prevention strategies should be appropriately targeted to each individual patient's anatomical needs and specific sexual practices. For example, nonpenetrative sexual activities with appropriate barrier protection (latex gloves, dental dams, nonmicrowaveable plastic wrap) or penetration with a dildo (covered by a condom) can be recommended for MTF patients who are taking feminizing hormones and are unable to sustain an erection sufficiently firm for condom use. To prevent condom breakage, supplemental lubrication should be recommended for MTFs who have had vaginoplasty (as the neovagina is not self-lubricating) and FTMs who take testosterone (as decreased estrogen can result in vaginal atrophy and dryness). Water-based lubricants only should be used with latex barriers, as oil-based products degrade latex and may therefore result in inadvertent transmission of infectious agents. For a more detailed discussion of STI prevention, please see Chapters 11 and 15.

The variable anatomy of transgender persons can affect diagnostic testing for some STIs. A urine-based test of a nonclean catch specimen of the first 25 ml of urine (eg, Gen-Probe™) can be used regardless of anatomy, making this the ideal testing method for chlamydia and gonorrhea in most transgender patients. Rectal and pharyngeal samples can be used in patients with symptoms in these areas. Hormone therapy does not affect treatment of STIs in the transgender individual. Some HIV medications increase or decrease serum estrogen levels, but there is no evidence that cross-sex hormones interfere with the effectiveness of HIV medication or negatively affect the progression of HIV/AIDS. Little has been published regarding the risks of reassignment surgery among patients with HIV/AIDS. HIV-infected persons have an increased risk of infection with any major surgery, with the number and severity of complications related to CD4 count. SRS outcomes appear to be good with adequate patient selection and preoperative preparation.[47]

Fertility Issues

Cross-sex hormones may reduce fertility, and this may be permanent even if hormones are discontinued. Cryopreservation of unfertilized ova is not generally available. Sperm banking is most useful prior to initiation of hormone therapy, as feminizing hormones can permanently impact fertility. Ideally, several samples should be banked. With the patient's permission, a letter of introduction should be sent to the collection center to ensure that the MTF patient who is already cross-living will be treated in a respectful manner.

FTMs may continue to ovulate on testosterone therapy, even if menses have stopped; the risk of pregnancy is reduced but not predictably. Additionally, testosterone can adversely affect a developing fetus. Depo-Provera®, barrier methods, and spermicides are possible contraceptive options for FTMs at risk of pregnancy who are receiving or considering testosterone therapy. Tubal ligation and intrauterine devices (IUDs) are effective, if less popular, alternatives for these patients.

Sexual Function

Testosterone therapy tends to increase libido among FTM patients, while feminizing hormone therapy tends to reduce libido, reduce erectile function, and decrease ejaculation among MTF patients. If an MTF patient is concerned about limiting erectile dysfunction while undergoing feminizing hormone therapy, the prescribing clinician should first consider adjusting the dose of hormones, while addressing the patient's desires regarding the degree of feminization and level of erectile function. If this is unsuccessful, erection-enhancing drugs (eg, phosphodiesterase inhibitors) may be considered. Following genital surgery, sexual function (libido, arousal, pain with sex, and orgasm) is variable and depends on preoperative sexual function, the type of surgery performed, and hormonal status. Sexual function is discussed further in *Endocrine Therapy for Transgender Adults in British Columbia: Suggested Guidelines*[48] and *Care of the Patient Undergoing Sex Reassignment Surgery.*[49]

Transgender Hormone Therapy

Transgender hormone therapy—the provision of exogenous endocrine agents to induce feminizing or masculinizing changes—is a strongly desired medical intervention for many transgender individuals. In addition to inducing physical changes, the act of using transgender hormones is itself an affirmation of gender identity—a powerful incentive for this population.[1] Studies of presurgical transsexuals indicate improved psychological adjustment and quality of life with hormone therapy.[50] There is great variation in the extent to which hormonal changes are undertaken or desired. Some individuals seek maximum feminization or masculinization, while others experience relief with an androgynous presentation resulting from hormonal minimization of existing secondary sex characteristics.

Transgender patients desiring hormone therapy may ask their primary care provider to offer this treatment. Primary care providers can increase their experience and comfort in providing transgender hormone therapy through a variety of means. First, simply caring for transgender patients improves understanding of transgender healthcare needs. In addition, familiarity with hormone regimens and the transition process is facilitated by comanaging care or consulting with a more experienced provider. Physicians who provide transgender hormone therapy come from many different specialties, including endocrinology, family medicine, internal medicine, obstetrics and gynecology, and psychiatry. There is no comprehensive list of experienced transgender hormone providers; physicians who publish in the medical literature and/or who are members of the Harry Benjamin International Gender Dysphoria Association (HBIGDA) are most easily identified. However, physicians who provide transgender hormone therapy undergo no specific training, and standard certification for this care does not exist. Thus, actual practices may vary significantly from provider to provider, making it difficult to discern which physicians are most qualified to serve as a mentor.

Ideally, the prescribing clinician and the patient will work with a psychotherapist trained in treating gender identity issues. As discussed in Chapter 12, psychotherapy is not a requirement prior to initiation of hormone therapy. However, the process of gender transition involves profound mental, social, emotional, economic, and legal changes in a patient's life. Hormone therapy can be both an enriching and complicating element in this transition, and "trans-competent" mental health professionals can provide a wide variety of resources to assist the transgender patient (and hormone provider) in this complex process. When a therapist is involved and with the patient's consent, regular communication is advised to ensure that the transition process is proceeding smoothly. The following section briefly explains the range of potential roles for the primary care provider in transgender hormone care. The TransCare Projects' *Endocrine Therapy for Transgender Adults in British Columbia: Suggested Guidelines*,[48] is an excellent resource for physicians providing any degree of hormone therapy.

Bridging

Patients may present for care already on hormones, whether obtained by prescription or through other means (eg, purchased over the Internet). If a clinician is uncomfortable providing long-term hormone therapy, a good option is to provide a one to three month prescription for hormones while assisting the patient in finding a clinician who can provide long-term follow-up care. Prior medical records should be requested and the history of hormone prescription documented in the current chart. The patient's current regimen should be assessed for safety and drug interactions; safer medications or doses should be substituted when indicated. Clear limits should be negotiated regarding the duration of bridging therapy.

Hormone Therapy Following Gonad Removal

Hormone replacement with estrogen or testosterone is usually continued lifelong after oophorectomy or orchiectomy, unless medical contraindications arise. In MTF patients, dosing is similar to that in postsurgical menopause in patients under 50 and in postnatural menopause in patients 50 and over. FTM patients should receive testosterone doses adequate to keeping free testosterone levels in the low to middle of the normal male range. Detailed dosing and laboratory monitoring guidelines can be found in *Endocrine Therapy for Transgender Adults in British Columbia: Suggested Guidelines*.[48] Laboratory monitoring can be done yearly for otherwise healthy patients.

Hormone Maintenance Prior to Gonad Removal

Once patients have achieved maximal feminizing or masculinizing benefit from hormones (typically two or more years), they remain on a maintenance dose. Maintaining body changes generally requires lower hormone doses compared to initial induction. The maintenance dose is then adjusted for change in health conditions, aging, or other considerations (eg, lifestyle changes). Patients should be monitored by physical exam and laboratory testing every six months. For MTFs over age 40, transdermal rather than oral estrogen is recommended due to increased thromboembolic risk. Based on the increased cardiovascular risk associated with estrogen in post-menopausal women, it may be appropriate to decrease the estrogen dose to 100 mcg twice per week or less in patients over 50, depending on the patient's health status (particularly cardiovascular risk).[31] For FTMs, testosterone doses should be sufficient to maintain free testosterone levels in the low-middle normal male range.

Patients may occasionally need to reduce or temporarily stop their hormone therapy in anticipation of upcoming medical procedures, such as surgery or sperm banking. MTF patients, in particular, should discontinue estrogen 2-4 weeks prior to any major surgery to reduce the risk of thromboembolic events. It is helpful to discuss any temporary interruption of hormones with the patient well in advance. *Endocrine Therapy for Transgender Adults in British Columbia: Suggested Guidelines*[48] provides detailed recommendations on adjusting and monitoring maintenance hormone therapy.

Initiating Hormonal Feminization or Masculinization

Primary care providers are well suited to provide safe and effective masculinizing or feminizing hormone therapy in the setting of comprehensive healthcare. It is not necessary for the prescribing clinician to be an endocrine expert, but it is important to be familiar with relevant medical and psychosocial issues. Hormone therapy must be individualized based on the individual's goals, the risk/benefit ratio of medications, the presence of other medical conditions, and consideration of social and economic issues. In general, hormone therapy should be consistent with the HBIGDA *Standards of Care* (SOC), available online at http://www.wpath.org. The SOC provides a flexible framework to guide the treatment of transgender individuals. Detailed recommendations regarding complete hormone therapy can be found in *Endocrine Therapy for Transgender Adults in British Columbia: Suggested Guidelines.*[48]

Surgical Interventions

Several surgical procedures exist to assist transgender persons in bringing their body into greater alignment with their gender identity. These procedures, in whole or part, are often referred to as sexual reassignment surgery (SRS). With some types of surgery (including but not limited to SRS), detailed protocols are used. HBIGDA's SOC contains recommendations to ensure that surgical treatment is appropriate and that the patient is a suitable candidate. Evaluation by a mental health professional is strongly advised prior to SRS, and the surgeon must not only understand the basis of the recommendation for genital surgery but also have specialized competence in SRS. A detailed description of the types of surgeries and their potential complications may be found in *Care of the Patient Undergoing Sex Reassignment Surgery* (SRS).[49]

Feminizing Procedures

Augmentation Mammaplasty
Breast augmentation, usually performed by a plastic surgeon, places saline-filled implants submuscularly via an incision under the breast (near the inframammary fold) or around the areola. Unless hormones are contraindicated, augmentation surgery is commonly delayed until after hormonal therapy has been undertaken for a period of 18 months to allow time for maximal hormonal breast development.

Vaginoplasty
The term vaginoplasty includes several procedures that transform the male external genitalia into female genitalia. Vaginoplasty includes orchiectomy, creation of a vaginal cavity and neoclitoris, labiaplasty (construction of labia) and penile dissection with partial penectomy. It is usually performed by the plastic surgeon in a single operative setting, although some surgeons prefer to perform labiaplasty and clitoroplasty as a second surgery following healing of the initial vaginoplasty. The penile inversion technique is most commonly used to create the neovagina.[51] In this technique the majority of skin from the shaft of the penis is inverted and used to line the inner walls.

Orchiectomy and Penectomy
Orchiectomy as a single procedure may be sought by patients who would like to reduce the risks and side effects of feminizing hormones by lowering the dosage needed to oppose endogenous testosterone.[52] Typically the testes are removed with preservation of scrotal skin in case vaginoplasty or labiaplasty are sought in the future, but there is risk of shrinkage or damage of the skin.

Some MTF patients seek penectomy without vaginoplasty as a less invasive alternative when vaginal penetration is not desired. A shallow vaginal dimple is created that does not require dilation (as in vaginoplasty), and a new urethral opening is created to allow the patient to urinate in a sitting position. Penectomy as a separate procedure is not recommended if the patient wishes to pursue vaginoplasty at a later date.

Facial Procedures
Facial feminizing surgeries include, but are not limited to, removal of supra-orbital bossing ("brow bossing"), brow elevation, rhinoplasty, ear pinning, augmentation of the lip vermilion area, cheek augmentation, chin/jaw

reduction, and reduction laryngochondroplasty (also known as "tracheal shave" or "Adam's apple reduction").

Silicone Injections

Injection of free (gelatinous) silicone is extremely hazardous. Use of free silicone is not legal in many countries (including Canada and the USA) but may be performed illicitly by nonmedical personnel.[53] Any patient who has undergone free silicone injection as part of breast augmentation or contouring of hips, buttocks, or the face should be referred for immediate medical evaluation, as effects of free silicone injection include severe disfigurement, neurological impairment, pulmonary disease (including embolism), and death.[54]

Masculinizing Procedures

FTM Chest Surgery

Subcutaneous mastectomy results in a chest that has a male contour, is fully sensate, and has minimal scarring.[55] The procedure consists of removal of most of the breast tissue, removal of excess skin, and removal of the inframammary fold. Reduction and repositioning of the nipple-areolar complex is often required to approximate male nipples. The choice of technique must be appropriately selected for the patient's breast size and skin quality: skin that is inelastic (often due to years of breast binding) can adversely affect the outcome and will influence (and limit) the surgeon's choice of technique. Some patients will choose a breast reduction in lieu of a subcutaneous mastectomy. Prior reduction affects options for reconstruction so should be approached cautiously for the patient who wants a full reconstruction in the future.

Hysterectomy and Oophorectomy

Patients may desire hysterectomy and oophorectomy to reduce gender dysphoria, to treat preexisting gynecological problems, to prevent menstrual bleeding in the patient who cannot tolerate testosterone, or to eliminate the need for regular Pap testing and pelvic exams in patients who cannot tolerate vaginal examination. Oophorectomy also allows reduction in testosterone dosage (and hence associated health risks and side effects).

Vaginectomy and Urethral Lengthening

Some patients may request vaginectomy concurrent with a vaginal or abdominal hysterectomy. This procedure includes excision of all vaginal mucosa and approximation of the levator ani muscles in order to obliterate the previous vaginal cavity. Vaginal mucosa is then recruited to lengthen the urethra, which will then carry urine through the neophallus in a metaidoioplasty or a phalloplasty.[56,57] If urethral extension is sought as part of future genital reconstruction (eg, phalloplasty) vaginectomy should not be performed, as vaginal mucosa is used to lengthen the urethra. These procedures are usually performed by the urologist and are a requisite part of a phalloplasty, but optional in metaidoioplasty.

Metaidoioplasty

Metaidoioplasty involves releasing the hormonally enlarged clitoris from its surrounding tissues.[58] A flap of skin from the labia minora is then "wrapped around" the stalk to add bulk, resulting in a small phallus which has erogenous sensation. In addition, the fixed part of the urethra can be extended and incorporated into the microphallus by recruiting tissue from the vaginal mucosa.[59] The procedure results in a small, sensate phallus that may allow for urination while standing.

The microphallus created by metaidoioplasty is typically not large enough for sexual penetration, and does not appear adult in size.[60] Despite the limits of size and sexual function, metaidoioplasty is an option for those FTM patients who do not want to undergo the lengthy phalloplasty procedure with its higher rate of complications and donor-site morbidity.

Phalloplasty

Phalloplasty is a long and complex microsurgical procedure that requires free tissue transfer, usually a forearm graft, to create the neophallus.[61] A small segment of the ulnar forearm is rolled into a tube to form the urethra. This is then rolled within a larger piece of the forearm (including fat and skin) to form a "tube within a tube." The procedure results in an adult male-size phallus that transmits urine, and may later achieve rigidity by insertion of an erectile prosthesis. The native clitoris is not removed but is de-epithelialized and covered by the base of the phallus to preserve erogenous sensation.[60] After anatomic and functional stability is ensured (approximately one year), an erectile prosthesis may be placed. Tattooing of the neoglans may be performed as a later procedure to help create a visible demarcation between the penile shaft and the glans.

Scrotoplasty

A scrotum facilitates life in the male role by more closely approximating male appearance in underwear and swim trunks. Performed by the urologist or plastic surgeon, the scrotoplasty uses tissue from the labia majora to create a pouch (neoscrotum), which is situated over the vaginal opening.[62] After full healing, testicular implants may be placed. Although the skin is initially tight, over time the weight of the prosthesis stretches the redraped labial skin to create a more natural appearance.[63]

Conclusion

Many healthcare providers across a variety of specialties provide excellent hormonal and surgical care for transgender patients. However, comprehensive healthcare for transgender patients should not be relegated exclusively to these clinicians; providing appropriate and sensitive care presents challenges and rewards for all healthcare providers. While not every primary care clinician will be able to offer all elements of comprehensive transgender care, with increasing availability of transgender-specific health information, every physician can become comfortable in working with transgender patients to meet their healthcare needs.

Summary Points

- When establishing care with a transgender patient, a thorough history of hormonal, surgical, or other gender-related interventions is essential. Risks and recommendations for preventive care often depend on the patient's hormonal and surgical status.
- Physical exams should be structured based on the organs present rather than the perceived gender of the patient.
- Screening mammography is advisable in MTF patients over age 50 with additional risk factors (eg, estrogen and progestin use > five years, positive family history, BMI > 35).
- Yearly chest wall and axillary exams, along with education regarding the small but possible risk of breast cancer, are recommended for FTM patients after chest reconstruction surgery.
- As testosterone therapy can result in atrophic changes to the cervical epithelium mimicking dysplasia, the cytopathologist reading a Pap smear should be informed of the FTM patient's hormonal status.
- The prostate is not removed in male-to-female genital surgery. Providers should consider PSA screening in high-risk patients only, but digital rectal exams should be performed as per natal males, along with education regarding the small but possible risk of prostate cancer.
- Regardless of hormone status, the transgender population as a whole has several risk factors for cardiovascular disease; feminizing or masculinizing hormone therapy further increases cardiovascular risks such as hypertension, diabetes and hyperlipidemia.
- Providers should screen all transgender patients for past and present tobacco use.
- MTF patients on any form of estrogen are at increased risk of venous thromboembolic events—potentially as high as a 20-fold increase.
- STI prevention strategies should be appropriately targeted to each individual patient's anatomical needs and specific sexual practices.

References

1. **Kammerer N, Mason T, Connors M, et al.** Transgender health and social service needs in the context of HIV risk. International Journal of Transgenderism, 1999;3. Available at http://www.symposion.com/ijt/hiv_risk/kammerer.htm. Accessed January 1, 2005.

2. **Feldman J, Goldberg J.** Transgender Primary Medical Care: Suggested Guidelines for Clinicians. Vancouver, BC: British Columbia Vancouver Coastal Health; 2006.

3. **Feldman J.** Preventive care of the transgendered patient: an evidence based approach. In: Ettner R, Monstrey S, Eyler E, eds. Principles of Transgender Medicine and Surgery. Haworth Press; 2006.

4. **Smith YLS, Van Goozen S H, Kuiper AJ, et al.** Sex reassignment: outcomes and predictors of treatment for adolescent and adult transsexuals. Psychological Medicine. 2005;35:89-99.

5. **Bosinski HAG, Peter M, Bonatz G, et al.** A higher rate of hyperandrogenic disorders in female-to-male transsexuals. Psychoneuroendocrinology. 1997;22:361-80.

6. **Lombardi EL, Wilchins RA, Priesing D, et al.** Gender violence: transgender experiences with violence and discrimination. Journal of Homosexuality. 2001;42:89-101.

7. **Sperber J, Landers S, Lawrence S.** Access to health care for transgendered persons: results of a needs assessment in Boston. International Journal of Transgenderism. 2005;8:75-91.

8. **Schlatterer K, Yassouridis A, von Werder K, et al.** A follow-up study for estimating the effectiveness of a cross-gender hormone substitution therapy on transsexual patients. Archives of Sexual Behavior. 1998;27:475-92.

9. **van Kesteren PJM, Asscheman H, Megens JAJ, et al.** Mortality and morbidity in transsexual subjects treated with cross-sex hormones. Clinical Endocrinology. 1997;47:337-42.

10. **Humphrey LL, Helfand M, Chan BK, et al.** Breast cancer screening: a summary of the evidence for the US Preventive Services Task Force. Annals of Internal Medicine. 2005;137:347-60.

11. **Deapen D, Hamilton A, Bernstein L, et al.** Breast cancer stage at diagnosis and survival among patients with prior breast implants. Plastic and Reconstructive Surgery. 2000;105:535-40.

12. **Eyler AE, Whittle S.** FTM breast cancer: community awareness and illustrative cases. Paper presented at: The 17th Biennial Symposium of the Harry Benjamin International Gender Dysphoria Association; Galveston, TX; 2001 [abstract]. Available at http://www.symposion.com/ijt/hbigda/2001/41_eyler.htm. Accessed January 1, 2005.

13. **Brinton LA, Persson I, Boice JD, et al.** Breast cancer risk in relation to amount of tissue removed during breast reduction operations in Sweden. Cancer. 2001;91:478-83.

14. **Lawrence AA.** Vaginal neoplasia in a male-to-female transsexual: case report, review of the literature, and recommendations for cytological screening. International Journal of Transgenderism. 2001;5. Available at http://www.symposion.com/ijt/ijtvo05no01_01.htm. Accessed January 1, 2005.

15. **Miller N, Bedard YC, Cooter NB, et al.** Histological changes in the genital tract in transsexual women following androgen therapy. Histopathology. 1986;10:661-9.

16. **Cibula D, Cifkova R, Fanta M, et al.** Increased risk of non-insulin dependent diabetes mellitus, arterial hypertension and coronary artery disease in perimenopausal women with a history of the polycystic ovary syndrome. Human Reproduction. 2000;15:785-9.

17. **Hage JJ, Dekker JJ, Karim RB, et al.** Ovarian cancer in female-to-male transsexuals: report of two cases. Gynecologic Oncology. 2000;76:413-5.

18. **Morgentaler A, Bruning CO III, DeWolf WC.** Occult prostate cancer in men with low serum testosterone levels. JAMA. 1996;276.23:1904-6.

19. **Thompson IM, Pauler DK, Goodman PJ, et al.** Prevalence of prostate cancer among men with a prostate-specific antigen level < or = 4.0 ng per milliliter. New England Journal of Medicine. 2004;350:2239-46.

20. **Guess HA, Heyse JF, Gormley GJ.** The effect of finasteride on prostate-specific antigen in men with benign prostatic hyperplasia. Prostate. 1993;22:31-7.

21. **Blanchard R.** A structural equation model for age at clinical presentation in nonhomosexual male gender dysphorics. Archives of Sexual Behavior. 1994;23:311-20.

22. **Biller J, Saver JL.** Ischemic cerebrovascular disease and hormone therapy for infertility and transsexualism. Neurology. 1995;45:1611-3.

23. **Rossouw JE, Anderson GL, Prentice RL, et al.** Risks and benefits of estrogen plus progestin in healthy postmenopausal women: principal results from the Women's Health Initiative randomized controlled trial. Journal of the American Medical Association. 2002;288:321-33.

24. **Grady D, Herrington D, Bittner V, et al.** Cardiovascular disease outcomes during 6.8 years of hormone therapy: Heart and Estrogen/Progestin Replacement Study follow-up (HERS II). Journal of the American Medical Association. 2002;288:49-57.

25. **Scarabin PY, Oger E, Plu-Bureau G.** Differential association of oral and transdermal oestrogen-replacement therapy with venous thromboembolism risk. Lancet. 2003;362:428-32.

26. **Grodstein F, Manson JE, Stampfer MJ.** Postmenopausal hormone use and secondary prevention of coronary events in the Nurses' Health Study: a prospective, observational study. Annals of Internal Medicine. 2001;135:1-8.

27. **Rhoden EL, Morgentaler A.** Risks of testosterone-replacement therapy and recommendations for monitoring. N Engl J Med. 2004;350.5:482-92.

28. **Meyer WJ, Webb A, Stuart CA, et al.** Physical and hormonal evaluation of transsexual patients: a longitudinal study. Archives of Sexual Behavior. 1986;15:121-138.

29. **New G, Timmins KL, Duffy SJ, et al.** Long-term estrogen therapy improves vascular function in male to female transsexuals. Journal of the American College of Cardiology. 1997;29:1437-44.

30. **The Writing Group for the PEPI Trial.** Effects of estrogen or estrogen/progestin regimens on heart disease risk factors in postmenopausal women. The Postmenopausal Estrogen/Progestin Interventions (PEPI) Trial. JAMA. 1995;273.3:199-208.

31. **Glueck CJ, Lang J, Hamer T, et al.** Severe hypertriglyceridemia and pancreatitis when estrogen replacement therapy is given to hypertriglyceridemic women. Journal of Laboratory and Clinical Medicine. 1994;123:59-64.

32. **Expert Panel on Detection, Evaluation, and Treatment of High Blood Cholesterol in Adults.** Executive Summary of the third report of the National Cholesterol Education Program (NCEP) expert panel on detection, evaluation, and treatment of high blood cholesterol in adults (Adult Treatment Panel III). JAMA. 2001;285:2486-97.

33. **McCredie RJ, McCrohon JA, Turner L, et al.** Vascular reactivity is impaired in genetic females taking high-dose androgens. Journal of the American College of Cardiology. 1998;32:1331-5.

34. **Pierpoint T, McKeigue PM, Isaacs AJ, et al.** Mortality of women with polycystic ovary syndrome at long-term follow-up. Journal of Clinical Epidemiology. 1998;51:581-6.

35. **Troisi R, Cowie CC, Harris MI.** Hormone replacement therapy and glucose metabolism. Obstetrics & Gynecology. 2000;96:665-70.

36. **Feldman J.** New onset of type 2 diabetes mellitus with feminizing hormone therapy: case series. International Journal of Transgenderism. 2002;6. Available at http://www.symposion.com/ijt/ijtvo06no02_01.htm. Accessed January 1, 2005.

37. **Nader S, Riad-Gabriel MG, Saad MF.** The effect of a desogestrel-containing oral contraceptive on glucose tolerance and leptin concentrations in hyperandrogenic women. Journal of Clinical Endocrinology & Metabolism. 1997;82:3074-7.

38. **Feldman J, Bockting WO, Allen S, et al.** Smoking cessation among transgender persons receiving hormone therapy. Paper presented at the 18th Biennial Symposium of

the Harry Benjamin International Gender Dysphoria Association, Ghent, Belgium; September 2003.

39. **Feldman J, Bockting WO.** Transgender health. Minnesota Medicine. 2003;86:25-32.

40. **Doeren, M, Samsioe G.** Prevention of postmenopausal osteoporosis with oestrogen replacement therapy and associated compounds: update on clinical trials since 1995. Human Reproduction Update. 2000;6:419-26.

41. **van Kesteren PJM, Lips P, Gooren LJG, et al.** Long-term follow-up of bone mineral density and bone metabolism in transsexuals treated with cross-sex hormones. Clinical Endocrinology. 1998;48:347-54.

42. **Turner A, Chen TC, Barber TW, et al.** Testosterone increases bone mineral density in female-to-male transsexuals: a case series of 15 subjects. Clinical Endocrinology. 2004;61:560-6.

43. **Scholes D, LaCroix AZ, Ichikawa LE, et al.** Injectable hormone contraception and bone density: results from a prospective study. Epidemiology. 2005;13:581-7.

44. **Tangpricha V, Turner A, Malabanan A, et al.** Effects of testosterone therapy on bone mineral density in the FTM patient. Paper presented at: The 17th Biennial Symposium of the Harry Benjamin International Gender Dysphoria Association; Galveston, TX; 2001. Abstract available at http://www.symposion.com/ijt/hbigda/2001/39_tangpricha.htm. Accessed January 1, 2005.

45. **Coleman E, Bockting WO, Gooren LJG.** Homosexual and bisexual identity in sex-reassigned female-to-male transsexuals. Archives of Sexual Behavior. 1993;22:37-50.

46. **Lawrence AA.** Sexuality before and after male-to-female sex reassignment surgery. Archives of Sexual Behavior. 2005;34:147-66.

47. **Kirk S.** Guidelines for selecting HIV positive patients for genital reconstructive surgery. International Journal of Transgenderism. 1999;3. Available at http://www.symposion .com/ijt/hiv_risk/kirk htm. Accessed January 1, 2005.

48. **Dahl M, Feldman J, Goldberg J, et al.** Endocrine Therapy for Transgender Adults in British Columbia: Suggested Guidelines. Vancouver, BC: Vancouver Coastal Health; 2006.

49. **Bowman C, Goldberg J.** Care of the Patient Undergoing Sex Reassignment Surgery (SRS). Vancouver Coastal Health; 2006.

50. **Leavitt F, Berger JC, Hoeppner JA, et al.** Presurgical adjustment in male transsexuals with and without hormonal treatment. Journal of Nervous and Mental Disease. 1980;168:693-7.

51. **Takata LL, Meltzer TR.** Procedures, postoperative care, and potential complications of gender reassignment surgery for the primary care physician. Primary Psychiatry. 2000;7: 74-8.

52. **Reid RW.** Orchidectomy as a first stage towards gender reassignment: a positive option. Paper presented at: Gendys '96: The Fourth International Gender Dysphoria Conference; Manchester, England; 1996.

53. **Israel GE, Tarver DEI.** Transgender Care: Recommended Guidelines, Practical Information, and Personal Accounts. Temple University Press; 1997.

54. **Gaber Y.** Secondary lymphoedema of the lower leg as an unusual side-effect of a liquid silicone injection in the hips and buttocks. Dermatology. 2004;208:342-4.

55. **Hage JJ, van Kesteren PJ.** Chest-wall contouring in female-to-male transsexuals: basic considerations and review of the literature. Plastic and Reconstructive Surgery. 2005;96:386-91.

56. **Hage JJ, Bouman FG, Bloem JJ.** Construction of the fixed part of the neourethra in female-to-male transsexuals: experience in 53 patients. Plastic and Reconstructive Surgery. 1993;91:904-10.

57. **Hage JJ, Torenbeek R, Bouman FG, et al.** The anatomic basis of the anterior vaginal flap used for neourethra construction in female-to-male transsexuals. Plastic and Reconstructive Surgery. 1993;92:102-8.

58. **Perovic SV, Djordjevic ML.** Metoidioplasty: a variant of phalloplasty in female transsexuals. BJU International. 2003;92:981-5.

59. **Hage JJ.** Metaidoioplasty: an alternative phalloplasty technique in transsexuals. Plastic and Reconstructive Surgery. 1996;97:161-7.

60. **Monstrey S, Hoebeke P, Dhont M, et al.** Surgical therapy in transsexual patients: a multi-disciplinary approach. Acta Chirurgica Belgica. 2001;101:200-9.

61. **Gottlieb LJ, Levine LA.** A new design for the radial forearm free-flap phallic construction. Plastic and Reconstructive Surgery. 1993;92:276-83.

62. **Sengezer M, Sadove RC.** Scrotal construction by expansion of labia majora in biological female transsexuals. Annals of Plastic Surgery. 1993;31:372-6.

63. **Hage JJ, Bouman FG, Bloem JJ.** Constructing a scrotum in female-to-male transsexuals. Plastic and Reconstructive Surgery. 1993;91:914-21.

Chapter 14

Disorders of Sex Development: Clinical Approaches

PETER A. LEE, MD, PhD
CHRISTOPHER P. HOUK, MD

F or many years, the term "intersex" has been used to describe those born with genital or reproductive anatomy that is neither clearly male or female. Recently, growing patient and parental concerns about the stigma associated with the term intersex, along with advances in treatment and diagnosis, have led to the adoption of the term disorders of sex development (DSD) in its place.[1,2] Although many people with DSD continue to refer to themselves as intersex in nonclinical settings, the term DSD is a more appropriate medical description. Similar to lesbian, gay, bisexual, and transgender (LGBT) individuals, many people with DSD have felt stigma and shame when dealing with the healthcare system. Moreover, intersex people (or people with DSD) have been considered a transgender subgroup by some,[3] and certain LGBT groups have included the intersex community in their advocacy work. But although people with DSD share several concerns with LGBT communities, the clinical and psychosocial challenges they and their families face from birth onward are unique.[4] This chapter is devoted to providing general clinicians with a basic understanding of the medical, surgical, ethical, and psychosocial complexities associated with DSD. The overarching goal will be to help promote patient-centered and responsive care to individuals with DSD and their families.

What Are Disorders of Sex Development?

Disorders of sex development encompass a diverse group of congenital conditions including atypical gonads, sex chromosomes, genitalia, and reproductive ducts. Because the definition of DSD is relatively broad and includes those with genitalia not consistent with the sex chromosomes, not all persons with DSD have abnormally appearing external genitalia. However, those formerly designated as intersex have genitalia that lie along the continuum between female and male. The 2006 International Consensus Conference on Intersex included all such conditions in the DSD definition and adopted an updated classification.[2a,b] In general, minor variations of genitalia, such as genital size, location of testes, or location of urethral opening (ie, mild hypospadias) are not considered to be DSD.

Disorders of sex development are conditions involving the following elements, modified from a listing in the *Clinical Guidelines for the Management of DSDs in Childhood*, published by the Intersex Society of North America (ISNA).[1] Because no one classification can accommodate all conditions, some conditions are contained in more than one category.

- *Congenital development of ambiguous genitalia*: as occurs in 46,XX persons with virilizing congenital adrenal hyperplasia (eg, fusion of the labia folds and clitoromegaly—see Figure 14-1); 46,XY persons with a urethral opening at the base of the penis associated with an incomplete fusion of embryonic folds that form the scrotum (see Figure 14-2). Note that the partial virilization shown in both Figures 1 and 2 may occur in 46,XX or 46,XY individuals, both reflecting the extent of androgen effect during the crucial time of external genital differentiation from seven to 12 weeks of fetal life. The presence of one or two palpable structures within the partially formed scrotum or inguinal canals make the presence of a Y chromosome more likely
- *Congenital disagreement between internal and external sexual anatomy*: Complete Androgen Insensitivity Syndrome (CAIS), in which testes are present, uterus is absent and external genitalia are female; persistent Müllerian duct syndrome, in which mutations in the MIS (Müllerian inhibiting substance) gene in 46,XY persons result in male external genitalia and a uterus; and 5ß-reductase deficiency, in which internal structures are male but external genitalia are usually considered female
- *Incomplete development of sexual anatomy*: 46,XY with micropenis; 46,XX with vaginal or uterine agenesis (Mayer-Rokitansky-Kuster-Hauser syndrome)
- *Sex chromosome anomalies*: Turner's syndrome (45X); Klinefelter syndrome (47,XXY); XXYY and XYY syndromes; and sex chromosome mosaicism
- *Disorders of gonadal development*: ovotestes or ovaries and testes in the same individual; mixed gonadal dysgenesis; and complete gonadal agenesis, in which both 46,XY and 46,XX persons having female external genitalia

Previously classified by gonadal histology, DSD are now divided into three main categories based on sex chromosome complement. The 3 main categories are 1) sex chromosome DSD (including those who have normal genital development); 2) 46,XX DSD; and 3) 46,XY DSD (including typical

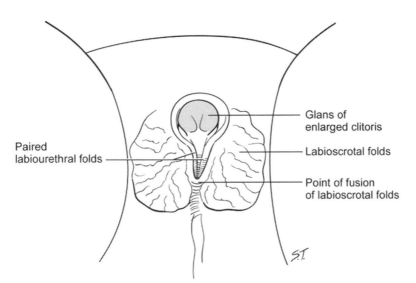

Figure 14-1 Female external genitalia virilized in utero showing clitoral enlargement, partial fusion of the labiourethral folds, and partial fusion of the labioscrotal folds. (From the collection of Peter A. Lee, MD. Used with permission.)

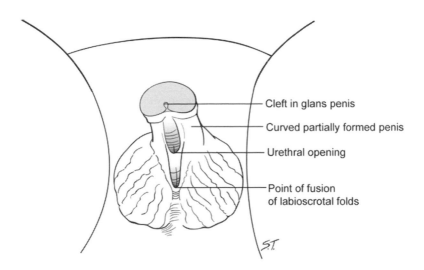

Figure 14-2 Example of incomplete virilization of male external genitalia as a consequence of inadequate androgen, showing incomplete formation of the penis involving incomplete tubularization of the labiourethral folds so that the urethral opening is along the shaft of the penis, and incomplete fusion of the scrotum showing the extent of fusion of the labioscrotal folds. (From the collection of Peter A. Lee, MD. Used with permission.)

female, male, and indistinct genital development). These main categories are subdivided further into disorders of gonadal differentiation and disorders of genital development (see Table 14-1).[2a,b]

Etiology

There are multiple causes of DSD, including chromosomal and specific gene mutations, as well as *in utero* exposure to sex hormones produced or ingested by the mother. The genes known to be involved in DSD are listed in the 2006 *Consensus Statement on Management of Intersex Disorders*.[2a,b] The etiology of some DSD conditions is unknown, while others are not well-characterized by any classification system. One of the most common DSD results from inadequate *in utero* androgen (testosterone) exposure in the 46,XY male or excessive androgen exposure in the 46,XX female during the crucial time window of sex differentiation (between 5 and 12 weeks of gestation). The most common DSD—46,XX congenital virilizing adrenal hyperplasia (CAH)—occurs because excessive androgens produced by the fetal adrenal gland masculinize the external genitalia; when CAH occurs in a 46,XY fetus, the excessive adrenal androgens have no effect on the normal virilization of male infants. Although there are multiple types of CAH, 21-hydroxylase–deficient CAH accounts for more than 90% of all cases.

During human fetal life, external genitalia develop from undifferentiated structures (see Figure 14-3) capable of developing into male or female

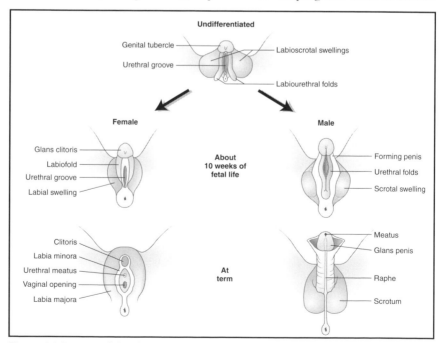

Figure 14-3   Typical development of male and female external genitalia.

Table 14-1   Disorders of Sex Development Classification*

Sex Chromosome Disorders of Sex Development

- 45,X (Turner syndrome and variants)
- 47,XXY (Klinefelter syndrome and variants)
- 45,X/46,XY (MGD, ovotesticular DSD)
- 46,XX/46,XY (chimeric, ovotesticular DSD)

46,XY Disorders of Sex Development

Disorders of gonadal development:

- Complete gonadal dysgenesis (Swyer syndrome)
- Partial gonadal dysgenesis
- Gonadal regression
- Ovotesticular DSD

Disorders in androgen synthesis or action:

- Androgen biosynthesis defects (eg, 17-hydroxysteroid dehydrogenase deficiency, 5RD2 deficiency, StAR mutations)
- Defects in androgen action (eg, CAIS, PAIS)
- Luteinizing hormone receptor defects (eg, Leydig cell hypoplasia, aplasia)

Disorders of anti-Müllerian hormone and anti-Müllerian hormone receptor (persistent Müllerian duct syndrome)

46,XX Disorders of Sex Development

Disorders of gonadal development:

- Ovotesticular DSD
- Testicular DSD
  - o SRY⁺
  - o SRY
  - o Duplicate SOX9
  - o SRY
  - o Gonadal dysgenesis

Androgen excess:

- Fetal
  - o 21-hydroxylase deficiency
  - o 11-hydroxylase deficiency
- Fetoplacental
  - o Aromatase deficiency
  - o POR (P450 oxidoreductase deficiency)
  - o Maternal
- Luteoma
- Exogenous

Additional disorders:

- Cloacal exstrophy
- Vaginal atresia
- MURCS (Müllerian renal-cervicothoracic somite abnormalities)
- Other syndromes

*Because of the complexity of DSD, there is no single classification that can accommodate all DSDs, and some diagnoses fall under more than one category. Although the major categories of the DSD classification are based upon chromosomes, it is important to recognize that the sex chromosomes present do not necessarily correlate with the gonadal or genital differentiation.

anatomy. In the typical female, paired genital swellings become the labia majora; in typical males, these fuse to form the scrotum. The erectile portions of both clitoris and penis develop from the genital tubercle. Paired genital folds fuse to form the urethra at the tip of the penis in the male, while in females these folds become the labia minora and the prepuce over the clitoris. Differentiation of the penis includes not only growth of the cavernous corpora (erectile paired structures) but also fusion of the inner pair of folds. In the female these folds remain unfused and become the labia minora.

Prevalence

The prevalence of DSD is unknown. Available data differ depending upon whether mild variations, such as coronal and glanular hypospadias (abnormal development of urethra) and cryptorchidism (undescended testis) are included. Overestimates may result from the incidence of cryptorchidism at birth, which ranges from two to five percent, but decreases to a prevalence of one percent with the spontaneous descension of testicles by four to six months of age. An estimate from a review including all conditions that "deviate from the ideal male or female"[5] suggests that the incidence may be as high as one in 1500 to one in 2000 births.[5] However, it is generally accepted that more than half of infants born with significant genital ambiguity have congenital adrenal hyperplasia. Since this occurs usually with a frequency of 0.08 per 1000 births, excluding the high prevalence in some relatively small ethnic populations, this suggests that the true incidence of medically significant DSD, those requiring decision concerning sex of rearing or genital surgery, are much less common than the all inclusive estimates.

While it is clear that a greater number of people are born with genital and/or reproductive anatomy that varies from what is strictly considered ideal, it is not clinically appropriate to consider these all as DSD. It is important to acknowledge a wide variety of shapes and size characteristics of all body parts. It must be recognized that individuals may become excessively concerned about minor variations, particularly of breast or penis development, and that concerns about such variation may be exacerbated by teasing and insinuations.

Some of the larger overall prevalence estimates include conditions that do not constitute the usual clinical challenges of DSD, are too subtle to have been detected at the neonatal examination, or do not present until puberty. Including conditions such as Turner and Klinefelter syndromes and late-onset congenital adrenal hyperplasia also results in an increased incidence of DSD over the conditions traditionally considered as intersex. In summary, the estimates of such a high incidence that include any "deviation from the ideal male or female"[5] must be considered all-inclusive and have limited usefulness clinically. However, if we extrapolate from these data to include only those traditionally considered intersex, the frequency is about 0.034 per 100 births or a prevalence of about one per 3500.

Clinical Approaches for Infants with DSD

Beginning at birth, the treatment and management of an individual with DSD presents great challenges to healthcare providers and to the parents of the newborn child. Clinical approaches to DSD continue to be debated, and the research on the medical, psychosocial, and psychosexual outcomes of those treated for DSD is limited. Currently, the two most crucial issues in the treatment of DSD are 1) how gender assignment in infants should be approached when it is unclear what the patient's eventual gender identity will be and 2) if genital surgery should be done and, if so, when. The following section presents a history of how these issues have been approached in the past, a review of some recent findings on these approaches, and finally, the most current recommendations for the clinical management of children born with DSD.

Historical Management of DSD

For centuries prior to the 1950s, gender assignment was based on the perception that all individuals have a "true sex" so that, in cases of DSD, the issue was to determine the "true sex" so that gender assignment could be made. Initially, the gonadal differentiation was felt to indicate the "true sex," the presence of ovaries or testes being the common basis for sex assignment or reassignment, regardless of external genital differentiation. The perception was that "true gender" would follow "true sex." By the middle of the 20th century, after chromosomal sex could be determined, the presence of male or female chromosomes together with gonadal sex was used to determine the "true sex."

The Optimal Gender Approach

The approach changed during the 1960s to what has been called the "optimal gender" approach, which recognized that assignment based on chromosomes and gonadal appearance was inadequate and that it was preferable to base gender assignment on the best (optimal) possible projected outcome.[6] Using this approach, sex assignment was based on genital anatomy, potential for fertility, and the projected quality of life, including what was considered optimal adult sexual function, defined in terms of the physical capability for traditional male-female intercourse. Hence, if an infant had ovaries that were expected to function normally at and after puberty and a well-developed uterus, but had external genitalia that would require surgery to exteriorize the vagina and permit penile penetration, the sex of rearing would be female, and surgery would be done. Unfortunately, surgical techniques and incomplete knowledge of genital nerve supply often resulted in a loss of genital sensitivity.

The tenets of this approach included the assumption that gender is a multifactorial process involving both prenatal and postnatal variables with gender not being firmly established at birth. It was assumed that prenatal factors could be overridden through the control of postnatal environmental or social influences. Sex of rearing during childhood was felt to be a dominant influence on gender identity, presuming that if parents and others interacted with a child as a girl, that the child would grow up identifying as a girl.

The application of the optimal gender approach to an infant with ovaries, female chromosomes and masculinized genitalia, as is seen in the most common type of DSD, 46,XX child with CAH, would be a female assignment and feminizing surgery. Since the internal reproductive development, including the ovaries and uterus, could be expected to support a pregnancy, and because puberty would be expected to occur spontaneously if the CAH was adequately treated, the child would be raised female. After genital surgery, intercourse and fertility would be expected to be possible. The goals of surgery were to create a normal appearance, allow for unobstructed urinary outflow, and allow for intercourse after maturity. Surgery typically involved reduction of the corpora of the clitoris and overlying redundant tissues, opening the fusion of the labial minora and majora, and exteriorizing the urethral and vaginal openings. Early surgical techniques, however, often resulted in damage to the neurovascular supply and genital sensitivity.

The application of the optimal gender approach to a 46,XY individual with incomplete genital development would take into consideration several criteria. If, as was commonly the situation, internal duct development was inadequate and hence expected to preclude normal maturation and delivery of sperm, and testicular function was compromised so that hormonal supplementation would be necessary at and after puberty, or, if the penis was considered inadequate for traditional male sexual function (ie, vaginal penetration), then a female sex of rearing was recommended. Feminizing surgery was undertaken to align with the sex assignment. Generally, it was felt to be inappropriate to raise a boy without a "functional" penis.

The optimal gender approach recognized three phases of development of gender identification. The attainment of the first, gender identity, as an internal sense of being male or female, was felt to be flexible during infancy. Hence, gender reassignment was deemed feasible at this age. The second phase, development of gender role, conduct, and behavioral patterns (such as rough-and-tumble childhood play among boys) attributed to one particular gender, are largely determined by an individual's response to society's expectations. For the child with gender assignment in infancy, it was expected that gender role would align with gender identity; that is, the child that was raised as a girl would learn to develop the role expected for a girl. The third phase, sexual orientation, which may not be realized until later, was felt to be most commonly manifested as heterosexual (considering the sex of rearing). In hindsight, while the relative impact of prenatal and postnatal factors on gender identity remain unclear, it appears that in some situations there are powerful prenatal influences, such as pre-natal androgen exposure on the central nervous system, that have major impact on the development of gender identity, perhaps overriding the impact of the sex of rearing. Also, with changes in society since the opti-mal gender approach was first advocated, gender roles attributed to one gender have become much more flexible and are must less stringent for an individual's social acceptance. The issue of sexual orientation, and the fac-tors determining it, while still unclear, are extraordinarily complex and resistant to one-dimensional modeling.

In part, problems associated with the optimal gender approach seem to extend from a narrowed perspective of human sexuality. The perspective that no one should be raised as a male who does not have an "adequately sized" functional penis is clearly flawed since individuals have chosen a male gender in spite of the lack of a penis.

The age-old dilemma of nature versus nurture, or genetics versus envi-ronment, with regard to sexual and gender issues persists. It is now clear that humans are not psychosexually neutral, blank slates at birth. However, since there is apparently no single or universal constellation of factors (such as chromosomes, hormones, or environment) that leads to one type of gen-der identity, it is impossible to predict gender identity with certainty.

Outcome-Based Evidence of Traditional Approaches

As noted previously, there are limited data on outcomes for children born with DSD. Most studies of long-term outcomes suffer from nonprobabilis-tic sampling methods and subjective interpretation. This lack of outcome data makes it more difficult for medical professionals to make strong rec-ommendations for gender assignment in children with DSD. As noted else-where, evidence from case series suggest that 46,XY patients with evidence of *in utero* androgen exposure will probably be better served with a male gender assignment even when the penis is judged to be inadequate for tra-ditional intercourse.[7,8] These include instances in which a specific diagnosis can be made, including 5α-reductase-2 deficiency and 17ß-hydroxysteroid dehydrogenase-3 deficiency.[9,10] There is no clinical or psychological evidence to support a reassignment to the female gender among patients born with normally formed but small penises who have palpable testes. While both male and female sex of rearing have been reported to result in "satisfactory" genito-sexual function, female sex of rearing requires more extensive surgery and is far more difficult to justify. There has been no doc-umentation of failure of assignment of such patients as males while there are multiple instances of failure in those assigned female.[11,12] Any consid-eration of a female sex assignment in these patients should be approached with extreme caution.

Among 46,XY individuals with incomplete genital development who are raised female, reasonable adjustment has been reported in a small series of people who had ongoing psychological counseling.[13] Another study of undervirilized 46,XY individuals[7] concluded that outcomes—including physician-rated cosmetic appearance of genitalia, satisfaction with body image, satisfaction with sexual function, experience with sexual partners, and perception of males as masculine and females as feminine—were similar, irrespective of gender assignment. In another report of this same study population, almost half of the 46,XY undervirilized participants indicated they were neither well informed nor satisfied with their clinical care, a seemingly clear mandate that the treatment approach needed to be modified.[14] Importantly, all of these patients identified ongoing problems and issues, such as dealing with the fact that they were born with undervirilized or overvirilized genitalia, being initially assigned a sex and then reassigned the opposite sex, having been told statements by family members or healthcare workers that implied they could never be well adjusted, and feeling stigmatized in the past by the healthcare system. This highlights that being born with genital ambiguity can be accompanied by a lifetime of concerns that may never be fully resolved. Clearly, while this is at least partly due to less than optimal medical care, lack of support, and lack of psychological counseling, it is impossible to determine whether resolution of these would result in an ideal situation because of the persistence of the underlying problem. Nevertheless, there are instances of excellent outcomes within these cohorts that suggest that DSD persons can be well-adjusted given excellent medical care and psychological support.[13]

Outcome data are likewise inadequate concerning gender assignment among genetic male patients born with cloacal exstrophy, a disorder resulting in lack of penis formation. In the past, these patients were often assigned female during infancy. Some patients have self-reassigned back to male in late childhood, while others appear to have adjusted to being female.[15]

Recent revelations in a famous case also highlight the challenges inherent in gender assignment. This case, popularly known as the "John-Joan case" (also explained in Chapter 12), is about a normally developed male infant who was reassigned female at 1.7 years of age following a botched circumcision at eight months of age.[16] The female reassignment was made because of the dilemma of raising a boy without a penis and because at the time (1967), gender development was believed to be malleable until two to three years of age. Feminizing genital surgery was done consistent with the sex reassignment. Although the initial literature on this case deemed the sex reassignment a success, it was revealed many years later that the child had numerous adjustment problems during childhood. At the age of 14, after he had learned what had happened to him as an infant, he self-reassigned as a male. He had masculinizing surgery and eventually married a woman and adopted her children. Sadly, he later committed suicide. Though this man was not born with atypical genitalia, his case has challenged the concept of gender malleability worldwide and is sometimes used as an argument against genital surgery in infants with DSD.

Impact of Hormonal Exposure on the Brain

The effect of fetal androgen exposure is crucial to understanding the challenges in gender identity assignment and development in some individuals with DSD. Unfortunately, these effects are not well defined. Nevertheless, this concept is most important for understanding two types of clinical scenarios, the incompletely virilized 46,XY child and the overly virlized 46,XX child. The prevailing hypothesis is that fetal androgen exposure leads to both anatomical and biochemical differences in the developing fetal brain, especially when this exposure occurs during crucial periods of embryonic growth, whether from androgens produced by the testes, by the adrenal glands in virilizing congenital adrenal hyperplasia, or from trans-placental passage of androgens from maternal circulation.[17] It is felt that these differences in androgen influence promote the development of neural circuits; in humans, these differences appear to be associated with the more aggressive, rough-and-tumble play behaviors commonly seen in boys. But while androgen seems to promote differences in gender role behaviors, its impact on gender identity and sexual orientation is far from clear. For example, 46,XX children born with an adrenal enzyme deficiency, congenital adrenal hyperplasia, are exposed to excessive androgen during fetal life. While this exposure manifests a clear influence on cognitive function and typical male gender-related childhood behavior, no clear influence has been demonstrated on gender identity and sexual orientation. This evidence of the impact of androgen upon the central nervous system provides a basis to explain the characteristics of overvirilized females who were exposed to excessive levels of fetal androgen exposure and who, for example, exhibit typical boy behaviors. Differences among undervirlized males are not well enough documented to suggest differences. In both instances, there is no accurate way to quantify fetal androgen exposure, indirect evidence being only the extent of undervirilization or overvirilization of the genitalia.

Genes and Genetic Action

Chromosomal sex is often seen as the major determinant of gender; those with a Y chromosome are considered male, and those with two X chromosomes are thought to be female. However, more current knowledge of the genome tells us that the determinants are actually at the gene level, and so it is possible for someone with 46,XX chromosomes to be male and someone with 46,XY chromosomes to be female. This is a consequence of an alteration or translocation of a crucial gene or genes. Examples include those with genetic mutations or deletions that result in a condition called 46,XX and 46,XY sex reversal, and in undervirilized 46,XY persons who were given a female sex assignment. Such people have typical internal and external genitalia of their gender, while gonadal function may be compromised so that fertility is not possible.

It is also apparent that the sex chromosomes, the X in the female and the Y in the male, have differing effects on gene expression involved in brain development. Such differences are determined by molecular biochemical methods of determining gene actions. Examples include the sex-determining region gene on the Y chromosome present only in male neuronal cells, as well as other X and Y linked genes. In addition to sex chromosomes, other chromosomes are also involved in gonadal determination and adult behaviors. It has generally also been understood that brain sexual differentiation and behavior determinants act primarily by sex hormone effects. However, in studies of the mouse brain, it has been shown that some genes are expressed by biochemical molecular changes before gonads are formed and capable of sex steroid hormone secretion. This suggests that some genetic factors independent of hormone secretion have roles in influencing brain differentiation.[18] It is still unknown what role such genetic factors may play and how they interact to influence the development of psychosexual components of gender.

Current Recommendations for the Care of Infants and Young Children

Reports by adults with DSD of the insensitive and inappropriate healthcare they received as children are all too common. Grievances include having been made to feel ashamed and freakish by their healthcare providers, having been denied access to medical records, not having been given the privacy afforded to other patients, and the loss of genital sensation as a consequence of genital surgery. Recent advocacy efforts by individuals and groups like the Intersex Society of North America (ISNA) have challenged the medical profession to reevaluate traditional approaches to treating DSD patients and to improve their overall quality of care. These situations have resulted in a call by adult DSD patients and the support groups representing them to do the following:

- Defer all genital surgery until the individual is old enough to consent to surgery for themselves.
- Avoid female reassignment for an underdeveloped penis.
- Provide full disclosure of all medical information to patients and parents of minors.
- Never conduct a medical examination in a setting that might make the child feel on display or embarrassed.

In response to these demands, as well as to recent outcome-based evidence, medical professionals have collaborated with patient advocates to develop patient-centered clinical guidelines on the management of DSD.[19]

These have been written up in the *Consensus Statement on Management of Intersex Disorders*,[2a,b] as well as in the *Clinical Guidelines for the Management of Disorders of Sex Development in Childhood*.[1] Both of these texts recommend a multidisciplinary team approach to help ensure that the patient receives expert and sensitive care focusing on the patient's overall well-being, including psychosocial and medical needs.

Although many children with DSD are quite healthy and will not need extensive medical management, it is appropriate to have a team of familiar caregivers available when needs do arise. Optimally, team members include pediatric subspecialists in surgery (urology, gynecology), endocrinology, child psychology or psychiatry, genetics, social work, nursing, and medical ethics. In addition, the team needs to coordinate with the primary care practitioner, who still serves an important function in the child's care. Team members will vary based on resource availability and diagnosis. In addition to providing support to parents and integrated care to patients, teams should aim to offer continuing education in DSD, ensure long-term follow-up of patients, provide education to other health professionals, and initiate peer support networks for patients and families.[1,2a,b]

It is also recommended that for proper functioning, each team should designate 1) a leader, typically a physician, who coordinates team efforts; 2) a coordinator, usually a nurse practitioner or social worker to ensures timeliness and continuity in case management; and 3) a liaison, preferably someone with excellent communication skills to keep parents informed of care and treatment options and to link them with resources and support services.[1]

Treatment and Management of Newborns with DSD

The initial reaction of parents when they first learn that their newborn child has been born with a DSD may be shock, shame, or sadness. It is crucial that parents be given supportive counseling, along with clear and complete information as their child's assessment progresses. Parents should be reassured that DSD do indeed occur, that they are not shameful, and that most individuals born with a DSD are healthy and well adjusted. This provides a basis for the parents to bond with their child and make informed decisions about gender assignment, treatment, and management. Because of the nature of DSD, extra care should be made to respect privacy and confidentiality. Communication should be honest and open, and the current provision for access to all medical information and records to patients and parents of minors must be followed.

Treatment protocols are suggested by the *Clinical Guidelines for the Management of Disorders of Sex Development in Childhood*[1] for managing the care of newborns with DSD. While ideally this is done by a multidisciplinary team approach, many institutions do not have a full complement of experienced individuals to constitute such a team. Protocols are summarized as follows:

1. The attending physician identifies the possible DSD, explains concerns to parents in a calm manner, and, if available, contacts the DSD multidisciplinary team.
2. The attending or team liaison explains initial information and support to the family and suggests resources for further support from individuals who have experience or a background that enables emotional reinforcement.
3. A conference designed specifically to review information concerning this patient in the context of knowledge of similar cases is scheduled.
4. The child is examined by designated healthcare workers or team members in the presence of the parents and, when available, the neonatologist or pediatrician. The physical findings should be demonstrated to the parents with sensitivity, using positive language. The goal is to avoid hesitancy by the parents in looking at and examining their child and to help them become comfortable doing this.
5. Designated healthcare workers or team members determine what tests should be done, explain these to the parents, and, with their permission, proceed with testing.
6. After sufficient data become available, a case conference is held to review and interpret findings and develop recommendations to be presented to the family to equip them to decide gender assignment and the treatment plan.
7. Team members discuss recommendations and options with the family.
8. After these options have been instituted, long-term care is planned, assigning appropriate roles for team members.[1]

Full disclosure is necessary at all times. An appropriate team member is responsible for providing the parents with the most up-to-date information on sexual and reproductive system development, together with available outcome data about adult adjustment, sexual function, and fertility. Information should be as specific as possible considering the child's diagnostic condition and should contain treatment, including surgical options, and, when appropriate, the option of no treatment. Of particular pertinence are physical and psychological outcome data related to surgery,[4,20] striving for the best balance between outcome data and differing opinions. While parents must receive an objective, realistic, and complete assessment including knowledge of causes, treatment, and outcome, care must be individualized based on all available information. At any point in time, however, parents or patients may not be prepared to hear all the details related to the DSD. At those times, the best approach is to wait until the parents say they are ready to learn more, while letting them know that they are allowed access to all medical data at all times.

Gender Assignment

All newborns should receive a gender assignment based on which gender the collective evidence suggests will most likely develop. This choice is ultimately the parents' right and responsibility and should be based on the information and recommendations given to them by their clinical team. Factors include the diagnosis and outcome data related to that diagnosis, family views, fertility potential, surgical and medical options, and genital appearance. So that parents can make fully informed and rational decisions, time and care should be taken to ensure understanding and interpretation of information is reached. Parents should realize that, while most people with DSD remain satisfied with their initial gender assignment, some may grow up to feel their gender assignment was incorrect. Commonly parents wonder if their child's DSD will affect their sexual orientation. They should realize that most individuals born with DSD are heterosexual, but as a group a greater portion are likely to be gay, lesbian, or bisexual. Nonetheless, homosexuality should not be interpreted by the parents as evidence of an incorrect choice of gender.

Genital Surgery

The ultimate decisions concerning surgery during infancy and childhood are, of course, the parents' responsibility. The team is obligated to honor the parents' desires. Parents should be given up-to-date, comprehensive information available in order to make a decision that is centered on their child's physical and psychosocial well-being. Surgery for variations in genital size or other cosmetic purposes, is discouraged. Today, parents are more accepting of genital variation and less likely to choose surgery for mild or moderate clitoromegaly.[21] While there is concern about loss of genital sensitivity with surgery, parents of children with severe genital ambiguity still usually seek surgery even after having been informed of various viewpoints concerning outcome data.[2a,2b,22] The consensus conference report recommends early surgery for 46,XX infants with significant virilization, in the context that genital surgery is usually not urgent. Urgent surgery is needed in rare cases, as for example when the urinary outflow tract is positioned so that there is retention of urine with risk of infection. All such surgery should be performed by experts only. It is also recommended that every effort should be made to discourage surgery for mild clitoral enlargement.

Many DSD support and advocacy groups and some medical professionals believe that because parents cannot possibly predict what will be best for their child in the future, they should defer all genital surgery (except those surgeries needed for immediate health reasons) until the patient is old enough to give informed consent. They feel that elective surgery, with its risks and potential harm, may be done to ease the distress of the parents rather than improve the patient's well-being. This position of avoiding any genital surgery is advocated because genital surgery may result in the loss of sexual responsiveness and because there is a risk that gender identity may not be consistent with the reconstructed genital appearance and that the potential to create genitalia of the opposite sex will be lost.

This discussion to discontinue genital surgery in infancy and childhood has developed because of grievances by adult DSD persons, many being virilized genetic females. Aspects of their care have included especially poor surgical results, lack of family participation in decisions regarding care, and difficulties in obtaining full disclosure of their medical histories. Both masculinizing and feminizing surgery have had poor results: among males, problems involve both curvature (chordee) of the penis and the creation of an intact patent tube opening at the end of the penis. In spite of repeat surgery, the cosmetic and functional outcome often has been unsatisfactory. After feminizing surgery, likewise, patients often have experienced poor cosmetic and functional outcomes,[23] particularly regarding compromised sexual function resulting from damaged neural supply after clitoral surgery with decreased sensuality and lack of orgasmic capability. Some studies have found more positive results regarding sexual development and activity,[24] in spite of the poor outcome of initial surgery and the need for re-operation in puberty. It appears that because there is now greater appreciation of female sexuality and genital variation, as well as a shift toward empowering the parents in decision-making, more parents are now refusing genital surgery in genetic females with relatively minor virilization but still choosing surgery for major virilization. Among those having surgery after puberty, it has been suggested that vaginal dilation using acrylic molds, when possible, results in better sexual satisfaction than subsequent surgery.

Current surgical techniques are designed to preserve function by avoiding, as much as possible, disruption of the neurovascular supply to the genitalia. Hence, there is an attempt to preserve sensory mechanisms while carefully reducing the excessive erectile tissue (corpora) by excision of a central section, preserving erectile capacity. This has become possible because of refined surgical techniques and studies that have delineated the clitoral nerve supply. Since the supply is primarily from above and beside the clitoris, the surgical approach from the underside of the clitoris minimally disrupts this.[25] Not only has the approach to surgery changed, but other practices have changed as well. For example, the use of vaginal dilators during childhood is now discouraged because of psychological impact and lack of efficacy in a nonestrogenized child. Although both cosmetic and functional outcomes of surgical techniques are expected to be considerably better, the collection of outcome data when the current patients reach adulthood will be necessary to document actual improvement.

When the external genitalia are neither predominantly male nor female, parents must weigh the potential issues their child will face by growing up with ambiguous genitalia against the risks of surgical complications. Parents must also keep in mind that the gender they assign their child may not be the gender identity their child eventually assumes. Hence, if they proceed with early surgical sex assignment, their child may eventually reassign gender and desire to have their genitalia reversed to accord with their gender identity. Because gender identity cannot be predicted, and surgeries have complications, there are advocates for delaying surgery until the individual is old enough to have formed a gender identity and give informed consent. At that point, the person may choose not to have surgery at all, or may choose to have feminizing or masculinizing surgery. Deferring surgery until the appropriate age of consent has many facets, including how to determine the age at which individuals are equipped to make such decisions. In one instance, an older teenager with a DSD chose to have feminizing genitoplasty; a few years later, this person identified as a man and desired to have masculinizing surgery. Unfortunately, this was impossible because of the previous resection of tissues.

Deferral of surgery also must take into account the impact of growing up with different genitalia, although the impact of this is unknown except for dramatic instances of ostracism from the past. Those who advocate for infant surgery argue that "normal" genital appearance decreases the risk of negative input from others and improves bonding between parents and child. Again, there is no systematic evidence to prove this. It is important not to underestimate the supportive role of parents and appropriate counseling and support, regardless of the physical problem. Children who have had surgery and later learn about their DSD may feel anger towards their parents, sensing that their condition implies shame. Whether or not surgery was chosen during infancy, it is clear that the proper approach is progressive disclosure to the child (disclosure is explained in more detail in the next section).

A 1999 opinion rendered by the Constitutional Court of Colombia[26] in South America provides a reasonable approach to the child for whom sex assignment and genital plastic surgery are being considered. The court recognized that parental surrogate consent for genital surgery in children with DSD is unique. Therefore, the courts required that further restrictions be put on consent in these cases, establishing a new category of consent called "qualified, persistent informed consent." Specifically, parents must be given access to complete and accurate information about the risks of surgery and about alternative treatment models. Verbal consent is not adequate. In order to ensure that parents have a complete understanding of all the implications of surgery, parents must give consent in written form, on multiple occasions, and over an extended period of time.

Disclosure of Condition to Children with DSD
Advice should be provided to the parents concerning how and when they should tell their children about their condition. It is recommended that

children be progressively told about their DSD in an age-appropriate manner throughout their lives, fitting information to the personality of the child, and taking advantage of opportunities and questions that inevitably arise.[27] This appears to avoid the negative emotions, including confusion, shame, isolation, and anger that may occur when people learn about their DSD in an inappropriate manner, often at an older age than childhood. Hopefully, this protects the confidentially about their condition without an inappropriate veil of secrecy, provides for acceptance of the alternatives concerning parenthood if fertility is impossible, and precludes any feelings of freakishness. This approach should also strengthen gender identity and minimize concerns about sexual function and satisfaction, and the ability to have intimate relationships. Parents can receive advice from experienced mental health professionals and through peer support groups on ways to share information with their children.

Table 14-2   Key Points for Clinicians to Discuss with Parents

- Review bi-potential primordial anatomic structures and basic developmental facts so parents can understand their child's development.
- Share all known physical findings and testing results.
  - o Demonstrate on genital examination, pointing out significant findings, including palpable genitalia
- Avoid making general statements about the significance of findings that might bias parents.
- If gender assignment is unclear, consider the following:
  - o Evidence of *in utero* androgen exposure greater than normal female or less than normal male levels upon the developing CNS
  - o Extent of knowledge concerning differentiation of gonads
  - o Likelihood of ovaries to contain follicles
  - o Presence or absence of spermatozoa in testes
  - o Probability of fertility as male or female utilizing existing techniques
- Discuss parents' preferences/inclinations concerning the sex of their child.
- Carefully discuss details of any specific diagnosis.
  - o For example, the virilization that is likely to occur in some conditions involving enzyme deficiencies, specifically 5-ß reductase deficiency, 3ß hydroxysteroid dehydrogenase deficiency, and the partial androgen insensitivity syndromes, or lack of virilization and feminization that occurs in complete androgen insensitivity syndrome. Such information can be used to predict physical responses to hormone stimulation that are expected to occur at puberty.
- If surgery is being considered:
  - o Do not imply that surgery will solve all issues.
  - o Discuss extent of surgery required for male versus female reconstruction, as well as risks and complications.
  - o Discuss reasons to defer surgery.

Discovery of DSD during Adolescence

DSD may not become apparent until the age of puberty. This situation can occur if an individual has generally normal-appearing external genitalia, either fully female or male, or if there has never been a complete enough genital examination to notice incomplete development, such as with vaginal dysgenesis. Inadequate gonadal function is usually not apparent until puberty does not happen. The default pattern of genital development is female, which occurs in the absence of any hormone stimulation. On the other hand, excessive androgen secreted by the adrenal glands in a 46,XX child may stimulate the development of male genitalia. Because this underlying cause is not recognized, a male sex is assigned at birth and not questioned until puberty. More commonly, attention leading to a diagnosis of DSD is associated with lack of puberty (because of lack of ovarian or testicular function). Other examples include inappropriate development, such as masculinizing changes in an apparent female, feminizing changes in a male such as marked breast development (gynecomastia), the discovery of the lack of a vagina or uterus in an apparent female, or blood in the urine of an assumed male, which is actually menstrual bleeding, a consequence of ovarian and uterine function.

When such situations occur and are found to be a consequence of DSD, there must be full, albeit sensitive and gradual, disclosure of all information to patients and, if they are still minors, to the parents. The patient (and parents) should be given information leading to a clear understanding of the reasons why the DSD developed and what therapies are possible, including the possibility of treatment with surgery and hormonal replacement. Particularly pertinent from a psychological standpoint is to provide information to enhance self-esteem, especially around issues of fertility and sexual activity.

Suggestions for the Care of
Youth and Adults with DSD

It is crucial to maintain a realistic long-term perspective concerning the care of the individual with DSD, since significant issues will continue to have an effect throughout the patient's life. Individual personality and psychological characteristics shape adjustment and quality of life. Clearly, individuals retain an awareness of their differences, including general body or genital appearance, decreased genital sensitivity, fertility problems as they understand them, and an attitude concerning how this impacts acceptance by new acquaintances. At times of stress, this may become acute. Hence, availability for support should always be present. Fundamental issues, such as the importance of sexual activity or biologically being able to be a parent, often change over time. Hence, no single specific approach will be applicable to all individuals at all times and construction of an algorithm may be unattainable. Nonetheless, there are certain points, summarized in Table 14-3, that clinicians should consider when caring for the older child, adolescent, or adult with DSD.

Primary Health Issues

To preserve and enable the development of the whole person, goals of comprehensive treatment within the realm of primary care, mental health and sexual health are to:

- Enhance abilities relating to life skills, creative and vocational talents, relationship and sexual abilities
- Maintain capability for sexual responsiveness, including medications such as hormone replacement
- Provide for fertility or parenthood, if desired, possibly utilizing current assisted fertility procedures.

General health practices should be encouraged, including nutrition, physical fitness, and social interactions. As long as basic hormonal treatments are provided and adjusted as indicated for the underlying condition, persons with DSD are expected to remain healthy. The need for individual

---

Table 14-3   Key Points for Caring for Teens and Adults with DSD

- Assess the following:
  - o Gender identity development
  - o Sexual experiences and intimate relationships
  - o External genital anatomy (considering any surgical changes)
  - o Internal genital anatomy (using ultrasound or MRI)
  - o Interest in fertility
- Evaluate pituitary-gonadal function (LH, FSH, Inhibin B, estradiol, testosterone and anti-Müllerian hormone) based on gonadal differentiation and physical development.
- Review medical records, including any previous genital surgery and, as pertinent, concerning specific etiologic causes.
- Discuss all treatment options and considerations with the patient.
- Recommend/arrange coordinated care with a team of specialists (endocrinology, urology, mental health, etc.), as appropriate to each patient's needs.
- Provide screening/surveillance as appropriate based upon reproductive system development, hormone replacement, and other therapy.
- Provide ongoing standard general medical care.

or group therapy sessions should be assessed and provided to support psychosocial and psychosexual adjustment. As with other chronic disorders, ongoing therapy is helpful and often necessary. With DSD, once medical therapy is established and surgery is completed, care usually primarily involves emotional and psychological support.

Sexual Function and Satisfaction

Data on sexual function and fulfillment in persons with DSD is sparse. Population-based studies are lacking and difficult to do because many people choose not to participate in research. Some do not want to reopen painful memories from the past; some are tired of focusing on their differences and would rather "get on" with their lives; and some are angry at the medical establishment. Thus, the very poignant cases that have been highly publicized may not be representative of all persons with DSD. Furthermore, outcome data from those treated during previous decades may not be applicable to current patients because of improvements in patient care and treatment. Namely, surgical procedures have changed, and parents and patients are now given full disclosure of medical information and invited to participate more in decisions concerning therapy. It is assumed that the current state-of-the-art surgery will be associated with much better sexual function, but only time can verify this. Finally, while sexual function in the past was primarily measured by ability to perform traditional intercourse, such a narrow definition of sex is inadequate to assess sexuality and sexual satisfaction, particularly in this patient population. In spite of limited studies concerning sexual satisfaction and function among individuals with DSD, sexual developmental milestones progress, as usual, from romantic interest to falling in love, kissing, petting, and intercourse.

Fertility

In the past, fertility was unlikely for many 46,XX and most 46,XY persons with DSD. 46,XY individuals with DSD usually have inadequate development of testes to produce sperm and incomplete development of the sperm ducts and reproductive system glands to provide for sperm maturation and delivery. While most 46,XX individuals with DSD had normal fetal internal development of the ovaries, fallopian tubes, and uterus, subsequent excessive androgen, as with those with adrenal hyperplasia, and difficulties creating an adequate vagina have been obstacles to fertility and carrying a pregnancy to term. Current assisted fertility techniques have increased the potential for fertility in both male and female patients with DSD. Eggs or sperm can be harvested from ovaries or testes, and procedures involving sperm injection and implantation of the fertilized egg (zygote) are now commonly done. If a patient's uterus is judged to be capable of maintaining a pregnancy, it may be feasible to implant a zygote using the patient's or a donated egg.

Healthcare: A More Sensitive Approach

Although most DSD patients are not at increased risk for acquiring chronic disease, it is very important that they have regular primary medical care. Unfortunately, in spite of decades of attempts to teach healthcare workers about using a sensitive approach with DSD patients, inappropriate insinuations continue to occur, often as a consequence of thoughtlessness or trivialization of issues of great importance to the DSD patient. There are examples of patients not returning for indicated medical care because of such interactions. Awareness leading to careful, thoughtful attitudes and interactions should be encouraged for healthcare workers. Clinicians should implement practices and policies that make the office environment welcoming for patients with DSD, as with all patients. Resources for learning more about caring for DSD patients can be found in Appendix A.

Conclusions

Part of the difficulties in caring for patients with DSD is that understanding human sexuality is elusive and complex. No one model will ever be able to predict or anticipate psychosexual outcomes, including gender identity and sexual orientation, in individuals with normal embryonic sexual development, much less in those with DSD. It is therefore important for clinicians to be leaders in changing social norms by recognizing and accepting the full spectrum of human sexual and gender expression. No other single perspective would do more to foster a high quality outcome in all individuals. Many people with DSD adjust well to life, in spite of the challenges they face. While it is the decision of such individuals whether to disclose their DSD to others, there are examples of persons who are highly successful that publicly proclaim their condition, and many others who no one would guess has a DSD.

Summary Points

- Disorders of sex development (DSD) are a diverse group of congenital conditions that include anomalies of the gonads, sex chromosomes, genitalia, and reproductive ducts. They most commonly present with problems of external genital development. While patients with DSD differ from transgender people, they may share some of the same social and psychosocial concerns.
- In spite of great strides in the understanding of the biology of DSD, management of those with DSD continues to be a complex topic at great risk of misunderstanding, confusion, and unsound perceptions.

- The standard of care for patients with DSD currently involves providing full disclosure and decision-making concerning all care, including surgery, to the patients and, for minors, to parents or legal caregivers.
- In spite of decades of attempts to sensitize healthcare workers to the needs of DSD patients and their families, awkwardness and inappropriate, thoughtless interactions continue to occur. Good patient-clinician communication is made more difficult by the persistent discomfort with sexuality and related issues.
- Because there is inadequate outcome data to direct the standard of care for DSD patients, experienced practitioners should assess care for patients on an individualized basis.
- Decisions concerning gender assignment and reassignment are very complex and must consider the impact of hormone exposures upon the developing brain, gonadal and genital development, probability of fertility (using current assisted techniques if necessary), and, of key importance, potential for sexual experiences and the preservation of genital sensitivity.
- Ideal care of the patient with DSD involves a team of experts in medical, surgical, and psychological care.
- The goals of primary care for adult patients with DSD are to enhance innate life skills, talents, relationship and sexual abilities; maintain capability for sexual responsiveness; and assist with fertility or parenthood, if desired.

References

1. **Consortium on the Management of Disorders of Sexual Development.** Clinical Guidelines for the Management of Disorders of Sexual Development. Intersex Society of North America; 2006.
2. a) **Lee PA, Houk CP, Ahmed SF, Hughes IA, and the International Consensus Conference on Intersex Working Group.** Consensus statement on management of intersex disorders. Pediatrics. 2006;118:e488-500.
   b) **Hughes IA, Houk C, Ahmed SF, Lee PA, and LWPES Consensus Group, ESPE Consensus Group.** Consensus statement on the management of intersex disorders. Arch Disease Child. 2006;91:554-63.
3. **Dean L, Mayer IH, Robinson K, et al.** Lesbian, gay, bisexual, and transgender health: findings and concerns. J Gay Lesbian Med Assoc. 2000;4:101-51.
4. **Lee PA.** A perspective on the approach to the intersex child born with genital ambiguity. J Pediatr Endocrinol Metab. 2004;17:133-40.
5. **Blackless M, Charuvasta A, Derryck A, et al.** How sexually dimorphic are we? Review and synthesis. Amer J Human Biol. 2000;12:151-66.
6. **Money J, Hampson J, Hampson J.** Hermaphroditism: recommendations concerning assignment of sex, change of sex, and psychologic management. Bull Johns Hopkins Hosp. 1995;97:284-300.
7. **Nicolino M, Bendelac N, Jay N, Forest MG, David M.** Clinical and biological assessments of the undervirilized male. BJU Int. 2004;93:20-5.

8. **Migeon CJ, Wisniewski AB, Gearhart JP, et al.** Ambiguous genitalia with perineo-scrotal hypospadias in 46,XY individuals: long-term medical, surgical, and psychosexual outcome. Pediatrics. 2002;110:e31.

9. **Cohen-Kettenis PT.** Gender change in 46,XY persons with 5-alpha-reductase deficiency and 17-beta-hydroxysteroid dehydrogenase-3 deficiency. Arch Sex Behav. 2005;34:399-410.

10. **Mendonca BB, Inacio M, Costa EMF, et al.** Male pseudohermaphroditism due to 5 alpha-reductase 2 deficiency: outcome of a Brazilian cohort. The Endocrinologist. 2003; 13:202-4.

11. **Mazur T.** Gender dysphoria and gender change in androgen insensitivity or micropenis. Arch Sex Behav. 2005;34:411-21.

12. **Bin-Abbas B, Conte FA, Grumbach MM, Kaplan SL.** Congenital hypogonadotropic hypogonadism and micropenis: effect of testosterone treatment on adult penile size why sex reversal is not indicated. J Pediatr. 1991;134:579-83.

13. **Mazur T, Sandberg DE, Perrin MA, Gallagher JA, MacGillivray MH.** Male pseudo-hermaphroditism: long-term quality of life outcome in five 46,XY individuals reared as female. J Pediatr Endocrinolo Metab. 2004;17:809-23.

14. **Migeon CJ, Wisniewski AB, Brown TR, et al.** 46,XY intersex individuals: phenotypic and etiologic classification, knowledge of condition, and satisfaction with knowledge in adulthood. Pediatrics. 2002;110:e32.

15. **Meyer-Bahlburg HF.** Gender identity outcome in female-raised 46,XY persons with penile agenesis, cloacal exstrophy of the bladder, or penile ablation. Arch Sex Behav. 2005;34:423-38.

16. **Calapinto J.** As Nature Made Him: The Boy Who was Raised as a Girl. HarperCollins Publishers, Inc.; 2000.

17. **Knickmeyer R, Baron-Cohen S.** Fetal testosterone and sex differences. Early Hum Dev. 2006;82:755-60.

18. **Dewing P, Shi T, Horvath S, Vilain E.** Sexually dimorphic gene expression in mouse brain precedes gonadal differentiation. Brain Res Mol Brain Res. 2003;21;118:82-90.

19. **Houk CP, Lee PA.** Intersexed states: diagnosis and management. Endocrine and Metabolic Clinics of North America. 2005;34:791-810.

20. **Myers C, Lee PA.** Communicating with parents with full disclosure: A case of cloacal extrophy with genital ambiguity. J Pediatr Endocrinol Metab. 2004;17:273-80.

21. **Lee PA, Witchel SF.** Genital surgery among females with congenital adrenal hyper-plasias: changes over the past five decades. J Pediatr Endocrinol Metab. 2002;15:1473-7.

22. **Dayner JE, Lee PA, Houk CP.** Medical treatment of intersex: parents' perspectives. J Urol. 2004;172:1762-5.

23. **Minto CL, Liao LM, Woodhouse CR, Ransley PG, Creighton SM.** The effect of clitoral surgery on sexual outcome in individuals who have intersex conditions with ambiguous genitalia: a cross-sectional study. Lancet. 2003;361:1252-7.

24. **Stikkelbroeck NM, Beerendonk CC, Willemsen WN, et al.** The long term outcome of feminizing genital surgery for congenital adrenal hyperplasia: anatomical, functional and cosmetic outcomes, psychosexual development, and satisfaction in adult female patients. J Pediatr Adolesc Gynecol. 2003;16:289-96.

25. **Baskin LS, Erol A, Li YW, Liu WH, Kurzrocl E, Cunha GR.** Anatomical studies of the human clitoris. J Urol. 1999;162:1015-20.

26. A summary of the opinion is available at http://www.isna.org.

27. **APA Online.** Answers to your questions about individuals with intersex conditions [publication online]. Available at http://www.apa.org/topics/intersx.html.

PATIENT COMMUNICATION AND THE OFFICE ENVIRONMENT

Chapter 15

Taking a Comprehensive History and Providing Relevant Risk-reduction Counseling

KELLY MCGARRY, MD
MEGAN R. HEBERT, MA
JOHN KELLEHER, MD
JENNIFER POTTER, MD

Introduction

Nationally, there is a call for action on the part of all healthcare providers to improve the care delivered to lesbian, gay, bisexual, and transgender (LGBT) patients. Given this impetus, healthcare professionals are beginning to actively educate themselves to provide individualized and optimal care to this population. In line with the American Medical Association's policy to encourage the Liaison Committee on Medical Education and the Accreditation Council for Graduate Medical Education to include LGBT health issues in the cultural competency curriculum for medical education,[1] the aim of this chapter is to offer healthcare providers some of the tools necessary to achieve the overall goal of providing the best care possible. Providers who learn to communicate more effectively through nonjudgmental interactions shaped by patient individuality and recognition of diversity will be better informed and in a position to improve quality of care for all patients, including those who are LGBT.

Barriers to Effective Patient-Clinician Communication

Barriers to effective communication exist on the part of both patient and provider. There is often fear on the part of the patient and inadvertent insensitivity or lack of knowledge or awareness on the part of providers. The most significant medical risk for LGBT individuals is the avoidance of routine healthcare.[2] Studies show that LGBT patients have more difficulty accessing healthcare than heterosexuals, often do not return to a provider after an initial visit,[3] and are more likely to leave their healthcare appointment before it is over because of feeling unsafe. A 1990 study revealed that due to negative experiences with providers, almost 50% of lesbians rarely or never sought care despite being professionals with adequate access to healthcare.[4] Fear of disclosure is common, with one study reporting that only 37% of lesbian, gay, and bisexual patients directly disclosed their sexual orientation to their provider. The two primary reasons for failure to disclose are lack of opportunity and fear that inadequate healthcare will result.[5] Unfortunately, fears are sometimes grounded in reality: Kenagy recently found that 26% of participants in a transgender health needs assessment had been denied medical care because of their transgender status.[6]

Another barrier to disclosure is that providers often do not include a comprehensive social and sexual history in the medical interview. Westerstahl found that only 28 of 76 general practitioners were aware of having a lesbian patient in their practice. [7] Four providers had inquired directly about their patient's sexuality, while 24 patients informed their provider. Of the providers who were unaware of having any lesbian patients, none had ever asked about a patient's sexuality. The most common reason cited for not asking was that sexuality was considered "unimportant" or that it was the patient's responsibility to mention. In a study of general practitioner attitudes toward discussing sexual issues with lesbian patients, physicians reported a lack of knowledge about sexual practices of lesbians;[8] another survey found that nearly 40% of surveyed physicians reported being sometimes or often uncomfortable providing medical care to gay patients.[9] Compounding the problem, studies show that when lesbians do seek screening such as Pap smears, providers often discourage them from having preventive exams based on the erroneous belief that they are unnecessary.[10]

Research has found that many LGBT patients would like their health providers to be aware of their sexual identity and orientation. In one study, 89% of lesbians reported that they would have come out to their providers if they had been given the opportunity, and 94% felt that it was important to do so in order to ensure more appropriate care, understanding, honesty, and inclusion of their partner.[11] Providers can do much to increase satisfaction and improve health outcomes for LGBT patients by creating welcoming office environments and facilitating open and comfortable communication.

Creating a Welcoming Environment

Every aspect of the healthcare environment contributes to patients' impressions about the office and the kind of welcome they can expect.

The experience begins with their initial telephone call to book an appointment, continues with the greeting they receive from the receptionist when they enter the office, includes messages conveyed by questions on intake forms and educational brochures in the waiting room, and culminates with the quality of interaction they have with their provider. LGBT patients seek a safe, nonjudgmental environment and validation of their lifestyle, just like their non-LGBT counterparts. Therefore, it is not surprising to learn that 95% of a lesbian, gay, and bisexual sample reported studying their provider's behavior for cues of acceptance and 85% assessed the environment of the office for signs of lifestyle affirmation.[5]

Fortunately, there are many opportunities to create a welcoming environment for LGBT patients (see Table 15-1). The prominent display of a statement that the office does not discriminate on the basis of sex, gender, and sexual orientation sets a reassuring tone (see Figure 15-1). Educational brochures that include information pertinent to LGBT populations convey the message that the provider a patient is about to see is knowledgeable about LGBT health issues and open to discussing related concerns. Appendix A contains a list of Web sites where good quality patient education materials for LGBT individuals can be found.

For LGBT patients, the way we ask questions, listen to responses, and address concerns determines whether they will be honest with us and if they will return for future care. The adoption of gender-neutral language and creation of intake forms that acknowledge the full range of gender identity and sexual expression signal acceptance and provide the foundation for a comprehensive health history. Ideally, forms should explicitly include questions about gender identity, sexual orientation, and a wide spectrum of sexual behaviors, in addition to the usual questions about other risk behaviors and past medical/surgical history. Appendix B contains

---

NON-DISCRIMINATION POLICY

We do not discriminate on the basis of:

Race/Ethnicity

Age

Sex/Gender

Sexual Orientation

Socioeconomic Status

Religion

Insurance Status

Country of Origin/Immigration Status

Physical Ability

Mental Ability

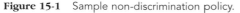

Figure 15-1 Sample non-discrimination policy.

Table 15-1   Providing an Inclusive and Welcoming Environment

Developing a Patient-Friendly Environment

Office Environment

- Have a non-discrimination policy visible to patients.
- Provide reading materials (magazines, health education pamphlets) that address the specific needs of LGBT patients.
- Ensure that the staff are comfortable with LGBT patients and their families.
- Ensure confidentiality.
- Make sure intake forms include options for non-married partners.

Interviewing (Questions can be modified from the sample intake form found in Appendix B and used in history-taking)

- Use gender-neutral language.
    "Do you have a significant other [or partner]?" "Are you in a relationship?"
- Ask the patient how they would like to be referred to and/or how to refer to their partner.
- Use language free of assumptions.
    Don't ask "Are you married?" or "What form of birth control do you use?"
    Avoid assumptions based on age, marital status, disability or other characteristics.
- Ask about specific sexual activities in a direct, nonjudgmental manner and assess risk behaviors.
- Normalize the discussion of sexual health by emphasizing that such discussion is routine with all patients.
    "Have you ever been sexually active with men, women, or both?"
    "Are you presently in a sexual relationship with a woman or a man or both?"
    "How many sexual partners have you had in the last six months?"
    "Do you have any sexual problems or questions?"
    "How do you protect yourself from STIs? Pregnancy?"
    "Have you ever been diagnosed with gonorrhea, chlamydia, syphilis, trichomonas, HIV, hepatitis, or any other STI?"
    "Have you ever had sex outside of your primary relationship?"
    "Do you use any recreational drugs when you have sex? Crystal meth? Cocaine? Alcohol? Others?"
- Ask who the patient lives with, who is important to them, who would care for them if they were sick. Consider asking, "Would you like to involve your partner or a friend or family member in your care?"
- Screen for mental health disorders. "Do you struggle at all with depression or feeling down?" "Do you struggle with anxiety?"
- Encourage patients to obtain legal documents that specify who can make medical and/or legal decisions for them (Durable Power of Attorney for Healthcare and Finances).

---

a sample intake form that includes broad designations of sex and gender (M, F, intersex, transgender), sexual orientation (attracted to men, women, transgender men, transgender women), sexual behavior (oral, vaginal, and/or anal sex with men, women, transgender men, and/or transgender women), and relationship status (single, partnered, married, divorced). Questions on this form can easily be adapted for use during interviewing.

Some providers believe that delving so thoroughly into "private" issues may turn patients away. On the contrary, patients believe it is appropriate to inquire about personal issues when it is relevant to their health.[12] Only through complete history-taking can we provide risk-reduction counseling that is pertinent to an individual patient. Providers need to explain that this extensive and sensitive information is asked of *all* patients and is asked *only* to ensure full, comprehensive care to all patients. Since some patients have concerns about the accessibility of such information to insurers, employers, or others, it is helpful to state explicitly that all information disclosed is confidential and will not be released unless a consent form is signed.

Beyond creating inclusive intake forms, providers and staff should be mindful of the language they use with patients. An unintentional assumption of heterosexuality is communicated to patients when we ask questions like "Are you married?" rather than, "Do you have a partner?" or "Are you in a relationship?" Questions that demonstrate preconceived ideas about a patient's behavior, whether about sexual practices, substance use, or other activities that impact health, make it more difficult for the patient to disclose information about actual behaviors, since he or she must actively correct the provider's assumptions. Using simple and quick educational sessions, healthcare providers can ensure that all office personnel learn to choose gender-neutral language and that communication during patient care is not heterosexually biased (see Table 15-1). Healthcare providers may be uncertain how to address transgender patients who have not legally changed their name and have not fully transitioned, yet have adopted the gender role consistent with their gender identity. In such cases, it is recommended that providers ask patients which name and pronoun they prefer and respect their choice.

Taking a Comprehensive History

LGBT patients have full and meaningful lives separate from their gender and sexual identities and their sexual behaviors and are at risk for contracting any of the illnesses that other patients develop. Therefore, it is important to perform a comprehensive review of systems and to obtain a thorough past medical and surgical history that includes attention to lifestyle risk factors, preventive behaviors, medications, allergies, history of abuse/violence, history of alcohol and other substance abuse, etc, just as one would do with any patient. As noted in other chapters, sexual minority populations have more risk factors for heart disease than the general population, as well as higher risk for depression and suicide, substance use (including tobacco), and both random violence and partner violence.

Asking pertinent questions about cardiac risk factors, including body image and perception of physical attractiveness in patients who are overweight, and performing a thorough mental health, substance use, and violence assessment may therefore be particularly important.

Selected LGBT populations also have higher risk for developing certain cancers as a result of health service utilization patterns (for example, development of later stage disease in persons who do not follow recommended screening protocols) or participation in specific risk behaviors (for example, development of HPV-associated anal cancer in men who practice anal-receptive sex). These latter examples underscore the importance of establishing a trusting patient-clinician relationship that supports adherence to health recommendations, performing a detailed review of risk behaviors, and providing pertinent risk-reduction counseling.

The medical literature is replete with information about how to obtain a comprehensive general health history, and most experienced clinicians know how to do this quite well: therefore, details about general history-taking will not be reviewed here. The reader is referred to the sample intake form for selected questions about body image, diet, exercise, mental health, and substance use; additional information about the latter two topics can also be found in this book's chapters on mental health and substance abuse. Most clinicians receive far less instruction and practice in obtaining a sexual history than in other aspects of the history; consequently, many feel uncomfortable and give this important area short shrift. For these reasons, the remainder of this section will review how to take a sensitive and thorough sexual history.

Taking a Sexual History

It is important to take a thorough sexual history from all patients, not just those who identify themselves as LGBT. Since patients can be uncomfortable discussing this topic, it is helpful to begin with a comprehensive social history. Asking patients about significant others or life partners, children, jobs, and hobbies demonstrates that we appreciate the breadth of their lives. This approach is especially useful with LGBT patients for two reasons. First, it prevents the sense of alienation a sexual minority patient tends to feel when a health provider zeroes in on a gender or sexual behavior topic after they reveal their LGBT status (for example, near-exclusive focus on HIV risk and testing after a gay or bisexual man discloses his sexual orientation). While we need to inquire about high-risk sexual behaviors (in all of our patients), validating the lives of our LGBT patients in their entirety allows us to build a trusting rapport and to assess health needs more effectively. Second, since many LGBT patients lose the support of family and friends after disclosing their identities, it is crucial to assess a patient's level of social adjustment and community support.

In taking a sexual history, it is important to distinguish between gender identity, sexual orientation, and sexual behavior. Gender identity refers to an individual's innate perception of their gender, which may or may not be consistent with their anatomical sex. Sexual orientation refers to emotional and sexual attraction to people of a particular sex. Heterosexuality is defined as sexual attraction to the opposite sex, homosexuality to the same sex, and bisexuality to both males and females. Gender identity is distinct from sexual orientation. For example, a person whose gender identity is female may exclusively date men and consider herself heterosexual even though she was born a biological male. Sexual orientation is distinct from sexual behavior, which refers to the specific sexual activities in which an individual engages, regardless of the individual's sexual orientation. Identity, orientation, and behavior are not always concordant. For example, only 30% of a sample of men who have sex with men (MSM) in a 1998 survey self-identified as gay, and 400 out of 7000 reported a history of having unprotected vaginal intercourse with women.[13] Similarly, studies of lesbian sexual behavior show that 75%-90% of self-identified lesbians report a history of heterosexual intercourse, sometimes with multiple partners.[14]

From the perspective of assessing risk for disease, sexual behavior is the most important concern. From a mental health perspective, all aspects of sexual identity and expression are important. Providers should make no assumptions—for instance, it cannot be assumed that a married man is not engaging in sex with other men. Many other commonly held notions need to be dismissed as well, including the belief that elderly patients cannot possibly be engaging in sexual activity, that all "sex" is penile-vaginal intercourse, and that sex outside committed relationships is rare. Making no assumptions about people's behavior and being clear and direct during history-taking will enable healthcare providers to provide outstanding care and to target risk-reduction counseling appropriately. Paramount to providing comprehensive medical care, it is also important to remember that sexual behavior, identity, and orientation can be dynamic and may change significantly over time. Hence, it is important for providers to assess this information each year or as the need arises.

As is the practice with heterosexual patients, the sexual history should begin by establishing whether an LGBT patient is sexually active, and, if so, by asking whom they are having sex with and what they know about their own and their partners' risks for sexually transmitted infections (STIs). Patients in monogamous relationships in which both partners are known to be free of STIs are at negligible risk for acquiring infections. Exploring sexual practices in these situations may be unnecessary except to ensure that the individual feels safe in the relationship and has an opportunity to disclose any sexual concerns he or she wishes to discuss. For any LGBT patient not in a monogamous relationship (or where monogamy is uncertain) or in a relationship with a partner who has STI risk factors or is currently infected with an STI, inquiry into sexual practices is critical to inform design of an appropriate risk-reduction and screening strategy.

Common sexual practices among women who have sex with women (WSW) include oral-vaginal contact, tribadism (genital to genital contact), digital stimulation, oral-anal contact, and sharing of sex toys. Tears or abrasions in skin or mucous membranes (in mouth, vagina, or anus) increase the risk of acquiring infections, such as herpes, human papillomavirus (HPV), contagious skin infections and, particularly for oral-anal contact, coliform bacteria, and hepatitis A. Importantly, women can acquire HPV from female partners without having had vaginal intercourse with men.[15] Lesbians, overall, may be less likely to use safer sex methods;[16] and while WSW may be at lower risk for STIs than gay men, bisexuals, transgender individuals, and heterosexuals, they are not risk-free and must be counseled according to their specific sexual practices. It is important to remember that WSW who engage in unprotected penile-vaginal or penile-anal sex with men are at high risk for acquisition of STIs; fertile WSW who engage in unprotected vaginal intercourse with men are also at risk for unintended pregnancy.

Sexual activities among men who have sex with men (MSM) include anal-receptive and anal-insertive intercourse, oral-genital and oral-anal contact, and digital stimulation of the rectum. Unprotected anal-receptive intercourse confers the highest risk of acquiring an STI. Oral-anal contact increases the risk of exposure to coliform bacteria and hepatitis A. MSM are also at increased risk for anal HPV, which is associated with an increase in anal cancers. Individuals who identify as bisexual may engage in any of the above high-risk behaviors and should be counseled appropriately. The same is true for transgender individuals; remembering to inquire about both sexual orientation *and* sexual behaviors helps to target counseling more effectively.

While transgender people have traditionally been described as belonging to one of two groups, characterized as biological females who identify as males (FTM) or biological males who identify as females (MTF), providers should appreciate that gender actually encompasses a much broader spectrum. Some transgender individuals identify as both male and female; some as neither, some identify as transgender before fully transitioning and later solely as their transitioned sex; and some always identify as transgender, gender variant, or gender queer. An individual may be a transgender FTM (transitioned or transitioning from female to male) but identify as gay (ie, seeking a male partner) and clinicians need to counsel around high-risk behaviors accordingly. Just as there are heterosexual, gay, and bisexual people who are traditionally male or female, there are heterosexual, gay, and bisexual transgender people as well. Once again, this highlights that sexual orientation reflects sexual attraction and possibly sexual behavior, whereas gender identity reflects an innate sense of self as male or female regardless of physical anatomy.

In summary, the traditional healthcare environment offers little sense of inclusiveness for LGBT patients; avoidance of routine medical care may be their most significant health risk.[2] As providers learn to recognize and address the specific needs of LGBT individuals in their practices, they can deliver optimal and much-needed healthcare experiences to this population. It is not possible to know everything about all aspects of the LGBT population, but a willingness to learn, to eliminate assumptions when asking questions, and to demonstrate concern and interest for patients are key to fostering open communication. Importantly, the process of increasing awareness of the variations in gender identity and human sexual expression, establishing a welcoming office environment, and learning how to discuss sensitive areas such as sexual history comfortably and openly will greatly enhance the healthcare provided to all patients.

Risk-reduction Counseling

A thorough sexual, behavioral, and psychological risk assessment at the initial exam, and all subsequent comprehensive exams, helps guide the clinician's efforts in providing appropriate risk-reduction counseling. LGBT patients should receive the same counseling that *all* patients receive regarding nutrition, exercise, weight management, cardiovascular health, substance abuse, risky sexual behavior, and a wide range of other risk- reduction topics. Several health issues and psychosocial risk factors, however, are unique to or more common in the LGBT population. The prevalence of cigarette smoking and the abuse of alcohol, marijuana, cocaine, and other recreational drugs are higher in gay men and lesbians.[17-19] The incidence of depression and anxiety disorders and risk for suicide are also more prevalent in the LGBT population.[20-21] Possible additional areas of higher risk include anal cancer for gay men and breast and endometrial cancer among lesbians, FTM patients, and bisexual women.[22-23] Lesbians may be at a higher risk of obesity and its health consequences than their heterosexual counterparts.[23] Smoking cessation counseling is of particular importance among transgender individuals, as smoking increases many risks associated with hormone therapy. Eating disorders are more likely in gay men than in heterosexuals, with one study reporting 17% of gay men with diagnosable eating disorders compared to 3.4% of heterosexual men.[24]

When discussing risk for STIs, it is important to identify and address the patient's perception of risk and to assess the validity and effectiveness of risk-reduction strategies they are already using. Misperceptions leave the patient with a false sense that they have eliminated their risk while continuing to engage in hazardous behavior. Among MSM, it is commonly believed that HIV and other STIs cannot be acquired by the "top" or insertive partner from the "bottom" or receptive partner, and that HIV cannot be acquired if the HIV-infected partner has a low viral load or is taking antiretroviral medications. More disturbingly, a popular drug combination known as "The Three V's"—Viread®, Viagra®, and Valium®—is commonly thought to reduce the risk of being infected with HIV while using crystal methamphetamine and engaging in risky sexual behavior. MSM may also engage in "serosorting," the belief that no protection is warranted if sexual partners are selected based on HIV status. Discussed more below, this practice has many risks for both HIV-infected and HIV-uninfected men. It is also necessary to assess for misconceptions among lesbians, such as the belief that STIs are not transmitted between female partners and that they are free from risk if they engage in unprotected anal sex, even if only using sex toys.

Patient education can have a profound effect on the way a patient manages his or her risk. Counseling should include accurate information about the relative risks of various sexual practices and guide the patient toward appropriate STI prevention strategies. In general, STI risk is highest with activities that involve contact with mucosal surfaces (anus/rectum > vagina > oral cavity) and secretions (semen, vaginal/cervical exudates). Risk-free and very low-risk activities include masturbation, Internet or telephone sex, dry kissing (no sores), and use of vibrators or sex toys that are not shared. Low-risk activities include wet (French) kissing, body-body rubbing (no fluids or skin lesions involved), sharing sex toys using a barrier, and hand-genital and hand-anal contact using a barrier. Medium-risk activities include hand-genital and oral-genital contact without a barrier. The highest-risk activities include sharing sex toys without a barrier, cunnilingus without a barrier during menses, deposition of vaginal secretions or semen in vagina or anus, rimming (mouth on anus) without a barrier, and fisting (fist in anus) without a barrier.

Behavioral risk-reduction strategies include abstinence, monogamy with an uninfected partner, avoiding sexual contact until partners have been screened, limiting the number of partners, practicing low-risk sexual activities, consistent and correct use of barrier methods, and avoidance of excessive alcohol and other substance use that could cloud judgment. It is important for patients to understand both the effectiveness and the limitations of barrier methods. In general, latex barriers provide reasonable protection against infections that are transmitted via fluids from mucosal surfaces (chlamydia, gonorrhea, trichomonas, HIV). In a study of HIV-discordant heterosexual couples, HIV seroconversion did not occur among those who used latex male condoms correctly and consistently for vaginal and anal intercourse, 10% seroconverted when condoms were used inconsistently, and 15% seroconverted when condoms were not used.[25] Latex barriers provide less protection against infections that are spread through skin-to-skin contact (HSV, HPV, syphilis, chancroid). In a study of HSV-2 serodiscordant heterosexual couples, latex male condom use during > 25% of sex acts prevented seroconversion in previously uninfected female, but not male, partners. This makes sense when we consider what is known about the most common sites of HSV shedding: penile skin (covered by the condom) versus vulva and perianal skin (where the condom affords less protection).[26] It is unclear to what extent latex male condoms protect against HPV transmission. While one meta-analysis of 20 studies provided no evidence that condom use is protective, a recent study suggested that latex condom use does provide some benefit.[27]

In light of this evidence, it is reasonable to recommend use of the latex male condom to cover the penis during oral, vaginal, and anal sex and to cover shared sex toys such as dildos. Limited data suggests that the female condom (worn by the receptive partner during either vaginal or anal intercourse) also provides protection against STI transmission.[28] While there are no specific studies to prove their utility, it makes theoretical sense to recommend use of plastic wrap (nonmicrowaveable, so there are no pores) or dental dams to cover the vulvar or vaginal opening and anus during oral-vaginal and oral-anal activity, and latex gloves during hand-genital or hand-anal stimulation. Choice of lubricant is an important consideration when using latex barriers: water-based and silicone-based products should be used exclusively, since oil-based lubricants are known to degrade latex. Use of the spermicide and microbicide Nonoxynol-9 (N-9) should be avoided, since a review of randomized trials demonstrated no significant reduction in risk for HIV, chlamydia, gonorrhea, or trichomoniasis in N-9 users, and genital erosions were more common, causing concern that this product might in fact increase, rather than decrease STI transmission.[29]

Obviously, barrier methods are far from perfect. First, many patients do not know how to use barrier methods correctly. For example, even though application of the male condom may seem straightforward and simple, one study showed that 80% of gay men did not know how to use a condom correctly.[30] Therefore, information about how to use both male and female condoms properly should always be provided (see Appendices C, D, and E for illustrations), and, when practical, opportunities to practice in the office (such as placing a male condom on a dildo or banana) can also be encouraged.

A second reason why barrier methods fail is that they are not always used consistently. There are a number of reasons why people fail to use barrier methods when their use is appropriate. These include: discomfort buying condoms, putting them on, or discarding them; concern that barriers will interfere with spontaneity and reduce or eliminate sensation; the belief that barriers are ineffective anyway because they can slip off, break, and provide incomplete protection against HSV and HPV; the perception that barriers are associated with casual sex, infidelity, and disease; discomfort advocating for barrier use with partner(s); lack of availability; and cost. It is helpful to assess patients' knowledge and comfort level by asking questions such as: "Have you tried using barrier methods like condoms?" "Have you had any problems using barrier methods?" "What kinds of problems?"

"Would you have any trouble getting a condom if you needed one?" and "Would you know how to put it on?"

It is important to respond in a thoughtful manner to a patient's concerns. Several practical tips can be suggested to enhance pleasure during barrier use. These include: practicing masturbation with a condom on; trying different types of condoms (latex or polyurethane only; lambskin condoms do not provide protection against HIV) that have bumps, ridges, etc; applying a layer of water-based lubricant under a dental dam or piece of plastic wrap; and eroticizing barriers by incorporating them into sexual activity in a playful and sexy manner. It is extremely important to help patients develop strategies for negotiating barrier use with partners: what to say, when to say it, and how they will respond if their partner(s) refuse(s). Use of methods within the patient's control (for example, use of the female condom by the receptive partner during anal intercourse) should be recommended for patients who have difficulty negotiating with their partners or whose partners are not cooperative.

Finally, even when barrier methods are used consistently and correctly, they are not foolproof, since they do not always cover areas of pathogen shedding and can either slip off the contact area or break. Therefore, it is imperative to utilize additional methods to prevent morbidity and mortality associated with STIs. Appropriate screening should be recommended at regular intervals for patients who are at risk for developing infection. The United States Preventive Services Task Force provides useful guidelines regarding optimal screening frequency (http://www.ahrq.gov/clinic/uspstfix.htm), and further detail on sexually transmitted infections can be found in Chapter 11. Appropriate vaccination should be provided, when available. This includes immunization against hepatitis A and B for individuals who practice high-risk sexual activities, particularly those that involve contact with the anus or rectum. In addition, the HPV vaccine can now be offered to young women ages 9-26; indications for men and older, uninfected women may soon be forthcoming. However, it should be noted that the first available vaccine (Gardasil™), only provide protection against two of the high-risk strains (HPV types 16 and 18);[31] thus, cervical cancer screening continues to be necessary in immunized individuals who are sexually active. Chemoprophylaxis is an additional option for prevention of HSV-2 transmission in serodiscordant couples, in whom daily administration of valacyclovir (500 mg per day) to the infected partner prevents seroconversion of the uninfected partner.[32]

Motivational Interviewing and Strategies for Change

A recent meta-analysis revealed that risk-reduction counseling and behavioral interventions reduce sexual risk, particularly if they include motivation and skills interventions.[33] The same analysis, however, concluded that members of the LGBT community have not benefited from existing risk-reduction counseling, largely because of poor communication between providers and their LGBT patients, as discussed above. Increasing health-care providers' comfort and knowledge around LGBT issues will improve the efficacy of risk-reduction counseling for LGBT patients.

It is important for the clinician to provide affirmation for whatever information the patient has disclosed, particularly if the patient has demonstrated discomfort in revealing the information. Statements like, "I'm glad you told me this," or "I know this wasn't easy for you to tell me, but I appreciate your honesty," provide much needed comfort to the patient and pave the way toward effective counseling. In particular, LGBT patients who are just beginning to "come out," who are working to resolve intense, conflicting feelings about their sexuality, and who may be facing negative reactions from family and friends, can benefit from simple and sincere affirming statements that recognize their struggle.

Risk-reduction counseling can be a defining aspect of the provider-patient relationship. Numerous strategies have been developed to change patient behavior, ranging from direct advice and outright shaming to more nonjudgmental approaches. Clinician-centered approaches, where the provider prescribes, for example, a drastic reduction in alcohol consumption, a minimum of 30 minutes of exercise per day, or better attention to glycemic control, have proven to be less effective than patient-centered approaches, where the provider attempts to meet the patient "where s/he's at." The latter approach is central to Prochaska and DiClemente's description of the stages of change, also known as the Transtheoretical Model, used extensively in treatment of alcoholism and tobacco abuse.[34-35] Motivational interviewing also adheres to a patient-centered approach, using the patient's own ambivalence about problem behaviors as a tool to affect change. Many healthcare professionals, however, feel ill-equipped to explore patients' feelings about behavioral change and find patient-centered risk-reduction counseling impossible to accomplish in a 15-20 minute office visit. The following steps provide a framework to discuss problem behaviors with patients efficiently and to assist them in adopting patterns of healthier living.

(1) *Develop an appreciation for the process of change.* As the saying goes, Rome was not built in a day. Providers use phrases like this to encourage their patients to be patient, for example, when allowing healing of a broken bone to proceed at a natural pace. Similarly, behavioral change needs to be understood as not occurring overnight, but rather as a series of predictable stages that patients must traverse. Prochaska and DiClemente proposed the following six stages:

Precontemplation Stage: During this stage, the patient is uninterested or unaware of the problem behavior or unwilling to consider changing the behavior. An alcoholic may perceive that she drinks only as much as everybody else does. A gay youth may erroneously believe that eventually all gay men will contract HIV and thus not see the importance of condom use. A lesbian may believe she is not at risk for cervical cancer and therefore has never been to a gynecologist and/or had a Pap smear. A young man who frequents bars and clubs may feel that ecstasy and crystal methamphetamine are indispensable for a fun night out.

Contemplation Stage: Patients in this stage express ambivalence about changing. They are able to perceive and discuss the potential benefits of change but give equal weight to the loss of an enjoyed behavior. Patients may begin to assess in a realistic way a cost-benefit analysis of embarking on a journey towards transformation, but they are still deeply invested in their present behavior. An alcoholic has located, perhaps even attended, a local AA meeting, but she has not decided a change is needed. A transgender individual engaging in unsupervised hormone therapy may be aware of some of the risks but at the same time struggle with potential prejudice and financial hardships associated with medical care.

Preparation Stage: Patients prepare to make a specific change during this stage. An alcoholic may experiment with small decreases in drinking as her ambivalence tips more towards recognizing a need for change. A cigarette smoker may buy a nicotine patch and set a quit date, and an overweight individual may join a gym. An HIV-infected individual may seek information about serosorting or may attempt to decrease unprotected anal-insertive sexual activity. A lesbian may ask her physician for a referral to a gynecologist, or a transgender individual may ask various sources to recommend transgender-friendly providers.

Action Stage: Commitment to change is supported by observable change and by a sense of momentum. An alcoholic enters rehab or makes a commitment to an AA sponsor, a smoker throws out his last cigarettes and puts on a patch, an overweight person begins an exercise regimen, and a transgender person stops sharing needles to inject hormones.

Maintenance Stage: The patient maintains the new behavior over an indefinite period of time, and the sense of momentum wanes. A recovering alcoholic proudly keeps track of the number of days of sobriety. A transgender individual continues ongoing and frequent consultation and care by a team of healthcare professionals. An HIV-infected individual never engages in unprotected sex. A previous dieter is now focused on maintaining weight loss. A cigarette smoker has quit for six months and is now devising strategies to maintain a life free from cigarettes.

Relapse Stage: The patient, for many reasons, may be unable to maintain the new behavior and slips into familiar and comfortable patterns. The patient, as well as the clinician, often view relapse as a "failure," and the patient usually feels demoralized. This stage should, however, be recognized as a normal part of the process of change. For example, smokers, on average, "fail" three to four times before quitting for good.

Practitioners who expect patients to change from being uninterested or unaware of their problematic behavior(s) to radically embracing healthier

habits will encounter few patients who can comply with their recommendations. Most patients progress slowly, with successes and slips that lead to
a steady improvement over time. Some individuals spend years in a single
stage; others may span more than one stage at a time. For example, a person with polysubstance abuse may be in the action stage for his heroin
addiction but in the precontemplation stage for marijuana. During the
process of change, regression is just as frequent an occurrence as progression, which can be frustrating for providers and patients alike.

(2) *Assess the current stage of the patient.* In order to offer a useful intervention, the provider must appreciate the stage at which he or she finds the
patient. It is pointless to give advice appropriate for a patient in the action
stage to a patient firmly entrenched in the precontemplation stage. Instead
of asking, "Why isn't this person motivated?" the provider might ask, "For
what *is* this person motivated?" The provider must not assume to understand the costs and benefits of the proposed behavior change for the
patient.[34] For change to occur, the patient must be ready, willing, and able
to commit to a change. Although providers feel most effective when a
patient feels ready for change, we must recognize that readiness presup-
poses a willingness (perceiving the change as *important*) and an ability
(perceiving self as *able*) to change.

Miller and Rollnick describe an algorithm for placing patients into categories regarding readiness for change.[36] In a simplified way, patients' willingness is assessed by the *importance* they assign to the change. The
confidence that they can actually make the proposed change is assessed by
their perception of their ability to change. Patients with *high importance*
and *high ability* are likely to be ready or near ready for change. Patients
may see the importance of a proposed change but see themselves as helpless to change their behaviors. Alternatively, patients may be confident in
their ability to change but assign no importance to change.

The following questions are useful for assessing patients' perceptions of
importance and confidence, and thus they help the provider to gain insight
into a patient's ambivalence.

(1) "How important would you say it is for you to _____? On
a scale from zero to ten, where zero is not at all important and ten is
extremely important, where would you say you are?"

(2) "How confident are you, that if you decided to _____, you
could do it? On the same scale from zero to ten, where zero is not at all
confident and ten is extremely confident, where would you say you are?"

Follow-up questions are then used to elicit the patient's perspectives on
importance and confidence:

"Why are you at a _____ and not 0?"

"What would it take for you to go from _____ to [a higher number, not 10]?"

The answers to these last two questions will provide a deeper understanding of the patient's ambivalence and place them in at least a provisional category of the stages of change. From there, the provider can

apply the principles of motivational interviewing to elicit change talk from the patient.

(3) *Apply the principles of motivational interviewing* based on where patient is in the process of change. This approach is based on a partnership with the patient rather than a confrontational style that imposes an "awareness and acceptance of 'reality' that the [patient] cannot see or will not admit."[36] This partnership takes as its foundation that the answers and motivations for change reside *in the patient*; the provider therefore attempts to draw out the patient's own perceptions, goals, and values. In order for this to occur, the patient must feel that the provider is *empathic* and *accepting* of the patient's ambivalence. The provider can then encourage the patient to explore the *discrepancy* between present behavior and deeply held values or goals. Patient resistance *should not be met with direct confrontation or arguments for change*, since these tactics merely cause the patient to defend their position more vehemently. The ultimate role of the provider is to resolve the patient's ambivalence and to *support self-efficacy*, because the patient's belief in the possibility of change is an essential motivator.

Precontemplation Stage: Providers often see patients in this stage as having a high level of resistance to changing their behavior, but it is less frustrating and more useful to think of these patients as being merely in the early stages of change. The provider can help to move the patient to the contemplation stage by using empathy and careful listening, providing a menu of behavioral options, and encouraging the patient to make small incremental changes rather than to espouse complete abstinence. Exploring barriers to change—hopelessness, cost, the fear and pain of withdrawal—can also be beneficial. These small interventions can be thought of as seeds that the precontemplator will slowly let germinate.

Contemplation Stage: Patients in this stage experience the most ambivalence and are often open to learning more information about the behavior but are unable to tip the balance toward change. Here the provider can explore the patient's investment in continuing the behavior.

Once a patient makes a commitment to change, ambivalence has been tipped in the direction of change, but it is important to remember that the ambivalence nevertheless persists. Some patients compare their addictions to elastic bands: the further they move away from the former behavior, the stronger the pull back. The provider can assist the patient by praising even the smallest change and making gentle evaluations and suggestions regarding the efficacy and feasibility of the proposed plan. For patients who are struggling to stay on track, it can be especially helpful to share experiences and obtain support from individuals who have succeeded in making difficult behavior changes.

Population-specific Examples

Two population-specific examples will now be described to demonstrate how providers can use increased awareness and knowledge of common behaviors to help individuals reduce health risks. The first example considers the pros and cons of "serosorting" as a means of reducing HIV transmission among gay men. The second example describes the importance of counseling to reduce the risks of unmonitored hormone use in transgender patients.

Many sexually active gay men undergo regular repeat HIV testing from every three months to annually; HIV testing is often sought during the early stages of a new relationship. It is postulated that the segment of the gay population that undergoes regular or frequent HIV testing often uses the information to select sexual partners who are seroconcordant.[37] Serosorting is a reasonable risk-reduction method when both partners are uninfected. However, effectiveness of this practice assumes that all sexual partners actually know their HIV status and will tell the truth, which is not always the case. Moreover, participants are sometimes unaware of the risks involved (co-infection with a drug-resistant strain of HIV or infection with another STI) in having unprotected sex when both parties are HIV-infected.[38] To complicate matters, many HIV-infected individuals mistakenly associate viral load with infectiousness and are unaware that viral loads in blood and those found in semen can differ significantly.[39] Gay men should be informed of the pros and cons of serosorting as a safer sex strategy; they can then incorporate this knowledge in the determination of acceptable personal risk limits.

As discussed more fully in Chapter 13, counseling regarding the risks of hormone therapy is especially important in the transgender community. Transgender individuals who inject street hormones and share needles are at increased risk for HIV transmission[40] and should be counseled and tested accordingly. Hormone treatment by any route may be associated with an increased risk of abnormal liver function, cardiovascular disease, diabetes, thromboembolism, osteoporosis, and certain cancers.[41] Patients receiving hormone therapy should be so advised, and a plan of care that includes regular monitoring and management of complications should be outlined. Comprehensive care for transgender patients, particularly those receiving hormones or requesting gender reassignment, often requires the involvement of experts from multiple specialties. Primary care providers can help tremendously by making appropriate referrals, coordinating care across disciplines, and ensuring that routine health maintenance, including age-appropriate and risk-appropriate screening, continues to occur.

Benefits to Improving the Healthcare Environment for LGBT Patients

The process of becoming an informed and informative, LGBT-friendly provider is personally, professionally, and financially rewarding. If as healthcare providers we simply avoid the assumption of heterosexuality by using gender-neutral language, we will make our offices much more welcoming to our LGBT patients. If we explore our patients' social histories in a gender-neutral manner, we will validate the importance of the significant people in their lives. Evidence suggests that LGBT populations experience higher rates of some harmful lifestyle factors than their heterosexual counterparts. Additionally, there are specific behaviors among subsets of the community that have health implications, for example, serosorting and recreational drug use among MSM and the unmonitored use of hormones in transgender patients. Being informed and being willing to ask our LGBT patients about these practices will enhance the care we provide.

If we are willing and able to discuss the risks associated with various behaviors, then we can better educate our patients about risk reduction. Motivational interviewing techniques can help us to understand our patients' readiness and ability to change and to assess their success on subsequent visits. Recognizing the significant psychosocial stressors faced by our LGBT patients, we should inquire specifically about stress and depression and make referrals when necessary. If we take an active role in the lives of our LGBT patients, we will help to provide them with the high quality healthcare that they need and deserve.

Summary Points

- The most significant medical risk for LGBT individuals is the avoidance of routine healthcare. Studies show that LGBT patients have more difficulty accessing healthcare than heterosexuals, often do not return to a provider after an initial visit, and are more likely to leave their healthcare appointment before it is over because of feeling unsafe.
- Research has found that many LGBT patients would like their health providers to be aware of their sexual identity and orientation. Nonetheless, a majority of lesbian, gay, and bisexual patients do not directly disclose their sexual orientation to their healthcare provider. Barriers to disclosure include the patient's fear of discrimination and the provider's failure to take a comprehensive social and sexual history.
- There are many opportunities to create a welcoming environment for LGBT patients, including prominently displaying a nondiscrimination statement, providing educational brochures that include information

pertinent to LGBT populations, and using language that is gender neutral and does not assume heterosexuality.

- Intake forms should acknowledge the full range of human identity and sexual expression. Ideally, they should explicitly include gender identity, sexual orientation, and a wide spectrum of sexual behaviors, in addition to the usual questions about other risk behaviors and past medical or surgical history.

- When taking a medical history, providers should acknowledge that LGBT people have full and meaningful lives separate from their gender and sexual identities and their sexual behaviors.

- Sexual minority populations are more at risk for certain health issues, such as depression and suicide, substance use (including tobacco), certain cancers and sexually transmitted infections, and both random and partner violence. Therefore, it is important for providers to ask pertinent questions related to these issues and to provide appropriate risk-reduction counseling.

- When taking a sexual history, it is important to understand that sexual identity, orientation and behavior may not correspond. For example, a man who identifies as heterosexual may engage in sex with men. Therefore, providers should remain open and nonjudgmental and should make no assumptions.

- Patient-centered approaches to risk-reduction counseling, where the provider attempts to meet the patient "where s/he's at," have proven more effective than other strategies. Motivational interviewing adheres to a patient-centered approach, using the patient's own ambivalence about problem behaviors as a tool to affect change.

References

1. **American Medical Association**. Available at http://www.ama-assn.org/ama/pub/category/14754.html. Accessed on June 28, 2006.
2. **Harrison AE, Silenzio VMB**. Comprehensive care of lesbian and gay patients and families. Prim Care. 1996;23:31-7.
3. **Diamant AL, Wold C, Spritzer K, et al**. Health behaviors, health status, and access to and use of health care. Arch Fam Med. 2000;9:1043-51.
4. **Zeidenstein L**. Gynecological and childbearing needs of lesbians. J Nurse Midwifery. 1990;35:10-8.
5. **Eliason MJ, Schope R**. Does "Don't ask, don't tell" apply to health care? Lesbian, gay, and bisexual people's disclosure to health care providers. J Gay Lesbian Med Assoc. 2001;5:125-34.
6. **Kenagy GP, Hsieh CM**. The risk less known: female-to-male transgender persons' vulnerability to HIV infection. AIDS Care. 2005;17:195-207.
7. **Westerstahl A, Segesten K, Bjorkelund C**. GPs and lesbian women in consultation: issues of awareness and knowledge. Scand J Prim Health Care. 2002;20:203-7.
8. **Hinchliff S, Gott M, Galena E**. 'I daresay I might find it embarrassing': general practitioners' perspectives on discussing sexual health issues with lesbian and gay patients. Health & Social Care in the Community. 2005;13:345-53.

9. **Mathews WC, Booth MW, Turner JD**. Physicians' attitudes toward homosexuality—survey of a California County Medical Society. West J Med. 1986;144:106.

10. **Brown R**. More Than Lip Service: Report on the Lesbian Health Information Project. Victoria BC: Royal Women's Hospital; 2000.

11. **Geddes VA**. Lesbian expectations and experiences with family doctors. Can Fam Physician. 1994;40:908-20.

12. **Stein GL, Bonuck KA**. Physician-patient relationships among the lesbian and gay community. J Gay Lesbian Med Assoc. 2001;5:87-93.

13. **Gay Men's Health Crisis**. Results of the 1998 beyond 2000 sexual health survey [pamphlet]. 1999.

14. **Bailey JV, Farquhar C, Owen C, et al**. Sexual behaviour of lesbians and bisexual women. Sex Transm Infect. 2003;79:147-50.

15. **Marrazzo JM, Stine K, Koutsky LA**. Genital human papillomavirus infection in women who have sex with women: a review. Am J Obstet Gynecol. 2000;183:770-4.

16. **Marrazzo JM, Coffey P, Bingham A**. Sexual practices, risk perception and knowledge of sexually transmitted diseases among lesbian and bisexual women. Perspectives on Sexual and Reproductive Health. 2005;37:6-12.

17. **Ryan H, Wortley PM, Easton A, et al**. Smoking among lesbians, gays, and bisexuals: a review of the literature. Am J Prev Med. 2001;21:142-9.

18. **Gruskin EP, Gordon N**. Gay/Lesbian sexual orientation increases risk for cigarette smoking and heavy drinking among members of a large Northern California health plan. BMC Public Health. 2006;6:241.

19. **Cochran SD, Ackerman D, Mays VM, et al**. Prevalence of non-medical drug use and dependence among homosexually active men and women in the US population. Addiction. 2004;99:989-98

20. **Cochran SD, Mays VM, Sullivan JG**. Prevalence of mental disorders, psychological distress, and mental health services use among lesbian, gay, and bisexual adults in the United States. J Consult Clin Psychol. 2003; 71:53-61.

21. **Clements-N K, Marx R, Guzman R, et al**. HIV prevalence, risk behaviors, health care use, and mental health status of transgender persons: implications for public health intervention. Am J Public Health. 2001;91:915-21.

22. **Breese PL, Judson FN, Penley KA, et al**. Anal human papillomavirus infection among homosexual and bisexual men: prevalence of type-specific infection and association with human immunodeficiency virus. Sex Transm Dis. 1995;22:7-14.

23. **Valanis BG, Bowen DJ, Bassford T, et al**. Sexual orientation and health: comparisons in the Women's Health Initiative sample. Arch Fam Med. 2000;9:843-53.

24. **Siever MD**. Sexual orientation and gender as factors in socioculturally acquired vulnerability to body dissatisfaction and eating disorders. J Consult Clin Psychol. 1994;62:252-60.

25. **De Vincenzi I**. A longitudinal study of human immunodeficiency virus transmission by heterosexual partner. N Engl J Med. 1994;331:341-6.

26. **Wald A, Langenberg AG, Link K, et al**. Effect of condoms on reducing the transmission of herpes simplex virus type 2 from men to women. JAMA. 2001;285:3100-6.

27. **Winer RL, Hughes JP, Feng Q.** Condom use and the risk of genital human papillomavirus infection in young women. N Engl J Med. 2006;354:2645-54.

28. **French PP, Latka M, Gollub, EL, et al**. Use-effectiveness of the female versus male condom in preventing sexually transmitted disease in women. Sex Transm Dis. 2003;30:433-9.

29. **Wilkinson D, Tholandi M, Ramjee G, et al.** Nonoxynol-9 spermicide for prevention of vaginally acquired HIV and other sexually transmitted infections: systematic review and meta-analysis of randomised controlled trials including more than 5000 women. Lancet Infect Dis. 2002;2:613-7.

30. **Martin DJ**. A study of the deficiencies in the condom-use skills of gay men. Public Health Rep. 1990;105:639-40.

31. **Widdice LE, Kahn JA**. Using the new HPV vaccines in clinical practice. Cleveland Clinic Journal of Medicine. 2006;73:929-35.

32. **Corey L, Wald A, Patel R, et al**. Once-daily valacyclovir to reduce the risk of transmission of genital herpes. N Engl J Med. 2004;350:11-20.

33. **Johnson BT, Carey MP, et al**. Sexual risk reduction for persons living with HIV: research synthesis of randomized controlled trials, 1993 to 2004. J Acquir Immune Defic Syndr. 2006;41:642-50.

34. **Prochaska JO, DiClemente CC**. Transtheoretical therapy: toward a more integrative model of change. Psychotherapy: Theory, Research and Practice. 1982;19:276-87.

35. **Prochaska JO, Velicer WF, Rossi JS, et al**. Stages of change and decisional balance for 12 problem behaviors. Health Psychol. 1994;13:39-46.

36. **Miller WR, Rollnick S**. Motivational Interviewing: Preparing People for Change. 2nd ed. Guilford Press; 2002.

37. **Leaity S, Sherr L, Wells H, et al**. Repeat HIV testing: high-risk behavior or risk redcution strategy? AIDS. 2000;14:547-52.

38. **Colfax GN, Guzman R, Wheeler S, et al**. Beliefs about HIV reinfection (superinfection) and sexual behavior among a diverse sample of HIV-positive men who have sex with men. J Acquir Immune Defic Syndr. 2004;36:990-2.

39. **Kalichman SC, Rompa D, Austin J, et al**. Viral load, perceived infectivity, and unprotected intercourse. J Acquir Immune Defic Syndr. 2001;28:3035.

40. **Nemoto T, Luke D, Mamo L, et al**. HIV risk behaviours among male-to-female transgenders in comparison with homosexual or bisexual males and heterosexual females. AIDS Care. 1999;11:297-312.

41. **Moore E, Wisniewski A, Dobs A**. Endocrine treatment of transsexual people: a review of treatment regimens, outcomes, and adverse effects. J Clin Endocrinol Metab. 2003;88: 3467-73.

LEGAL ISSUES AND THE LGBT COMMUNITY

Chapter 16

Legal Issues of Importance to Clinicians

DENISE MCWILLIAMS, ESQ
DEBORAH FOURNIER, ESQ
BETHANY A. BOOTH, ESQ
PAUL BURKE, ESQ
JOYCE KAUFFMAN, ESQ

LGBT Rights and Patient Rights

Introduction

The history of homophobia is much longer and better known than the history of gay rights. Throughout most of western history, same-sex relationships have been prohibited, stigmatized, and often punished, forcing lesbian, gay, bisexual, transgender (LGBT) persons to hide their sexuality or gender identity in order to survive. This experience varies historically in different cultures. It is only in the years following World War II that LGBT people in the United States began moving to cities, forming their own communities, and leading more open lives. And it is only since 1969, when the police raided the Stonewall Inn, a gay bar in New York City, and encountered violent resistance from its patrons, that the modern gay rights movement was born. Since the Stonewall riots, the gay rights movement has grown to encompass other sexual minorities, including lesbians, bisexuals and transgender persons. The AIDS movement was rooted in the experiences of the gay rights movement, as was the women's health movement. More recently, some states have begun to recognize LGBT rights by enacting hate crime laws and antidiscrimination laws that include sexual orientation, and by offering civil unions, domestic partnerships, or marriage for same-sex couples.

Even with these advances, however, LGBT people continue to face many barriers. Large numbers of LGBT people across much of the country still feel a need to hide their identity as sexual and gender minorities in order to get by in homophobic environments. Virtually every LGBT person today has known someone or has themselves been the victim of job discrimination, ostracism, a bashing, or denial of needed services. Federal laws do not yet prohibit discrimination based on sexual orientation or gender identity. In some states, having sexual relations with someone of the same gender is still an illegal act. The federal Defense of Marriage Act (DOMA), enacted in 1996, defines marriage only as a union between one man and one woman and provides that states need not recognize same-sex marriages; taking this one step further, the majority of states have enacted their own statutory Defense of Marriage Acts.

For the clinician, the role that LGBT rights plays in patient care may not be immediately evident. However, because the lives and well-being of LGBT patients can be affected by these issues, it is important for clinicians to become more familiar with certain rights, laws, and policies that concern LGBT people. These include the need for advance healthcare directives, the right of confidentiality around disclosure of sexual orientation in medical records, and policies that formalize relationships and allow second-parent adoption. Laws vary from state to state, but this chapter will introduce some of the major issues faced by all clinicians in practice. Ultimately, whenever a person is unable to express his or her true identity openly and proudly because of a legal or perceived restriction of the basic human rights provided to heterosexuals, that person's mental or physical health can be significantly affected.

Healthcare Decision-making

Because the partners and families of LGBT individuals are not uniformly recognized by states or communities, clinicians should strongly encourage LGBT patients to complete advance directives that make explicit their medical decision-making wishes should they become incapacitated. The basic rule across the country is that a competent patient makes the decisions necessary for his healthcare. If the patient is not competent, whether the incompetence is temporary or permanent, most jurisdictions turn to the spouse or next of kin, or rely upon a "substituted judgment" determination to ascertain what the patient would have decided. This can leave a great deal of uncertainty as to whether the patient's wishes were correctly assessed and can exclude the unmarried partner or other close companion of an LGBT patient from making any healthcare decisions despite knowing the patient's wishes best. Fortunately, two types of advance directives have been developed that memorialize an individual's wishes before the need arises and thus legally protect against such scenarios. These are the living will and the healthcare proxy (also known as durable healthcare power of attorney).

A living will allows a person to formally declare the type of medical care to be pursued should she be incompetent to make the decision at the time (eg, life support or organ donation). Executed with the same formality as a last will and testament, such documents are given great weight by medical professionals and courts and will usually be considered determinative. There are some states that do not recognize living wills. Even in these, however, the living will has great value as evidence of what the person would have decided had they been able to do so.

A healthcare proxy designates someone to act as the patient's "proxy," or healthcare decision maker, in the event of incapacitation. A healthcare proxy document can include instructions as to what the proxy should do in particular circumstances, but in most cases it simply names the proxy and gives them the power to make decisions based on what they believe the patient would want (a living will helps guide these decisions).

Forms for both the living will and healthcare proxies are readily available—in fact all hospitals are required to offer forms to patients upon admission. Some examples of forms are included in Appendix F and Appendix G. These are just samples of language and are presented as a framework; they should be adapted to the specific needs and wishes of each person, rather than used verbatim. Also, technical requirements differ among jurisdictions, and care should be taken to comply with all such requirements (see Appendix A for more resources).

Persons signing these documents should understand that the forms themselves are not the most important part of the process. The critical part is understanding all the potential decision points and all the situations in which the need for advance directives can arise. At a minimum, patients should consider what level of discomfort and/or disability they are willing to tolerate and what would constitute a "meaningful life" if exceptional measures were needed to keep them alive. Legal counsel can be helpful. In addition, it is critical that patients review these decisions periodically. As life changes occur, so too can views on medical decision making. These decisions are seldom a matter of right or wrong, but rather of being more or less informed. Finally, healthcare proxies should be kept aware of the patient's thoughts on all of these matters.

Patient Rights

There are certain, long-established rights that people have when they interact with the healthcare system and, more recently, the healthcare financing system. Some of those are established by specific statutes. Others are found in the common law (law derived through judicial decision). Still others are guaranteed by "Patients' Bills of Rights"—omnibus statutes purporting to establish a full array of legal protections for people interacting with healthcare providers, facilities, or private or public insurers (note that typically patients' bills of rights have little more than symbolic import). Finally, there are rights based in contract law that arise out of the agreements people have with their providers and health plans.

The following are the rights most often guaranteed to people across the country that can have a direct impact on LGBT people in the context of the healthcare system. Note that this is a rapidly evolving area of law. Also note that many patient rights are contractual and can be overridden by certain factors; for example, patients may not have their healthcare wishes realized if they do not communicate them in a living will or if they sign consent forms that conflict with their wishes. Therefore, it is very important that patients always be given fully informed consent, be aware of the benefits of advance directives, and be encouraged to use appropriate legal counsel if they need help understanding what they are signing, as clinicians are not generally trained in the finer points of law.

Right of Confidentiality

LGBT patients have the same concerns as anyone else with regard to protection of personal information; in addition, LGBT patients can have concerns about potential advertent or inadvertent disclosure to others of their sexual orientation or gender identity. There are federal and state constitutional and statutory protections of health privacy (See Fourteenth Amendment of the US Constitution; see also http://www.healthprivacy.org for a review). Such statutes provide protection against the intentional or negligent breach of confidentiality. Virtually all professional organizations also have a standard requiring members to respect patient privacy (for example, the American Medical Assocation: http://www.ama-assn.org). Additionally, the Joint Commission on Accreditation of Health Care Organizations—the professional body which established minimum standards for healthcare organizations and audits compliance with them—has established a standard for the protection of the medical record (see http://www.jointcommission.org).

Although the vast majority of healthcare and related organizations have policies to protect patient information, there is not always enough done to ensure those protections are followed carefully. For example, some research, government, and healthcare organizations have enormous data banks of health information with personal identifiers that are not properly secured and can be accidentally or purposively released to the public. The last 10 years have seen numerous examples of this. In 1997, a CD-ROM containing the names of approximately 4000 people with HIV/AIDS in Pinellas County Florida was sent to newspapers by the disgruntled boyfriend of a health department employee.[1] In 2005, a researcher's laptop containing the names of people with HIV/AIDS who received services from a clinic in Sacramento was stolen in a burglary from his home.[2] In 2006, a laptop containing personal information, including the medical records, of 28 million veterans was stolen from a Veterans Affairs employee.[3] Few employers do background checks on employees who have access to such data, and oversight of the personnel involved with the data is virtually nonexistent.

It is therefore of utmost importance that clinicians protect their patients' confidential information and train office staff to do the same. Some steps that clinicians can take include discussing with patients why it is sometimes important to include sexual orientation or gender identity information in the medical record (eg, certain routine screenings are recommended for sexually active gay and bisexual men) and how that information will be used and protected. Some LGBT individuals may still request that their sexual orientation or gender identity be kept out of their medical records. These patients may fear discrimination by insurers, clinicians, or other healthcare workers or may worry about disclosure of this information to family members. Patients should be reassured to the extent possible (some fears may be warranted) and also given the chance to request this information be left out of the record. Be aware that the ability of clinicians to edit already-written medical reports is sharply limited by legal requirements, so editing after the fact is almost never an option.

Patients should be informed that they can request and review their medical records so that if they are asked for copies, they can make an informed decision as to which parts, if any, they feel comfortable releasing. For example, they may authorize release only of laboratory results or certain parts of the narrative. Most institutions spell out this right in their patient's bill of rights. Finally, if patients suspect a breach of confidentiality, they should be able to pursue a variety of remedies, be it an internal complaint, a complaint to the licensing or accrediting body, or litigation.

Right to Services

Although protection for LGBT people against discrimination varies across the country, many states do provide such protection in places of public accommodation, including protection for medical treatment in hospitals and clinics (a review of state protections can be found at http://www.glad.org or http://www.lambdalegal.org). Even where state law provides no protection, many professional organizations, such as the American Medical Association and the American Nurses Association, have prohibited discrimination against LGBT people, and aggrieved persons can look to these organizations for redress. In theory, this means that people cannot be denied medical services because of their sexual orientation and that designees of LGBT patients must be afforded the same access to participate in their healthcare (eg, access to medical records and involvement in treatment decisions) as those of all patients.

Right to Informed Consent

In simplest terms, informed consent is the process whereby, in the name of treatment, a person agrees to certain procedures to cure or alleviate an injury, disease, or condition. Treatment is defined broadly and includes just about anything one could imagine a healthcare provider offering to a patient. Although the standards for informed consent vary greatly among states, there are two basic approaches. Approximately half the the states use a "reasonable person" approach, ie, the information about risks that must be disclosed is that which a reasonable person in the patient's position would want to know.[4] In other states, people are entitled to all significant medical information that a healthcare provider possesses or reasonably should possess that is material to an intelligent decision by the patient.[5]

Historically, many states have enacted specific statutes requiring separate consent for HIV testing. In an attempt to decrease the steady annual incidence of 40 000 new cases of HIV each year in the United States, in 2006, the Centers for Disease Control issued guidelines which called for removal of separate consent and recommended routine HIV testing with the right to "opt out" of being tested.[6] Although the guidelines do not have the force of law, many states are now reconsidering their requirement for specific consent for an HIV test.

Dispute Resolution

Clinicians who have a good rapport with their patients, who are open, non-judgmental, and familiar with LGBT health and identity issues, will be less likely to encounter disputes from their patients. Throughout the process of care for their patients, clinicians can help prevent litigation by carefully explaining issues as they arise. However, even among the most competent and sensitive of providers, disputes can still occur. In these cases, there are some steps that clinicians and patients can take to resolve the issue as smoothly as possible. Litigation should always be the last resort. It is expensive and complicated, and it takes far too much time to be useful to an individual trying to solve, rather than be compensated for, a problem.

It can be helpful for patients to have an advocate involved, particularly when patients are limited in their ability to ask questions, to make sure they have appropriate and complete information. The advocate does not necessarily need to be a professional—a friend may do. Even conversations about routine information can become adversarial if conducted in a state of high emotionality. Having someone present who can detach from the emotion of the conversation can be invaluable in finding a rapid solution.

In very difficult situations, most practices and facilities have internal mechanisms, such as an ombudsperson, that can help resolve disputes. Frequently problems can be resolved simply by finding someone with either distance from the original dispute or sufficient authority to overrule a decision.

While it is rarely necessary, if the internal process fails, patients can attempt to mediate or arbitrate the dispute. Many communities have dispute resolution centers that maintain lists of mediators. Frequently a skillful mediator can assist in coming to an agreement at a significant savings in time and money.

Hate Crimes and Antidiscrimination Laws

Hate Crimes

"Hate crime" is a term widely used; however, its meaning is not commonly understood. A discussion of hate crimes often evokes images of brutal violence and blatant bigotry, such as the infamous 1998 murder of Matthew Shepard, a young man targeted because he was gay. Advocacy organizations describe the impact of hate crimes as hurting not only the victim of the crime but also creating an environment of fear and intimidation that affects every member of that group or community.

According to LAMBDA (http://www.lambda.org), a hate crime may be described as a criminal action that is committed due to (or motivated in part by) a bias against the victim's particular race, religion, ethnicity, sexual orientation, gender, gender identity, or other characteristic.[7] That is to say, a hate crime is a crime in which the perpetrator specifically chooses the victim because of his or her real or perceived race, religion, color, disability, sexual orientation, etc.

The function of a hate crime law is to increase or enhance the punishment for criminal actions when it can be shown that those criminal actions are motivated, at least in part, by a bias or hatred of a particular characteristic of the victim. Hate crime laws are not the same as antidiscrimination laws; they do not civilly prohibit behavior that has not been previously designated as a criminal act by that jurisdiction. In some instances trespass, intimidation, threats, or verbal harassment may constitute crimes under state laws; what is considered a criminal act will vary from state to state, depending on the different criminal codes of each state. Physical assault, destruction of property, robbery, arson, and homicide generally are considered criminal acts. All laws criminalizing behavior can be applied to any crime committed against an LGBT person. Whether or not it will be considered a hate crime will be dictated by whether the conduct is proscribed as criminal conduct in that jurisdiction, whether that jurisdiction has a hate crime statute, and whether there is evidence that the victim was chosen because he or she is believed to be an LGBT person.

Federal hate crime law does not include sexual orientation as a protected class. Current federal hate crime law covers only those crimes committed on the basis of race, religion, color, or national origin. Additionally, current federal hate crime law requires proof that the crime was committed because the victim was exercising a federally protected activity. There have been legislative proposals to amend the federal hate crime statute to include sexual orientation, gender, or disability in the protected classes and to remove the federally protected activity proof requirement, but to date none have been passed. The Justice Department is required to collect data on hate crimes, including those motivated by bias against sexual orientation, from law enforcement agencies across the country and publish the results annually. In the latest statistics available from the FBI, racially and ethnically motivated crimes remain the most predominant hate crimes reported. However, the number of reported crimes based on sexual orientation have steadily increased since 1991.[8]

Not every state in the union has a hate crime law. State hate crime laws vary from state to state in terms of which groups are included in the lists of protected categories. Sexual orientation and gender identity are not explicitly included in the list of protected groups in every state that has a hate crime statute (see Table 16-1). However, case law in some states may expand protection for sexual orientation or gender identity–motivated crimes despite the failure to explicitly delineate them as protected classes in the legislation.

It is debated whether hate crime laws infringe on free speech or expression. There have been two Supreme Court cases regarding the constitutionality of hate crime legislation, *R.A.V. v. City of St. Paul* and *Wisconsin v. Mitchell*. Essentially, these cases together hold that legislation that enhances the penalty for committing a crime because the crime is bias-motivated and which uses the perpetrator's speech as evidence of his or her motive or intent are not violations of the First Amendment's protection of free speech. However, statutes that criminalize symbolic speech or bias-motivated speech in and of themselves may in fact be violations of the First Amendment. Neither case dealt specifically with the constitutionality of including sexual orientation as a protected class in such legislation. Some activist groups oppose including sexual orientation or gender identity in hate crime legislation because they believe it will prohibit their ability to oppose homosexuality. However, it appears that hate crimes do not criminalize thought or speech and would pose no legal limitation on speech in the absence of a commission of a crime. Only a criminal act can become a hate crime.

Table 16-1   Hate Crime Laws by State (including District of Columbia)[9]

States with hate crime laws that include sexual orientation as a protected category	AZ, CA, CO, CT, DE, FL, HI, IL, IA, KS, KY, LA, ME, MD, MA, MN, MO, NE, NV, NH, NJ, NM, NY, OR, PA, RI, TN, TX, VT, WA, WI, DC
States with hate crime laws that include gender identity as a protected category	CA, CO, CT, HI, MD, MN, MO, NM, PA, VT, DC
States with hate crime laws that *do not* include sexual orientation or gender identity	AL, AK, ID, MI, MS, MO, NC, ND, OH, OK, SD, VA, WV
States with hate crime laws that do not list any categories	UT
States with no hate crime laws of any kind	AR, GA, IN, SC, WY

Sexual Orientation and Gender Identity Antidiscrimination Laws

There are 17 states that prohibit employment discrimination on the basis of sexual orientation (CA, CT, HI, IL, MA, MD, ME, MN, NH, NJ, NM, NV, NY, RI, VT, WA, WI);[10] seven states have laws that prohibit private sector employment discrimination on the basis of gender identity (CA, IL, ME, MN, NM, RI, WA).[11] Many of the states that prohibit employment discrimination on the basis of sexual orientation also prohibit sexual orientation discrimination in public employment, public accommodations, education, housing, credit, and labor practices.[11] Hundreds of cities and counties prohibit sexual orientation discrimination in public and private employment as well.

Sexual orientation is not included in the federal laws that prohibit discrimination on the basis of race, color, sex, religion, national origin, age, and disability. There is proposed federal legislation, the Employment Non-Discrimination Act, or ENDA, that would prohibit sexual orientation by employers. In its current form, ENDA would not provide protection against gender identity employment discrimination. As of the date of this writing, ENDA has not been successfully passed.[12]

However, federal law and many state laws make sexual harassment illegal as a form of sex discrimination. Some courts have interpreted laws prohibiting sex discrimination and sexual harassment as extending their protections to gender identity discrimination. The vast majority of states offer no discrimination protection for sexual orientation or gender identity in any of these sectors.

Implications of Formalized LGBT Relationships

There are a range of vehicles whereby same-sex couples can have their relationships legally sanctioned. These include marriage, civil union, and domestic partnership. Each have legal implications that can impact the rights of individuals to receive and access healthcare. In the United States, all forms of legally sanctioned relationships have occurred at the state level. Federal laws which apply to legally sanctioned relationships among heterosexuals do not apply.

Same-sex Marriage

When the Supreme Judicial Court ruled in the *Goodridge v. Department of Public Health* case (Goodridge) in 2003, Massachusetts became the first state to allow marriage between couples of the same sex. Currently, federal law does not recognize Massachusetts same-sex marriages, and many other states have passed constitutional amendments and laws that invalidate same-sex marriages, despite their current legitimacy in Massachusetts. Because same-sex marriage laws are extremely fluid, a patient in a same-sex marriage should always check with a local attorney prior to making any healthcare decisions based on marital status.

With the legality of same-sex marriage in Massachusetts, many rights improved for same-sex couples in that state, including benefits in the workplace, inheritance rules, medical decision-making policies, and income tax laws. At the same time, marriage also has some legal and financial costs. Some of these disadvantages are common to all marriages, while some pertain only to same-sex couples. For example, prior to the *Goodridge* case, many employers already provided domestic partnership benefits, such as health and dental insurance, to employees' unmarried different-sex and same-sex partners. If a domestic partner plan requires employees to be unmarried in order to be eligible, then marriage may disqualify them, although they may then be eligible for benefits for married employees.[13,14] Individuals should always check with their employers to ensure coverage if their marriage status changes. This is just one example of the complexities that individuals need to be aware of even when embracing the many joys of marriage.

Medical Decision-making

When individuals cannot communicate their healthcare wishes, standard practice is for medical providers to go to the next of kin to make decisions. Unmarried partners are rarely considered next of kin and are therefore denied the rights to make these decisions, unless they have been designated as the healthcare proxy. In Massachusetts, same-sex spouses are considered next of kin for their incapacitated spouses, so not having a healthcare proxy would not affect their decision-making role. Nonetheless, it is still wise for same-sex married couples to draft healthcare proxies in the event that the medical emergency or decision takes place out of Massachusetts, where the marriage is not recognized as valid. All unmarried couples should draft healthcare proxies to ensure decision-making authority.

Transgender Marriages [15,16]

People who are transgender can encounter unique difficulties in obtaining a legally validated marriage. The validity of the marriage depends on a number of factors, including the birth sexes of the couple, the couple's state of residence, and whether or not a person has legally "transitioned" from one sex to another. If one partner has transitioned from one gender to the other *prior* to the marriage, the prevailing rule used to be that a marriage was valid if 1) a court determined that the individual had successfully fulfilled the relevant legal benchmark for changing gender in that particular state, and 2) the individual wished to marry someone of the (current) opposite gender. More recently, however, many courts have adopted the "Corbett rule," which holds that biological sex is set at birth and cannot be altered by either natural physical development or medical and surgical procedures. Courts in Florida, Kansas, Texas, and Ohio have adopted the

Corbett rule. In these states, even if individuals have taken extensive measures to transition to the opposite sex, they cannot change their sex *legally* throughout their lives; consequently, transgender individuals may only marry persons of the opposite birth sex. Note, however, that this also means that if the couple is of opposite birth sex from each other, then they can marry, even if they express their gender as the same.

If a person transitions to the opposite sex *after* marrying, the transition should have no impact on the validity of a legally recognized marriage in any state. With a legally recognized marriage, only divorce or death can end it. Because the Defense of Marriage Act centers on state and federal power to disregard marriages *entered into* by same-sex couples, it should have no impact on a marriage where a different-sex couple marries and subsequently one spouse transitions to the opposite sex (therefore making the marriage into a union between same-sex individuals). It should be noted, however, that there have not been any court decisions about this situation yet.

Civil Unions and Domestic Partnerships

Civil unions provide same-sex couples with the same state-based legal benefits, protections, and responsibilities available to married spouses under that state's laws. Civil unions are currently legal in Vermont, Connecticut, and New Jersey. As with same-sex marriage in Massachusetts, couples in civil unions only receive benefits from the state; federal laws applicable to married couples do not apply.

California allows same-sex couples to register as domestic partners, akin to civil unions. Registered domestic partners have all the same rights, protections, and benefits and are subject to the same responsibilities, obligations, and duties under state law as are granted to and imposed upon spouses. Unlike civil unions in other states, California's domestic partnership law does not require an official ceremony. For Web sites that provide further details on civil unions and domestic partnerships, see Appendix A.

Other Legal Protections

As state-legalized protections are not available uniformly, are not recognized by federal laws, and often are not recognized by states other than the one where the relationship was legally sanctioned, many couples choose to protect their relationships by entering into legal agreements. Even in states where legal unions exist, some couples will choose to prepare the necessary legal documents to make sure there is no question about their wishes. Given the ever-changing legal landscape, it is best to be too prepared than not prepared enough.

Advanced legal planning can protect patients, their families, and their property. It can make sure that patient wishes are carried out and can prevent disputes between patients and their partners. The unfortunate reality is that without the necessary legal documents, unmarried partners may have no legal right to visit their partners in the hospital or to receive their property in the event they die. The law still favors biological families and therefore will turn to those definitions in the absence of legal documents clearly expressing the patient's wishes.

Basic legal planning includes preparing documents such as a will, a healthcare proxy, and a living will. Some individuals also put together other documents such as a cohabitation agreement, which clearly states what property each individual owns separately and jointly, a couple's expectations and responsibilities regarding the relationship, and how material goods would be distributed if a relationship ends. Additional documents can also specify the rules both members of a couple wish to govern relationships with children. It is often helpful for clinicians to know about a couple's wishes so they can provide optimal support if any changes do occur.

Adoption

Becoming Parents

Without question, parenting has become commonplace within the gay community. Better access to reproductive technology and adoption and advancements in the legal landscape have made it possible for more lesbians and gay men to become parents. Respected professional organizations such as the American Academy of Pediatrics, the American Psychological Association, the Child Welfare League of America, and the North American Council on Adoptable Children have all formally expressed their support of the right of lesbians and gay men to raise children.

Lesbians and gay men, of necessity, have to be very creative and thoughtful in their efforts to become parents. Many people choose to have biological children. For lesbians, anonymous donor sperm is available from several reputable sperm banks. Some lesbians choose to have children with a known donor, entering into arrangements with a friend or relative in order to bear children. For gay men, traditional or gestational surrogacy arrangements can be made either informally or formally through agencies who work with single men or couples to find egg donors and surrogates. Some lesbian couples elect to have children through *in vitro* fertilization, where one of them is the egg donor and the other the birth-mother.

Others choose to adopt, either domestically or internationally. "Private" domestic adoptions are most often "identified adoptions," in which birth-parents are presented with several potential adoptive families from which they select the family into which their child will be placed. "Public" domestic adoptions are through a state child welfare agency and involve the adoption of children who have been placed in the custody of the agency, usually due to neglect and/or abuse by their parents.

International adoption can be a challenging, though certainly not impossible, option. There is no country that allows openly lesbian or gay foreigners to adopt. Each country has its own internal regulations and restrictions concerning adoption, some of which may make it impossible for lesbian and gay individuals to adopt. For example, in order to adopt from China, single people who wish to adopt must sign an affidavit in which they confirm that they are not homosexual. Restrictions on the percentage of adoptions by unmarried persons exist in several countries. Further, the adoption policies of foreign countries are subject to political change; programs sometimes shut down altogether for lengthy periods of time. Couples are advised not to formalize their relationships through marriage, civil union, or domestic partnership if they are considering international adoption, as an adoption agency may be obligated to ask for that information, which would likely prevent the couple from being eligible to adopt internationally.

Adoption laws vary widely from state to state, but generally speaking, all adoptions (domestic and international) begin with a home study, an investigation by a licensed adoption agency which must approve the home as an appropriate placement for a child. Applicants will be required, among other things, to submit to criminal record checks and to supply references, financial documentation, and medical information. Those seeking international adoptions will be fingerprinted and must submit to record checks by the Federal Bureau of Investigation. The adoptive parent will also have to obtain the necessary permission to bring a child into the country from the US Citizenship and Immigration Services (USCIS, formerly the Immigration and Naturalization Service or INS).

There are a number of states that explicitly prohibit lesbians and gay men from adopting and others that, while they may not explicitly prohibit such adoption, may make it quite difficult to traverse the system (see Table 16-2).

Second-parent Adoption

Regardless of how children come into the home of a same-sex couple, it is strongly recommended that the parents create a legal relationship between the children and the parent who is not the biological or adoptive parent. Without creating that legal relationship, the children are vulnerable to losing their relationship with that parent in the event of the death of the legal parent or the end of the couple's relationship. This dilemma has plagued the lesbian/gay community for decades, often resulting in lengthy and costly litigation concerning support, visitation, and custody. Even aside from the most stark situations, there are numerous scenarios in which non-legal lesbian and gay parents face difficulty on a daily basis. They may be

Table 16-2	States that Explicitly Prohibit Adoption by Lesbian and Gay People
Florida	Bans all adoption by lesbians and gay men
Nebraska	Bans adoption by "known" gay and lesbian people
North Dakota	Law allows discrimination for "religious reasons"
Utah	Bans adoption by lesbian and gay couples
Oklahoma	In 2004, enacted a statute stating that will not recognize second-parent adoptions by lesbian and gay couples. That statute has been successfully challenged, although the state has appealed the decision.

prevented from visiting a sick child in the hospital, they may be unable to access medical or educational records; unable to interface with medical professionals and schools to advocate for their children, or not permitted to travel outside the country with the child. This individual's role as a parent is unacknowledged and devalued on a regular basis. The only way to remedy this situation is to create a legal relationship between the child and that parent, either through second-parent adoption, judgment of parentage, or guardianship.

On September 23, 1993, the Massachusetts Supreme Judicial Court, in a landmark decision, upheld entry of an adoption decree allowing the joint adoption of a child by her biological mother and the mother's lesbian partner, both of whom had planned for and raised the child from birth. In so doing, the court found that nothing in the Massachusetts adoption statute prevented joint adoption by unmarried cohabitants.[17] Shortly before the Massachusetts decision, the Vermont Supreme Court upheld a nonbiological parent's right to adopt the biological children of her female partner while keeping the parental rights of the biological mother intact. The court found that this would be in the best interest of the children.[18] In 1999, not long after the Connecticut appellate court determined that the then-existing adoption statute did not allow for the joint petition of a lesbian couple,[19] the Connecticut legislature enacted a statute, effective in 2000, that created a process for second-parent adoption. In addition to Massachusetts, Connecticut, and Vermont, several other appellate courts and/or legislatures have confirmed the right of lesbian and gay individuals to adopt the biological or adoptive children of their same-sex partners. These include California, the District of Columbia, Illinois, Indiana, New York, New Jersey, and Pennsylvania.

Trial courts in many other jurisdictions throughout the country have similarly allowed second-parent adoption. This means that second-parent adoption is available in certain counties in Indiana, Iowa, Louisiana, Maryland, Minnesota, Nevada, New Mexico, Oregon, Rhode Island, Tennessee, Texas, and Washington. Other appellate courts have concluded that second-parent adoptions are not permissible under the law. These include Colorado, Nebraska, Ohio, and Wisconsin.

Access to second-parent adoption has made it possible for thousands of unmarried same-sex and heterosexual couples to legalize their relationships with their children. Once such an adoption has been approved, both parents have the same legal rights and responsibilities. In the event of the death of one parent, the surviving parent would have legal custody. In the event of the dissolution of the relationship, both parents would have legal standing to seek custody, support, and visitation through the courts.

Even in states with formal recognition of same-sex relationships, it is recommended that legally recognized same-sex couples pursue second-parent adoptions. Although there is a legal presumption that the children born into a legally recognized partnership, civil union, or marriage are the legal children of that relationship, that relationship may not be viewed as valid elsewhere. The federal government and any state that has a Defense of Marriage Act (DOMA) will not recognize either the validity of the partnership, civil union, or marriage or any state-based legal rights that flow from the partnership or marriage.

Another reality in lesbian and gay families is that many children have more than two parents, for example, when a lesbian couple enters into an agreement with a gay man to parent a child together or a woman and a gay male couple have a child together. It can also occur if there has been a breakup of one relationship and the subsequent involvement of other individuals as parents to the child (similar to a stepparent situation). In a very few jurisdictions, it has been possible to legally recognize these family constellations through three-parent adoptions. This author is aware of three-parent adoptions having been allowed in Alaska, California, and Massachusetts.

For obvious reasons, lesbian and gay parents are often concerned about the finality of the adoption even once it has been granted. Under the US Constitution's "full faith and credit clause," which provides that all states recognize the judgments of all other states, adoption decrees should be fully recognized by other jurisdictions. Absent fraud or a timely appeal by a parent who had no notice of the filing of a petition, it is highly unusual for an adoption decree to be later vacated. Many states have specific statutes addressing the recognition of adoptions finalized in another state or country.

The concern, however, is not entirely unfounded. The Mississippi legislature, in 2000, narrowly defeated proposed legislation that not only would have banned lesbians and gay men from adopting but also would have refused to recognize foreign adoptions by lesbians and gay men. In 2004, the Oklahoma legislature passed an amendment to its adoption law prohibiting the recognition of the validity of adoptions of children by same-sex couples approved by other states. On May 19, 2006, the US District Court ruled that this amendment was unconstitutional; the state of Oklahoma is appealing this ruling.

Another possibility is the challenge by a former partner of the validity of a co-parent adoption. In *Starr v. Erez*, no. COA99-1534 (North Carolina

Appellate Court, 14th District, April 13, 2004), a former lesbian partner sought the revocation of an adoption decree, but that request was denied. To date, no such challenge has succeeded.

In the several years since second-parent adoption has become available, thousands of children have been adopted by lesbian and gay couples. Not only has this had a profound impact on lesbian and gay families, but it has also had a profound impact on the courts, which have had a unique opportunity to learn about lesbian and gay families through the adoption process. Access to second-parent adoption, as well as the growing recognition and acceptance of the relationships between lesbians and gay men and their children, has not only made a tremendous difference to the children in lesbian and gay families, it has also made a tremendous difference to their parents, granting them full parental status where, only a short time ago, there was none.

Alternatives to Adoption

Even in states where second-parent adoption is available, the circumstances of a particular family may make it impossible to accomplish. For example, if the children have another parent who refuses to surrender his or her rights, it will be virtually impossible to pursue an adoption. For these families and for others who live in states where lesbian, gay, or second-parent adoption is not permissible, other ways of creating either legal relationships between parents and children or other legal protections must be explored.

In some jurisdictions, it may be possible to petition the court to appoint the parents as legal guardians of the children; this will grant the previously nonlegal parent at least some of the legal authority he or she must have in order to care for a child. The difference between guardianship and adoption is that adoptions are "final and irrevocable"; guardianships end on the child's 18th birthday and can be revoked by further petition to the court. Note, however, that if the children have another legal parent and that parent does not assent to the guardianship, this, too, may be unavailable.

In a few jurisdictions, same-sex couples have successfully obtained "judgments of parentage" from the courts under a law known as the Uniform Parentage Act (UPA). The UPA has a more expansive definition of who is a parent, and creative lawyers in California and Colorado have been able to secure such judgments so that both parents are considered to be legal parents. Courts in Massachusetts have similarly entered judgments of parentage in situations where, for example, a lesbian couple had a child through IVF, where one of the women is the egg "donor" and the other carries the child or, more recently, where a married gay couple arranged to have a child through gestational surrogacy. One of the men was the sperm "donor," eggs from an anonymous donor were used, and the gestational carrier desired no parental rights.

Where none of these options—second-parent adoption, parentage judgment, and guardianship—is available to same-sex parents, it is essential that families create other forms of protection through estate planning documents, parenting agreements, donor agreements, authorizations for medical treatment, and the like. Because lesbian and gay families do not often have legal sanction, they need to draft agreements that reflect a family's intentions about their parenting arrangements. These agreements may be important down the road if disputes arise concerning custody or support. Parenting agreements should outline the agreement to jointly parent and speak to how custody, visitation, and support issues would be resolved in the event of a separation. If a lesbian couple is using a known sperm donor, a donor agreement can define what the relationship(s) will or will not be between the couple and the donor and between the donor and the child. For men entering into gestational or traditional surrogacy agreements, it is essential to draft contracts using reputable agencies to make the necessary arrangements.

Because relationships between same-sex partners are most often legally unrecognized, it is especially important to execute a will that designates who will be the guardian of that person's children. Without a will, the relatives of the decedent will in many cases have a superior claim to be appointed as guardian of any minor children.

Summary Points

- LGBT rights have seen many advances in current years. These include the right to formalize relationships, adopt children, and be protected against discrimination based on sexual orientation or gender identity. The granting or denial of these rights can have a direct impact on LGBT patients' access to care, healthcare decision-making, and overall well-being.
- Because recognition of LGBT partners and families varies by community, clinicians should strongly encourage LGBT patients to complete advance directives (living wills and healthcare proxies) that make explicit their medical decision-making wishes.
- Confidentiality rights include protection of information regarding sexual orientation or gender identity. Clinicians should explain to patients why it might be important to include this information in the medical record and how that information will be used and protected. Patients should be given the chance to request this information be left out of the record.
- Sexual orientation is not included in the federal laws that prohibit discrimination on the basis of race, color, sex, religion, national origin, age, and disability. However, some states prohibit employment discrimination on the basis of sexual orientation, and many states and

medical organizations prohibit sexual orientation discrimination in public accommodations (including hospitals), education, housing, credit, and labor practices.

- A hate crime is a crime in which the perpetrator specifically chooses the victim because of his or her real or perceived race, religion, sexual orientation, etc. Hate crime laws increase the punishment for criminal actions when those actions are shown to be motivated by a bias or hatred of a particular characteristic of the victim. Federal hate crime law does not include sexual orientation as a protected class, but many states laws do.

- Only a few states allow same-sex couples to legally sanction their relationships by marriage, civil union, or domestic partnership. Each formal relationship has legal implications that can impact the rights of individuals to receive and access healthcare. All same-sex couples are encouraged to complete advance legal planning to protect their interests.

- It is strongly recommended that same-sex couples with children seek to create a legal relationship between the children and the person who is not the biological or adoptive parent, either through second-parent adoption, judgment of parentage, or guardianship. Otherwise, the nonbiological or adoptive parent is vulnerable to losing the role as parent if the legal parent dies or if the couple ends their relationship.

- Respected professional organizations such as the American Academy of Pediatrics, the American Psychological Association, and the Child Welfare League of America have all formally expressed their support of the right of lesbians and gay men to raise children.

- Patient rights and LGBT rights are regional and always evolving. When in any doubt, patients should be encouraged to consult a legal professional.

References

1. Health worker gets probation in leak of AIDS records. AIDS Policy Law. 1997;12:2.
2. **Milbourn T.** California: stolen laptop contains files on HIV patients. Sacramento Bee. February 23, 2006. Available at http://www.aegis.org/news/ads/2006/AD060335.html.
3. **Associated Press.** IDs of active personnel on stolen laptop. USAToday.com. June 3, 2006. Available at http://www.usatoday.com/news/washington/2006-06-03-vets-id -theft_x.htm.
4. *Canterbury v Spence*, 464 F.2d 772 (DC Cir 1972).
5. *Martin v Lowney*, 401 Mass. 1006, 517 NE2d 162 (1988).
6. **Branson BM, Handsfield HH, Lampe MA, et al.** Revised recommendations for HIV testing of adults, adolescents, and pregnant women in health-care settings. MMWR Recomm Rep. 2006;55:1-17.
7. **Lambda GLBT Community Services.** Lambda Gay and Lesbian Anti-Violence Project (AVP): what is a hate crime? Available at http://lambda.org/hatecr1.htm.
8. **Anti-Defamation League.** Hate crimes: offenders reported motivations. Available at http://www.adl.org/99hatecrime/offenders_Motivations.asp.

9. **Human Rights Campaign Foundation.** Statewide hate crime laws. Available at http://www.hrc.org.

10. **Human Rights Campaign Foundation.** The state of the workplace for gay, lesbian, bisexual and transgender Americans 2005-2006. Available at http://www.hrc.org/workplace.

11. **Lambda Legal.** Summary of states which prohibit discrimination based on sexual orientation. Available at http://www.lambdalegal.org/cgibin/iowa/news/resources.html ?record=185.

12. **Workplace Fairness.** Sexual orientation discrimination, workplace fairness. Available at http://www.workplacefairness.org/sexualorientation#2.

13. **Human Rights Campaign Foundation.** Frequently asked questions on domestic partnership benefits. Available at http://www.hrc.org/Content/NavigationMenu/Work_Life/Get_Informed2/Frequently_Asked_Questions/Frequently_Asked_Questions.htm#1.

14. **Gay and Lesbian Advocates and Defenders (GLAD).** Domestic partnership benefits still matter in the age of equal marriage: marriage does not mean instant equality for lesbian and gay employees. Available at http://www.glad.org/rights/DPpostgoodridge.pdf.

15. **Levi JL.** Advising transgender clients. In: Triantafillou K, et al, eds. Representing Nontraditional Families. 2nd ed. MCLE, Inc.; 2006: 397-9.

16. **Gay and Lesbian Advocates and Defenders (GLAD).** Transgender legal issues in New England. Available at http://www.glad.org/rights/Transgender_Legal_Issues.PDF.

17. Adoption of Tammy, 416 Mass. 205, 619 NE2d 315 (1993).

18. Adoptions of BLVB and ELVB, 628 A2d 1271, 160 Vt. 368 (1993).

19. Adoption of Baby Z, A2d 1035, 247 Conn. 474, 724 (1999).

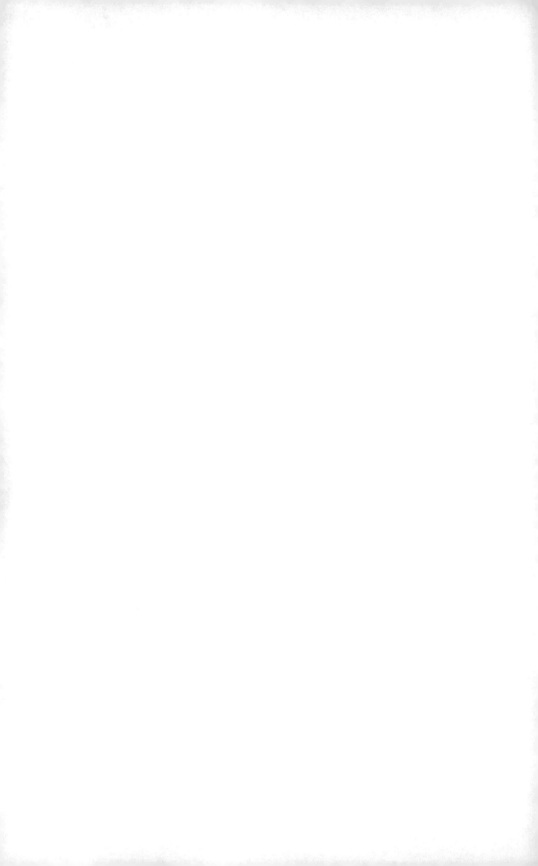

Appendix A

Resources for Clinicians and Patients

We recommend that clinicians use the following resources for further learning, as well as for providing referrals and support for patients. Resources are organized by chapter topic.

Chapter 1: Clinicians and the Care of Sexual Minorities, and Chapter 2: Demography and the LGBT Population

Literature on LGBT Health and Healthcare

American Public Health Association. Lesbian, gay, bisexual, and transgender health issues. selections from the American Journal of Public Health. American Public Health Association; 2001.

Bonvicini KA, Perlin MJ. The same but different: clinician-patient communication with gay and lesbian patients. Patient Education and Counseling. 2003;51:115-22.

Centers for Disease Control and Prevention. Sexual behavior and selected health measures: men and women 15-44 years of age, United States, 2002. Available at http://www.cdc.gov/nchs/products/pubs/pubd/ad/361-370/ad362.htm.

Dean L, Meyer IH, Robinson K, et al. Lesbian, gay, bisexual, and transgender health: findings and concerns. Journal of the Gay and Lesbian Medical Association. 2000;4:101-51.

Diamant AL, Wold C, Spritzer K, et al. Health behaviors, health status, and access to and use of health care: a population-based study of lesbian, bisexual, and heterosexual women. Archives of Family Medicine. 2000;9:1043-51.

Gay and Lesbian Medical Association. Healthy People 2010: Companion Document for Gay, Lesbian, Bisexual, and Transgender Health. San Francisco, CA; 2001. Available at http://www.glma.org.

Harcourt J, ed. Current Issues In Lesbian, Gay, Bisexual, and Transgender Health. Haworth Press; 2004.

Institute of Medicine, Solarz AL, eds. Lesbian Health: Current Assessment and Directions for the Future. The National Academies Press; 1999.

Kaiser Permanente National Diversity Council and the Kaiser Permanente National Diversity Department. A Provider's Handbook on Culturally Competent Care: Lesbian, Gay, Bisexual and Transgendered Population. San Francisco CA; 2000.

Knight D. Health care screening for men who have sex with men. Am Fam Physician. 2004;69:2149-56.

Makadon HJ. Improving health care for the lesbian and gay communities. N Engl J Med. 2006;354:895-7.

Makadon H. Primary care of gay men. UpToDate 2006, Version 14.2.

Makadon HJ, Mayer KH, Garofalo R. Optimizing primary care for men who have sex with men. JAMA. 2006;296:2362-5.

Meyer IH. Prejudice, social stress, and mental health in lesbian, gay and bisexual populations: conceptual issues and research evidence. Psychological Bulletin. 2003;129:674-7.

Meyer IH, Northridge ME, eds. The Health of Sexual Minorities: Public Health Perspectives on Lesbian, Gay, Bisexual and Transgender Populations. Springer; 2006. Includes: Mayer K, Mimiaga M, VanDerwarker R, et al. Fenway Community Health's model of integrated community-based LGBT care, education and research.

National Lesbian and Gay Health Association and Mautner Project for Lesbians with Cancer. Removing barriers to health care for lesbian, gay, bisexual, and transgendered clients: a model provider education program; 1997.

Peterkin A, Risdon C. Caring for Lesbian and Gay People: A Clinical Guide. University of Toronto Press; 2003.

Potter JE. Do ask, do tell. Annals Internal Medicine. 2002;137:341-3.

White J, Levinson W. Primary care of lesbian patients. J Gen Int Med. 1993;8:41-7.

Wolitski R, Stall R, Valdiserri R, eds. Unequal Opportunity: Health Disparities Among Gay and Bisexual Men in the United States. Oxford University Press; in press.

Background Reading on LGBT Populations

Faderman L. Odd Girls and Twilight Lovers: A History of Lesbian Life in the Twentieth Century. Penguin; 1992.

Duberman M. About Time: Exploring the Gay Past. Plume; 1991.

Feinberg L. Transgender Warriors: Making History from Joan of Arc to Dennis Rodman. Beacon Press; 1997.

Hutchins L, Kaahumanu L, eds. Bi Any Other Name: Bisexual People Speak Out. Alyson Publications; 1991.

Ochs R, Rowley SE. Getting Bi: Voices of Bisexuals Around the World. Bisexual Resources Center; 2005.

General LGBT Health Web Sites

GayHealth
http://www.gayhealth.com

GLBT Health from the Department of Public Health, Seattle and King County, WA
http://www.metrokc.gov/health/glbt

Gay and Lesbian Medical Association
http://www.glma.org

LGBTHealthChannel
http://www.lgbthealthchannel.com

The Mautner Project
http://www.mautnerproject.org

National Coalition for LGBT Health
http://www.lgbthealth.net

General LGBT Information and Support Web Sites

Bisexual Resource Center
http://www.biresource.org

Gaydata.org
http://www.gaydata.org

Human Rights Campaign
http://www.hrc.org

National Gay and Lesbian Task Force
http://www.thetaskforce.org

National Association of LGBT Community Centers
http://www.lgbtcenters.org

Parents, Families, and Friends of Lesbians and Gays
http://www.pflag.org

LGBT Health Centers

The following list of health centers have a principal mission to provide primary care to LGBT communities. Please note that this is a partial list and that many more healthcare facilities, clinical practices, and hospitals across the nation have expertise, or are developing expertise, in LGBT care.

Fenway Community Health, Boston, Mass
http://www.fenwayhealth.org
(617) 267-0900

Callen-Lorde Community Health Center, New York, NY
http://www.callen-lorde.org
(212) 271-7200

Whitman-Walker Clinic, Washington, DC
http://www.wwc.org
(202) 797-3500

Chase-Brexton Health Services, MD
http://www.chasebrexton.org

Howard Brown Health Center, Chicago, Ill
http://www.howardbrown.org
(773) 388-1600

Montrose Clinic, Houston, TX
http://www.montroseclinic.org
(713) 830-3000

L.A. Gay and Lesbian Center, Los Angeles, Calif
http://www.lagaycenter.org
(323) 993-7400

Resources for LGBT Racial and Ethnic Minorities

FO' brothas.com
http://www.fobrothas.com

The Gay and Lesbian Latino AIDS Education Initiative, Philadelphia, Penn
http://www.galaei.org

Gay Asian Pacific Support Network, San Francisco, Calif
http://www.gapsn.org

Gay Asian Pacific Alliance
http://www.gapa.org

Hispanic AIDS Forum, New York, NY
http://www.hafnyc.org

Latin American Health Institute, Boston, Mass
http://www.lhi.org

Latino Gays and Lesbians Online
http://www.latinoglo.com

List of organizations that specialize in healthcare for black gay men and lesbians
http://www.blk.com/resources/o-health.htm

QV Magazine: Links to Latino LGBT agencies and support organizations
http://www.qvmagazine.com/gaylatinolinks.html

Utopia: Asian Gay and Lesbian Resources
http://www.utopia-asia.com/

LGBT Support Hotlines

Gay, Lesbian, Bisexual and Transgender Helpline
(888) 340-4528
Monday through Friday, 6pm-11pm, Eastern Time
Serves all ages. Provides information, referrals, and support on coming
out, HIV/AIDS, safer sex and relationships, and locating GLBT groups
and services

Peer Listening Line (staffed by youth 25 and under)
(800) 399-PEER
Monday through Friday, 6pm-11pm, Eastern Time
Staffed by youth 25 and under. Provides information, referrals, and support on coming out, HIV/AIDS, safer sex and relationships, and locating GLBT groups and services

GLBT National Help Center Hotline
(888) the-GLNH
Monday through Friday, 4pm-midnight, Eastern Time
Saturday, 12pm-5pm, Eastern Time
Serves all ages. Provides peer counseling, information and local resources

GLBT National Youth Hotline
(800) 246-PRIDE
Monday through Friday, 8pm-midnight, Eastern Time
Staffed by youth 25 and under. Provides peer counseling, information and
   local resources

Chapter 3: Coming Out:
The Process of Forming a Positive Identity

Books About the Coming Out Experience

Bass E, Kaufman K. Free Your Mind: The Book for Gay, Lesbian, and Bisexual Youth and
   Their Allies. HarperCollins; 1996.
Boenke M, ed. Trans-Forming Families: Real Stories about Transgendered Loved Ones.
   Walter Trook; 1999.
Borhek MV. Coming Out to Parents: A Two-way Survival Guide for Lesbians and Gay Men
   and Their Parents. The Pilgrim Press; 1993.
Fortunato J. Embracing the Exile: Healing Journeys for Gay Christians. Seabury Press; 1982.
Fricke A. Reflections of a Rock Lobster: A Story of Growing up Gay. Consortium Book Sales
   & Dist, 1995.
Griffin CW, Wirth MJ, Wirth AG. Beyond Acceptance: Parents of Lesbians & Gays Talk
   About Their Experiences. St. Martin's Press; 1996.
Holmes S, Tust J. Testimonies: Lesbian and Bisexual Coming Out Stories. Alyson
   Publications; 2002.
Kailey M. Just Add Hormones: An Insiders Guide to the Transsexual Experience. Beacon
   Press; 2005.
Miner J, Connoley JT. The Children Are Free: Reexamining the Biblical Evidence on Same-
   sex Relationships. Jesus Metropolitan Community Church; 2002.
Penelope J, Wolfe SJ. The Original Coming Out Stories. Crossing Press; 1989.
Pierce Buxton A. The Other Side of the Closet: the Coming Out Crisis for Straight Spouses
   and Families. John Wiley and Sons; 1994.
Signorili M. Outing Yourself: How to Come Out As Lesbian or Gay to Your Family, Friends
   and Coworkers. Fireside; 1995.

Coming Out: Organizations and Web sites

Parents, Family and Friends of Lesbians and Gays (PFLAG)
http://www.pflag.org

Human Rights Campaign—Coming Out Pages
http://hrc.org/Template.cfm?Section=Coming_Out

Web sites with coming out stories:
http://www.comingoutstories.com
http://www.rslevinson.com/gaylesissues/comingoutstories/blcoming.htm
http://www.avert.org/comingoutstories.htm
http://www.lesbianworlds.com/out/
http://www.outpath.com/
http://www.bibble.org/gay/stories/comingout.html

Chapter 4: Addressing LGBTQ Youth in the Clinical Setting

Literature on the Care of LGBTQ Youth

Ryan CC, Futterman D. Lesbian and Gay Youth: Counseling and Care. Columbia University Press; 1998.
Perrin E. Sexual Orientation in Child and Adolescent Health Care. Springer; 2002.

Organizations and Web Sites for Youth

Afraidtoask.com
http://www.afraidtoask.com

Advocates for Youth
http://www.advocatesforyouth.org
(202) 419-3420

Campus Pride
http://www.campuspride.org
(704) 277-6710

Gay, Lesbian & Straight Education Network (GLSEN)
http://www.glsen.org
(212) 727-0135

Gay-Straight Alliance Network
http://www.gsanetwork.org
(415) 552-4229

The Hetrick-Martin Institute, Home of the Harvey Milk High School
http://www.hmi.org
(212) 674-2400

Lavender Youth Recreation and Information Center (LYRIC)
http://www.lyric.org
(415) 703-6150

The National Youth Advocacy Coalition (NYAC)
http://www.nyacyouth.org
(800) 541-6922
Office: (202) 319-7596

Sexual Minority Youth Assistance League (SMYAL)
http://www.smyal.org
(202) 546-5940

Youth Resource
http://www.youthresource.com
(202) 419-3420

Teenwire.com
http://www.teenwire.com

Youth Guardian Services
http://www.youth-guard.org
(877) 270-5152

Hotlines for Youth

GLBT National Youth Hotline
(800) 246-PRIDE
Monday through Friday, 8pm-Midnight, Eastern Time

National Runaway Switchboard
(800) 231-8946
24 hour; 7 days/week

Peer Listening Line
(800) 399-PEER
Monday through Friday, 6pm-11 pm, Eastern Time

Trevor Helpline Crisis Intervention for LGBTQ Youth
(800) 850-8078
24 hour; 7 days/week

Chapter 5: LGBT Couples and Families with Children

Literature on LGBT Couples and Families

LGBT Couples
Boyd H. My Husband Betty: Love, Sex, and Life with a Crossdresser. Thunder Mouth's Press; 2003.
Clunis DM, Green GD. Lesbian Couples: A Guide to Creating Healthy Relationships. Seal Press; 2005.
Erhardt V. Head Over Heels: Wives Who Stay with Cross-Dressers and Transsexuals. The Hayworth Press; 2007.
Lahey KA, Alderson K. Same-Sex Marriage: The Personal and the Political. Insomniac Press; 2004.

LBGT Parents and Prospective Parents
Aizley H. Buying Dad: One Woman's Search for the Perfect Sperm Donor. Alyson Publications; 2003.

Aizley H. Confessions of the Other Mother: Non-Biological Lesbian Mothers Tell All. Beacon Press; 2006.

Alternative Families Project. Children, Lesbians, and Men: Men's Experiences as Known and Anonymous Sperm Donors. Men's Resource Center of Western Massachusetts; 1994. To order, write to The Alternative Families Project, 442 Warren Wright Road, Belchertown, MA 01007.

Benkov L. Reinventing the Family: The Emerging Story of Lesbian and Gay Parents. Crown Trade Paperbacks; 1994.

Boenke M. Trans Forming Families: Real Stories about Transgendered Loved Ones. Walter Trook Publishing; 1999.

Brill S. The New Essential Guide to Lesbian Conception, Pregnancy & Birth. Alyson Books; 2006.

Brill S. The Queer Parent's Primer; A Lesbian and Gay Families' Guide to Navigating the Straight World. New Harbinger Publications; 2001.

Chan RW, Raboy B, Patterson CJ. Psychosocial adjustment among children conceived via donor insemination by lesbian and heterosexual mothers. Child Development. 1998;69:443-57.

Coll CG, Surrey JL, Weingarten K, eds. Mothering Against the Odds: Diverse Voices of Contemporary Mothers. The Guilford Press; 1998.

Ehrensaft D. Mommies, Daddies, Donors, Surrogates: Answering Tough Questions and Building Strong Families. The Guilford Press; 2005.

Galluccio J, Galluccio M. An American Family. St. Martin's Press; 2001.

Garner A. Families Like Mine: Children of Gay Parents Tell It Like It Is. HarperCollins; 2004.

Hicks S, McDermott J. Lesbian and Gay Fostering and Adoption: Extraordinary Yet Ordinary. Jessica Kingsley Publishers; 1999.

Howey N, Samuels E. Out of the Ordinary: Essays on Growing Up with Gay, Lesbian, and Transgender Parents. St. Martin's Press; 2000.

Johnson S, O'Connor E. For Lesbian Parents: Your Guide to Helping Your Family Grow Up Happy, Healthy, and Proud. Guilford Press; 2001.

Lev A. The Complete Lesbian and Gay Parenting Guide. Berkley Books; 2004. (More inclusive of transgender parents than many other books on the subject.)

Mallon GP. Gay Men Choosing Parenthood. Columbia University Press; 2004.

McGarry K. Fatherhood for Gay Men: An Emotional and Practical Guide to Becoming a Gay Dad. Haworth Press; 2003.

Melina L. Making Sense of Adoption: Conversations and Activities for Families Formed Through Adoption, Donor Insemination, Surrogacy and In Vitro Fertilization. Harper & Row; 1989.

Pepper R. The Ultimate Guide to Pregnancy for Lesbians: How to Stay Sane and Care for Yourself from Preconception Through Birth. Cleis Press Inc.; 2005.

Pies C. Considering Parenthood. Spinsters, Inc.; 1988.

Rizzo C, et al, eds. All The Ways Home: Parenting and Children in the Lesbian and Gay Communities: A Collection of Short Fiction. New Victoria Publishers, Inc.; 1995.

Saffron L. It's A Family Affair: The Complete Lesbian Parenting Book. Diva Books; 2001.

Savage D. The Kid: What Happened After My Boyfriend and I Decided To Go Get Pregnant. Penguin Putnam, Inc.; 2000.

Slater S. The Lesbian Family Life Cycle. Free Press; 1995.

Snow JE. How It Feels to Have Gay and Lesbian Parents: A Book by Kids for Kids of All Ages. Harrington Park Press; 2004.

Strah D, Margolis S. Gay Dads: A Celebration of Fatherhood. Penguin Group; 2003.

Children of LGBT Parents

Elwin R, Paulse M. Asha's Mums. Women's Press; 1990.
Jeness A. Families: A Celebration of Diversity, Commitment and Love. Houghton Mifflin; 1990.
Newman L, Crocker R. Gloria Goes to Gay Pride. Alyson Press; 1991.
Newman L. Heather Has Two Mommies. Alyson Publications; 1990.
Valentine J. One Dad, Two Dads, Brown Dads, Blue Dads. Alyson Press; 1994.
Valentine J. The Daddy Machine. Alyson Press; 1992.
Valentine J. Two Moms, The Zark, and Me. Alyson Press; 1993.
Willhoite M. Daddy's Roommate. Alyson Press; 1990.

Videos on LGBT Couples and Families

Both of My Moms' Names Are Judy. Lesbian and Gay Parents Association; 1995. Available from (415) 522-8773, lgpasf@aol.com
Lifetime Commitment: A Portrait of Karen Thompson. Kiki Zeldes; 1994. Available from New Day Films, 22-D Hollywood Avenue, Ho-ho-kus, NJ 07423, (201) 652-6590:
It's Elementary: Talking About Gay Issues in School. Debra Chasnoff & Helen S. Cohen; 1996.
That's a Family! Debra Chasnoff & Helen S. Cohen; 2000.

Organizations and Web Sites for LGBT Couples and Families

Alternative Family Matters
http://www.alternativefamilies.org
(617) 576-6788

COLAGE: Children of Lesbians and Gays Everywhere
http://www.colage.org
(415) 861-KIDS

Families like Ours
http://www.familieslikeours.org
(206) 441-7602

Family Diversity Projects Inc.
http://www.familydiv.org
(413) 256-0502

Family Pride Coalition
http://www.familypride.org
(202) 331-5015

Freedom to Marry
http://www.freedomtomarry.org
(212) 851-8418

Human Rights Campaign—FamilyNet
http://www.hrc.org/familynet
(202) 628-4160

Organization of Parents Through Surrogacy (OPTS)
(847) 782-0224
http://www.opts.com

Parents, Family and Friends of Lesbians and Gays (PFLAG)
http://www.pflag.org
(202) 467-8180

Prospective Queer Parents
http://www.queerparents.org

Rainbow Families
http://www.rainbowfamilies.org
(612) 827-7731

Straight Spouse Network
http://www.ssnetwk.org
(510) 595-1005

Women's Educational Media
http://www.womedia.org
(415) 641-4616
(800) 405-3322

Alternative Insemination Resources

Fenway Community Health, Alternative Insemination Program
http://www.fenwayhealth.org
(617) 927-6243

California Cryobank Inc.
http://www.cryobank.com

New England Cryogenic Center
http://www.necryogenic.com

The Sperm Bank of California
http://www.thespermbankofca.org

Xytex Corporation
http://xytex.com

Chapter 6: Late Adulthood and Aging:
Clinical Approaches

Organizations and Web Sites on Aging

American Society on Aging: Lesbian & Gay Aging Issues Network
http://www.asaging.org/LGAIN

The Gay and Lesbian Association of Retiring Persons TM (GLARP)
http://www.gaylesbianretiring.org
(310) 709-8743 or (310) 722-1807

Gay and Lesbian Elder Housing
http://www.gleh.org
(323) 954-3900

The LGBT Aging Project: Older Lesbian Energy
http://www.lgbtagingproject.org/ole.php
(781) 275-7701

National Gay and Lesbian Task Force: Aging Issues
http://www.ngltf.org

Primetimers
http://members.aol.com/gendervariant/prime/

Senior Action in a Gay Environment (SAGE)
http://www.sageusa.org
(212) 741-2247

Stonewall Communities (senior housing)
http://www.stonewallcommunities.com
(617) 369-9090

Chapter 7: Health Promotion and Disease Prevention

Health Promotion Organizations and Web Sites

US Preventive Services Task Force (USPSTF)
http://www.ahrq.gov/clinic/uspstfix.htm

Guide to Community Preventive Services: Evidence-based recommendations for programs and policies to promote population health.
http://www.thecommunityguide.org

The Mautner Project, the National Lesbian Health Center
http://www.mautnerproject.org

Put Prevention Into Practice: A Step-by-Step Guide to Delivering Clinical Preventive Services: A Systems Approach
http://www.ahrq.gov/ppip/manual

LGBT Smoking Cessation Programs

Gay American Smokeout
http://www.gaysmokeout.net
(206) 938-8828

The Last Drag, San Francisco
http://www.lastdrag.org
(415) 339-7867

The LGBT Smoke-Free Project, LGBT Community Center
http://www.gaycenter.org
(212) 620-7310

QueerTIPs for LGBT Smokers, A Stop Smoking Class for LGBT Communities
Contact Greg Greenwood at (415) 597-9164 or email ggreenwood@psg.ucsf.edu.

Smoking Cessation Program, LA Gay and Lesbian Center
http://www.lagaycenter.org
(323) 860-7305

Chapter 8: Mental Health: Epidemiology, Assessment, and Treatment

Literature on LGBT Mental Health

Browning C, Reynolds AL, Dworkin SH. Affirmative psychotherapy for lesbian women. The Counseling Psychologist. 1991;19:177-95.

Cabaj RP, Stein TS, eds. Textbook of Homosexuality and Mental Health. American Psychiatric Publishing; 1996.

Davies D, Neal C. Therapeutic Perspectives on Working with Lesbian, Gay and Bisexual Clients. Open University Press; 2000.

Domenici T, Lesser RC, eds. Disorienting Sexuality. Routledge; 1995.

Drescher J. Psychoanalytic Therapy and the Gay Man. Analytic Press; 1998.

Group for Advancement of Psychiatry (GAP), Committee on Human Sexuality. Homosexuality and the Mental Health Professions: The Impact of Bias. Analytic Press; 2000.

Jones BE, Hill MJ, eds. Mental Health Issues in Lesbian, Gay, Bisexual and Transgender Communities. Review of Psychiatry. 2002;21:4. Oldham JM, Riba MB, series editors, American Psychiatric Publishing.

Magee M, Miller DC. Lesbian Lives: Psychoanalytic Narratives Old & New. Analytic Press; 1997.

Martell C, Safren S, Prince S. Cognitive Behavioral Therapy with Lesbian, Gay and Bisexual Clients. The Guilford Press; 2004.

Omoto A, Kurtzman H. Sexual Orientation and Mental Health. American Psychological Association; 2006.

Perez R, DeBord K, Bieschke K. Handbook of Counseling and Psychotherapy with Lesbian, Gay and Bisexual Clients. American Psychological Association; 2000.

Shannon JW, Woods WJ. Affirmative psychotherapy for gay men. The Counseling Psychologist. 1991;19:197-215.
Shidlo A, Schroeder, M, Drescher J, eds. Sexual Conversion Therapy: Ethical, Clinical, and Research Perspectives. Haworth; 2001.

Mental Health Organizations and Web Sites

American Psychological Association (APA)
Lesbian, Gay, & Bisexual Concerns Office
http://www.apa.org/pi/lgbc
(202) 336- 6041

Association for Gay, Lesbian, & Bisexual Issues In Counseling
http://www.aglbic.org

Association of Gay and Lesbian Psychiatrists (AGLP)
http://www.aglp.org
(215) 222-2800

Gay and Lesbian International Therapist Search Engine (GLITSE)
http://www.glitse.com

National Association of Social Workers (NASW)
National Committee on Lesbian, Gay, & Bisexual Issues
http://www.socialworkers.org
(202) 408-8600

Chapter 9: Substance Use and Abuse

Literature on Substance Abuse

A Provider's Introduction to Substance Abuse Treatment for Lesbian, Gay, Bisexual, and Transgender Individuals. US Department of Health and Human Services. Substance Abuse and Mental Health Services Administration, Center for Substance Abuse Treatment. 2001. DHHS Publication No. (SMA) 01-3498. Available at http://www.nalgap.org/PDF/Articles/csat.pdf.
Kettelhack G. Vastly More Than That: Stories of Lesbians & Gay Men in Recovery. Hazelden; 1999.
Kominars K. Accepting Ourselves and Others—A Journey Into Recovery From Addictive and Compulsive Behaviors for Gays, Lesbians, and Bisexuals. Hazelden; 1996.
NALGAP 1994 Prevention Policy Statement and Prevention Guidelines. National Association for Gay and Lesbian Addiction Professionals; 1994. Available at http://www.nalgap.org/PDF/Resources/NALGAP_94_Prev_Policy_Guidelines.pdf

Substance Abuse Organizations and Web Sites

National Association for Gay and Lesbian Addiction Professionals
http://www.nalgap.org
(703) 465-0539

National Institute on Drug Abuse
http://www.nida.nih.gov
(301) 443-1124

Substance Abuse & Mental Health Services Administration
http://www.samhsa.gov
(202) 619-0257

Alcohol and Drug Treatment Facilities Specializing in LGBT Populations

Alternatives: Gay treatment of drugs and alcohol abuse, depression, mental illness, or anxiety, Los Angeles, CA
http://www.alternativesinc.com
(800) Dial-Gay

Fenway Community Health: Mental health and addiction services, Boston, MA
http://www.fenwayhealth.org
(617) 927-6202
Includes counseling, acupuncture detox program, and support groups.

Freedom Rings at Lakeview Health, Jacksonville, FL
http://www.gay-rehab.com
(800) 231-1820
Drug and alcohol rehabilitation for LGBT people.

Pride Institute (multiple locations)
http://www.pride-institute.com
(800) 547-7433
Hours: 24 hours/day, 7 days/week
Chemical dependency/mental health referral and information hotline for lesbian, gay, bisexual, and transgender communities.

Chapter 10: Trauma and Violence: Recognition, Recovery, and Prevention

Literature on Violence Prevention

Domestic Violence
Island D, Letellier P. Men Who Beat the Men Who Love Them. Haworth Press; 1991.
Leventhal B, Lundy S, eds. Same-Sex Domestic Violence: Strategies for Change. Sage; 1999.
Lobel K, ed. Naming the Violence: Speaking out about Lesbian Battering. Seal Press; 1986.
McClennen JC, Gunther J, eds. A Professional Guide to Understanding Gay and Lesbian Domestic Violence. Edwin Mellen Press; 1999.
Pitt E, Dolan-Soto D. Clinical considerations in working with victims of same-sex domestic violence. Journal of the Gay and Lesbian Medical Association. 2001;5(4):163-9.

Renzetti CM. Violent Betrayal: Partner Abuse in Lesbian Relationships. Sage Publications; 1992.

Ristock JL. Responding to lesbian relationship violence: an ethical challenge. In: Tutty L, Goard C, eds. Reclaiming Self: Issues and Resources for Women Abused by Intimate Partners. Fernwood Publishing; 2002.

Ristock J. Relationship violence in lesbian/gay/bisexual/transgender/queer communities: moving beyond a gender-based framework. Violence Against Women Online Resources, 2005. Available at http://www.mincava.umn.edu/documents/lgbtqviolence/lgbtqviolence .html

Walker L. The Battered Woman. Harper & Row; 1979.

Hate Crimes

DeCecco JP, ed. Bashers, Baiters & Bigots: Homophobia in American Society. Harrington Park Press; 1985.

Herek GM, Berrill KT, eds. Hate Crimes: Confronting Violence Against Lesbians and Gay Men. Sage; 1992.

Herek GM, Cogan JC, Gillis JR. Victim experiences in hate crimes based on sexual orientation. Journal of Social Issues. 2002;58:319-39.

Forum with Michael Krasny on Hate Crimes Against Gays, Lesbians, Bisexuals, and Transgenders, Featuring Greg Herek, Podcast on KQED-FM Northern California. Broadcast on July 18, 2006. Available at http://www.kqed.org/epArchive/R607180900.

Sexual Assault

Scarce M. Male on Male Rape: The Hidden Toll of Stigma and Shame. Basic Books; 1997.

When Men Are Raped. Columbus OH: Ohio State University Rape Education and Prevention Program; 1997. Available from 464 Ohio Union, 1739 High Street, Columbus OH 43210.

Violence Prevention Organizations and Web Sites

Family Violence Prevention Fund
http://www.fvpf.org
(415) 252-8900

Fenway Community Health, Violence Recovery Program.
http://www.fenwayhealth.org.
(617) 927-6250

Gay Men's Domestic Violence Project
http://www.gmdvp.org
(617) 354-6056

Hatecrime.org
http://www.hatecrime.org

MaleSurvivor
http://www.malesurvivor.org

National Coalition of Anti-Violence Programs, New York, NY
http://www.ncavp.org
(212) 714-1184

National Domestic Violence Hotline
1-800-799-7233 (24 hours)
http://www.ndvh.org

National Gay and Lesbian Task Force
http://thetaskforce.org
(202) 393-5177

The Network/La Red: Ending abuse in lesbian, bisexual women's and transgender communities.
http://www.thenetworklared.org
(617) 695-0877

Rape, Abuse, Incest National Network
http://www.rainn.org
(202) 544-1034

Sexual Assault Hotline
(800) 656-HOPE (24 hours)

Chapter 11: Sexual Health

Literature on Sexual Health

Caster W, Kramer BR, May J. The Lesbian Sex Book: A Guide for Women Who Love Women. 2nd ed. Alyson Publications; 2003.

Massachusetts Department of Public Health, The Fenway Institute. Prevention and management of sexually transmitted diseases in men who have sex with men: a toolkit for clinicians, 2004. Available at www.aidsetc.org/pdf/p02-et/et-17-00/msm_toolkit.pdf.

Silverstein C, Picano F. The Joy of Gay Sex: Revised and Expanded. 3rd ed. HarperCollins; 2004.

Sexual Health Organizations and Web Sites

The Body: The Complete HIV/AIDS Resource.
http://www.thebody.com
Safer sex guidelines and resources: http://www.thebody.com/safesex/safer.html

Centers for Disease Control and Prevention
Sexually Transmitted Infections, including updated treatment guidelines: http://www.cdc.gov/std
Revised guidelines for HIV testing, counseling and referral: http://www.cdc.gov/MMWR/preview/mmwrhtml/rr5019a1.htm

GayHealth.com
http://www.gayhealth.com
STI information: http://www.gayhealth.com/templates/sex/std/index.html

HIVInsite
http://www.hivinsite.ucsf.edu

LesbianSTD.com
http://www.lesbianstd.com

National and state AIDS hotlines from aidshotline.org (list)
http://www.aidshotline.org/crm/asp/refer/state_hotlines.asp

National Minority AIDS Council
http://www.nmac.org
(202) 483-6622

National CDC STD/HIV Hotline
(800) 342-2437

National Center for HIV/AIDS, Viral Hepatitis, STD, and TB Prevention
http://www.cdc.gov/nchstp/od/nchstp.html

Project Inform
http://www.projectinform.org
Hotline: 800-822-7422

Chapter 12: Introduction to Transgender Identity and Health; and Chapter 13: Medical and Surgical Management of the Transgender Patient

Literature on Transgender Health

Brown ML, Rounsley CA. True Selves: Understanding Transsexualism—For Families, Friends, Coworkers, and Helping Professionals. Jossey-Bass; 2003.

Feldman JL, Goldberg J. Transgender Primary Medical Care: Suggested Guidelines for Clinicians in British Columbia Vancouver Coastal Health. Vancouver, BC; 2006. Available at http://www.vch.ca/transhealth/resources/library/tcpdocs/guidelines-primcare.pdf.

Harry Benjamin International Gender Dysphoria Association. The standards of care for gender identity disorders. 6th Version, 2001. Available at http://www.wpath.org/Documents2/socv6.pdf.

Israel GE, Tarver DE. Transgender Care: Recommended Guidelines, Practical Information and Personal Accounts. Temple University Press; 1997.

International Journal of Transgenderism. The official journal of the World Professional Association for Transgender Health. Available at http://www.haworthpress.com/store/product.asp?sku=J485.

Leli U, Drescher J, eds. Transgender Subjectivities: A Clinician's Guide. Haworth Press; 2004.

Lev AI. Transgender Emergence: Therapeutic Guidelines for Working with Gender-Variant People and Their Families. Haworth Press; 2004.

Transgender Personal Stories

Bornstein K. Gender Outlaw: On Men, Women, and the Rest of Us. Vintage; 1995.

Finney Boylan J. She's Not There: A Life in Two Genders. Broadway Books; 2003.
Green J. Becoming a Visible Man. Vanderbilt University; 2004.

Transgender Health Organizations and Web Sites

Fenway Community Health: Transgender Health Program
http://www.fenwayhealth.org
(617) 927-6223

Notes on Gender Role Transition by Ann Vitale, PhD
http://www.avitale.com

International Foundation for Gender Education
http://www.ifge.org
(781) 899-2212

Transgender Care
http://www.transgendercare.com

Transsexual Women's Resources
http://www.annelawrence.com/twr

The World Professional Association for Transgender Health, Inc. (formerly HBIGDA)
http://www.wpath.org
(612) 624-9397

Transgender Education and Advocacy Organizations and Web sites

Alliance for Gender Awareness
http://www.genderawareness.com
(877) GENDER 1

Gender Public Advocacy Coalition
http://www.gpac.org
(202) 462-6610
http://www.gender.org

National Center for Transgender Equality
http://www.nctequality.org
(202) 903-0112

Transgender Law and Policy Institute
http://www.transgenderlaw.org
Email: query@transgenderlaw.org

Transgender Support Organizations and Web Sites

Compass (New England female-to-male transgender group)

http://geocities.com/ftmcompass
(781) 899-2212

Becky Allison, MD, Friends and Family Issues
http://www.drbecky.com/trans.html

FTM International
http://www.ftmi.org

Hudson's FTM Comprehensive Resource Guide
http://www.ftmguide.org

Society for a Second Self (cross-dressers)
http://www.tri-ess.org

Transsexual Roadmap
http://www.tsroadmap.com

Transgender Crossroads
http://www.tgcrossroads.org

The Transitional Male
http://www.thetransitionalmale.com

Transgender Forum's Community Center (list of local community groups in the US)
http://www.transgender.org

Chapter 14: Disorders of Sex Development: Clinical Approaches

Literature on Disorders of Sex Development/Intersex Health

Balen AH, Creighton SM, Davies MC, et al, eds. Pediatric and Adolescent Gynecology: A Multidisciplinary Approach. Cambridge University Press; 2004.

Consortium on the Management of Disorders of Sex Development. Clinical guidelines for the management of disorders of sex development. Intersex Society of North America; 2006. Available at http://www.dsdguidelines.org.

Consortium on the Management of Disorders of Sex Development. Handbook for parents. Intersex Society of North America; 2006. Available at http://www.dsdguidelines.org.

Dreger, Alice. Intersex in the Age of Ethics. University Publishing Group; 1999.

Hughes IA, Houk C, Ahmed SF, Lee PA, LWPES Consensus Group, ESPE Consensus Group. Consensus statement on the management of intersex disorders. Arch Disease Child. 2006; 91:554-63.

Lee PA, Houk CP, Ahmed SF, Hughes IA, the International Consensus Conference on Intersex Working Group. Consensus statement on management of intersex disorders. Pediatrics. 2006;118:e488-500.

Parens E. Surgically Shaping Children: Technology, Ethics, and the Pursuit of Normality. The Johns Hopkins University Press; 2006.

Preves S. Intersex and Identity: The Contested Self. Rutgers University Press; 2003.

Systma SE. Ethics and Intersex. Springer; 2006.

Videos on Intersex

Discovery Channel (Phyllis Ward). Is it a Boy or a Girl? First broadcast March 26, 2000.
   Available for purchase from http://www.isna.org.
NOVA. Sex: Unknown. First broadcast October 30, 2001. Available for purchase from WGBH
   Boston Video at 1-800-255-9424.

Intersex Organizations and Web Sites

American Association for Klinefelter Syndrome Information and Support (AAKSIS)
http://www.aaksis.org
(888) 466-KSIS

American Psychological Association Online: Answers to Your Questions About Individuals with Intersex Conditions
http://www.apa.org/topics/intersx.html

Androgen Insensitivity Support Group
http://www.medhelp.org/ais

Bodies Like Ours: Intersex Information and Peer Support
http://www.bodieslikeours.org /forums/

CARES Foundation, Inc. (Congenital Adrenal Hyperplasia Research Education & Support)
http://www.caresfoundation.org
(973) 912-3895

Intersex Initiative
http://www.intersexinitiative.org

Intersex Society of North America
http://www.isna.org

Turner Syndrome Society
http://www.turner-syndrome-us.org
(832) 249-9988
(800) 365-9944

xyTurners
http://www.xyxo.org

Chapter 15: Taking a Comprehensive History and Providing Relevant Risk-Reduction Counseling

Education and Awareness Materials

CDC Division of Viral Hepatitis: MSM Information Center
http://www.cdc.gov/ncidod/diseases/hepatitis/msm

Includes:
- Prevent STDs among MSM pocket cards and posters
- Protect Yourself from Hepatitis booklet

Fenway Community Health
http://www.fenwayhealth.org
Resources section includes the following brochures:
- Safer Sex (inclusive of LGBT people)
- Safer Sex for Bisexuals and their Partners
- Talking about Safer Sex with Your Patients

Gay and Lesbian Medical Association
http://www.glma.org
Resources for Patients section includes:
- List of top 10 things gay men, lesbians, and transgendered patients should discuss with their healthcare provider

Resources for Providers and Researchers section includes:
- Guidelines for the care of lesbian, gay, bisexual, and transgender patients

Gay, Lesbian, Bisexual, and Transgender Health Access Project
http://www.glbthealth.org
Includes:
- Community Standards of Practice for the Provision of Quality Health Care Services to Lesbian, Gay, Bisexual, and Transgender Clients
- Materials (such as posters and stickers) to create welcoming healthcare environments

Lesbian Resource Center
http://www.trianglerc.org
Includes:
- Safer sex kit and brochure
- Healthcare provider training in culturally competent care

Web Sites: How to Put on Male and Female Condoms

http://www.friendtofriend.org/condom/usage.html
http://www.phoenixcenteronline.com/reality.htm
http://www.ripnroll.com/femalecondoms.htm

Chapter 16: Legal Issues of Importance to Clinicians

LGBT Rights: Organizations and Web Sites

American Civil Liberties Union Lesbian and Gay Rights and AIDS Project

http://www.aclu.org/lgbt
(212) 549-2627

Gay and Lesbian Advocates and Defenders (GLAD)
New England-based, but has national resources, including standards
concerning custody disputes in the LGBT community.
http://www.glad.org
GLAD Legal infoline (legal questions related to sexual orientation, gender
identity, or HIV status):
Boston Area: (617) 426-1350
New England: 1-800-455-GLAD
Monday-Friday, 1:30-4:30pm, Eastern Standard Time, English and Spanish

Gay and Lesbian Alliance Against Defamation (GLAAD)
http://www.glaad.org
(323) 933-2240

Gender Public Advocacy Coalition
http://www.gpac.org
(202) 462-6610

Human Rights Campaign
http://www.hrc.org
(202) 628-4160
(800) 777-4723

Human Rights Watch (on LGBT rights)
http://www.hrw.org/doc/?t=lgbt
(212) 290-4700

LAMBDA Legal Defense and Education Fund (LLDEF)
http://www.lambdalegal.org
(212) 809-8585

National Black Justice Coalition
http://www.nbjcoalition.org
(202) 349-3755

National Center for Lesbian Rights
http://www.nclrights.org
(415) 392-6257

National Center for Transgender Equality
http://www.nctequality.org
(202) 903-0112

Hate Crimes: Organizations and Web Sites

Federal Bureau of Investigation Hate Crime Statistics
http://www.fbi.gov/ucr/hc2005

HateCrime.org
http://www.hatecrime.org

Matthew Shepard Foundation
http://www.matthewshepard.org
(307) 237-6167

National Coalition of Anti-Violence Programs, New York, NY.
http://www.ncavp.org
(212) 714-1184

Marriage and Partnership Rights: Organizations and Web Sites

Freedom to Marry Coalition
http://www.freedomtomarry.org
(212) 851-8418

Marriage Equality USA
http://www.marriageequality.org
(510) 496-2700

Partners Task Force for Gay and Lesbian Couples
http://www.buddybuddy.com/partners.html

California Domestic Partnership Registry
http://www.ss.ca.gov/dpregistry/

Connecticut Civil Unions:
http://www.infoline.org/InformationLibrary/Documents/civilunionsct.asp

Vermont Civil Unions:
http://www.sec.state.vt.us/otherprg/civilunions/civilunions.html

Parental Rights: Organizations and Web Sites

American Psychological Association: Lesbian and Gay Parenting
http://www.apa.org/pi/parent.html

COLAGE: Children of Lesbians and Gays Everywhere
http://www.colage.org
(415) 861-KIDS

Family Pride Coalition
http://www.familypride.org
(202) 331-5015

Human Rights Campaign—FamilyNet
http://www.hrc.org/familynet
(202) 628-4160

Advance Directives: Web Sites

Financial Planning Toolkit: Statutory Power of Attorney and Medical Treatment Forms
http://www.finance.cch.com/tools/poaforms_m.asp
Provides proxy forms for all states

Time Magazine Online Edition: Living Will Resources.
http://www.time.com/time/covers/1101050404/schiavo_webguide.html
Provides a state-by-state directory of laws governing living wills.

US Living Will Registry
http://www.uslivingwillregistry.com
Individuals can complete and store their advance directives with the
registry, which will then distribute the directives to health care
providers when requested.

Appendix B

Sample New Patient Intake Form

Date: _____

Patient Intake Form

We'd like to welcome you as a new patient. Please take the time to fill out this form as accurately as possible so we can most appropriately address your health needs.

The confidentiality of your health information is protected in accordance with federal protections for the privacy of health information under the Health Insurance Portability and Accountability Act (HIPAA).

You will notice that we ask questions about race and ethnic background. We do this so we can review the treatment that all patients receive and make sure everyone gets the highest quality of care.

While this clinic recognizes a number of sexes/genders, many insurance companies and legal entities do not. Please understand that the legal name and sex listed on your insurance must be used on documents pertaining to insurance and billing. If your preferred name and pronouns are different from these, please let us know.

Please print all responses.

Name: _____   Date of Birth: _____

Address: _____   Sex/Gender: M F Intersex Transgendered

_____   Race (eg, African-American, Latino, Asian, etc)

_____

Home Tel (___) ___ - ____   Ethnicity (eg, Mexican, Hawaiian, Irish, etc)
OK to leave a message? Y N   _____

Work Tel (___) ___ - ____   Education Level: _____
OK to leave a message? Y N

Cell Tel (___) ___ - ____   Occupation: (Do you work outside the home?
OK to leave a message? Y N   Please be specific in describing your work)

_____

1

Email Address: _____

Number of Hours Worked per Week: _____

OK to contact by email: Y   N

Religious/Spiritual Beliefs: _____

Insurance Type: _____

ID#: _____

Relationship/Marital Status: (eg, single, married, partnered, living together, divorced)

_____

Subscriber: _____

Name of Your Partner or Spouse: (if applicable)

Secondary Insurance: _____

_____

ID#: _____

Do You Live with Anyone? Y   N

Subscriber: _____

_____

Language Spoken Most Often:
At Home: _____

Number of Children: _____   Ages _____

At Work: _____

Do You Feel Safe at Home?: Y   N   Sometimes

Do You Need an Interpreter?
Y   N

Have you felt threatened, controlled by, or afraid of a partner, family member, or caregiver?
Y   N

2

Medical History

Please check all that apply

___ Emphysema
___ Tuberculosis
___ Pneumonia
___ Bronchitis
___ Asthma
___ Allergies
___ Heart Disease
___ Stroke
___ High Blood Pressure
___ Elevated Cholesterol
___ Diabetes
___ Venous Thrombosis
___ Hepatitis A
___ Hepatitis B
___ Hepatitis C
___ Cirrhosis
___ Anemia
___ Thyroid Trouble
___ Gallbladder Disease
___ Ulcers
___ Frequent Urinary Tract Infections
___ Sexually Transmitted Infections
___ Prostate Trouble
___ Cancer
___ Arthritis
___ Osteoporosis
___ Fractures
___ Migraines
___ Depression
___ Anxiety or Panic Disorder
___ Posttraumatic Stress Disorder
___ Alcohol or Substance Use Problem
Other: _____

3

Systems Review

Please check any of the following symptoms that you have recently experienced or are a concern to you.

General:

___recent weight loss   ___recent weight gain   ___fatigue

___fever   ___changes in appetite   ___night sweats

Skin:

___rashes   ___lumps   ___itching

___dryness   ___color change   ___hair or nail change

Head:

___headaches   ___head injuries   ___dizziness

Eyes: Date of last exam: ___/___/___

___glasses   ___contacts

___pain   ___double vision   ___redness

___glaucoma   ___cataracts

Nose:

___frequent colds   ___nasal stuffiness   ___hay fever

___nosebleeds   ___sinus trouble   ___dust/animal allergies

Ears:

___hearing loss

Mouth & Throat: Date of last dental exam: ___/___/___

___bleeding gums   ___frequent sore throats ___hoarseness

Neck:

___goiter   ___lumps/swollen glands ___pain

Breasts: Date of last mammogram: ___/___/___

___lumps   ___pain   ___nipple discharge

4

Respiratory:

___cough   ___wheezing   ___shortness of breath

___coughing up blood

Cardiac:

___heart murmur   ___chest pain   ___palpitations

___swelling of feet   ___shortness of breath

Gastrointestinal:

___trouble swallowing   ___heartburn or gas   ___nausea

___vomiting   ___rectal bleeding   ___constipation

___diarrhea   ___abdominal pain   ___hemorrhoids

___jaundice (skin or whites of eyes turning yellow)

Urinary:

___frequent urination   ___painful urination   ___blood in urine

___stones   ___difficulty urinating or difficulty holding
                            urination

___waking up to go to the bathroom several times at night

Musculoskeletal:

___joint stiffness   ___arthritis   ___gout

___backache   ___muscle pains   ___muscle cramps

Peripheral Vascular:

___leg cramps while walking   ___varicose veins
                                                           ___thrombophlebitis

Neurological:

___fainting   ___blackouts   ___seizures

___weakness   ___numbness   ___tremors

___tingling hands or feet ___change in memory

Psychiatric/Psychological:

___anxiety   ___depression   ___phobias
___family problems   ___eating disorder

5

Have you ever been hit, slapped, kicked, or otherwise physically hurt by someone?

___Yes, in the past year ___Yes, prior to this past year   ___No

Has anyone ever forced you into having any type of sexual activity?

___Yes ___No

Hematologic:

___anemia   ___easy bruising or bleeding

___blood transfusions: Year(s) _____

Endocrine:

___heat or cold intolerance   ___excessive sweating

___excessive hunger   ___excessive urinating

Do you experience chronic pain?   Yes   No

If YES, how is your pain managed (ie, physical therapy, medication, etc)?

_____

On a scale of zero to ten, with ten being the worst and zero being no pain, how would you rate your current pain? ____

Operations and/or Hospitalizations: (Please list surgeries and/or hospitalization reasons and dates)

_____

_____

_____

Current Medications: (Please include any non-prescription drugs as well, eg, vitamins, aspirin, etc.)

Medication Name   Dose   Frequency of Use

1. _____   _____   _____

2. _____   _____   _____

3. _____   _____   _____

If you need more room, please list additional medications on back of last page.

Allergies: (Please list any allergies you may have to medications and food)

_____

Family Medical History

Please check all that apply.
___ Stroke
___ Heart Disease
___ High Blood Pressure
___ Thyroid Disease
___ Kidney Disease
___ Diabetes
___ Arthritis
___ Osteoporosis
___ Migraine Headaches
___ Alcoholism
___ Asthma
___ Depression
___ Anxiety
___ Cancer/Type(s): _____

Vaccinations/Prevention

Date of Last Tetanus Vaccination: ___/___/ _____

Have you received any of the following vaccines:

Hepatitis A?   Yes   No   Not Sure

Hepatitis B?   Yes   No   Not Sure

Pneumo vax?   Yes   No   Not Sure

Have you had a blood test for Rubella (German Measles)?
Yes   No   Not Sure

Date of Last Colonoscopy: ___/___/____   ___ Check here if not
                                             applicable

How often do you wear seatbelts? _____

Are there any firearms kept in your home?   Yes   No

Does someone have power of attorney or healthcare proxy giving them the power to make decisions about your care in life-threatening situations?

No   Yes: (*name of person and their relationship to you*)

_____

Do you have an advanced health directive, such as do not resuscitate?
Yes   No

7

Gender Identity

Please list any questions, concerns, or comments you have, if any, about your gender or gender identity (sense of your femaleness/maleness).

_____

_____

_____

_____

_____

_____

Sexual Orientation & Sexual History

How do you identify in terms of sexual orientation?

_____

Are you attracted to (*check all that apply*):

___Men   ___Women   ___Transgendered Men   ___Transgendered Women

Have you had sex with (*check all that apply*):

___Men   ___Women   ___Transgendered Men   ___Transgendered Women

When you have sex, do you have (*check all that apply*):

___Oral Sex   ___Vaginal Sex   ___Anal Sex

How often do you use condoms when having:

Oral Sex: _____

Vaginal Sex: _____

Anal Sex: _____

When is the last time you had sex without using a condom?

_____

Do you have a primary (main) sexual partner?   Yes   No

Do you have any casual sexual partners?   Yes   No

When was the last time you were tested for HIV?

_____

What were the results? _____

8

Please check any of the following infections that you have had:

___Syphilis   ___Gonorrhea   ___Pelvic Inflammatory
                                             Disease

___Herpes   ___Trichomonas   ___Genital Warts

___ Yeast Infections ___Chlamydia   ___Crabs

___ Bacterial Vaginosis

For each of the above that you checked, please note: 1) when the infection was, 2) if you completed treatment, 3) if your partner(s) were informed, and 4) if you need help telling your partners.

1) _____   2) _____   3) _____   4) _____

1) _____   2) _____   3) _____   4) _____

1) _____   2) _____   3) _____   4) _____

1) _____   2) _____   3) _____   4) _____

Do you know or believe that any of your partners have had HIV or another sexually transmitted infection?

Yes   No   I'm not sure

Have your current partners been tested for HIV and other sexually transmitted infections?

Yes   No   I'm not sure

What were the results? _____

Are you satisfied with your sexual life?   Yes   No   I'm not sure

Please describe any sexual concerns you may have:

_____
_____
_____
_____
_____
_____

9

Gynecologic History

If not applicable due to sex and/or gender please check here ___ and skip to Hormones section

Age of First Period: ___

Date of Last Pap: ___/___/___   Results: ___Normal   ___Abnormal

Have you *ever* had:

An abnormal Pap?   Yes   No   Ovarian Cysts?   Yes   No

Fibroids?   Yes   No   DES Exposure?   Yes   No

Have you had a hysterectomy?   Yes   No

If YES: Why was it performed?

_____

Were your ovaries removed?   Yes, both   Yes, one   No

If menopausal/postmenopausal, please check here ___ and skip to below the dotted line

Date of Last Period: ___/___/___

Frequency of Periods: (*eg, every 28 days*) _____
Average Length of Period: ___days

Bleeding: ___Light   ___Moderate   ___Heavy

Other Bleeding: ___No   ___Yes, between periods ___Yes, after penetrative sexual activity

Do you experience any of the following symptoms with your period? *Check all that apply.*

___Headaches   ___Weight Gain ___Swelling ___Cramps ___Anxiety

___Depression   Other: _____

Are you currently using birth control?   Yes   No

If YES: Which type are you using:

___Pills   ___IUD   ___Condoms   ___Foam   ___Foam & Condoms

___Patch   ___Diaphragm   ___Ring   ___Depo   ___Tubal Ligation

___Vasectomy   Other: _____

10

Have you *ever* taken birth control pills?

Yes, for _____(how long?)   No

Are you currently pregnant or planning to become pregnant?

Yes   No

If you have not begun menopause, please check here ___ and continue to the next section

Age at menopause: ___

Have you *ever* taken estrogen replacement?   Yes   No

If YES: What was the name of the estrogen replacement?

_____

Age when estrogen replacement was started: _____

How long was estrogen replacement used? _____

What was your estrogen dose? _____

Have you *ever* taken progesterone?   Yes   No

If YES: How many days per month? _____

How long was progesterone replacement used? _____

What was your progesterone dose? _____

Please check any of the following symptoms of menopause you are having:

___ Hot Flashes   ___Fatigue   ___Anxiety

___Depression   ___Insomnia   ___Irregular Bleeding

___Vaginal Burning/Itching   ___Vaginal Dryness

___Pain during Vaginal Penetration   Other: _____

11

Obstetric History

How many times have you been pregnant? _____

How many miscarriages have you had? _____

How many pregnancy terminations have you had? _____

How many vaginal deliveries have you had? _____

How many caesarean sections have you had? _____

Have you had any ectopic pregnancies?   Yes   No

Have you had gestational diabetes?   Yes   No

Do you have a history of infertility?   Yes   No

Hormones for Gender/Sex Transitioning

If not applicable, please check here ___ and skip to the next section.

Are you currently taking hormones for gender or sex transitioning purposes?   Yes   No

If YES: How long have you been taking them? _____

What hormones are you taking?

_____

Have you ever used transitioning hormones in the past?   Yes   No

If YES to past or current hormone use, what types of complications, if any, have you experienced?

_____
_____
_____
_____

What types, if any, of sex reassignment surgery have you had?

_____
_____
_____

What types, if any, of other feminizing or masculinizing procedures have you had?

_____
_____
_____

12

What types of complications, if any, have you experienced following such surgeries and/or procedures?

_____

_____

_____

_____

What concerns or questions, if any, do you have regarding gender/sex transitioning?

_____

_____

_____

_____

Lifestyle & Health Habits

Do you follow a special diet?   Yes   No

If YES, please check appropriately:

___Vegetarian   ___Vegan   ___Low Fat

___Low Carb   ___High Fiber   ___Calorie Restriction

Other: _____

Have you ever binged, purged, or restricted your food intake?

No   Yes, I have _____
              (please describe)

What concerns, if any, do you have about your eating practices?

_____

_____

_____

How often do you exercise at a moderate or vigorous level for 30 minutes or more? _____

What type of exercise(s) and/or sports do you engage in?

_____

_____

_____

_____

On a typical day, how many cups of caffeine containing beverages (coffee, tea, soda, energy drinks, etc) do you have? _____

13

On a typical day, how many portions of calcium enriched food do you eat? _____

Portion = one cup of milk = one slice of cheese = one cup yogurt = 1/2 cup of ice cream

On a daily basis, how much calcium do you consume through tablets or chews?

<500 mg   600-1200 mg   Not Sure

Substance Use History

How many drinks containing alcohol do you have, on average, per week?
_____

Have you ever been concerned about your drinking?   Yes   No   Not Sure

Has anyone, including a family member, friend, or healthcare worker been concerned about your drinking or suggest you cut down?

Yes   No   I'm not sure

How many cigarettes do you smoke per day? _____

How old were you when you first started smoking? ____

Have you ever tried to quit smoking?   Yes   No   NA

Are you interested in quitting smoking?   Yes   No   NA

If you are a former smoker, how long ago did you quit?
_____

Please check any of the substances listed below that you have used, even if it was only once:

___ Marijuana

When was the last time you used it? _____

How frequently do you/did you use it? _____

___Cocaine

When was the last time you used it? _____

How frequently do you/did you use it? _____

How do/did you use it (ie, smoke, inject, sniff)? _____

14

___Crystal Meth

When was the last time you used it? _____

How frequently do you/did you use it? _____

How do/did you use it (ie, smoke, inject, etc)? _____

___Heroin

When was the last time you used it? _____

How frequently do you/did you use it? _____

How do/did you use it (ie, smoke, inject, etc)? _____

___Other Opiates (oxycontin, vicodin, percodan, etc)

When was the last time you used it? _____

How frequently do you/did you use it? _____

How do/did you use it (ie, orally, smoke, inject, etc)? _____

___Ecstasy/Mushrooms/LSD

When was the last time you used it? _____

How frequently do you/did you use it? _____

Other Substance(s):

_____

When was the last time you used it? _____

How frequently do you/did you use it? _____

How do/did you use it (ie smoke, inject, etc)? _____

Have you *ever* injected any type of substance?   Yes   No

Did you ever share your needle, cooker, cotton, rinse water, or any other part of your set?

Yes   No   I'm not sure

What types of problems has drug use caused for you (ie, relationships with others, problems at work, depression, anxiety, physical health, etc)?

_____

_____

_____

_____

15

What concerns, if any, do you have about either your past or current drug use?

_____

_____

_____

_____

Thank you for answering this comprehensive health history form. Your answers are confidential and will help us provide more complete and knowledgeable care of you.

16

Appendix C

How to Put on a Male Condom

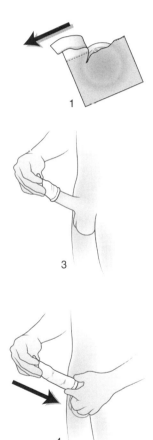

1. Carefully open package to avoid tearing.
2. Put the condom on when the penis is erect and before any contact between penis and partner's body.
3. Hold the tip of the condom between your forefinger and thumb to squeeze out the air (air trapped inside a condom could cause it to break).
4. Use your other hand to unroll the condom all the way over the erect penis. Make sure the roll is on the outside.
5. Leave some space at the tip to hold the ejaculate (cum).
6. After sex, withdraw when the penis is still erect. Hold the condom at the rim while pulling out slowly. Do not remove condom before fully with-drawn.
7. Use a new condom every time you have sex.

Appendix D

How to Put on a Female Condom (For Vaginal Sex)

1. Carefully open package to avoid tearing.
2. At the closed end of the condom, squeeze the flexible inner ring between your thumb and second or middle finger so that the ring becomes long and narrow.
3. Gently insert the inner ring into the vagina.
4. With your index finger inside the condom, push the inner ring up as far as it will go. Be sure the condom is not twisted. When inserted properly, the outer ring of the condom will remain on the outside of the vagina.
5. Add lubricant to inside of condom or to the penis or sex toy. The female condom is made of polyurethane and therefore can be used with any kind of lubricant.
6. To remove the condom, squeeze and twist the outer ring and gently pull the condom out. Remove the condom before standing up to avoid spillage.
7. Wrap the condom in the package or tissue, and throw it in the garbage. Do not put it into the toilet.

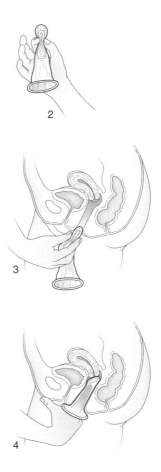

Additional Notes

- It is recommended that you practice placing and removing the female condom a few times before using it for the first time during sexual intercourse.
- Make sure that the penis or sex toy enters *inside* the center of the condom and *not* on the side, between the condom and the vaginal wall.
- You may notice that the condom moves around during sex. This is normal.
- Do not use the male and female condoms at the same time.

Appendix E

How to Put on a Female Condom (For Anal Sex)

These are provisional guidelines for using the female condom for anal sex. The female condom was not originally designed for anal sex, and more research is needed to determine the safety, effectiveness, or acceptability of the female condom for anal sex.

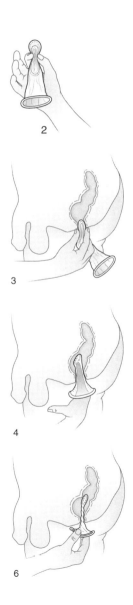

1. Carefully open package to avoid tearing.
2. At the closed end of the condom, squeeze the flexible inner ring between your thumb and second or middle finger so that the ring becomes long and narrow.
3. Gently insert the inner ring into the anal opening.
4. With your index finger inside the condom, push the inner ring up the anal cavity (for maximum protection, the inner ring should be inserted past the sphincter muscle). Be sure the condom is not twisted. When inserted properly, about one inch of the outer ring of the condom will hang out of the anal opening.
5. Add more lubricant to inside of condom or to the penis or sex toy. The female condom is made of polyurethane and therefore can be used with any kind of lubricant.
6. To remove the condom, squeeze and twist the outer ring and gently pull the condom out.
7. Wrap the condom in the package or tissue, and throw it in the garbage. Do not put it into the toilet.

Additional Notes

- It is recommended that you practice placing and removing the condom a few times before using it for the first time during sexual intercourse.
- Extra lubrication is strongly recommended.
- Make sure that the penis or sex toy enters *inside* the center of the condom and is *not* underneath or beside the condom.
- You may feel the condom slipping up and down in the anal cavity, riding on the penis. This is normal as long as the outer ring does not get pushed into the anal cavity. If this happens, stop immediately, remove and discard the condom, and insert a new one.
- Do not use the male and female condoms at the same time.
- Another way to use the female condom for anal sex is for the insertive partner to wear it like a male condom. 1) Add extra lubricant inside the female condom. 2) Place the condom over the penis. 3) Add extra lubricant on the outside of the condom.

Appendix F

Sample Living Will

Below is an example of language used for a living will. It is strongly recommended that individuals adapt the language to meet their own needs and check the specific laws of their state of residence (a helpful Web site is http://www.finance.cch.com/tools/poaforms_m.asp).

Sample: Living Will

I, _____, of _____, willfully and voluntarily making known my desire that my dying shall not be artificially prolonged under the circumstances set forth below, do hereby declare:

If at any time I should have an incurable injury, disease, or illness certified to be a terminal condition by two physicians who have personally examined me, one of whom shall be my attending physician, and the physicians have determined that my death will occur whether or not life-prolonging procedures would serve only to prolong the moment of death artificially, I direct that such procedures be withheld or withdrawn, and that I be permitted to die naturally with only the administration of medication or the performance of any medical procedure deemed necessary to provide me with comfort care.

In the absence of my ability to give directions regarding the use of such life-sustaining procedures, it is my intention that this declaration shall be honored by my family and physicians as the final expression of my legal right to refuse medical or surgical treatment and accept the consequences from such refusal.

In testimony whereof I hereunto set my hand and in the presence of two witnesses declare this to be my declaration this _ day of 200_ .

Sample Healthcare Proxy Form

Below is an example of language used for a Massachusetts healthcare proxy form. It is strongly recommended that individuals adapt the language to meet their own needs and check the specific laws of their state of residence (a helpful Web site is http://www.finance.cch.com/tools/poaforms_m.asp).

MASSACHUSETTS HEALTHCARE PROXY

OF

(CLIENT NAME)

TO ALL PEOPLE CONCERNED WITH MY MEDICAL CARE:

A. APPOINTMENT

I, **(client name)**, residing at **(address)**, _____County, Massachusetts, being a competent adult of at least 18 years of age, of sound mind, and under no constraint or undue influence, hereby appoint the following person to be my HEALTHCARE AGENT under the terms of this document:

NAME:
Address:
Telephone:

    In so doing, I create a Healthcare Proxy according to Chapter 201D of the General Laws of Massachusetts. I hereby give my Healthcare Agent the authority to make any and all healthcare decisions on my behalf, subject to any limitations that I state in this document, in the event that, in the future, I should become incapable of making healthcare decisions for myself.

    If my original Healthcare Agent is unable or unwilling to serve, I hereby appoint the following person as my Healthcare Agent:

NAME:
Address:
Telephone:

1

B. POWERS OF HEALTHCARE AGENT

1. I give my Healthcare Agent full authority to make any and all health-care decisions for me, including decisions about life-sustaining treatment, subject only to any limitations that I state below.

2. My Healthcare Agent shall have authority to act on my behalf only if, when and for so long as a determination has been made that I lack the capacity to make or to communicate healthcare decisions for myself. This determination shall be made in writing by my attending physician accord-ing to accepted standards of medical judgment and the requirements of Chapter 201D of the General Laws of Massachusetts.

3. The authority of my Healthcare Agent shall cease if my attending physician determines that I have regained capacity. The authority shall recommence if I subsequently lose capacity and consent for treatment is required.

4. I shall be notified of any determination that I lack capacity to make or communicate healthcare decisions where there is any indication that I am able to comprehend this notice.

5. My Healthcare Agent shall make healthcare decisions for me only after consultation with my healthcare providers and after consideration of acceptable medical alternatives regarding diagnosis, prognosis, treatments, and their side effects.

6. My Healthcare Agent shall make healthcare decisions for me in accor-dance with his/her assessment of my wishes, my moral or religious beliefs, or, if such factors are unknown, then in accordance with my Healthcare Agent's assessment of my best interests.

7. My Healthcare Agent shall have the right to receive any and all med-ical information necessary to make informed decisions regarding my healthcare, including any and all confidential medical information that I would be entitled to receive.

8. If I object to a healthcare decision made by my Healthcare Agent, my decision shall prevail unless it is determined by court order that I lack capacity to make healthcare decisions.

9. The decisions made by my Healthcare Agent on my behalf shall have the same priority as my decisions would have if I were competent over decisions by any other person, except for any limitation I state below or a specific court order overriding this proxy.

10. Nothing in this proxy shall preclude any medical procedure deemed necessary by my attending physician to provide comfort care or pain alle-viation including but not limited to treatment with sedatives and pain-killing drugs, non-artificial oral feeding, suction, and hygienic care.

C. COURT-APPOINTED GUARDIAN

If it is deemed necessary to seek the appointment by a probate court of a guardian of my person, I hereby nominate the persons named herein as my

2

appointed Healthcare Agent and alternate Healthcare Agent for appointment by such court to serve as such fiduciary.

D. HIPAA RELEASE AUTHORITY

I hereby grant my Healthcare Agent release authority that applies to any information governed by the Health Insurance Portability and Accountability Act of 1996 (HIPAA), 42 U.S.C. 1320d, as now in effect, and as such law may from time to time hereafter be amended. I intend that my Healthcare Agent be treated as I would be, with respect to my rights regarding the use and disclosure of my individually identifiable health information and/or other medical records.

I hereby authorize any physician, healthcare professional, dentist, health plan, hospital, clinic, laboratory, pharmacy, or other covered healthcare provider, any insurance company or healthcare clearinghouse that has provided treatment or services to me, that has paid for or that is seeking payment from me for such services, to give, disclose and release to my Healthcare Agent, without restriction, all of my individually identifiable health information and medical records regarding any past, present or future medical or mental health condition.

The authority given to my Healthcare Agent under this Section D supercedes any prior agreement that I may have made with my healthcare providers with respect to disclosure of my individually identifiable health information.

As long as this Healthcare Proxy remains in full force and effect, the HIPAA release authority given under this Section D has no expiration date and shall expire only in the event that I revoke the authority in writing and deliver it to my healthcare provider.

E. REVOCATION

This Healthcare Proxy shall be revoked upon any one of the following events:

a. my execution of a subsequent Healthcare Proxy
b. my divorce or legal separation from my spouse where my spouse is named as my Healthcare Agent
c. my notification to my Healthcare Agent or a healthcare provider orally or in writing or by any other act evidencing a specific intent to revoke the Healthcare Proxy

SIGNATURE OF PRINCIPAL
I hereby sign my name on this _____ day of _____,
_____, to this Healthcare Proxy in the presence of two witnesses.
_____   Client Name

3

If the principal is physically incapable of signing:
I hereby sign the name of the principal at the principal's
direction and in the presence of the principal and two witnesses.
Name of Principal: _____
Name of Signatory: _____
Date: _____
Address of Signatory: _____
_____

WITNESSES:
We, the undersigned, have witnessed the signing of this document by the principal or at the direction of the principal and state that to the best of our knowledge, the principal is at least 18 years of age, of sound mind, and under no constraint or undue influence. We, the witnesses, have not been named as Healthcare Agents.

1. _____   _____
                Witness (Sign)   Date

_____
                Print Name

_____
                Address

2. _____   _____
                Witness (Sign)   Date

_____
                Print Name

_____
                Address

Notarization
Commonwealth of Massachusetts
County of _____

On this _____ day of _____, _____, before me, the undersigned, a notary public of the Commonwealth of Massachusetts, personally appeared **(client name)**, proved to me through satisfactory evidence of identification, which was _____, personally known to me or proven on the basis of satisfactory evidence to be the person whose name is subscribed to this instrument, a Healthcare Proxy, and acknowledged that he executed it voluntarily and for its stated purpose.

4

I declare under the penalty of perjury that the persons whose names are subscribed to this instrument appear to be of sound mind and under no duress, fraud, or undue influence.

_____

My Commission Expires: _____

Index